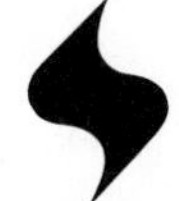

Stedman's PSYCHIATRY WORDS

FOURTH EDITION

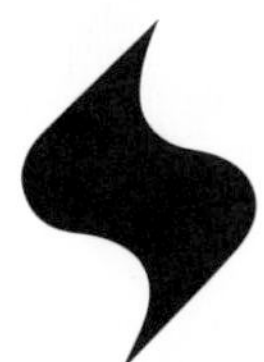

Stedman's PSYCHIATRY WORDS

FOURTH EDITION

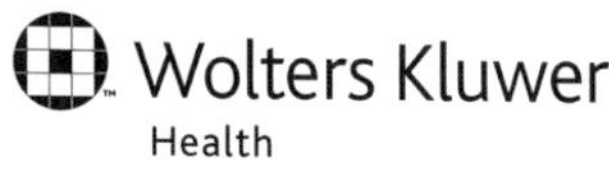

Lippincott Williams & Wilkins

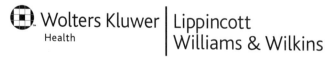

Publisher: Julie K. Stegman
Senior Product Manager: Eric Branger
Managing Editor: Amy Millholen
Typesetter: Josephine Bergin
Printer & Binder: Malloy Litho, Inc.

351 West Camden Street
Baltimore, Maryland 21201-2436

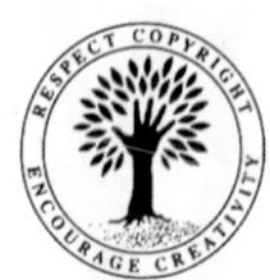

Printed in the United States of America

2007

Library of Congress Cataloging-in-Publication Data
Stedman's psychiatry words. -- 4th ed.
p. ; cm. -- (Stedman's word books)
Includes bibliographical references.
ISBN-13: 978-0-7817-6191-8 (alk. paper)
ISBN-10: 0-7817-6191-3 (alk. paper)
1. Psychiatry—Dictionaries. 2. Neurology—Dictionaries. 3. Nervous system—Surgery—Dictionaries. I. Stedman, Thomas Lathrop, 1853-1938. II. Title: Psychiatry words. III. Series.
[DNLM: 1. Psychiatry—Terminology—English. WM 15 S812 2007]
RC437.S753 2007
616.89001'4--dc22

2006025715

06 07 08
1 2 3 4 5 6 7 8 9 10

Contents

Acknowledgements

An important part of our editorial process is the involvement of medical transcriptionists—as advisors, reviewers, and editors.

We extend special thanks to Pat Forbis and Kathy Hess for editing the manuscript and helping to resolve many difficult questions. We are grateful to editorial advisory board members Deanna Frosty, CMT, FAAMT, Janet West, and Robin Koza, who shared their valuable judgment, insight, and perspective.

Our appreciation goes to Pat Forbis and Robin Koza, who helped to enhance the A-to-Z content for this edition. We also extend thanks to Jo-Ann Clarke for her contributions to the Sample Reports appendix. Thanks to Helen Littrell for performing the final prepublication review.

We thank Barb Ferretti, who played an integral role in the process by reviewing the content files for format and updating the manuscript.

As with all our *Stedman's* word references, this resource incorporates the suggestions and expertise of our many contacts in the medical transcriptionist community. Thanks to all of our advisory board participants, reviewers, and editors; AAMT meeting attendees; and others who have written us with requests and comments—keep talking, and we'll keep listening.

Acknowledgments

Editor's Preface

It is easy to acknowledge that change for medical transcriptionists is standard operating practice these days, but some things are not likely to change. The support given to MTs, our profession, and the healthcare industry by Lippincott Williams & Wilkins and Stedman's seems to have no limit. The staff is always eager to assist, discuss new ideas, or make a correction where it is needed. In a word: Thanks! And, special thanks to Julie Stegman and Amy Millholen for providing valuable resources for all of us who are involved in ensuring patient safety through documentation and continuing to take a personal interest in MTs.

Psychiatry remains a curious and fascinating subspecialty of medicine. The user of this 4th edition of *Stedman's Psychiatry Words* will find useful words and phrases from the 1800s and before intermingled with terminology specific to today's practices. Together it creates a unique and often colorful vocabulary. New terms continue to be introduced as our society and culture evolve. Terms such as "starter marriage," "hanging game," and "torture survivor" remind us that more human complexities and personal issues exist than ever before.

Because we have become a nation of great diversity, spellings of various nations, their peoples, and religions have been entered into this edition in an effort to simplify the exercise of searching. You will find easily misspelled words, such as Hmong, Buddhism, Caribbean, The Philippines, but Filipino (male) or Filipina (female) for their people.

The appendices have again been set apart from the A to Z contents to make referencing sample reports, phobias (by clinical name and by definition), tests, drugs, and the DSM-IV Diagnoses and Codes more easily accessible. As it is in the A to Z portion of the book, the appendices have many new entries.

Last, but certainly not least, it is important to say that books are not created in a vacuum. It takes many eyes and hands to go from initial idea to finished product, so my sincere appreciation is extended to Kathy Hess and Barb Ferretti and other individuals named on the Acknowledgements page for their part in making this a better resource. Your help with this project and your contribution to the working medical transcriptionist does not go unnoticed.

Pat Forbis

Publisher's Preface

Stedman's Psychiatry Words, Fourth Edition, offers an authoritative assurance of quality and exactness to the wordsmiths of the healthcare professions—medical transcriptionists, medical editors and copyeditors, health information management personnel, court reporters, and the many other users and producers of medical documentation.

In *Stedman's Psychiatry Words, Fourth Edition,* users will find tests, disorders, treatments, and drugs; slang terms; and other key terminology in psychiatry and psychology. Users will also find terms related to new developments in these areas: fear and anxiety associated with bioterrorism and war, child and adolescent issues and treatment, drug and alcohol addiction, and technology-related issues. The appendix sections include an alphabetical listing of DSM-IV diagnoses and codes, sample reports, common terms by procedure, slang terms, psychiatric and psychological tests, drugs, phobias listed by clinical name, and phobias listed by abnormal fear.

This new edition contains more than 5,000 new terms. The extensive A-Z list was developed from manufacturers' literature, scientific reports, books, journals, CDs, and websites (please see list of References on page xvii).

We at Lippincott Williams & Wilkins strive to provide you with the most up-to-date and accurate word references available. Your use of this *Word Book* will prompt new editions, which we will publish as often as updates and revisions justify. We welcome your suggestions for improvements, changes, corrections, and additions—whatever will make this Stedman's product more useful to you. Please complete the postage-paid card in this book for future suggestions and recommendations, or visit us online at www.stedmans.com.

Explanatory Notes

Medical transcription is an art as well as a science. Both approaches are needed to correctly interpret the dictation of a physician, whose language is a product of education, training, and experience. This variety in medical language means that there are several acceptable ways to express certain terms, including jargon. *Stedman's Psychiatry Words, Fourth Edition*, provides variant spellings and phrasings for many terms. These elements, in addition to complete cross-indexing, make *Stedman's Psychiatry Words, Fourth Edition*, a valuable resource for determining the validity of terms as they are encountered.

Alphabetical Organization

Alphabetization of main entries is letter by letter as spelled, ignoring punctuation, spaces, prefixed numbers, or other special characters. For example:

daymare
3-day schizophrenia
daytime
day-to-day

Terms beginning or ending with Greek letters show the Greek letters spelled out and listed alphabetically. For example:

beta
b. amyloid protein
b. arc
b. blocker

In subentry alphabetization, the abbreviated singular form or the spelled-out plural form of the noun main entry word is ignored.

Format and Style

All main entries are in **boldface** to expedite locating a sought-after term, to enhance distinction between main entries and subentries, and to relieve the textual density of the pages.

Irregular plurals and variant spellings are shown on the same line as the singular or preferred form of the word. For example:

continuum, pl. continua
akinesia, akinesis

Hyphenation

As a rule of style, multiple eponyms (e.g., Mears-Rubash approach) are hyphenated. Also, hyphens have been added between a manufacturer and one or more eponyms (e.g., Vital-Metzenbaum dissecting scissors). Please note that in many cases, hyphenation is a question of style, not of accuracy, and thus is a matter of choice.

Possessives

Possessive forms have been dropped in this reference for the sake of consistency and conformance with the guidelines of the American Association for Medical Transcription (AAMT) and other groups. Please note, however, that in many cases, retaining the possessive, like hyphenating, is a question of style, not of accuracy, and thus is a matter of choice. To form the possessive of a word, simply add the apostrophe or apostrophe "s" to the end of the word.

Cross-indexing

The word list is in an index-like main entry–subentry format that contains two combined alphabetical listings:

(1) A *noun* main entry–subentry organization, which is typical of the A–Z section of medical dictionaries like *Stedman's:*

caregiver
family c.
home c.

guidance
spiritual g.
vocational g.

(2) An *adjective* main entry–subentry organization, which lists words and phrases as you hear them. The main entries are the adjectives or modifiers in a multiword term. The subentries are the nouns around which the terms are constructed and to which the adjectives or modifiers pertain:

critical
c. age
c. analysis

educational
e. acceleration
e. achievement

This format provides the user with more than one way to locate and identify a multiword term. For example:

dangerous
d. activity

activity
dangerous a.

fanatic
f. personality

personality
fanatic p.

fantasized
f. sexual experience

experience
fantasized sexual e.

It also allows the user to see together all terms that contain a particular descriptor, as well as all types, kinds, or variations of a noun entity. For example:

flashback
acid f.
combat f.
f. hallucinosis

ill
i. at ease
chronically mentally i.
mentally i.

Wherever possible, abbreviations are separately defined and cross-referenced. For example:

CAPTA
Child Abuse Prevention and Treatment Act

child
C. Abuse Prevention and Treatment Act (CAPTA)

act
Child Abuse Prevention and Treatment A. (CAPTA)

References

In addition to the lists of our MT Editorial Advisory Board members (from their daily transcription work), we used the following sources for new terms in *Stedman's Psychiatry Words, Fourth Edition.*

Books

Agronin ME. Dementia: A Practical Guide. Philadelphia: Lippincott Williams & Wilkins, 2004.

American Heritage Dictionary of the English Language. 4th Ed. Boston: Houghton Mifflin, 2000.

Beers MH, Berkow R, and Burs M (eds.). Merck Manual of Diagnosis & Therapy. Whitehouse Station, NJ: Merck & Co., 1999.

Dorland's Illustrated Medical Dictionary, 29th Ed. Philadelphia: Saunders, 2000.

Drake E, Drake R. Saunders Pharmaceutical Word Book. Philadelphia: Saunders, 2002.

Fadem B, Simring S. High-Yield Psychiatry, 2nd Ed. Baltimore: Lippincott Williams & Wilkins, 2003.

Forbis P. The Psychiatry Word Book with Street Talk Terms. Philadelphia: FA Davis, 1993.

Garcia KS, Lin TL (eds.). The Washington Manual Psychiatry Survival Guide. Philadelphia: Lippincott Williams & Wilkins, 2003.

Keltner NL, Folks DG. Psychotropic Drugs, 3rd Edition. St. Louis, MO: Mosby, 1998.

Kohut J. The Little Book of Phobias. Philadelphia: Running Press, 1994.

Petit JR. Handbook of Emergency Psychiatry. Philadelphia: Lippincott Williams & Wilkins, 2004.

Rhodes SB, Walsh A (eds.). Dorland's Psychiatry Word Book for Medical Transcriptionists. St. Louis, MO: Elsevier, 2004.

Sadock BJ, Sadock VA (eds.). Kaplan & Sadock's Comprehensive Textbook of Psychiatry, 8th Ed. Volumes 1 and 2. Philadelphia: Lippincott Williams & Wilkins, 2005.

Schiffer RB, Rao SM, Fogel BS (eds.). Neuropsychiatry, 2nd Ed. Philadelphia: Lippincott Williams & Wilkins, 2003.

Stedman's Abbreviations, Acronyms & Symbols, 3rd Ed. Baltimore: Lippincott Williams & Wilkins, 2003.

Stedman's Medical Dictionary, 28th Ed. Baltimore: Lippincott Williams & Wilkins, 2006.

Journals

Addictive Disorders & Their Treatment. Philadelphia: Lippincott Williams & Wilkins, 2004-2006.

Alternative Therapies in Health and Medicine. Aliso Viejo, CA: Innovision Communications, 2002.

The American Journal of Psychiatry. Washington, DC: American Psychiatric Press, 2000-2006.

Clinical Psychiatry News. Rockville, MD: International Medical News Group, 1999-2001.

Cognitive and Behavioral Neurology. Baltimore: Lippincott Williams & Wilkins, 2005-2006.

Current Opinion in Psychiatry. London: Lippincott Williams & Wilkins, 2004-2006.

Journal of the American Academy of Child and Adolescent Psychiatry. Baltimore: Lippincott Williams & Wilkins, 2000-2006.

Journal of Clinical Psychopharmacology. Philadelphia: Lippincott Williams & Wilkins, 2004-2006.

The Journal of Nervous and Mental Disease. Philadelphia: Lippincott Williams & Wilkins, 2004-2006.

Journal of Psychiatric Practice. Philadelphia: Lippincott Williams & Wilkins, 2004-2006.

Psychiatric Annals. Thorofare, NJ: Slack, Inc., 2000-2006.

Psychiatric Genetics. London: Lippincott Williams & Wilkins, 2004-2006.

Psychosomatic Medicine. Hagerstown, MD: Lippincott Williams & Wilkins, 2004-2006.

CD-ROMs

Stedman's Plus 2006 Medical/Pharmaceutical Spellchecker. Baltimore: Lippincott Williams & Wilkins, 2006.

Web Sites

http://aroundrtp.com/PED84.htm

http://healthweb.org/browse.cfm?subjectid=79

http://pni.med.jhu.edu

http://www.aacap.org/Web/aacap/clinical/psychLinks.htm

http://www.aagpgpa.org

http://www.apa.org

http://www.athealth.com/Consumer/rcenter/

http://www.behavior.net

http://www.cfah.org

http://www.csuniv.edu/Academics/Behavioral/psichi/links.htm

http://www.dna.com

http://www.drbobmentalhealth.org

http://www.drugs.com/newdrugs.html

http://www.hoptechno.com/book48.htm

http://www.hypnosis.edu/glossary/a.asp

http://www.mentalhealth.com

http://www.mentalhealth.gov.au/

http://www.nami.org

http://www.nimh.nih.gov

http://www.panic-and-anxiety.com/general_4.html

http://www.psych.org/

http://www.psychiatry.ox.ac.uk/cebmh/

http://www.psycom.net/depression.central.html.org

http://www.pubmed.gov
http://www.saferchild.org/mental.htm
http://www.stoeltingco.com/tests/products2/intellearnpage.htm
http://www.uic.edu/labs/hprl/About%20Us/Professional_links.html
http://www.usdoj.gov/ndic/pubs07/708/
http://www.virtualdrugstore.com
http://www.yorku.ca/psycenter/tests/aptitude.html
http://www4.rmwc.edu/plesson/intelligence.htm

a
a posteriori
a priori criterion
AA
academic alertness
achievement age
Alcoholics Anonymous
anticipatory avoidance
AAA
acute anxiety attack
AAAP
American Academy of Addiction Psychiatry
AABT
Association for Advancement of Behavior Therapy
AACAP
American Academy of Child and Adolescent Psychiatry
AACD
American Association for Counseling & Development
AACI
American Association for the Cure of Inebriates
AACP
American Academy of Clinical Psychiatrists
AACRC
American Association of Children's Residential Centers
AADPRT
American Association of Directors of Psychiatric Residency Training
AAF
altered auditory feedback
AAGP
American Association for Geriatric Psychiatry
AAGT
Arizona Association for the Gifted and Talented
Association for the Advancement of Gestalt Therapy
Austin Association for the Gifted and Talented
AAI
adolescent alienation index
AAMFT
American Association for Marriage and Family Therapy
AAMI
age-associated memory impairment
AAMR
American Association of Mental Retardation
AAO
awake, alert, and oriented
AAP
Administrators in Academic Psychiatry
American Academy of Pediatrics
American Academy of Psychoanalysis
American Academy of Psychotherapists
Association for the Advancement of Psychoanalysis
Association for the Advancement of Psychotherapy
AAPAA
American Academy of Psychiatrists in Alcoholism and Addictions
AAPDP
American Academy of Psychoanalysis and Dynamic Psychiatry
AAPL
American Academy of Psychiatry and Law
AAPM
American Academy of Pain Medicine
AAPP
American Academy on Physician and Patient
AAPSC
American Association of Psychiatric Services for Children
AAS
American Association of Suicidology
anabolic-androgenic steroid
AASM
American Academy of Sleep Medicine
AB, ab
abortion
ABA
applied behavioral analysis
abactio
abactus venter
A/B/A design
abalienate
abalienatio mentis
abandon
abandoned
a. child
a. during battle
abandonment
child a.
a. concern
emotional a.
fear of a.
feeling of a.

abandonment *(continued)*
imagined a.
perceived emotional a.
real a.
spouse a.
abase
abasement
abash
abasia
atactic a.
ataxic a.
hysterical a.
paralytic a.
paroxysmal trepidant a.
spastic a.
trembling a.
a. trepidans
abasia-astasia
abatardissement
abate
abatement
abating
abbau
ABC
assessment of basic competency
atomic, biological, chemical
ABC warfare
ABCs
affect, behavior, cognition
Abderhalden-Fauser reaction
abdicate
abdomen
gridiron a.
abdominal
a. distress
a. migraine
a. pain
abduct
abduction
abed
aberrancy
aberrant
a. behavior
a. behavior checklist
a. cycle
a. gene
a. motivational syndrome
a. parental characteristic
a. parental environment
a. regeneration
aberration
autosomal a.
chromosomal a.
mental a.
a. of perception
semantic a.
sexual a.
aberrometer
abet
abetted
abetting
abeyance
ABFP
American Board of Forensic Psychiatrists
ABFPN
American Board of Forensic Psychiatry and Neurology
abhor
abhorrent
abidance
abiding
law a.
abient
abilitator
change a.
ability
a. to abstract and calculate
abstracting a.
abstraction a.
abstractive a.
attentional a.
attention shift a.
auditory a.
cognitive a.
communication a.
a. to con
conceptual a.
concrete abstractive a.
construction a.
coping a.
crystallized a.
disturbance in perceptual motor a.
drawing a.
eidetic a.
focal a.
general learning a.
impaired abstraction a.
impaired concentration a.
impaired driving a.
impaired thinking a.
intellectual a.
language a.
learning a.
a. to manage money
mathematical a.
memory a.
mental a.
motor a.
nonverbal abstractive a.
nonverbal synthesizing a.
occupational a.
oral sensory a.
parenting a.
perceptual motor a.
poor reasoning a.
premorbid a.
primary mental a.
psychic a.

psycholinguistic a.
reality testing a.
reasoning a.
reduced attention a.
self-regulatory a.
sequencing a.
shift a.
spatial a.
synthesizing a.
a. to take criticism
thinking a.
thoroughness, reliability, efficiency, analytic a.
verbal conceptualization a.
visuoconstructional a.
visuomotor a.
visuospatial a.
word-finding a.
writing a.

ab initio

abiotic

abiotrophy

abject

ablate

ablation

Amytal a.

ABLB

alternate binaural loudness balance

able-bodied

ablution

ablutomania

ABMS

American Board of Medical Specialties

abnegate

abnegation

abnormal

a. appetite
a. asymmetry
a. behavior during sleep
a. brain structure
a. calorie consumption
a. circumstance
a. development
a. EEG tracing
a. energy intake
a. eye movement
a. food consumption
a. food intake
a. food intake pattern
a. gait
a. habitus
a. illness behavior
a. involuntary movement
a. involuntary movement disorder (AIMD)
a. metabolism
a. mood
a. motor behavior
a. muscle response (AMR)
a. pathologic condition
a. perception
a. personality
a. physiological event during sleep
a. position of distal limb
a. psychology
a. reaction
a. response
a. responsiveness
a. sleep-wake schedule
a. stoppage of sound
a. tactile sensation
a. taste sensation
a. thinking
a. trait

abnormality

a. of affect
anatomic a.
attentional a.
autosomal a.
behavioral a.
brain a.
chromosomal a.
cranial nerve a.
electrolyte a.
eye movement a.
food intake a.
gait a.
immunologic a.
inherited a.
insulin a.
laboratory a.
lateralizing a.
mental a.
metabolic a.
morphometric a.
motoric a.
movement a.
neuroendocrine a.
neurotransmitter a.
nonspecific a.
peculiar breathing a.
perceptual a.
performance a.
personality a.
polysomnographic a.
psychomotor a.

NOTES

abnormality *(continued)*
pursuit a.
sleep a.
sleep-wake a.
abnormalities in sleep-wake timing mechanism
startle a.
structural brain a.
subcortical-frontal lobe a.
trait-level region a.
vocal pitch a.
X-linked genetic a.
aboiement
abolish
abominable
abomination
aboriginal therapy
abort
abortifacient
abortion (AB, ab)
criminal a.
elective a.
induced a.
missed a.
spontaneous a.
a. technique
therapeutic a. (TAB)
aboulia (*var. of* abulia)
about
bandy a.
a. face
set a.
above-average
a.-a. intelligence
a.-a. student
aboveboard
ABP
American Board of Psychiatry
ABPN
American Board of Psychiatry and Neurology
ABR
auditory brainstem response
ABR audiometry
abradant
Abraham
A. theory of depression
A. view of depressive disorder
abrasive
abreact
abreaction
drug a.
hypnotic a.
motor a.
abreactive drug
abrogate
abrosia
abrupt
a. onset
a. shift in affective expression
a. topic shift
a. withdrawal phenomenon
ABS
acute brain syndrome
aloin, belladonna, strychnine
abscess
brain a.
abscise
abscissa
abscission
abscond
ABSEG
atlas-based segmentation
absence
atypical a.
automatic a.
complex a.
a. of depressed mood
a. of eating plan
a. of elevated mood
a. of emotional responsiveness
enuretic a.
a. epilepsy
epileptic a.
a. episode
fantasy a.
a. of feeling
hypertonic a.
a. of insight
leave of a. (LOA)
myoclonic a.
pure a.
retrocursive a.
a. seizure
simple a.
a. status
subclinical a.
a. syndrome
typical a.
unauthorized a. (UA)
vasomotor a.
absent
a. ataxia
a. drive
a. eye contact
a. parent
a. sexual desire
a. speech
a. state
a. without leave (AWOL)
absenteeism
work a.
absentia
a. epileptica
in a.
absent-minded
absent-mindedness

absinthe, absinth
a. addiction
a. dependence
absinthism
absolute
a. agraphia
a. bioavailability
a. bliss
a. diet
a. field
a. flow
a. impression
a. inversion
a. measurement
a. metabolic activity
a. pitch
a. quantity
a. rating scale
a. scotoma
a. sensitivity
a. systemic availability
a. threshold
a. unconsciousness
absolution
absolutism
cultural a.
phenomenal a.
absolve
absorb
absorbance
absorbed mania
absorbefacient
absorbent
absorption
drug a.
erratic a.
a. of inhalant
intramuscular a.
transdermal a.
abstain
abstainer
abstemious
abstention
abstinence
alcohol a.
alimentary a.
caffeine a.
a. delirium
drug a.
a. group
long-term a.
nicotine a.
opiate a.
a. phenomenon
rule of a.
sexual a.
smoking a.
a. symptom
a. syndrome
total a.
abstinent
a. days per month
a. tobacco smoker
abstract
a. attitude
a. concept
a. conceptualization
a. expression
a. idea
a. intelligence
a. interpretation
a. logical thinking
a. logical thought
a. modeling
a. perception
a. reasoning
a. term
a. theory
a. versus representational dimension
a. wit
abstracting
a. ability
a. disability
abstraction
a. ability
a. ladder
level of a.
selective a.
a. skill
abstractive ability
abstruse
absurd
absurdity
abubble
abulia, aboulia
cyclic a.
social a.
abulic mental change
abulomania
abundance
abundant motives
abuse
adolescent a.
adult a.
aerosol spray a.
a. of aged

NOTES

abuse *(continued)*
alcohol a.
amphetamine a.
amyl nitrate a.
analgesic a.
animal a.
antidepressant a.
anxiety due to substance a.
anxiolytic a.
barbiturate a.
benzodiazepine a.
caffeine a.
cannabis a.
a. case (AC)
cathartic a.
chemical of use and a.
a. in childhood
childhood sexual a.
child physical a.
child sexual a.
chronic alcohol a.
chronic drug a.
cocaine a.
Committee on Family Violence and Sexual A.
comorbid substance a.
concurrent alcohol and substance a.
continued a.
a. counseling
credit card a.
a. criterion
diet drug a.
domestic partner a.
drug a.
early a.
elder a.
emotional a.
episodic substance a.
ethanol a.
exposure to a.
extent of a.
extrafamilial sexual a.
fetal a.
a. field
financial a.
geriatric a.
hallucinogen a.
history of a.
hypnotic a.
illicit drug a.
index episode of sexual a.
index of spouse a.
inhalant a.
institutional a.
intrafamilial sexual a.
intravenous drug a. (IVDA)
IV drug a.
laxative a.
a. of leave time
liability a.
a. liability
long-term course of a.
maladaptive pattern of substance a.
maternal a.
a. measure
medication a.
mental a.
methamphetamine a.
mixed substance a.
narcotic a.
National Institute on Drug A. (NIDA)
newborn a.
nicotine a.
nondependent adult a.
a. of nonprescribed drug
nonprescription drug a.
opioid a.
over-the-counter drug a.
parent a.
parental a.
patent medicine a.
paternal a.
patient a.
peer a.
perpetrator of a.
pharmacology of a.
physical a.
polydrug a.
polysubstance a.
a. potential
prescription drug a.
problem related to a.
psychoactive drug a.
psychoactive substance a.
psychological a.
recurrent a.
repeated a.
reporting a.
ritual a.
sadistic sexual a.
sedative a.
sexual a.
solvent a.
spousal a.
spouse a.
12-step program for substance a.
stimulant a.
substance a.
survivor of a.
sympathomimetic a.
tobacco a.
tranquilizer a.
traumatic childhood a.
verbal a.
victim a.
victimology in a.
vocal a.

abused
being a.
a. child hotline
a. child syndrome
a. partner
a. spouse hotline
a. wife hotline
abuse/neglect
suspected child a./n. (SCAN)
abuser
anxious substance a.
child sexual a.
drug a.
ethanol a.
remitted substance a.
repeat a.
sedative a.
spouse a.
substance a.
abusive
being a.
a. dating behavior
a. father
a. language
a. mother
a. parent
a. partner
a. sibling
abysm
abyss
emotional a.
AC
abuse case
alcoholic cirrhosis
alternating current
ACA
American Counseling Association
academic
a. alertness (AA)
a. asset
a. difficulty
a. dysfunction
a. failure
a. inhibition
a. medical center
a. organizational skill
a. orientation (AO)
a. performance
a. preparation
a. problem
a. psychiatrist
a. psychiatry
a. skills disorder
a. underachievement disorder
Academy
American Family Therapy A. (AFTA)
A. of Certified Social Workers (ACSW)
A. of Organizational and Occupational Psychiatry (AOOP)
A. of Psychosomatic Medicine (APM)
acalculia
aphasic a.
visuospatial a.
acamprosate calcium
acanthesthesia
acatalepsia
acatamathesia
acataphasia
acatastasia
acatastatic
acathexis
acathisia (*var. of* akathisia)
ACCA
American College Counseling Association
accede
accelerant
accelerated
a. heart rate
a. interaction
a. reaction
a. speech
acceleration
educational a.
positive a.
accelerator
accelerometer
accentuation
acceptability
suicide a.
acceptable
a. behavior
a. treatment plan
acceptance
a. of aging
a. and commitment therapy
group a.
a. of self
social a.
a. strategy
acceptant
acceptation

NOTES

accepted
a. behavior
a. belief
a. ritual
access
a. to gun
a. to healthcare services
a. to weapon
accessing cue
accession
accessory
a. chromosome
a. cramp
a. to crime
a. sign
a. symptom
accident
alcohol-related risk for a.
a. behavior
fatal a.
a. neurosis
a. prevention
a. reduction
a. repeater
a. risk
a. victim
accidental
a. affair
a. autoerotic asphyxiation
a. crisis
a. death
a. error
a. experience
a. hanging
a. hypothermia
a. image
a. injury
a. overdose
a. pregnancy
a. psychosis
a. shooting
a. stimulus
a. suicide
accident-prone behavior
acclamation
acclimate
acclimation
cold a.
acclimatize
accolade
accommodate
accommodation
auditory a.
interpersonal a.
mutual a.
a. of nerve
passive a.
visual a.
accommodationist
accommodative
accompaniment
psychopathologic a.
accompli
fait a.
accomplished suicide
accomplishment quotient (AQ)
accordance
accost
accoucheur's hand
account
emotion-consistent a.
narrative a.
accountability
accountable for action
accredit
accretion
accrual
accrue
acculturate
acculturation
a. difficulty
a. problem
a. problem with expression of habit
a. problem with expression of political value
a. problem with expression of religious value
psychological a.
accumulated
accumulation
accuracy of memory
accurate empathy (AE)
accursed
accusation
false a.
accusative
accusatory hallucination
accuse
accustom
AC/DC
alternating current and/or direct current bisexual
ACE
acute care of elderly
ace
acedia
acenesthesia
ACER
Australian Council for Educational Research
acerb
acerbate
acervuline
acervulus
acetate
amyl a.
acetonemia

acetonemic
acetous
acetum
acetylcholinesterase (AChE)
achalasia
AChE
acetylcholinesterase
ache
brain a.
acheiria
Achenbach system of empirically based assessment
achieved
highest grade a.
achievement
a. age (AA)
assessment of academic a.
a. battery
a. behavior
a. drive
educational a.
a. ethics
exaggerated a.
expected level of a.
a. identification measure
mathematics a.
a. motivation
motive a.
a. motive
a. need (n-Ach)
a. oriented
a. quotient (AQ)
a. ratio (AR)
reading a.
school a.
a. through counseling and treatment (ACT)
vocational a.
achiever
high academic a.
Achilles
A. heel
A. jerk
achromatic
a. color
a. color response
achromatism
achromatopsia
acid
clorazepic a.
deoxyribonucleic a. (DNA)
a. flashback
gamma amino benzoic a. (GABA)
homovanillic a. (HVA)
ibotenic a.
ribonucleic a. (RNA)
a. rock
vanillylmandelic a. (VMA)
vanillylmandelic a. (VMA)
acid-base
a.-b. balance
a.-b. disturbance
acidic
acidifiable
acidification treatment
acidify
acidism
acidity
acidogenic
acidosis
lactic a.
metabolic a.
acid-sensing ion channel
acidulate
acidulous
aciduria
acknowledged victim
acknowledgment
ACLU
American Civil Liberties Union
acme
acmesthesia
ACN
acute conditioned neurosis
acne-like rash
acne vulgaris
ACO
alert, cooperative, and oriented
ACOA
adult child of alcoholic
aconative
aconite
aconitine
aconuresis
acoria
acosmia
Acosta
A. disease
A. syndrome
acoupedic rehabilitation
acousma
acousmatagnosis
acousmatamnesia
acoustic
a. agnosia
a. agraphia

NOTES

acoustic *(continued)*
a. ambiguity
a. analysis
a. aphasia
a. area
a. center
a. energy
a. evoked potential
a. feedback
a. input
a. interface
a. irritability
a. nerve
a. neurasthenia
a. phonetics
a. pressure
a. radiation
a. reflex threshold
a. resonance
a. signal
a. spectrum
a. startle
a. stria
a. trauma
a. trauma deafness
acousticomotor epilepsy
acoustico-optic
ACP
American College of Psychiatrists
acquaint
acquaintance
sexual assault by a.
acquaintanceship procedure
acquiesce
acquiescence
response a.
social a. (SA)
acquiescent response set
acquirable
acquire
failure to a.
acquired
a. agraphia
a. character
a. drive
a. dyslexia
a. epilepsy
a. epileptic aphasia
a. fluent aphasia
a. folie morale
a. immunodeficiency syndrome (AIDS)
a. knowledge
a. paranoia
a. reflex
a. sexual disorder
a. sexual dysfunction
a. situational narcissism
acquisition
language a.
psychosocial skill a.
reading skill a.
acquisitive
a. instinct
a. spirit
acquittal
acrasia
acrescentism
acrid
acrimonious
acrimony
acroagnosis
acroanesthesia
acroataxia
acrocentric chromosome
acrocinesia, acrocinesis
acrocinetic
acrocyanosis
acrodynia
acrodysesthesia
acroesthesia
acrognosis
acrolein
acromania
acromegaloid personality
acromegaly, acromegalia
acromial reflex
acromicria
acroparesthesia syndrome
across identity state
ACS
acute confusional state
ACSW
Academy of Certified Social Workers
ACT
achievement through counseling and treatment
adaptive control of thought
American College of Testing
anxiety control training
act
Adoption and Safe Families A.
aggressive a.
Americans with Disabilities A. (ADA)
assaultive a.
autoerotic a.
biologic a.
Child Abuse Prevention and Treatment A. (CAPTA)
compulsive a.
consummatory a.
Controlled Substances A. (CSA)
criminal sexual a.
a. of disrespect
Drug-Induced Rape Prevention and Punishment A.

Elder Justice A.
frequency of violent a.'s
future suicidal a.
a. of God
habitual a.
Harrison Antinarcotic A.
heinous a.
heroic a.
imperious a.
impulsive a.
innocent a.
instrumental avoidance a.
intervening a.
mental a.
motive for violent a.
overt aggressive a.
past suicidal a.
predisposition to suicidal a.
promiscuous a.
psychology a.
rape a.
A. & React test system
reflex a.
sadistic rape a.
self-harming a.
self-soothing a.
sensorimotor a.
serious assaultive a.
Sexually Dangerous Persons A.
Sexually Violent Persons Commitment A.
speech a.
suicidal a.
suicide a.
symptomatic a.
terrorist a.
trivial a.
a. up
a. utilitarianism
a. of violence
violent a.
a. and volition

Actigraph

A. device
A. zero-crossing mode

acting

a. in
a. out
play a.
a. up

acting-out

a.-o. behavior
a.-o. defense mechanism
a.-o. potential
a.-o. tendency

action

accountable for a.
aggressive a.
amphetamine-like a.
antiaggressive a.
antigonadal a.
antipsychotic a.
a. of arrest
automatic a.
calorigenic a.
chance a.
chemical a.
coercive legal a.
compulsive a.
consensual a.
consequence of a.
cumulative drug a.
a. current
disciplinary a.
drug a.
dual mechanism of a.
duration of drug a.
effective a.
a. group
a. group process
a. guide
hypnotic a.
independent a.
initiation of a.
intensified a.
a. interpretation
irrational a.
a. level
local vasoconstrictive a.
a. location
missing in a. (MIA)
moral a.
morphine-like a.
a. organization
a. painting
a. pattern
a. potential
raptus a.
a. recipient
a. research
semiautomatic a.
seriously wounded in a. (SWA)
a. system
tendency of a.
thermogenic a.
toxic a.

NOTES

action *(continued)*
a. tremor
unacceptable a.
uncontrollable a.
vasoconstrictive a.
willed a.
wounded in a.
actionless
action-oriented personality
activa
oneirodynia a.
activated
a. epilepsy
a. sleep
a. state
activating condition
activation
amygdala a.
brain a.
cerebellar a.
disturbance of behavioral a.
EEG a.
emotion-related a.
a. factor
functional a.
hippocampal a.
limbic a.
metabolic a.
neural a.
neuronal a.
a. pattern
phasic a.
prefrontal cortex a.
semantic a.
a. technique
a. theory of emotion
transient channel a.
activator
active
a. algolagnia
a. analysis
a. analytic psychotherapy
a. antidepressant medication
a. bilingualism
a. castration complex
a. compound
a. concretization
a. coping
a. daydream technique
a. delirium
a. desire
a. displacement of emotive energy
a. euthanasia
a. fantasizing
a. filter
a. friendliness
a. general medical condition
a. hostility index (AHI)
a. imagining
a. immunity
a. incontinence
a. intervention
a. metabolite
a. mode of consciousness
a. modification
a. movement
a. negativism
a. nymphomania
a. passivity
a. pathophysiologic process
a. phase
a. placebo
a. psychoanalysis
a. psychosis
a. psychotic symptom
a. recreation
a. risk factor
sexually a.
a. sleep
a. state
a. therapist
a. therapy
a. transport
a. treatment
a. trigger
a. vocabulary
a. voice
actively
a. aggressive reaction type
a. phrased question
a. suicidal
active-passive model
active-phase
a.-p. symptom
a.-p. symptom of schizophrenia
activism
activist
activity
absolute metabolic a.
adolescent sexual a.
aimless motor a.
alpha a.
antisocial a.
anxiolytic a.
a. and attention disturbance
autonomic a.
a. and behavior
biochemical a.
blocking a.
brain opioid a.
brain wave a.
a. catharsis
cerebral a.
cholinergic a.
constricted a.
cortical a.
cortical-subcortical network a.
criminal a.

activities of daily living (ADL)
dangerous a.
decreased interest in a.
delta a.
a. deprivation
diminished pleasure in everyday activities
a. displacement
disruption of normal a.
diversionary a.
a. drive
dynamic physical a.
electrocortical a.
electrooculographic a.
emotional a.
excessive motor a.
experience with criminal a.
experimental sexual a.
exposure to terrorist a.
fad a.
fast a.
fine motor a.
forced sexual a.
frenzied psychomotor a.
functional a.
gambling a.
goal-directed a.
graded a.
gross motor a. (GMA)
group a.
a. group psychotherapy
a. group therapy (AGT)
hedonistic a.
high-risk sexual a.
hypnotic a.
impulsive a.
inappropriate a.
intellectual a.
a., interest, options (AIO)
intergenerational a.
late-night a.
leisure a.
a. level
limited a.
locomotor a.
a. log
loss of interest in usual activities
major life a.
masochistic sexual a.
masturbatory a.
mental a.
metabolic a.
motor a.
neuronal a.
nighttime a.
nonproductive a.
occupational a.
online sexual a.
orbitofrontal a.
organized a.
orogenital a.
outside a.
oxygen-depriving a.
paroxysmal a.
peak level of drug a.
perilous a.
peripheral cholinergic a.
persistent motor a.
physical a.
planned after-school a.
play therapy a.
a. pleasure
polyphasic a.
psychomotor a.
purposeless a.
a. quotient
random a.
rapid change in a.
a. record
religious a.
REM sleep a.
repetitious a.
repetitive motor a.
restricted a.
a. restriction
risky sexual a.
safe sex a.
seizure a.
self-care a.
sentinel a.
serotonergic a.
sexual a.
sleep a.
slow-frequency EEG a.
social a.
solitary a.
solo sexual a.
spiritual a.
stereotyped a.
stream of mental a.
supervised after-school a.
synaptic a.
a. system
thalamocortical a.
a. theory of aging
a. therapist

NOTES

activity *(continued)*
thermoeffector a.
vacuum a.
a. of violence
voyeuristic a.
a. wheel
activity-interview group psychotherapy (A-IGP)
activity-reactivity
autonomic a.-r.
actograph
actometer
actor
bad a.
actual
a. derailment
a. mortality
a. neurosis
a. self
a. or threatened death
actualization
actuarial
actuate
actus reus
ACU
acute care unit
acuity
auditory a.
sensory a.
visual a.
aculalia
acumen
acuology
acupressure
acupuncture
acupuncturist
acute
a. adolescent inpatient unit
a. affective reflex
a. alcoholic delirium
a. alcoholic mania
a. alcoholic myopathy
a. alcohol intoxication
a. alcoholism
a. amnesia
a. amphetamine poisoning
a. anxiety attack (AAA)
a. anxiety depression
a. anxiety reaction
a. ataxia
a. atrophic paralysis
a. bipolar mania
a. brain syndrome (ABS)
a. care of elderly (ACE)
a. care unit (ACU)
a. cerebral tremor
a. change in mental status
a. conditioned neurosis (ACN)
a. confusion
a. confusional insanity
a. confusional migraine headache
a. confusional state (ACS)
a. danger
a. decompensation
a. delusional psychosis
a. distress
a. drug toxicity
a. drunkenness
a. dystonia
a. exacerbation
a. extrapyramidal event
a. foot-shock stress
a. hallucinatory mania
a. hallucinatory paranoia
a. hallucinosis
a. head trauma
a. hysterical psychosis
a. idiopathic polyneuritis
a. impairment
a. infective psychosis
a. ingestion
a. intensive treatment (AIT)
a. lead poisoning
a. maladjustment situation
a. manic episode
a. melancholia
a. neuropsychologic disorder
a. onset
a. organic brain syndrome
a. organic reaction
a. paranoid disorder
a. paranoid reaction
a. paranoid schizophrenic reaction (APSR)
a. phase
a. posttraumatic neurosis
a. posttraumatic organic psychosis
a. posttraumatic stress syndrome
a. primary dementia
a. psychiatric symptomatology
a. psychogenic paranoid psychosis
a. psychoorganic syndrome
a. psychopathology
a. psychotic aggressive behavior
a. psychotic break
a. psychotic episode
a. psychotic inpatient
a. schizophrenic attack
a. schizophrenic episode
a. sedation
a. seizure
a. shock psychosis
a. simple-type schizophrenia
a. situational crisis
a. situational depression
a. situational disturbance
a. situational maladjustment reaction
a. situational stress reaction

a. sleep problem
a. stabilization
a. stabilization inpatient care
a. state
a. stress disorder (ASD)
a. stress reaction
a. stress response
a. suicide risk
a. suicide threat
a. symptom
a. therapy
a. tolerance
a. toxic encephalopathy
a. treatment
a. undifferentiated schizophrenia
a. undifferentiated schizophrenic reaction (AUSR)

acutely
a. abstinent tobacco smoker
a. agitated
a. manic
a. psychotic schizophrenic patient
a. symptomatic

acute-phase treatment

acyanotic

acyclic

AD
addict
adherent
admitting diagnosis
Alzheimer disease

ad
ad hominem
ad lib
ad nauseam

ADA
American Diabetes Association
American Dietetic Association
Americans with Disabilities Act
ADA diet

ADAA
Anxiety Disorders Association of America

adage

ADAM
arrestee drug abuse monitoring
ADAM system

adamant

ADAMHA
Alcohol, Drug Abuse, and Mental Health Administration

Adams-Stokes syndrome

Adapin

adaptability
cultural a.
environmental a.
a. profile
a. to stress

adaptation
air pollution a. (APA)
a. approach
autoplastic a.
brightness a.
cross a.
cross-cultural a.
dark a.
disease a.
a. dynamic
failure in social a.
a. level theory
a. to life
a. mechanism
migration a.
a. period
positive a.
a. reaction
reality a.
sexual a.
a. skill
social a.
a. syndrome
a. syndrome of Selye
a. time

adaptational
a. approach
a. psychodynamic

adaptation-promoting therapy

adaptedness

adaptive
a. approach
a. behavior
a. capacity
a. clothing
a. control of thought (ACT)
a. control of thought system
a. coping
a. defense mechanism
a. delinquency
a. device
a. ego mechanism
a. functioning
a. hypothesis
a. involuntary coping mechanism
a. nature
a. process
a. response

NOTES

adaptive *(continued)*
a. skill
a. skill domain
a. style
a. technique
a. testing
adaptiveness
aging a.
ADC
affective disorders clinic
aid to dependent children
AIDS dementia complex
ADD
attention deficit disorder
AD-DBD
attention deficit and disruptive behavior disorder
ADD-HA
attention deficit disorder with hyperactivity
addict (AD)
computer a.
drug a.
exercise a.
food a.
a. friend
gambling a.
heroin a.
narcotic a.
object a.
opiate a.
sex a.
shopping a.
street a.
work a.
addiction
absinthe a.
alcohol a.
American Academy of Psychiatrists in Alcoholism and A.'s (AAPAA)
barbiturate a.
behavioral a.
biologic root of a.
care management for chronic a. (CMCA)
a. center
chemical a.
cocaine a.
computer a.
cross a.
cybersex a.
drug a.
dual a.'s
enema a.
ethyl alcohol a.
exercise a.
food a.
gambling a.
heroin a.
iatrogenic a.
inhalant a.
Internet a.
laxative a.
methadone a.
methamphetamine a.
methylated spirit a.
morphine a.
narcotic a.
nicotine a.
nonprescription drug a.
object a.
online sexual a.
opiate a.
a. organic psychosis
over-the-counter drug a.
polydrug a.
polysubstance a.
polysurgical a.
a. potential
prescription drug a.
proneness to a.
a. psychiatry
psychological a.
relationship a.
a. relationship
a. root
sedative a.
a. severity
sexual a.
shopping a.
a. specialist
substance a.
surgical a.
sympathomimetic a.
a. syndrome
a. theory
tobacco a.
a. treatment
true a.
a. withdrawal
work a.
addictionist
addiction-prone personality (APP)
addiction-related problem
addiction-type organic psychosis
addictive
a. behavior
a. disease unit (ADU)
a. disorder
a. personality
a. potential of drug
a. risk
a. syndrome
addictologist
addictology
additional drug dependence
addition articulation

additive
a. environmental influence
food a.
a. genetic influence
addle
add-on drug
addressability
content a.
adduce
adductor spasmodic dysphonia
adenoid type
adenosine
endogenous a.
a. monophosphate
a. receptor
adept
adequacy
nutritional a.
adequate
a. care
a. diet
a. stimulus
a. treatment
ADH
antidiuretic hormone
ADHD
attention deficit hyperactivity disorder
ADHD ritual
ADHD-PI
attention deficit hyperactivity disorder-predominantly inattentive
adherence
adherent (AD)
adhesive
socially a.
adiadochokinesis, adiadochocinesia, adiadochocinesis
adiaphoria
adience
adient behavior
adipometer
adiposis
adiposity
adiposogenitalis
dystrophia a.
adiposogenital syndrome
adipsia, adipsy
adjudge
adjudicate
adjunct
neuroleptic a.
a. to treatment
adjunctive
a. amphetamine
a. benzodiazepine
a. individual session
a. intervention
a. medication
a. mental health service
a. strategy
a. therapy
a. treatment
a. use
adjuration
adjure
adjustment
attitude a.
Bonferroni a.
cultural a.
a. depression
a. disorder, chronic
a. disorder with angry mood
a. disorder with anxiety
a. disorder with anxious mood
a. disorder with disturbance of conduct
a. disorder with mixed anxiety and depressed mood
a. disorder with mixed disturbance of emotions
elective mutism a.
emotional a.
environmental a.
a. following migration
a. interface disorder
inventory a.
life-cycle a.
marital a.
a. measure
a. mechanism
a. method
modified Bonferroni a.
occupational a.
partial a.
personal a.
premorbid a.
a. process
psychological a.
a. reaction of adolescence
a. reaction of childhood
a. reaction conduct disorder
a. reaction disturbance
a. reaction of infancy
a. reaction of later life
a. reaction of menopause

NOTES

adjustment *(continued)*
a. reaction of middle age
a. reaction physical symptom
a. reaction physical syndrome
school a.
sexual a.
a. situational reaction
social a.
stimulation a.
a. therapy
vocational a.
withdrawal a.
adjust repetitive behavior
adjuvanticity
adjuvant therapy
ADL
activities of daily living
adlerian
a. psychoanalysis
a. psychology
a. psychotherapy
a. theory
Adler theory
ADLS
activities of daily living skills
administration
Alcohol, Drug Abuse, and Mental Health A. (ADAMHA)
anal a.
avenue of a.
chronic a.
compulsive drug a.
drug a.
Drug Enforcement A. (DEA)
ECT a.
enema drug a.
Food and Drug A. (FDA)
intramuscular a.
method of a.
methylphenidate a.
nicotine a.
oral a.
parenteral drug a.
Social Security A. (SSA)
standard dose a.
Substance Abuse Mental Health Services A.
systematic drug a.
unsanitary drug a.
Veteran's A. (VA)
administrative
a. psychiatry
a. segregation
a. therapy
administrator
A.'s in Academic Psychiatry (AAP)
American Association of Psychiatric A.'s
third-party a.
admirable
admiration
excessive a.
need for a.
admissible
a. admission
a. evidence
admission
admissible a.
a. criterion
elective a.
first a.
hospital a.
informal a.
involuntary a.
prior to a. (PTA)
psychiatric a.
temporary a.
voluntary a.
admitting diagnosis (AD)
admonish
admonition
ADMSEP
Association of Directors of Medical Student Education in Psychiatry
adnata
alopecia a.
adolescence
adjustment reaction of a.
anxiety disorder of a.
avoidant disorder of a.
body dysmorphic disorder in a.
complication of a.
crisis of a.
crush in a.
delinquency in a.
disorder of infancy, childhood, or a.
early stage in a.
emancipation disorder of a.
emotional disturbance of a.
ethical issue in a.
fearfulness disorder of a.
gender identity disorder in a.
identity disorder of a.
introverted disorder of a.
late stage in a.
middle stage in a.
oppositional disorder of a.
overanxious disorder of a.
reaction of a.
relaxation training in a.
sensitivity reaction of a.
a. in special population
Tanner stage in a.
withdrawal reaction of a.

adolescent
a. abuse
alcoholic a.
a. alcohol use
a. alienation index (AAI)
a. anger management
antidepressant for a.'s
antisocial a.
a. antisocial behavior
a. anxiety
at-risk a.
a. at risk
a. attitude toward death
a. attitude toward dying
autistic presymbiotic a.
communication with a.
a. counseling
a. criminal
a. crisis
a. culture
delinquent a.
a. depression
a. depression symptom
a. depressive symptom
a. developmental stage
disturbed a.
a. diversion project
a. drug use
a. educational need
emancipated a.
a. environment
evaluation of a.
a. gambler
a. gang member
a. group therapy
a. guardedness
high school a.
inner city a.
a. inpatient unit
a. insanity
Internet-addicted a.
a. language quotient
a. limitation
limit-setting for a.
a. mania
a. medication
middle school a.
a. moral development
a. negativism
a. neurotic delinquency
obese a.
a. onset
out-of-control a.
a. pedophilia
a. personal identity
a. pharmacotherapy
a. population
a. pregnancy
a. psychiatry
a. psychology
a. psychopharmacology
a. psychotherapy
a. rapist
a. rebellion
a. recovery
a. risk for violence
self-destructive a.
a. self-esteem
a. sex offender
a. sexual activity
a. sexual behavior
a. sexual change
a. sexual ideation
a. sexual identity
a. skepticism
a. socialization
socially dysfunctional a.
a. suicide
a. support group
a. support system
a. thinking
traumatized a.
troubled a.
troublesome a.
a. turmoil
a. turmoil reaction
a. use of Internet
violent a.
a. voice
a. voyeurism

adolescent-onset conduct disorder
adolescent-parent interview
adopt
adoptable
adopted
a. child
a. father

adoptee
a. family method
putative a.

adoption
closed a.
a. from foster care
international a.
A. and Safe Families Act

NOTES

adoption *(continued)*
a. study
transracial a.
adoptive
a. care
a. caregiver
a. family
a. father
a. parent
ADP
adenosine diphosphate
ADP ribosylation factor
ADR
adverse drug reaction
adrenal
a. disorder
a. hyperplasia
a. segment
adrenalin
adrenarche
adrenergic response state
adrenoceptor
adrenocortical insufficiency
adrenogenital syndrome (AGS)
adrenomedullary component
adrenopathy
adrenopause
adrift
adroit
adromia
ADU
addictive disease unit
adulate
adult
a. abuse
a. child of alcoholic (ACOA)
consenting a.
a. depressive disorder
a. depressive episode
a. development
a. diagnostic and treatment center
a. dissociation
a. ego state
a. environment
a. foster home
gender identity disorder in a.'s
a. group therapy
a. life
a. major depression
a. motivation
nonconsenting a.
A. Protective Services (APS)
a. psychopathology
a. schizophrenia
a. self-harm behavior
a. self-injury
sexual abuse of a.
a. sexual assault
a. situational stress reaction (ASSR)
a. social dysfunction
a. socialization
stress effect on a.
a. survivor of neglect
a. unit
adult-child sex
adulterant
adulterate
adulteration
adulterer
adulterous
adultery
adulthood
a. developmental stage
early a.
a. and elderly parent
fifth individuation in late a.
friendship in a.
gender identity disorder of a.
late a.
middle a.
a. psychiatry
young a.
adult-life psychosexual identity disorder
adultomorphism
adult-onset
a.-o. obesity
a.-o. proband
advance
a. directive
phase a.
sexual a.
unwanted sexual a.
advanced
a. dementia
a. education
a. sleep-phase pattern
a. sleep-phase syndrome (ASPS)
advantage
economic a.
a. by illness
law of a.
psychometric a.
take a.
therapeutic a.
adventitious
a. motor flow
a. movement
a. reinforcement
adventurousness
sexual a.
adversarial relationship
adversary model
adverse
a. autonomic response
a. background factor
a. childhood experience

a. drug effect
a. drug reaction (ADR)
a. medication effect
a. negative immunosuppressive effect
a. neurologic complication
a. psychological response
a. psychosocial environment
a. race-related event
a. selection
a. working conditions

adversity
childhood a.

advertising psychology

advice
against medical a. (AMA)
discharged against medical a. (DAMA)
face-to-face a.
medical a.
signed out against medical a. (SOAMA)
spiritual a.

advisor
school a.
spiritual a.

advocacy research

advocate
child a.
devil's a.
mental health a.
patient a.

ADW
assault with a deadly weapon

adynamia episodica hereditaria

adynamic

AE
accurate empathy
anoxic encephalopathy

AEA
autoerotic asphyxiation

AEP
auditory evoked potential

AEq
age equivalent

aerobic exercise

aerodynamic speech analysis

aeroneurosis

aerophagia, aerophagy

aerosialophagy

aerosol
a. inhalant
a. propellant
a. spray abuse
a. spray dependence

AESP
applied extrasensory perception

aesthetic, esthetic
environmental a.'s
environmentally a.
a. pleasure
a. sensibility
a. value

aestheticism

aeternus
puer a.

AF
alleged father

affability
surface a.

affable

affair
accidental a.
Department of Veteran A.'s
extramarital a.
instrumental a.
love a.
multiple a.'s
unhappy love a.
withdrawal from social a.

affect
abnormality of a.
ambivalent a.
angry a.
apathetic a.
appropriate a.
assessment of a.
a., behavior, cognition (ABCs)
bland a.
a. block
blunted a.
broad a.
charge of a.
cognitive generation of a.
congruent a.
constricted a.
cooling of a.
depressed a.
diffuse a.
diminution of a.
disorder of a.
a. displacement
a. display
dramatic a.
dull a.
dysphoric a.

NOTES

affect *(continued)*
elated a.
a. elicitation
emptiness of a.
energy a.
euphoric a.
evoked a.
facial a.
a. fantasy
a. fixation
flat a.
fluctuating a.
full a.
garrulous a.
generation of a.
hostile a.
a. hunger
hyperactive a.
hypoactive a.
impaired a.
inappropriate a.
incongruous a.
infantile a.
a. instability
intense a.
a. intensity measure
a. intensity problem
a. inversion
isolation of a.
labile range of a.
a. memory
modulated a.
a. modulation
mood and/or a. (M/A)
negative a.
normal a.
painful a.
pervasive a.
pleasurable a.
predominant a.
preservation of a.
range of a.
removed a.
a. response
restricted range of a.
reversal of a.
schizophrenic a.
shallow a.
short-lived schizophrenic a.
silly a.
solemn a.
a. spasm
a. state
strangulated a.
superficial a.
transformation of a.
transposition of a.
a. trauma model
unstable a.
vacuous a.
a. within normal range

affectation

affected
a. by feeling
germinally a.
a. individual
proportion of survivors a. (PSA)

affection
gesture of a.
masked a.

affectional
a. attachment
a. bond
a. drive

affectionate transference

affective
a. alcoholic psychosis
a. ambivalence
a. amnesia
a. arousal
a. arousal theory
a. bipolar disorder
a. blunting
a. cathexis
a. charge
a. constriction
a. dependence
a. depressive reaction
a. determined disorder
a. discharge
a. disease
a. disharmony
a. disorders clinic (ADC)
a. disorder syndrome
a. disturbance
a. dyscontrol
a. dysregulation
a. epilepsy
a. episode
a. experience
a. expression
a. feeble-mindedness
a. flattening
a. function
a. hallucination
a. illness
a. imagery
a. incontinence
a. insanity
a. instability
a. intensity
a. interaction
a. lability
a. melancholia
a. modulation of startle
a. monomania
a. need
a. neurotic personality disorder

a. paranoid organic psychosis
a. and paranoid state
a. personality
a. process
a. processing
a. property
a. ratio
a. reaction type
a. reactivity
a. responsiveness
a. rigidity
a. schematic mental model
a. schizophreniform psychosis
a. separation
a. significance
a. slumber
a. spectrum disorder
a. stupor
a. suggestion
a. symptom
a. temperament
a. tone
a. value

affectivity
characteristic pattern of a.
a. ratio

affect-laden
a.-l. delusion
a.-l. paranoia

affectomotor pattern

affect-related
a.-r. meaning
a.-r. processing
a.-r. schematic mental model

affectualization

afferent
a. feedback
a. input
a. motor aphasia
a. relation
a. stimulus interaction
a. thermosensory information

affiliation
a. bonding
a. drive
history of cult a.
intense a.
lifelong a.
a. need
political a.
religious a.

affinal

affined

affinity
receptor a.

affinous

affirmation

afflict

affliction

affluence

affluent

affordance

affright

affront

AFI
amaurotic familial idiocy

aforementioned

aforethought

AFPMH
ASEAN Federation for Psychiatry and Mental Health

African American, African-American

AFTA
American Family Therapy Academy
American Family Therapy Association

after
a. glide
morning a.

afteraction

aftercare
a. group
a. worker

after-effect
a.-e. of drinking
figural a.-e.

afterimage
memory a.
positive a.
Purkinje a.

afterimpression

afterlife

aftermath
a. of attack
a. of trauma

afterperception

aftersensation

aftershock
psychic a.

aftersound

aftertaste

afterthought

aftertouch

afunction

against medical advice (AMA)

agape

agapism

NOTES

age
achievement a. (AA)
adjustment reaction of middle a.
anatomic a.
appearance for a.
a. at first intercourse
a. at onset
basal mental a.
a. bias
Binet a.
biologic a.
bone a. (BA)
calendar a.
ceiling a.
characteristic a.
childbearing a.
chronologic a. (CA)
climacteric a.
a. of consent
a. correction
a. correction procedure
critical a.
a. critique
developmental a. (DA)
a. discrimination
educational a. (EA)
a. effect
emotional a.
a. equivalent (AEq)
functional a.
a. group
legal a.
maternal a.
mean a.
mental a. (MA)
middle a.
new a.
a. norm
old a.
paternal a.
a. peer
physiologic a.
a. prejudice
a. ratio
a. of reasoning
a. regression
relation to a.
school a.
a. score
social a. (SA)
stated a.
stress effect in old a.
test a. (TA)
a. transition
typical a.
well adjusted for a.
age-adjusted
a.-a. genome screen
a.-a. logistics regression
age-appropriate
a.-a. behavior
a.-a. cognitive change
a.-a. societal norm
a.-a. strategy
age-associated memory impairment (AAMI)
aged
abuse of a.
a. person
age-grade scaling
age-inappropriate
a.-i. cognitive change
a.-i. knowledge of sexual behavior
ageism
ageist belief
age-level behavior
age-matched individual
agency
A. for Health Care Policy and Research
health systems a. (HSA)
home service a.
law enforcement a.
social service a.
agency-centered consultation
agenda
hidden a.
personal a.
sociopolitical a.
agenesis
gonadal a.
agent
a., action, and object
alkylating a.
alpha receptor blocking a.
anabolic a.
antianxiety a.
antidepressant a.
antidyskinetic a.
antihypertensive a.
antipanic a.
antipsychotic a.
anxiolytic a.
atypical antipsychotic a.
beta adrenergic-blocking a.
blocking a.
butyrophenone a.
catalytic a.
causative a.
a. of change
change a.
chelating a.
chemical a.
conventional neuroleptic a.
etiological a.
excitatory a.
fast-acting a.
first-line a.

heterocyclic a.
5-HT releasing a.
hypnotic a.
lacing a.
MAOI-serotonergic a.
MAOI-tricyclic a.
mood stabilizing a.
neuroleptic a.
noxious a.
offending a.
A. Orange
paralyzing a.
pharmacological a.
possessing a.
psychedelic a.
psychopharmacologic a.
psychotropic a.
reinforcing a.
second-line a.
sedative-hypnotic a.
serotonergic a.
short-acting hypnotic a.
sympathomimetic a.
therapeutic a.
traditional antipsychotic a.
traditional neuroleptic a.
transforming a.
transmissible a.
typical antipsychotic a.

agentry
double a.
multiple a.

agerasia

age-related
a.-r. brain change
a.-r. cognitive decline
a.-r. comorbidity
a.-r. decline
a.-r. deterioration
a.-r. developmental process
a.-r. feature
a.-r. genomic change
a.-r. hearing loss
a.-r. pharmacodynamics
a.-r. pharmacokinetic change
a.-r. trend

age-specific
a.-s. cumulative incidence rate
a.-s. feature
a.-s. risk factor

ageusia, ageustia

ageusic aphasia

agglutination
image a.

aggrandize

aggravate

aggravated
a. battery
a. sexual assault

aggregate

aggregation
familial a.
a. problem

aggression
a. against property
a. against self
antipredatory a.
antisocial a.
authoritarian a.
constructive a.
destructive a.
domestic a.
early a.
externally directed a.
a. factor
general anger disorder with a.
general anger disorder without a.
healthy a.
hostile a.
husband-to-wife a.
identifying with a.
impulsive a.
indirect a.
instrumental a.
inward a.
juvenile a.
a. level
lifetime a.
moment of a.
oral a.
parent-to-child a. (PTCA)
passive a.
pattern of a.
a. to people and animals
physical a.
a. replacement training
retaliatory a.
self-directed a.
self-reported a.
sexual a.
situational anger disorder with a.
situational anger disorder without a.
target of a.
territorial a.

NOTES

aggression *(continued)*
a. toward objects
a. toward people
unassertive a.
undirected a.
verbal a.
wife-to-husband a.
a. without provocation

aggressive
a. act
a. action
a. attributional style
a. behavior theory
a. drive
a. episode
a. fantasy
a. hostility
a. impulse
a. instinct
a. invasion
a. objectionable behavior
a. obsession
a. outburst
a. personality
a. predatory type
a. psychotic behavior
a. psychotic inpatient
a. response
a. thought
a. undersocialized reaction

aggressively boisterous

aggressive-type undersocialized conduct disorder

aggressor
identification with a.

aggrieved

aghast

aging
acceptance of a.
activity theory of a.
a. adaptiveness
biologic change associated with a.
coping with a.
cybernetic theory of a.
dementia and a.
a. effect on sleep
ethnoracial issue in a.
eversion theory of a.
gender issue in a.
intimacy in a.
a. issue
menopause and a.
normal a.
parental a.
precocious a.
role transition in a.
sleep change in a.
a. theory

agitated
acutely a.
a. behavior
a. depression
a. melancholia
a. patient
a. reaction
a. state

agitation
drug-induced a.
early manic a.
emotional a.
extreme a.
frank a.
a. level
manic a.
marked motor a.
mental a.
nighttime a.
nocturnal a.
onset of a.
overlapping a.
overt a.
physical a.
psychomotor a.
psychotic a.
purposeless a.
reduced a.
a. response
unpredictable a.
unrelieved a.
untriggered a.
verbal a.
violent a.
visible a.

agitative feature

agitographia

agitolalia

agitophasia

aglutition

agnea

agnosia
acoustic a.
apperceptive visual a.
associative visual a.
auditory a.
body image a.
color a.
corporal a.
facial a.
finger a.
generalized auditory a.
ideational a.
integrative a.
landmark a.
localization a.
motion a.
object a.
optic a.

position a.
selective auditory a.
spatial a.
tactile a.
time a.
topographical a.
verbal a.
verbal-auditory a.
verbal-visual a.
visual a.
visuospatial a.

agnostic
a. alexia
a. behavior
self-described a.

agonadal

agonadism

agonal

agonist
dopamine a.
5-HT a.
inverse a.
a. medication
partial a.
a. therapy

agonize

agony
intellectual a.
personal a.
private a.

agoramania

agoraphobia
panic disorder with a.
panic disorder without a.
a. without history of panic disorder

agoraphobic

agouti-related protein

agrammatica

agrammatic speech

agrammatism

agrammatologia

agranulocytosis
drug-induced a.

agraphia
absolute a.
acoustic a.
acquired a.
alexia with a.
alexia without a.
amnemonic a.
a. amnemonica
aphasic a.
apraxic a.
atactic a.
cerebral a.
developmental a.
jargon a.
lexical a.
literal a.
mental a.
motor a.
musical a.
optic a.
phonological a.
pure a.
spatial a.
verbal a.

agraphic

agreeableness

agreed-on
a.-o. pattern
a.-o. routine

agreement
contractual a.
reciprocal a.
separation a.

agriothymia hydrophobica

agroterrorism

agrypnia

agrypnotic

AGS
adrenogenital syndrome
audiogenic seizure

AGT
activity group therapy

agyria

AH
alcoholic hepatitis

AHCPR
Agency for Health Care Policy and Research

AH1 Forms X and Y

AHI
active hostility index
anterior horn index

ahistorical

ahylognosia

AI
allergy index
anxiety index
autoimmune

Aicardi syndrome

aid
daily living a.
a. to dependent children (ADC)

NOTES

aid *(continued)*
eating a.
electronic a.
emergency psychiatric first a.
ergogenic a.
first a.
functional a.
sexual fantasy a.
Unisom Nighttime Sleep A.
Unisom with Pain Relief Sleep A.
visual a.

aide
childcare a.
home health a.
nurses' a.

aidoiomania

AIDS
acquired immunodeficiency syndrome
AIDS dementia complex (ADC)
AIDS encephalopathy
person with AIDS (PWA)

AIDS-related complex (ARC)

A-IGP
activity-interview group psychotherapy

aigu
délire a.

AIHQ
American Institute for Healthcare Quality
A. hostility bias-accidental
A. hostility bias-ambiguous
A. hostility bias-intentional

ailment
functional a.

ailurophilia

AIM
artificial intelligence in medicine

aim
a. inhibition
instinctual a.
partial a.
a. transference

AIMD
abnormal involuntary movement disorder

aimless
a. behavior
a. motor activity
a. wandering

AIN
American Institute of Nutrition

Ainsworth strange situation assessment

AIO
activity, interest, options

air
complemental a.
a. conduction
a. conduction deafness
a. conduction test
a. drinking
a. encephalopathy
a. hunger
a. pollution adaptation (APA)
a. pollution index
a. pollution syndrome (APS)
a. pressure effect
recycled a.
a. swallowing
a. wastage

air-blade sound

airplane glue dependence

AIT
acute intensive treatment

AK-47

AKA
alcoholic ketoacidosis
also known as

akathisia, acathisia
neuroleptic dose-dependent a.
neuroleptic-induced a.
treatment-emergent a.

akinesia, akinesis
a. amnestica
neuroleptic-induced a.
psychic a.

akinesia/diminished emotional expression

akinesic

akinesis (*var. of* akinesia)

akinesthesia

akinetic
a. apraxia
a. autism
a. depression
a. epilepsy
a. mania
a. mutism
a. patient
a. psychosis
a. seizure
a. stupor

akinetic-abulic syndrome

AL
annoyance level

alacrity

alalia
a. cophica
a. organica
a. physiologica
a. prolongata

alalic

alanine aminotransferase (ALT)

Al-Anon

alar flutter

alarm
a. reaction (AR)
a. reaction stage

alarmism

alarmist

alaryngeal speech

Alateen

A

albedo
Albert's Famous Faces
ALC
alcohol
approximate lethal concentration
alcohol (ALC)
a. abstinence
a. abstinence syndrome
a. abuse
a. addiction
allyl a.
a. amnestic syndrome
amyl a.
a. anxiety disorder
a. as cause of seizure
a. binge
blood a. (BA)
a. consumption
a. consumption behavior
a. counseling
a. craving
a. dependence
a. dependence syndrome
a. dependence with tolerance
a. dependent
a. derivative
a. detoxification
a. drinking
A., Drug Abuse, and Mental Health Administration (ADAMHA)
fetal effect of a.
a. habit
intermediate brain syndrome due to a.
a. intolerance
a. intoxication
a. intoxication-related disorder
a. level
lifetime risk for a.
a. metabolism
a. metabolizing system
a. misuse
a. mood disorder
a. offense
a. on breath (AOB)
a. paranoid state
pathologic reaction to a.
a. persisting dementia
a. poisoning
prenatal exposure to a.
a. problem
a. relapse prevention
a. related (AR)
saliva screen for a.
screening for a.
a. sensitivity
a. sleep disorder
tolerance to a.
toxic effect of a.
a. toxicity
a. treatment program
a. use
a. use disorder
a. withdrawal delirium
a. withdrawal hallucinosis
a. withdrawal seizure
a. withdrawal syndrome
a. withdrawal tremulousness
alcohol-Antabuse reaction
alcohol-associated dementia
alcoholate
chloral a.
alcohol-dependent
a.-d. individual
a.-d. patient
a.-d. sleep disorder
alcoholic
a. adolescent
adult child of a. (ACOA)
a. amblyopia
a. amentia
a. amnesia
a. amnestic disorder
A.'s Anonymous (AA)
a. ataxia
a. beverage
a. blackout
a. brain syndrome
a. cardiomyopathy
child of a. (COA)
a. cirrhosis (AC)
a. classification
closet a.
a. coma
a. confusional state
a. delirium
a. dementia
a. deterioration
detoxified a.
a. drunkenness
a. epilepsy
a. family
a. gastritis
genetics of a.'s
a. hallucination
a. hallucinosis

NOTES

alcoholic *(continued)*
a. hepatitis (AH)
inactive a. (IA)
a. insanity
a. jealousy
a. ketoacidosis (AKA)
a. Korsakoff psychosis
a. liver damage
a. liver disease (ALD)
a. liver disease-type organic psychosis
a. malabsorption syndrome
a. mania
a. myocardiopathy
a. myopathy
newly abstinent a.
a. organic mental disorder
a. pancreatic encephalopathy
a. pancreatitis
a. paralysis
a. paranoia
a. paranoid psychosis
a. paranoid state
a. paraplegia
a. parent
a. paresis
a. pellagra encephalopathy
a. peripheral neuropathy
a. poisoning
a. polyneuritic psychosis
a. pseudoparesis
a. rehabilitation
a. smoker
a. stupor
a. symptom
a. tremulousness
a. twilight state
type I, II a.
a. withdrawal tremor

alcoholica
amblyopia a.

alcoholicum
delirium a.

alcohol-induced
a.-i. anxiety
a.-i. delirium
a.-i. dementia
a.-i. depression
a.-i. nighttime sleep
a.-i. organic mental syndrome
a.-i. paranoid state
a.-i. peripheral neuropathy
a.-i. psychotic disorder
a.-i. psychotic disorder with delusions
a.-i. psychotic disorder with hallucinations
a.-i. sexual dysfunction

alcoholism
acute a.
alpha a.
antisocial a.
a. associated with dementia
beta a.
chronic a.
comorbid past a.
culture and a.
delta a.
dementia associated with a.
developmentally cumulative a.
developmentally limited a.
early-onset a.
epsilon a.
essential a.
Feighner criteria for a.
gamma a.
genetic a.
a. in isolation
mental disorder due to a.
negative-affect a.
past a.
prenatal a.
psychiatric disorder associated with a.
reactive a.
regressive a.
a. risk

alcoholization

alcohol-methadone interaction

alcoholomania

alcoholophilia

alcohol-positive history (APH)

alcohol-precipitated epilepsy

alcohol-related
a.-r. behavior
a.-r. birth defect (ARBD)
a.-r. cerebellar degeneration
a.-r. diagnosis
a.-r. harm
a.-r. injury
a.-r. insomnia
a.-r. offense
a.-r. phenotype
a.-r. physical problem
a.-r. psychiatric problem
a.-r. risk for accident
a.-r. risk for suicide
a.-r. risk for violence
a.-r. seizure
a.-r. tremor
a.-r. use disorder, NOS

ALD
alcoholic liver disease

alert
a. awake state
a., cooperative, and oriented (ACO)

A

a. inactivity
a. and oriented
alerting
a. effect
a. mechanism
a. stimulus
alertness
academic a. (AA)
a. level
level of a.
mental a.
state of a.
visual a.
alexia
agnostic a.
a. allochiria
anterior a.
auditory a.
central a.
cortical a.
incomplete a.
literal a.
motor a.
musical a.
optical a.
posterior a.
pure a.
sensory a.
subcortical a.
tactile a.
verbal a.
visual a.
a. with agraphia
a. without agraphia
alexic
alexithymia
alexithymic
a. behavior
a. personality
algedonic
algesia
algesic
algesichronometer
algesiogenic
algesthesia, algesthesis
algetic
algica
synesthesia a.
algogenesis
algogenic psychosyndrome
algolagnia
active a.
passive a.
algolagniac
algolagnist
algometer
algophilia, algophily
algopsychalia
algorithm
confusion assessment method diagnostic a.
diagnostic a.
algospasm
alias
use of a.
alibi
Alice in Wonderland syndrome
alien
ego a.
a. hand
a. obsession
a. thought
alienate
alienated
socially a.
alienatio mentis
alienation
body a.
a. coefficient
sense of a.
social a.
alienism
alienist
aliment
alimentary
a. abstinence
a. obesity
alimentation
forced a.
parenteral a.
alimentotherapy
alive
buried a.
alkali
alkaline phosphatase
alkaloid
belladonna a.
ergot a.
hydrogenated a.
alkalosis
metabolic a.
tetany of a.
alkylating agent
allachesthesia
Allah
all-American

NOTES

allay
allegation
  child molestation a.
alleged father (AF)
allegiance
allegorical
allegorization
allegory
allele frequency
allele-specific polymerase chain reaction
allelic
allelism
allelomorph
allergen
allergenic
allergic
  a. psychogenic disorder
  a. reaction
allergy
  drug a.
  immediate a.
  a. index (AI)
alleviating violence
alley
  blind a.
alliance
  contractual a.
  dysfunctional a.
  relational a.
  therapeutic a.
  treatment a.
  working a.
allied
  a. health professional
  a. reflex
alliterate
alliteration
allobarbital
allocentric
allochiria, allocheiria
  alexia a.
allocortex
allocortical cortex
allodynia
alloerotic
alloerotism, alloeroticism
alloesthesia
allogamy
allogrooming
allokinesis
allolalia
allomorph
allopath
allopathic
allopathist
allopathy
allopatric species
allophasis
allophone
alloplasty
allopsyche
allopsychic delusion
allopsychosis
all-or-none reaction
allosteric manner
allotoxin
allotriogeustia, allotriogeusia
allotriophagia, allotriophagy
allotriorhexia
allotriosmia
allotropic personality
allowable
allowance
  recommended daily a. (RDA)
Allport
  A. A-S reaction study
  A. group relations theory
  A. personality trait theory
Allport-Vernon-Linzey study of values
allure
allurement
allusion in wit
allusive thinking
all-women group
allyl alcohol
alma
  perdida del a.
alogia
aloneness
aloof
alopecia
  a. adnata
  androgenic a.
  a. areata
  a. celsi
  Celsus a.
  cicatricial a.
  a. cicatrisata
  a. circumscripta
  a. congenitalis
  congenital sutural a.
  a. disseminata
  a. dynamica
  a. hereditaria
  a. leprotica
  male pattern a.
  a. marginalis
  a. medicamentosa
  a. mucinosa
  a. neurotica
  a. parviculata
  a. pityrodes
  postoperative pressure a.
  postpartum a.
  a. prematura
  premature a.
  a. presenilis
  psychogenic a.

self-induced a.
a. senilis
stress-induced a.
a. symptomatica
syphilitic a.
a. syphilitica
a. totalis
a. toxica
traction a.
traumatic a.
trichotillomania-induced a.
a. universalis

alpha
a. activity
a. adrenergic-blocking drug
a. adrenergic receptor
a. adrenergic-stimulating drug
a. alcoholism
a. apparent
a. arc
a., beta, gamma hypotheses
a. block
a. blocking
a. cell
a. coefficient
coefficient a.
Cronbach a.
a. error
a. examination
a. factor
a. feedback
a. frequency
a. index
a. level
a. methyldopa-induced mood disorder
a. movement
a. receptor blocking agent
a. rhythm
a. state
a. synuclein protein
a. wave

alpha-2
a.-2 adrenergic receptor
a.-2 antagonist

alphabet
initial teaching a.

alphalytic
alphamimetic
alphaprodine
alpha-wave training
alpidem
alpinism

ALSD
Alzheimer-like senile dementia

alseroxylon
also known as (AKA)

ALT
alanine aminotransferase

alter
a. ego
a. egoism
a. ego theory
a. ego transference

alterable

alteration
behavior a.
identity a.
a. in identity
ionic transduction a.
a. of memory structure
neurocognitive a.
neuropathological a.
a. in rate of speech
reactive ego a.
receptor a.
selective speech perception a.
signal transduction a.
speech processing a.
speech tracking a.
stress-induced immune system a.
a. in time perception

alterative
altercation

altered
a. appetite
a. auditory feedback (AAF)
a. cognition
a. emotion
a. function
a. level of consciousness
a. life circumstance
a. memory network
a. menses
a. mental status
a. mentation
a. mind-body perception
a. personality
a. sensation
a. sensory perception
a. sleep schedule
a. state
a. state of consciousness (ASC)
a. tau processing
a. time perception

NOTES

altered *(continued)*
a. vision
a. voice
alternate
a. binaural loudness balance (ABLB)
a. form reliability coefficient
a. hemianesthesia
a. identity
a. monaural loudness balance (AMLB)
a. motion rate (AMR)
alternating
a. behavior
a. bipolar disorder
a. current (AC)
a. current and/or direct current (AC/DC)
a. insanity
a. mydriasis
a. personalities
a. perspective
a. psychosis
a. pulse
a. role
a. tremor
alternation
alternative
a. alter ego
a. approach
a. behavior
a. criterion B for dysthymic disorder
a. diagnosis
a. dimensional descriptor for schizophrenia
a. explanation
a. intervention
least restrictive a.
a. lifestyle
a. lifestyle community
a. medicine
a. method
a. perspective
pharmaceutical a.
a. psychosis
psychotherapy a.
a. school
a. strategy
a. therapy
a. treatment
viable a.
a. viewpoint
altitude
a. anoxia
a. disease
a. sickness
altrigenderism
altruism
altruistic
a. behavior
a. personality
a. role
a. suicide
aluminum exposure
alveolar hypoventilation syndrome
alymphoplasia
Alzheimer
A. dementia
A. disease (AD)
A. disease neuropathology
A. Disease and Related Disorders Association
A. psychosis
A. syndrome
Alzheimer-like senile dementia (ALSD)
AM
amplitude modulation
attitude to medication
AMA
against medical advice
amalgam
dental a.
emotional a.
emotional object a.
Amanita
A. muscaria
A. panthera
A. phalloides
A. verna
amanitin
amanitoxin
amasesis
amative
amativeness
amatory
amaurosis
epileptoid a.
hysterical a.
toxic a.
amaurotic
a. axonal idiocy
a. familial idiocy (AFI)
amaxoapraxia
ambageusia
AMBHA
American Managed Behavioral Healthcare Association
ambiance
family a.
sociocultural a.
ambidexterity, ambidextrism
ambidextrous
ambient
a. air pressure
a. behavior
a. noise
a. temperature

ambiguity
acoustic a.
diagnostic a.
lexical a.
role a.
structural a.
a. tolerance
ambiguous
a. external stimulus
a. figure
a. genitalia
ambilaterality
ambilevous
ambisexual
ambisinister, ambisinistrous
ambitendency
ambitieux
délire a.
ambivalence
a. about living
affective a.
dual a.
a. of intellect
a. of will
ambivalent
a. affect
a. attachment style
a. feeling
a. quotient
ambiversion
ambivert
amblyaphia
amblygeustia
amblyopia
alcoholic a.
a. alcoholica
arsenic a.
color a.
hysterical a.
nutritional a.
tobacco a.
toxic a.
traumatic a.
ambulance chaser
ambulans
paroniria a.
ambulation index
ambulatory
a. automatism
a. care
a. mental health service
a. schizophrenia
a. status
ambush
sudden a.
ameboidism
ameliorate
amelioration
tendency toward a.
amenable to treatment
amenia
amenomania
amenorrhea
dietary a.
dysponderal a.
emotional a.
nutritional a.
pathologic a.
physiologic a.
premenopausal a.
secondary a.
stress-related a.
amenorrheic
ament
amentia
alcoholic a.
a. attonita
isolation a.
nevoid a.
a. paranoides
phenylpyruvic a.
primary a.
Stearns alcoholic a.
amential
Amerasian
America
Anxiety Disorders Association of A. (ADAA)
Big Brothers of A.
Big Sisters of A.
Child Welfare League of A. (CWLA)
Radiological Society of North A.
americamania
American
A. Academy of Addiction Psychiatry (AAAP)
A. Academy of Child and Adolescent Psychiatry (AACAP)
A. Academy of Clinical Psychiatrists (AACP)
A. Academy on Physician and Patient (AAPP)
A. Academy of Pain Medicine (AAPM)
A. Academy of Pediatrics (AAP)

NOTES

American *(continued)*
A. Academy of Pediatrics Task Force on Violence
A. Academy of Psychiatrists in Alcoholism and Addictions (AAPAA)
A. Academy of Psychiatry and Law (AAPL)
A. Academy of Psychoanalysis (AAP)
A. Academy of Psychoanalysis and Dynamic Psychiatry (AAPDP)
A. Academy of Psychosomatic Medicine
A. Academy of Psychotherapists (AAP)
A. Academy of Sleep Medicine (AASM)
African A.
Asian A.
A. Association of Chairmen of Departments of Psychiatry
A. Association of Children's Residential Centers (AACRC)
A. Association of Community Psychiatrists
A. Association for Counseling & Development (AACD)
A. Association for the Cure of Inebriates (AACI)
A. Association of Directors of Psychiatric Residency Training (AADPRT)
A. Association of Emergency Psychiatry
A. Association of General Hospital Psychiatrists
A. Association for Geriatric Psychiatry (AAGP)
A. Association for Marriage and Family Therapy (AAMFT)
A. Association of Mental Retardation (AAMR)
A. Association of Psychiatric Administrators
A. Association of Psychiatric Services for Children (AAPSC)
A. Association of Psychotherapists
A. Association of Suicidology (AAS)
A. Board of Forensic Psychiatrists (ABFP)
A. Board of Forensic Psychiatry
A. Board of Forensic Psychiatry and Neurology (ABFPN)
A. Board of Medical Specialties (ABMS)
A. Board of Professional Psychology
A. Board of Psychiatry (ABP)
A. Board of Psychiatry and Neurology (ABPN)
A. Board of Sleep Medicine
A. Civil Liberties Union (ACLU)
A. College Counseling Association (ACCA)
A. College of Forensic Psychiatry
A. College of Neuropsychiatrists
A. College of Psychiatrists (ACP)
A. College of Testing (ACT)
A. Counseling Association (ACA)
A. Diabetes Association (ADA)
A. Diabetes Association diet
A. Dietetic Association (ADA)
European A.
A. Family Therapy Academy (AFTA)
A. Family Therapy Association (AFTA)
A. Foundation for Suicide Prevention
A. Indian
A. Institute for Healthcare Quality (AIHQ)
A. Institute of Nutrition (AIN)
Latin A.
A. Law Institute formulation of insanity
A. Law Institute rule
A. Managed Behavioral Healthcare Association (AMBHA)
Native A.
A. Occupational Therapy Association (AOTA)
A. Orthopsychiatric Association (AOA)
A. Pain Society (APS)
A. Pharmaceutical Association (APhA)
A. Physical Therapy Association (APTA)
A. Psychiatric Association (APA)
A. Psychiatry Association-Center for Mental Health Services
A. Psychoanalytical Association (APA)
A. Psychological Association (APA)
A. Psychological Society (APS)
A. Psychosomatic Society
A. Public Health Association (APHA)
A. Society of Addiction Medicine (ASAM)
A. Society for Adolescent Psychiatry
A. Society of Group Psychotherapy and Psychodrama (ASGPP)

A. Society of Psychoanalytic Physicians (ASPP)
A.'s with Disabilities Act (ADA)

americanize

ametamorphosis

amiable
socially a.

amicable

amide
lysergic acid a.

amimia
amnesic a.
ataxic a.
expressive a.

amine
biogenic a.
a. tricyclic antidepressant
tricyclic secondary a.
tricyclic tertiary a.

amino

aminotransferase
alanine a. (ALT)
aspartate a. (AST)

amitriptyline hydrochloride

amitriptyline-induced mood disorder

AMLB
alternate monaural loudness balance

ammonium
a. bromide
a. salicylate

amnalgesia

amnemonic
a. agraphia
a. aphasia

amnemonica
agraphia a.

amnesia
acute a.
affective a.
a. after trance
alcoholic a.
amnesic a.
anterograde a.
asymmetrical a.
audioverbal a.
auditory a.
autohypnotic a.
axial a.
Broca a.
catathymic a.
childbirth a.
a. in children
chronic a.
circumscribed a.
complete a.
concussion a.
continuous a.
cortical a.
degree of a.
dissociative a.
emotional a.
episodic a.
epochal a.
evidence of a.
generalized a.
global a.
hippocampal a.
hypnotic a.
hysterical a.
ictal a.
infantile a.
Korsakoff a.
lacunar a.
localized a.
neurologic a.
nonpathological a.
olfactory a.
organic a.
partial a.
patchy a.
polyglot a.
postconcussion a.
post-ECT a.
postelectroconvulsive a.
posthypnotic a.
posttraumatic a. (PTA)
profound a.
psychogenic a.
residual a.
retroactive a.
retroanterograde a.
retrograde a.
reversible a.
selective a.
shrinking retrograde a.
a. for sleep and dreaming
a. for sleep terror event
subsequent a.
systematized a.
tactile a.
toxin-provoked a.
transient global a. (TGA)
a. for trauma
traumatic a.
a. traumatica
true a.

NOTES

amnesia *(continued)*
verbal a.
visual a.
amnesic, amnestic
a. amimia
a. amnesia
a. aphasia
a. apraxia
a. color blindness
a. memoration
a. patient
a. state
a. syndrome
amnestica
akinesia a.
amok, amuck
amor
amoral
a. psychopathic personality
a. trend
amorist
amorous paranoia
amorphagnosia
amorphism
amorphosynthesis
amotivated behavior
amotivation
amotivational syndrome
amount
maximum tolerable a.
amour
amour-propre
ampere
ampheclexis
amphetamine (AMT)
a. abuse
adjunctive a.
a. delirium
a. delusional disorder
a. dependence
a. inhaler
a. intoxication
a. intoxication with perceptual disturbance
a. look-alike
a. overdose
a. poisoning
a. psychosis
racemic a.
substituted a.
a. use disorder
a. withdrawal
amphetamine-induced
a.-i. anxiety
a.-i. psychotic disorder
a.-i. psychotic disorder with delusions
a.-i. psychotic disorder with hallucinations
a.-i. sexual dysfunction
amphetamine-like
a.-l. action
a.-l. substance
amphetamine-related disorder
amphetamine-type stimulant (ATS)
amphicrania
amphierotism
amphigenesis
amphigenic inversion
amphigonadism
amphimixis
amphitypia
amphoriloquy
amphorophony
amphotonia, amphotony
amplification
memory a.
symptom a.
amplitude modulation (AM)
amputee
AMR
abnormal muscle response
alternate motion rate
AMS
auditory memory span
amuck (*var. of* amok)
amulet
amusia
expressive a.
motor a.
sensory a.
vocal a.
amusing aspect
amygdala, pl. **amygdalae**
a. activation
a. atrophy
a. damage
a. nucleus group
a. response
a. subnucleus
a. volume
a. volumetric loss
amygdala-fear circuitry
amygdala-prefrontal cortex-locus ceruleus interaction
amygdaloid stimulation
amyl
a. acetate
a. alcohol
a. chloride
a. nitrate abuse
a. nitrate inhalant
a. salicylate
a. valerate
amylase
amylene

amylobarbitone
amyloid
a. plaque
a. plaque formation
a. precursor protein
amylophagia
amyoesthesia, amyoesthesis
amyostasia
amyosthenia
amyotaxy, amyotaxia
Amytal
A. ablation
A. interview
AN
anorexia nervosa
anabolic
a. agent
a. steroid
anabolic-androgenic steroid (AAS)
anabolism
anacatesthesia
anachronism
anachronobiology
anaclasis
anaclitic
a. depression
a. psychotherapy
a. relationship
a. therapy
Anaconda
Operation A.
anacusis
anagogic
a. interpretation
a. symbolism
a. tendency
anagogy
anal
a. administration
a. canal
a. character
a. eroticism
a. fissure
a. humor
a. impotence
a. intercourse
a. masturbation
a. personality
a. phase
a. phase of infancy
a. rape
a. rape fantasy
a. retentive
a. sadism
a. sex
a. stage
a. stage psychosexual development
a. trauma
anal-aggressive character
analeptic
anal-expulsive stage
analgesia
a. dolorosa
hypnotic a.
patient-controlled a. (PCA)
analgesic
a. abuse
controlled a.
a. cuirass
narcotic a.
nonnarcotic a.
pharmaceutical a.
analgesimeter
analgetic
analis
coitus a.
anality
analog, analogue
a. experiment
I-labeled cocaine a.
libido a.
a. marking
a. of meperidine
a. of phencyclidine
prion a.
a. study
analogic change
analogous brain mechanism
analogue (*var. of* analog)
analogy
anal-retentive personality
anal-sadistic love
analysand
analysis, pl. **analyses**
acoustic a.
active a.
aerodynamic speech a.
applied behavioral a. (ABA)
auditory a.
behavior a.
blind a.
cephalometric a.
chain a.
character a.
child a.
classical a.

NOTES

analysis *(continued)*
clinical a.
cluster a.
complex segregation a.
content a.
contrastive a.
control a.
conventional factor a.
a. of coping style
cost-benefit a.
cost-reward a.
a. of covariance (ANCOVA)
Cox regression a.
critical a.
Dasein a.
a. in depth
didactic a.
discriminant a.
distal distinctive feature a.
distinctive feature a.
distributive a.
ego a.
error a.
existential a.
expectant a.
factor a.
fate a.
feature a.
feeling a.
final a.
focused a.
Fourier a.
fractional a.
functional a.
furthest-neighbor a.
gait a.
genetic linkage a.
group a.
handwriting a.
harmonic a.
hierarchical regression a.
holistic a.
immunoblot a.
impact a.
individual a.
intent-to-treat a.
interaction process a.
item a.
job a.
kinesthetic a.
kinetic a.
latent class a.
lay a.
logistic regression a.
method a.
minor a.
molecular genetic a.
morphometric a.
motivation a.
multiple analyses
multivariate a.
neurometric a.
occupational a.
passive a.
pattern a.
percept a.
perception a.
perceptual a.
personal document a.
phenomenological a.
philosophical a.
phonemic a.
phonetic a.
phonological a.
policy a.
post hoc a.
preliminary a.
principal-component a. (PCA)
a. procedure
regression a.
resistance a.
a. of resistance
Schicksal a.
script a.
segmental a.
sequential multiple analyses (SMA)
shape a.
situs a.
solution a.
sound a.
state-of-the-art a.
substitution a.
suprasegmental a.
a. by synthesis
a. and synthesis
task performance and a.
taxometric a.
therapeutic group a.
toxicological a.
traditional phonetic a.
training a.
transactional a. (TA)
a. of transference
trial a.
a. of variance (ANOVA)
variance components a.

analyst

analytic
a. approach
a. boundary
a. couch
a. exegesis
a. frame
a. group psychotherapy
a. insight
a. interpretation
a. method
a. neurosis

a. object
a. patient
a. psychiatry
a. psychology
a. rule
a. stalemate
a. therapy
a. treatment
analytical
a. breakdown
a. philosophy
a. play therapy
a. process
a. psychology
analyzer
breath a.
noise a.
wave a.
analyzing new information disturbance
anamnesis
associative a.
anamnestic response
ananastasia
anancasm
anancastia
anancastic
a. depression
a. neurosis
a. personality
anandamide
anandria
anaphia, anhaphia
anaphor
anaphoric pronoun
anaphrodisia
anaphrodisiac
anaphrodite
anaphylaxis
psychiatric a.
psychic a.
anaptic
anarchic behavior
anarchism
anarithmia
anarthria
anatomic
a. abnormality
a. age
a. brain change
a. correlate
a. evidence
a. impotence
a. site of pain
anatopism
anatripsis
anatriptic
anaudia
ancestral
a. spirit
a. worship
ancestry
anchone
anchor
collapsing a.
firing an a.
a. sign of withdrawal
stacking a.
stealing an a.
a. symptom
anchoring
perceptual a.
ancillary care
ANCOVA
analysis of covariance
Andes disease
Andreasen positive and negative symptoms of schizophrenia
androgen
a. insensitivity syndrome
a. level
androgenesis
androgenic alopecia
androgenization
androgenous
androgynoid
androgynous individual
androgyny
android
andrology
andromania
andromimetic
andromorphous
androphilia
androsterone
anecdotal
a. data
a. evidence
a. method
anecdote
clinical a.
Anectine
anelectrotonic zone
anelectrotonus
anemia
anepia
anepithymia

NOTES

anerethisia
anergasia
anergastic
a. organic psychosis
a. reaction
anergic
a. depression
a. schizophrenic
a. stupor
anergy, anergia
denial of a.
physical a.
anesthesia
block a.
central a.
closed a.
combined a.
compression a.
conversion a.
crossed a.
cutaneous a.
diagnostic a.
dissociative a.
a. dolorosa
electric a.
emotional a.
first stage of a.
gauntlet a.
general a.
girdle a.
glove a.
gustatory a.
Gwathmey a.
halogenated inhalation a.
hypnotic a.
hysterical a.
infiltration a.
inhaled a.
insufflation a.
insulation a.
laryngeal a.
mental a.
muscular a.
neuroleptic a.
olfactory a.
painful a.
perineural a.
peripheral a.
pressure a.
primary a.
segmental a.
sensory a.
sexual a.
spinal a.
splanchnic a.
stocking a.
stocking-and-glove a.
tactile a.
thermal a.
traumatic a.
unilateral a.
visceral a.
anesthetic
a. conversion reaction
dissociative a.
medical a.
anethopath
anetic
A9 neuron
angel-of-death hallucination
angel's trumpet
Angelucci syndrome
anger
a. attack
a. behavior
chronic state of a.
constant a.
controlled a.
deeply buried a.
difficulty controlling a.
a. dysregulation
externalized a.
feeling of a.
fit of a.
ineffective a.
intense a.
internalized a.
inwardly directed a.
irrational a.
a. mallet
a. management
marked a.
a. outburst
outburst of a.
overt sign of a.
quick to a.
a. reaction
redirecting a.
suppressed a.
transient state of a.
trigger for a.
a. and violence psychiatric syndrome
withdrawal-related a.
anger-related personality trait
angiography
angiopathic neurasthenia
anglicize
Anglo
anglomania
anglophile
angor
a. animi
a. ocularis
a. pectoris
angry
a. affect
a. behavior

a. memory
a. outburst
a. reaction
a. reaction to minor stimulus
a. temperament
a. woman syndrome
a. word exchange

anguish
existential a.
personal a.
postbinge a.

anhalonine

anhaphia (*var. of* anaphia)

anhedonia
orgasmic a.
pervasive a.
social a.

anhedonia-asociality

ani (*pl. of* anus)

anileridine

anilinction

anilinctus

anilingus

anility

anima

animal
a. abuse
aggression to people and a.'s
a. companionship
cruelty to a.'s
history of abusing a.'s
a. loss grief
a. magnetism
skin of a.'s

animal-assisted therapy

animalize

animal-like

animated

animation
suspended a.

animatism

animi
angor a.
demissio a.

animism

animist

animistic thinking

animosity

animus

ankh

ankle
a. clonus
a. jerk
a. restraint

anlage, pl. **anlagen**

annihilation anxiety

annihilator

anniversary
a. date
a. excitement
a. hypothesis
personally significant a.
a. reaction

annoyance level (AL)

annulment

ano
coitus in a.
in a.

anodyne

anoetic

anogenital

anomalies (*pl. of* anomaly)

anomalotrophy

anomalous
a. movement
a. parental vocal pattern
a. result
a. sexual behavior
a. sexual urge

anomaly, pl. **anomalies**
Aristotle a.
autosomal a.
cranial a.
metabolic a.
sexual a.
structured interview for assessing perceptual anomalies

anomia
color a.
finger a.
tactile a.

anomic
a. aphasia
a. error
a. suicide

anomie

anonymity

Anonymous
Alcoholics A. (AA)
Cocaine A. (CA)
Codependents A. (CODA)
Gamblers A. (GA, GamAnon)
Narcotics A. (NA, NarcAnon)
Overeaters A. (OA)
Parent's A.

NOTES

Anonymous *(continued)*
Schizophrenics A. (SA)
Sex Addicts A. (SAA)
Sexaholics A. (SA)
Workaholics A. (WA)
anorchism
anorectal
a. physiological dysfunction
a. spasm
anorectic, anoretic, anorexic
anorexia
elective a.
a. nervosa (AN)
social a.
anorexiant
anorexic (*var. of* anorectic)
a. behavior
a. fast
anorexigenic
anorgasmic
anorgasmy, anorgasmia
secondary a.
SSRI-induced a.
anosmia
essential a.
functional a.
mechanical a.
respiratory a.
true a.
anosodiaphoria
anosognosia
anosognosic
anosphrasia
ANOVA
analysis of variance
anoxemia
anoxia
altitude a.
cerebral a.
fulminating a.
hypokinetic a.
metabolic a.
transitory a.
anoxic encephalopathy (AE)
ANS
autonomic nervous system
Anstie rule
answer
bizarre a.
false-positive a.
irrelevant a.
syndrome of approximate relevant a.'s
syndrome of deviously relevant a.'s
yes-no a.
antagonism
antagonist
alpha-2 a.
benzodiazepine a.
beta adrenergic a.
beta noradrenergic a.
dopaminergic a.
D_4-receptor a.
a. drug
high-potency D_2 a.
5-HT a.
low-potency D_2 a.
a. medication
mid-potency D_2 a.
narcotic a.
opiate a.
opioid a.
antagonistic
a. behavior
a. muscle strength
a. reflex
a. thermoeffector
antagonize
antalgic gait
antaphrodisiac
antaphroditic
antapoplectic
antasthenic
antecedent
cognitive a.
early childhood identifiable a.
a. event
identifiable a.
a. variable
a. of violence
antecedent-consequence variable
antepartum
anterior
a. alexia
a. aphasia
a. capsulotomy for treatment of OCD
a. cingulate
a. cingulate flow
a. cingulate pathway
a. cingulotomy for treatment of OCD
a. feature English phoneme
a. horn index (AHI)
a. hypothalamus
a. insula region
a. nucleus
a. nucleus of thalamus
a. speech zone
a. vermis
a. vertical canal
anterograde
a. amnesia
a. loss of memory
a. memory interference
anterotic
anthomania

A

anthrax
a. anxiety
a. exposure
anthropocentric
anthropocentrism
anthropogenic
anthropography
anthropoid
anthropological
a. linguistics
a. philosophy
anthropology
applied a.
criminal a.
cultural a.
medical a.
physical a.
social a.
anthropometric identification
anthropometry
anthropomorphic
anthropomorphism
anthropomorphize
anthroponomy
anthropopathism
anthropopathy
anthropophagus
anthropophilic
anthroposophy
anthypnotic (*var. of* antihypnotic)
anthysteric (*var. of* antihysteric)
antiabortion
antiadrenergic effect
antiaggressive
a. action
a. effect
antiaging
antiamericanism
antianaphylaxis
antiandrogen therapy
antianxiety
a. agent
a. medication
antibody
antibrain
anticatalyst
anticipatory a.
anticathexis
anticephalalgic
antichrist
anticipated emotional suffering
anticipation
a. of role
a. of trigger
anticipatory
a. anticatalyst
a. anxiety
a. autocastration
a. avoidance (AA)
a. coarticulation
a. error
a. grief
a. guidance
a. maturation principle
a. response
a. and struggle behavior
a. worry
anticlimactic
anticlimax
anticonvulsive
anticrime
antidepressant
a. abuse
a. for adolescents
a. agent
amine tricyclic a.
atypical a.
a. compound
a. inhibition
a. medication
monocyclic a.
a. monotherapy
a. response
serotonergic a.
somatic a.
tetracyclic a.
a. therapy
a. treatment
antidepressant-resistant
antidiuretic hormone (ADH)
antidotal
antidote
antidromic
antidyskinetic agent
antiemetic
antienergic
antiepileptic
a. drug
a. medication
antierotica
antiestablishment
antiestrogenic
antiexpectancy speech
antifeminist

NOTES

antifetishism
antigen
H-Y a.
antigen-antibody reaction
antigonadal action
antigovernment feeling
antihallucinatory
antihistamine
sedative a.
antihistaminergic effect
anti-5-HT_2
antihypertensive
a. agent
a. medication
antihypnotic, anthypnotic
antihysteric, anthysteric
antiimpulse effect
antiinflammatory therapy
antiinstinctual force
anti-Lewisite
British a.-L. (BAL)
Antilirium
antimanic
antimotivational syndrome
antimuscarinic effect
anti-Muslim sentiment
antimyasthenic
antinarcotic
antinauseant
antinomianism
antinomy
antioxidant therapy
antipanic agent
antipathetic
antipathetical
antipathy
antipersonnel
antiphobic
antiphony
antiposia
antipredatory aggression
antipsychiatry
antipsychomotor
antipsychotic
a. action
atypical a.
a. compound
conventional dopamine receptor-blocking a.
depot a.
a. drug
a. drug therapy
a. drug treatment
a. effect
high-potency a.
low-dose a.
a. medication
a. medication exposure
new-generation a.
novel a.
a. pharmacotherapy
a. preparation
a. response
thioxanthene a.
traditional a.
a. treatment
tricyclic a. (TCA)
typical a.
antipsychotic-associated sexual dysfunction
antipsychotic-induced weight gain
antipsychotic-related hyperkinesis
antipyretic
antiresonance
antiretroviral medication
antireward system
antiruminant
antiseizure
a. drug
a. medication
antisemite
antisemitic
antisemitism
antiserotonergic effect
antislavery
antisocial (AS)
a. activity
a. adolescent
a. aggression
a. alcoholism
a. behavior
a. child
a. compulsion
a. feature
a. juvenile
a. lifestyle
a. neurotic personality
a. patient
a. personality (ASP)
a. personality disorder (APD, ASPD)
a. psychopathic Q factor
a. reaction
a. teenager
a. tendency
a. trends psychopathic personality
antispasticity
antisyphilitic
antiterrorism
antiterrorist
antitetanic
antithesis
antithetical
antitonic
antitoxin
antitragus
antitrismus
antitussive

antivivisection
antiwar
Anton syndrome
antrophose
antsy
anum
- per a.

anus, pl. **ani**
anxietas
- a. presenilis
- a. tibiarum

anxiety
- a. adjustment disorder
- adjustment disorder with a.
- adolescent a.
- alcohol-induced a.
- amphetamine-induced a.
- annihilation a.
- anthrax a.
- anticipatory a.
- anxiolytic-induced a.
- a. attack
- authority a.
- basic a.
- caffeine-induced a.
- cannabis-induced a.
- castration a.
- catastrophic a.
- childhood separation a.
- chronic a.
- clinically significant a.
- cocaine-induced a.
- a. comorbidity
- a. control technique
- a. control training (ACT)
- covert a.
- death a.
- debilitating a.
- delusional a.
- dental a.
- a. depression
- desertion a.
- a. diagnosis
- diffuse a.
- disabling a.
- a. discharge
- disintegration a.
- a. disorder of adolescence
- a. disorder of childhood
- A. Disorders Association of America (ADAA)
- a. disturbance
- a. dream
- a. due to physical disorder
- a. due to substance abuse
- a. during pregnancy
- ego a.
- eighth-month a.
- elementary a.
- environmentally induced a.
- erotized a.
- examination a.
- excessive social a.
- existential a.
- extreme a.
- feeling of a.
- a. fixation
- a. fluctuation
- focus of a.
- free-floating a.
- frequency of a.
- gender difference in a.
- generalized a.
- heightened a.
- heterosexual a.
- a. hierarchy
- high a. (HA)
- high impulsiveness high a. (HIHA)
- high impulsiveness low a. (HILA)
- hypnotic-induced a.
- hyposomnia associated with a.
- a. hysteria
- id a.
- immediate a.
- increased a.
- a. index (AI)
- insomnia associated with a.
- instinctual a.
- intense a.
- intercourse a.
- intercurrent a.
- internal sensation of a.
- level of a.
- a. level
- low a. (LA)
- a. management
- a. management training (AMT)
- manifest a.
- marked a.
- masked a.
- means for a.
- moral a.
- morbid a.
- a. neurosis
- neutralized a.
- noetic a.

NOTES

anxiety *(continued)*
nonpathological a.
nonpsychotic a.
normal a.
a. object
objective a.
obsessional a.
oral a.
organic a.
overwhelming a.
pain-type a.
panic attack neurotic a.
a. panic reaction
panic-type a.
paradoxical a.
peer a.
performance a.
persecutory a.
persistent episodic a.
pervasive a.
phobic a.
prenatal a.
a. preparedness
a. prevention
primal a.
primary a.
a. profile
profound a.
prominent a.
provoked a.
psychic a.
psychogenic a.
a. psychogenic disorder
a. psychoneurosis
a. psychoneurotic reaction
a. reaction, mild (ARM)
reactive depression and a.
real a.
reality a.
reduced a.
a. reduction
relaxation-induced a. (RIA)
a. relief response
a. resolution
sedative-induced a.
self-disclosure a.
self-induced a.
self-reported a.
a. sensitivity (AS)
separation a.
severe a.
sexual a.
signal theory of a.
situation a.
situational a.
sleeplessness associated with a.
social a.
a. source
a. state (AS)
a. state neurotic disorder
stranger a.
substance-induced a.
superego a.
symbolic a.
a. symptom
a. syndrome
a. tension state (ATS)
test a.
theory of a.
a. tolerance
total phobic a. (TPA)
trait a.
transformation theory of a.
trauma-specific a.
traumatic a.
true a.
a. typology
uncontrollable a.
undue social a.
urethral a.
virginal a.

anxiety-avoiding personality disorder
anxiety-blissfulness psychosis
anxiety-induced impaired social functioning
anxiety-like behavior
anxiety-mood comorbidity
anxiety-producing situation
anxiety-provoking
a.-p. cue
a.-p. event
a.-p. situation

anxiety-related
a.-r. mental disorder
a.-r. psychiatric syndrome
a.-r. sensation
a.-r. tremor
a.-r. word

anxiety-sensitivity theory
anxiolytic
a. abuse
a. activity
a. agent
a. amnestic disorder
a. delirium
a. dependence
a. disinhibition
a. drug
a. effect
a. intoxication
a. medication
a. response
serotonergic a.
a. stimulus
a. substance
a. substance-use disorder
a. use disorder
a. withdrawal

anxiolytic-induced
a.-i. anxiety
a.-i. persisting dementia
a.-i. psychotic disorder with delusions
a.-i. psychotic disorder with hallucinations
a.-i. sexual dysfunction
anxious
a. arousal
a. delirium
a. expectation
a. mania
a. mood
a. mood adjustment reaction
a. new mother
a. rumination
a. somatic depression
a. substance abuser
a. thought
anxious-fearful cluster
anxiousness
anxious-neurotic personality trait
AO
academic orientation
avoidance of others
AOA
American Orthopsychiatric Association
AOB
alcohol on breath
AOOP
Academy of Organizational and Occupational Psychiatry
AOTA
American Occupational Therapy Association
APA
air pollution adaptation
American Psychiatric Association
American Psychoanalytical Association
American Psychological Association
apallesthesia
apallic
a. state
a. syndrome
apandria
apanthropia, apanthropy
apareunia
apartness
apastia
apastic
apathetic
a. affect
a. attitude
a. thyrotoxicosis
a. withdrawal
apathetic-type personality disorder
apathic
apathism
apathy
avolition a.
euphoric a.
a. syndrome
APD
antisocial personality disorder
avoidant personality disorder
aperient
aperiodic
a. reinforcement
a. wave
aperitif
apertive
apertural hypothesis
APH
alcohol-positive history
APHA
American Public Health Association
APhA
American Pharmaceutical Association
aphagia
psychogenic a.
aphasia
acoustic a.
acquired epileptic a.
acquired fluent a.
afferent motor a.
ageusic a.
amnemonic a.
amnesic a.
amnestic a.
anomic a.
anterior a.
associative a.
ataxic a.
auditory a.
Bastian a.
Benson-Geschwind classification of a.
Broca a.
callosal disconnection syndrome a.
central a.
childhood a.
combined transcortical a.
commissural a.
complete a.
conduction a.

NOTES

aphasia *(continued)*
contiguity a.
cortical a.
developmental a.
a. disorder
dynamic a.
efferent motor a.
epileptic a.
executive a.
expressive a.
expressive-receptive a.
fluent a.
frontocortical a.
frontolenticular a.
functional a.
gibberish a.
global a.
graphic a.
graphomotor a.
Grashey a.
hypophonic a.
ideomotor a.
impressive a.
infantile a.
intellectual a.
isolation a.
jargon a.
Kussmaul a.
lenticular a.
lethica a.
Lichtheim a.
major motor a.
mixed a.
motor a.
nominal a.
nonfluent a.
optic a.
parietooccipital a.
partial nominal a.
pathematic a.
pictorial a.
pragmatic a.
primary progressive a.
psychogenic a.
psychosensory a.
pure a.
a. quotient (AQ)
receptive a.
semantic a.
sensory a.
similarity disorder of a.
simple a.
speech-reading a.
subcortical motor a.
syndrome a.
syntactic a.
tactile a.
total a.
transcortical a.
traumatic a.
true a.
verbal a.
visual a.
Wernicke a.

aphasic, aphasiac
a. acalculia
a. agraphia
a. disturbance
a. error
a. migraine
a. patient
a. phonological impairment
a. seizure

aphemesthesia

aphemia
pure a.

aphilopony

aphonia
conversion a.
functional a.
hysterical a.
intermittent a.
paralytica a.
a. paranoica
spastic a.
tactile a.

aphonic episode

aphonous

aphorize

aphose

aphrasia paranoica

aphremia

aphrodisiac

aphrodisia phrenitica

aphrodisiomania

aphthongia

aphylactic

aphylaxis

apical

apicalization

aplomb

APM
Academy of Psychosomatic Medicine

apnea
central sleep a.
narcolepsy-associated sleep a.
obstructive sleep a.

apneic
a. pause
a. period
a. seizure

apneustic
a. breathing
a. period

apocalypse

apocalyptic

apocalypticism

apocryphal

apodictic
ApoE genotyping
apogee
apolitical
apologetic behavior
apopathetic behavior
apophysary point
apoplectic
a. coma
a. dementia
a. type
apoplectica
dementia a.
apoplectiform
a. convulsion
a. seizure
apoplexy
functional a.
apoptotic cell death
apostasis
apostasy
apostate
apostatize
apotemnophilia
apotheosis
apotreptic therapy
apotropaic
APP
addiction-prone personality
apparatus, pl. **apparatus**
autonomic a.
disk-over-water a.
heat-loss a.
mental a.
psychic a.
apparent
alpha a.
a. competence
a. death
apparition
appeal
a.'s court
fear a.
inspirational a.
sex a.
snob a.
appearance
a. for age
asthenic a.
body a.
a. deterioration
disheveled a.
emaciated a.
exaggerated defect in physical a.
haggard a.
inappropriate a.
peculiar a.
physical a.
a. preoccupation
preoccupation with a.
sloppy a.
unkempt a.
appeaser
appendicular ataxia
apperception
feeling a.
tendentious a.
apperceptive
a. distortion
a. mass
a. visual agnosia
appersonification
appetite
abnormal a.
altered a.
change in a.
a. change
a. control
a. disturbance
increased a.
insatiable a.
a. for life
a. loss
loss of a.
perverted a.
poor a.
a. psychogenic disorder
a. suppressant
voracious a.
appetitive
a. behavior
a. center
a. drive
a. phase
a. state
applicable
not a. (N/A)
application
biofeedback a.
diverse medicinal a.
ritualized makeup a.
applicator
applied
a. anthropology
a. behavioral analysis (ABA)
a. extrasensory perception (AESP)

NOTES

applied *(continued)*
a. extrasensory projection
a. psychoanalysis
a. psychology
a. relaxation (AR)
a. research
a. science
appraisal
conflict management a. (CMA)
inflated a.
manager-style a.
vocational a.
apprehend
apprehensible
apprehension
a. expectation
intense a.
irresistible a.
sensation-focused a.
sense of a.
a. span
a. state
apprehensive
apprehensiveness
social a.
apprise
approach
adaptation a.
adaptational a.
adaptive a.
alternative a.
analytic a.
assertive community treatment a.
basal reader a.
behavioral a.
bottom-up a.
carrot-and-stick a.
categorical a.
checklist a.
cholinergic a.
client-centered a.
clinical a.
cluster a.
cognitive appraisal a.
cognitive-behavioral a.
community reinforcement a.
comprehensive therapeutic a.
constructive a.
contemporary a.
continuous a.
cross-culture a.
descriptive a.
dimensional a.
economic a.
empirical a.
environmental a.
ethical a.
ethnographic a.
evidence-based a.
flexible treatment a.
freudian a.
functional a.
fundamental a.
a. gradient
healthy a.
here-and-now a.
high-risk a.
holistic a.
idiographic a.
insight-oriented a.
integrative a.
interdisciplinary a.
language experience a. (LEA)
legal a.
linguistic a.
mechanistic a.
mixture a.
molar a.
motivational enhancement a.
multimodal therapeutic a.
multiple-tracer a.
multisystemic therapy a.
Mutt and Jeff a.
neuroimaging a.
nomothetic a.
nondirective a.
organic a.
patient-centered a.
person-situation-interaction a.
pharmacologic a.
pharmacological a.
primary pharmacological a.
priori a.
psychodynamic a.
psychotherapeutic a.
qualitative a.
quantitative a.
regressive-reconstructive a.
religious a.
self-efficacy and outcome expectation a.
sensate focus a.
serial problem-solving a.
spiritual a.
targeted a.
task-oriented a.
therapeutic a.
there-and-then a.
unifactorial a.
yawn-sign a.
approachable
approach-approach conflict
approach-avoidance
a.-a. conflict
a.-a. stance
approbation
appropriate
a. affect

a. behavior
culturally a.
a. facial expression
a. in gender
a. relationship
a. response
a. treatment
appropriately talkative
appropriateness of emotional response
approval
a. loss
social a.
approximate
a. answer syndrome
a. lethal concentration (ALC)
approximation
a. conditioning
a. method
successive a.
word a.
appurtenance
apractagnosia
apractic (*var. of* apraxic)
apragmatism
apraxia
akinetic a.
amnesic a.
amnestic a.
cerebral mapping of a.
classic a.
construction a.
constructional a.
cortical a.
developmental a.
disconnection a.
dressing a.
facial a.
gait a.
ideational a.
ideatory a.
ideokinetic a.
ideomotor a.
innervation a.
kinesthetic a.
Liepmann a.
limb kinetic a.
magnetic a.
motor a.
ocular a.
oculomotor a.
optic a.
oral a.
orolingual a.
sensory a.
speech a.
transcortical a.
verbal a.
apraxic, apractic
a. agraphia
a. behavior
a. disorder
aproctia
aprophoria
apropos
aprosexia
aprosodic speech
aprosody
speech a.
APS
Adult Protective Services
air pollution syndrome
American Pain Society
American Psychological Society
apselaphesia
apsithyria
APSR
acute paranoid schizophrenic reaction
apsychia
apsychognosia
apsychosis
APTA
American Physical Therapy Association
aptitude
learning a.
mechanical a.
numerical a. (N)
A. Research Project (ARP)
spatial a.
AQ
accomplishment quotient
achievement quotient
aphasia quotient
aqueduct veil
AR
achievement ratio
alarm reaction
alcohol related
applied relaxation
Arab
A. Federation of Psychiatrists
A. Gulf Psychiatric Association
arachnoid
a. layer
a. tissue
ARBD
alcohol-related birth defect

NOTES

arbiter
arbitrament
arbitrary
arbitrate
arborization
ARC
AIDS-related complex
arc
alpha a.
beta a.
a. de cercle
reflex a.
sensorimotor a.
archaic
a. brain
a. inheritance
a. paralogical thinking
a. residue
a. thought
archenemy
archetype
archfiend
architectural barrier
architecture
a. of brain
sleep a.
Archives of General Psychiatry
Arctic hysteria
arcuate movement
ardanesthesia
ardent
ardor
veneris a.
arduous
area
acoustic a.
association a.
auditory cortical a.
auditory projection a.
basic skill a.
body surface a.
brain a.
Broca a.
Brodmann a. 6
Brodmann a. 7
Brodmann a. 9
Brodmann a. 24
Brodmann a. 32
Brodmann a. 41
Brodmann a. 43
Brodmann a. 44
Brodmann a. 46
Brodmann a. 47/11
a. CA4-1
callosal a.
catchment a.
conflict-free a.
cortical a.
cross-sectional a. (CSA)
cultural a.
dominant hemisphere parietal a.
dominant hemisphere temporal a.
epidemiological catchment a. (ECA)
formed response of colored a. (FC)
frontocortical a.
gray matter a.
hypothalamic a.
language a.
lateral rostral supplementary motor a.
medial rostral supplementary motor a.
mesial prefrontal cortical a.
motor a.
National Institute of Mental Health-Epidemiologic Catchment A. (NIMH-ECA)
neocortical association a.
neuropsychologic a.
occipital association cortical a.
orbitofrontal a.
parabrachial a.
paracentral gray a.
parietal neocortical association a.
parietotemporal a.
periventricular gray matter a.
prefrontal cortical a.
premotor a.
processing a.
rostral supplementary motor a.
a. sampling
sclerotic a.
sclerotome a.
sensory association a.
sensory processing a.
septal a.
shading response to black a.'s (Fc)
shading response to gray a.'s (Fc)
silent a.
skill a.
somatesthetic a.
somesthetic a.
subcortical gray matter a.
superior temporal auditory cortical a.
supplementary motor a. (SMA)
temporal neocortical association a.
trigger a.
visual cortical a.
watershed a.
Wernicke 22, 39, 40 a.
areata
alopecia a.
arecoline
areflexia
arenacea
corpus a.

argentophilic plaque
argot
argument
irrational a.
semantic a.
argumentative
argumentativeness
aristocrat
aristogenic
aristotelian method
Aristotle anomaly
arithmetic
a. developmental delay disorder
a. grade equivalent
a. mean
a. problem
a. sign
arithmetical
a. reasoning
a. skills learning retardation
arithmomania
Arizona Association for the Gifted and Talented (AAGT)
ARM
anxiety reaction, mild
arm
fixed dosing a.
a. phenomenon
armamentarium
clinical a.
pharmacological a.
armed combat
Armenian
A. genocide
A. Psychiatric Association
armistice
armor
character a.
Army
US A.
aromatherapy
around
hang a.
kick a.
turn a.
around-the-clock observation
arousability factor
arousal
affective a.
anxious a.
autonomic a.
a. boost mechanism
a. category
conditional a.
confusional a.
a. detection
deviant a.
a. disorder
a. dysfunction
emotional a.
erotic a.
a. from sleep
a. function
hanging a.
high a.
hyperactive sexual a.
hypoactive sexual a.
impaired a.
increased a.
inhibited sexual a.
intense autonomic a.
a. jag
level of a.
mental a.
nonspecific a.
object of a.
oxygen-deprived sexual a.
penile a.
physiologic a.
psychological-physiological a.
a. reaction
a. reduction mechanism
a. reduction technique
sense of a.
sexual a.
sleep a.
sleeplessness associated with conditional a.
a. state
a. symptom
a. theory
aroused
a. motive
a. state of disturbed behavior
ARP
Aptitude Research Project
arranged marriage
arrangement
change in living a.
contractual a.
family sleeping a.
gene a.
living a.
picture a.
arranging
ordering and a.

NOTES

array of symptoms
arrest
action of a.
cardiac a.
cardiopulmonary a.
false a.
a. history
house a.
locomotor a.
multiple a.'s
a. reaction
a. of schizophrenia
a. of speech
a. for violence
arrested development
arrestee drug abuse monitoring (ADAM)
arrhigosis
arrhythmia
cardiac a.
ventricular a.
arriere-pensée
arrogance
arrogant
a. behavior
a. style
arseniasis
arsenic (As)
a. amblyopia
a. compound
a. exposure
arsenic-induced tremor
arsenotherapy
arsine
arson
arsonist
incendiary a.
art
black a.
language a.'s
martial a.'s
a. therapy
artefacta
self-induced dermatitis a.
Artemisia vulgaris
arteriopalmus
arteriosclerotic
a. brain disease-type organic psychosis
a. brain disorder
a. dementia confusional state
a. depression
a. paranoid state
a. psychosis confusional state
artery
a. occlusion
a. stenosis
arthropodiasis
articular sensibility
articulate
articulation
addition a.
a. developmental delay disorder
garbled a.
a. index
infantile a.
a. of speech
articulator
articulatory
a. loop component
a. tic
artifact
edge a.
statistical a.
artifactitious
artifactual
artificial
a. assist
a. disorder
a. dream
a. fecundation
a. insemination
a. intelligence in medicine (AIM)
a. language
a. life support
a. neural network
a. neurosis
a. penis
artificialism
artist
confidence a.
escape a.
artlessness
arylcyclohexylamine intoxication
AS
antisocial
anxiety sensitivity
anxiety state
As
arsenic
as
also known as (AKA)
as necessary
as needed (p.r.n., PRN)
as soon as possible (ASAP)
ASAM
American Society of Addiction Medicine
ASAP
as soon as possible
asaphia
asapholalia
ASC
altered state of consciousness
ascendance-submission
ascending
a. degeneration
a. neurotransmitter system
a. paralysis

a. pitch break
a. reticular activating system
a. technique
ascension phase
ascertainment
method of a.
asceticism
Asch situation
ascriptive responsibility
ASD
acute stress disorder
ASEAN Federation for Psychiatry and Mental Health (AFPMH)
asemia, asemasia
a. graphica
a. mimica
a. verbalis
aseptic
asexual
ASGPP
American Society of Group Psychotherapy and Psychodrama
ashamed
Asian
A. alcohol flush reaction
A. American
A. American Pacific Islander
aside
set a.
thinking a.
as-if
a.-i. hypothesis
a.-i. performance
a.-i. personality
pseudo a.-i.
asinine
asitia
asocial
a. acting out
a. trend psychopathic personality
asociality
premorbid a.
schizophrenia with premorbid a. (SPA)
asonia
asoticamania
ASP
antisocial personality
aspartame-restricted diet
aspartate aminotransferase (AST)
ASPD
antisocial personality disorder
aspect
amusing a.
associative a.
diagnostic a.
executive a.
immunologic a.
integrative a.
ironic a.
normative a.
perceptual a.
physiologic a.
prominent a.
speech a.
Asperger disorder
aspermia
psychogenic a. (PA)
asphalgesia
asphyctic syndrome
asphyxia
autoerotic a.
chemical a.
mechanical a.
traumatic a.
asphyxiant
asphyxiation
accidental autoerotic a.
autoerotic a. (AEA)
erotic a.
asphyxiophilia
aspiration
Cheyne-Stokes a.
a. level
level of a.
aspirational group
aspirin
a. combination
a. effect
a. poisoning
ASPP
American Society of Psychoanalytic Physicians
ASPS
advanced sleep-phase syndrome
assail
assassination
character a.
assault
adult sexual a.
aggravated sexual a.
a. and battery
brain a.
caretaker a.
child sexual a.

NOTES

assault *(continued)*
civilian sexual a.
drug-facilitated sexual a.
grievous a.
a. gun
indecent a.
military sexual a.
misdemeanor a.
personal a.
physical a.
a. precaution
psychiatric patient a.
a. rifle
sexual a.
verbal a.
violent personal a.
a. weapon
a. with a deadly weapon (ADW)
witness to a.
assaulter
serial a.
assaultive
a. act
a. behavior
assay
a. buffer
chloride channel flux a.
cocaethylene a.
drug a.
enzyme-linked immunoabsorbent a. (ELISA)
immunofluorescence a.
immunosorbent a.
assembly
cell a.
object a. (OA)
picture a.
assertion-structured therapy
assertive
a. behavior
a. community treatment
a. community treatment approach
a. conditioning
a. outreach
a. training
assertiveness
a. skill
a. training
assess
assessment
a. of academic achievement
Achenbach system of empirically based a.
a. of affect
Ainsworth strange situation a.
automated a.
baseline a.
a. of basic competency (ABC)
behavior a.
behavior-oriented a.
a. of bizarre idiosyncratic thinking
child and adolescent psychiatric a. (CAPA)
cocaine symptom severity a. (CSSA)
cognitive a.
communication skills a.
community a.
a. of competence
competency a.
complement symptom-focused a.
comprehensive a.
criminal responsibility a.
cross-sectional a.
cultural a.
developmental a.
a. and diagnosis
diagnostic a.
disorganized speech a.
environmental a.
family a.
fantasy a.
functional a.
general personality a.
home a.
individual comprehensive a.
language a.
longitudinal a.
luteal phase a.
a. in mathematics
a. measure
mental status a.
a. method
moral a.
multidimensional a.
multidisciplinary a.
multiple-choice a.
neurobehavioral a.
neuroimaging a.
neurolinguistic a.
neurophysiological a.
neuropsychologic a.
objective a.
outcome a.
performance a.
personality a.
play-based a.
a. procedure
projective personality a.
psychiatric a.
psychosocial a. (PA)
quality of life rehabilitation a.
quantified cognitive a.
rehabilitation a.
risk-benefit a.
self-report a.
social and health a.
specialized language a.

spiritual a.
standardized a.
suicide risk a.
symptom a.
task-oriented a.
asset
academic a.
assets-liabilities technique
assiduity
assign blame
assigned
a. responsibility
a. sex
assignment
random a.
sex a.
a. therapy
writing a.
assimilable
assimilated nasality
assimilating
a. information
a. information disturbance
assimilation
cultural a.
double a.
a. effect
information a.
law of a.
progressive a.
reciprocal a.
regressive a.
reproductive a.
a. rule
velar a.
vowel a.
assimilative factor
assist
artificial a.
assistance
medical a.
social a.
assistant
physician's a. (PA)
psychiatric a.
research a.
assisted suicide
associate
a. learning
paired a.'s
Science Research A.'s (SRA)
verbal paired a.'s
associated
a. descriptive feature
a. disability
a. disorder
a. idea
a. intervention
a. laboratory finding
a. movement
a. physical examination finding
association
A. for Academic Psychiatry
A. for Advancement of Behavior Therapy (AABT)
A. for the Advancement of Gestalt Therapy (AAGT)
A. for the Advancement of Psychoanalysis (AAP)
A. for the Advancement of Psychotherapy (AAP)
Alzheimer Disease and Related Disorders A.
American College Counseling A. (ACCA)
American Counseling A. (ACA)
American Diabetes A. (ADA)
American Dietetic A. (ADA)
American Family Therapy A. (AFTA)
American Managed Behavioral Healthcare A. (AMBHA)
American Occupational Therapy A. (AOTA)
American Orthopsychiatric A. (AOA)
American Pharmaceutical A. (APhA)
American Physical Therapy A. (APTA)
American Psychiatric A. (APA)
American Psychoanalytical A. (APA)
American Psychological A. (APA)
American Public Health A. (APHA)
Arab Gulf Psychiatric A.
a. area
Armenian Psychiatric A.
backward a.
causal a.
a. center
characteristic a.
a. characteristic
A. for Child Psychiatrists

NOTES

association *(continued)*
a. coefficient
conditioned fear a.
consequence a.
contextual a.
controlled a.
co-occurring a.
A. of Correctional Psychologists
a. cortex
a. deficit pathology
Depression and Related Affective Disorders A. (DRADA)
direct a.
A. of Directors of Medical Student Education in Psychiatry (ADMSEP)
a. disease
dominant a.
dream a.
Eastern Psychiatric Research A.
Egyptian Psychiatric A.
etiological a.
false a.
fear a.
a. fluency
free a.
freudian free a.
A. for Frontotemporal Dementia
genetic a.
guilt by a.
idea a.
a. index
indirect a.
induced a.
International Psychoanalytical A. (IPA)
International Transactional Analysis A. (ITAA)
law of a.
a. learning
loose a.
looseness of a.
loosening of a.'s (LOA)
Louisiana Psychiatric Medical A.
meaningless word a.
a. mechanism
Mental Health A. (MHA)
multiple a.'s
National Depressive and Manic-Depressive A. (NDMDA)
National Mental Health A. (NMHA)
National Rehabilitation A. (NRA)
a. neurosis
occipital a.
phoneme-grapheme a.
preceding a.
psychosis of a.
a. reaction time
schizophrenia with premorbid a. (SPA)
a. of sounds and symbols
sound-symbol a.
subordinate a.
tangential a.
temporal a.
verbal a.
word a.
World Psychiatric A. (WPA)

associationism

association-sensation ratio

associative
a. anamnesis
a. aphasia
a. aspect
a. facilitation
a. fluency
a. inhibition
a. learning
a. linkage
a. memory
a. play
a. reaction
a. shifting
a. strength
a. thinking
a. visual agnosia

associativity
criterion of a.

assonance

assortative, assortive
a. mating

ASSR
adult situational stress reaction

assuasive

assumed
a. mean
a. similarity

assumption
cultural a.
gentle a.
a. of new identity
reality a.
theoretical a.

assumptive

assurance

assuredness

AST
aspartate aminotransferase

astasia

astasia-abasia

astatic

Astemizole

astereognosis, astereocognosy, astereognosia

asteric seizure

asterixis

asthenia
heat-induced a.
mental a.
neurocirculatory a.
psychogenic a.
treatment-emergent a.
asthenic
a. appearance
a. constitutional type
a. delirium
a. diathesis
a. neurosis
a. personality
a. personality disorder
a. reaction
asthenopia
asthenospermia
asthma
bronchial a.
intrinsic a.
nervous a.
sleep-related a.
asthmogenic
astomia
astral
a. body
a. projection
astray
astrobiology
astrology chart
astrotravel
astute
astyphia
asyllabia
asylum
asymbolia
asymmetrical amnesia
asymmetric motor neuropathy
asymmetry
abnormal a.
cerebral a.
facial a.
functional a.
interhemispheric a.
leftward a.
mental a.
metabolic a.
a. and order effect
perception a.
perceptual a.
reflex a.
skull a.
asymptomatic
a. neurosyphilis
a. seizure
asymptotic wish fulfillment
asynchronously
asynchrony
asyndesis
asyndetic thinking
asynergy, asynergia
asynesia
asynodia
at
being stared at
at large
at risk
tear at
atactic
a. abasia
a. agraphia
a. ataxia
atactilia
ataque de nervios
ataractic drug
ataralgesia
ataraxia, ataraxy
ataraxic
atavism
atavistic regression
ataxia, ataxy
absent a.
acute a.
alcoholic a.
appendicular a.
atactic a.
autonomic a.
Briquet a.
Bruns a.
cerebellar a.
choreic a.
conversion a.
crural a.
equilibratory a.
Friedreich a.
hysterical a.
intrapsychic a.
ipsilateral cerebellar a.
kinesigenic a.
kinetic a.
Leyden a.
locomotor a.
Marie a.
mental a.
mild a.

NOTES

ataxia *(continued)*
moderate a.
moral a.
motor a.
neurotoxicant-related a.
noothymopsychic a.
optic a.
psychogenic a.
sensory a.
severe a.
spinal a.
static a.
trunk a.
ataxiadynamia
ataxiagram
ataxiagraph
ataxiameter
ataxiamnesic
ataxiaphasia
ataxic
a. abasia
a. amimia
a. aphasia
a. diplegia
a. dysarthria
a. feeling
a. gait
a. speech
a. writing
ataxiophemia, ataxophemia
ataxy (*var. of* ataxia)
atelectasis
atelesis
atelia
ateliosis
atheist
atheoretical
atheromata
athletic constitutional type
athrepsia, athrepsy
athymia
athymic
athymism
athyreosis
atlas-based segmentation (ABSEG)
atman
atmosphere
a. effect
emotional a.
optimistic a.
situationally appropriate a.
situationally optimistic a.
therapeutic a.
a. of trust
atmospheric
a. condition
a. perspective
a. pollution exposure
atocia
atolide
atom
social a.
atomic
a., biological, chemical (ABC)
a., biological, chemical warfare
atomism
atomistic psychology
atone
atonement
atonia, atony
atonic
a. absence seizure
a. impotence
atonicity
atony (*var. of* atonia)
atopognosia, atopognosis
ATP
adenosine triphosphate
atrabiliary
atrabilious
atraumatic
atremble
atretic
at-risk
a.-r. adolescent
a.-r. high school student
a.-r. middle school student
a.-r. patient
a.-r. youth
atrocious
atrocity
participated in a.'s
witnessed a.'s
atrophedema
atrophic dementia
atrophoderma neuriticum
atrophy
amygdala a.
brain a.
cerebral a.
diffuse brain a.
frontotemporal brain a.
multiple-system a.
neuritic a.
neurogenic a.
neurotrophic a.
nutritional-type cerebellar a.
Pick a.
structural a.
whole brain a.
atropine
a. coma therapy
a. psychosis
atropinic
ATS
amphetamine-type stimulant
anxiety tension state

attachment
affectional a.
avoidant a.
a. behavior
a. bond
Bowlby theory of a.
clearcut a.
continuity of a.
a. disorder
a. disorder of infancy
disorganized form of a.
disoriented form of a.
a. dynamic
a. fantasy
feeling of a.
a. figure
grief-based a.
a. in infancy
insecure a.
a. learning
liquidation of a.
locality a.
a. in making
maternal a.
mother-child a.
mother-infant a.
object a.
oscillation of a.
poor a.
predisposition to a.
a. relationship
resistant a.
secure a.
selective a.
sense of a.
social a.
a. style
suffocating a.
symbiotic a.
a. theory
unstable a.

attachment-separation disorder

attack
acute anxiety a. (AAA)
acute schizophrenic a.
aftermath of a.
anger a.
anxiety a.
attitude of a.
bioterrorist a.
biting a.
bound panic a.
character a.
clawing a.
crying a.
cued panic a.
dream anxiety a.
drop a.
full-blown panic a.
gang a.
glottal a.
limited symptom a.
nocturnal panic a.
obsessive a.
panic a.
physical a.
position of a.
psychomotor a.
psychotic a.
quiet biting a.
rage a.
recurrent panic a.'s
refreshing sleep a.
savage a.
schizophrenic a.
schizophreniform a.
situationally bound panic a.
situationally predisposed panic a.
sleep a.
spontaneous panic a.
terrorist a.
twilight a.
uncinate a.
uncontrollable sleep a.
uncued panic a.
unexpected panic a.
vagal a.
vasovagal a.
vocal a.
word a.
World Trade Center a.

attacked with weapon

attacker role

attacking behavior

attainment
educational a.
emotional a.
goal a.
scholastic a.

attaint

attempt
a. at reconciliation
current suicide a.
failed suicide a.
future suicide a.
hanging a.

NOTES

attempt *(continued)*
history of suicide a.
home life, education level, activities, drug use, sexual activity, suicide ideation or a.'s (HEADSS)
impending suicide a.
past suicide a.
previous a.
reconciliation a.
remote suicide a.
repeated suicide a.'s
risk of suicide a.
suicide a. (SA)
attempted intercourse
attempter
remote a.
suicide a.
attended death
attending
a. behavior
a. to language stage
a. physician
attention
a. blink paradigm
center of a.
a. and concentration
controlled a.
covert visuospatial a.
a. deficit
a. deficit disorder (ADD)
a. deficit disorder, residual type
a. deficit disorder with hyperactivity (ADD-HA)
a. deficit disorder without hyperactivity
a. deficit and disruptive behavior disorder (AD-DBD)
a. deficit hyperactivity disorder (ADHD)
a. deficit hyperactivity disorder, combined type
a. deficit hyperactivity disorder, predominantly hyperactive-impulsive type
a. deficit hyperactivity disorder-predominantly inattentive (ADHD-PI)
a. deficit symptom
a. disorder
disturbance of a.
divided a.
fix and focus a.
a. fluctuation
a. focus
focus of clinical a.
focus-execute component of a.
a. focusing procedure
free-floating a.
heightened a.
impaired a.
a. impairment
impairment of a.
a. lapse
medical a.
need for constant a.
a. network
a. overload
a. problem
quest for a.
raptus of a.
a. reflex
selective a.
selectivity of a.
a. shift
a. shift ability
a. to sound
span of a.
a. span
state of heightened a.
sustained a.
a. testing
a. time
a. training
unwanted sexual a.
vigility of a.
visual a.
visuospatial a.
wandering a.
attentional
a. ability
a. abnormality
a. circuit
a. control
a. demand
a. disturbance
a. dysfunction
a. failure
a. functioning
a. impairment
a. measure
a. mechanism
a. performance
a. problem
a. processing
a. skill
attention-getting
attention-information processing
attention-seeking behavior
attenuation
attitude
abstract a.
a. of active friendliness
a. adjustment
apathetic a.
a. of attack
catatonoid a.
categorical a.

change of a.
complacent a.
concrete a.
concretizing a.
condescending a.
counterphobic a.
crucifixion a.
cultural a.
a. to death
defeatist a.
a. defense
defense a.
deferential a.
deviant a.
devil-may-care a.
Dionysian a.
dog-eat-dog a.
do-not-care a.
eating a.
emotion a.
emotional a.
emotionally charged a.
exposition a.
fatalistic a.
feminine a.
forced a.
gambling a.
gender-based a.
gender-linked a.
holier-than-thou a.
illogical a.
inappropriate a.
inflexible a.
ingratiating a.
judgmental a.
listening a.
masculine a.
maternal a.
a. to medication (AM)
mistrustful a.
moral a.
mummy a.
negative a.
neutral a.
nonjudgmental a.
object a.
objectifying a.
oppositional a.
overdependent a.
passionate a.
a. passionelle
paternal a.
pessimistic a.
phobic a.
positive mental a. (PMA)
preadaptive a.
primary oppositional a.
punitive psychologic a.
realistic a.
a. reassessment
referential a.
religious a.
restrictive a.
a. restructuring
rigid a.
self-centered a.
self-critical a.
self-medicating a.
sexual a.
shift in a.
spiritual a.
stereotyped a.
stilted a.
a. theory
a. therapy
third-person a.
a. tic
a. type
unsympathetic a.

attitudinal
a. group
a. pathosis
a. reflex
a. risk factor
a. type

attitudinize

attonita
amentia a.
cephalea a.
melancholia a.

attonity

attorney
durable power of a.
medical power of a.

attract

attraction
fatal a.
gain-loss theory of a.
magnetic a.
sexual a.
social a.

attractiveness

attributable risk

attribute
behavioral a.
a. entity

NOTES

attribution
controllability a.
environmental a.
a. error
false a.
personal a.
situational a.
social a.
a. theory
attributional style
attrition rate
attune
atypia
atypical
a. absence
a. absence seizure
a. affective disorder
a. antidepressant
a. antipsychotic
a. antipsychotic agent
a. antipsychotic drug
a. antipsychotic preparation
a. anxiety disorder
a. behavior
a. bipolar disorder
a. child
a. childhood psychosis
a. conduct disorder
a. course
a. delusional experience
a. depression
a. development
a. dissociative disorder
a. eating disorder
a. factitious disorder with physical symptoms
a. feature
a. gender identity disorder
a. impulse control disorder
a. mania
a. or mixed organic brain syndrome
a. mixed or other personality disorder
a. neuralgia
a. neurotic anxiety state
a. pain
a. paranoid disorder
a. paraphilia
a. personality trait
a. pervasive developmental disorder
a. presentation
a. psychosexual dysfunction
a. puberty
a. schizophrenia
a. somatoform disorder
a. specific developmental disorder
a. stereotyped movement disorder
a. tic disorder
atypicality
atypism
au courant
audacious
audacity
audible
a. blocking in speech
a. speech blockade
a. thought
audience effect
audile
audiogenic
a. epilepsy
a. seizure (AGS)
audiogram
audiologist
audiology
audiometry
ABR a.
automatic a.
behavioral observation a. (BOA)
audiophile
audioverbal amnesia
audiovisual
a. brain stimulation
a. cue
a. training
audit
medical a.
patient-care a.
personal a.
stress a.
audition
chromatic a.
gustatory a.
mental a.
auditive
auditognosis
auditory
a. ability
a. accommodation
a. acuity
a. agnosia
a. alexia
a. amnesia
a. analysis
a. aphasia
a. aura
a. blending
a. brainstem response (ABR)
a. bulb
a. canal
a. closure
a. comprehension
a. continuous performance task
a. cortical area
a. discrimination
a. disorientation
a. distance cue

a. distortion
a. evoked potential (AEP)
a. evoked response
a. fatigue
a. feedback
a. hallucination
a. hyperalgesia
a. hyperesthesia
a. imagery
a. learner
a. localization
a. memory
a. memory span (AMS)
a. nerve
a. pathway
a. perceptual disorder
a. processing
a. projection area
a. radiation
a. region
a. seizure
a. sequencing
a. skill
a. space perception
a. span
a. stimulus
a. symptom
a. synesthesia
a. system
a. threshold
a. training

auditory-verbal dysgnosia
auditory-visual synesthesia
augment
augmentation
a. agent overactivity in OCD
breast a.
drug a.
a. strategy
thyroid a.

augmentative communication
augury
aura, pl. **aurae**
auditory a.
cephalic a.
electric a.
epigastric a.
epileptic a.
gustatory a.
hysterical a.
intellectual a.
a. intelligence
a. interpretation
jamais vu a.
kinesthetic a.
migraine with a. (MA)
migraine without a.
motor a.
olfactory a.
a. procursiva
reminiscent a.
sensory a.
status a.
visual a.

aural pathology
AUSR
acute undifferentiated schizophrenic reaction

austere
austerity
Austin Association for the Gifted and Talented (AAGT)
Australian Council for Educational Research (ACER)
autarky, autarchy
autemesia
authenticate
authentication
patient a.
therapist a.

authenticity
authoritarian
a. aggression
a. character
a. conscience
a. leader
a. leadership pattern
a. personality
a. rejecting-neglecting parent
a. submission

authoritarianism
right wing a. (RWA)

authoritative manner
authority
a. anxiety
a. complex
a. confusion
a. figure
a. figure fixation
prescriptive a.
a. principle
rebel against a.
rejection of a.

authorization
away without a. (AWA)
treatment a.

authorized leave
autia

NOTES

autism
akinetic a.
childhood a.
a. criteria
early infantile a.
high-functioning a. (HFA)
infantile a.
Kanner a.
primary a.
secondary a.
semantics of a.
a. spectrum disorder
susceptibility locus for a.
traditionally defined a.
autisme pauvre
autism-like condition
autismus infantum
autistic
a. behavior
a. child
a. disorder
a. enterocolitis
a. fantasy
a. isolation
a. phase
a. presymbiotic adolescent
a. proband
a. psychopathy
a. psychosis
a. thinking
autistic-spectrum children
autoactivation
autoaggression
autoaggressive behavior
autoanalysis
autoanamnesis
autobiographical
a. information
a. life chart
autobiographic memory
autobiography
autocastration
anticipatory a.
autocatharsis
autochthonous
a. delusion
a. gestalt
a. idea
a. variable
autoclitic operant
autocorrelation
autocrat
autodestruct
autodidact
autoecholalia
autoechopraxis
autoerogenous
autoerotic
a. act
a. asphyxia
a. asphyxiation (AEA)
a. behavior
a. death
a. fatality
a. massage
a. pleasure
a. practice
autoerotism, autoeroticism
secondary a.
autogenic training
autogenital stimulation
autogenous depression
autognosis
autognostic
autohypnosis
autohypnotic amnesia
autohypnotism
autoimmune (AI)
a. deficiency
a. illness
a. obsessive-compulsive tic disorder
autointoxication
autokinetic effect
autolesion
autologous
autolysis
automania
automanipulation
automated
a. assessment
a. clinical record
automatic
a. absence
a. action
a. audiometry
a. behavior
a. chorea
a. drawing
a. epilepsy
a. gain control
a. judgment
a. language
a. memory
a. movement
a. obedience
a. phrase level
a. psychological process
a. reactivity
a. seizure
a. speech
a. thought
a. volume control
a. writing
automaticity of performance
automation
automatism
ambulatory a.
chewing a.

command a.
epileptic a.
facial expression a.
gestural a.
ictal a.
immediate posttraumatic a.
mumbling a.
primary ictal a.
swallowing a.
verbal a.

automatograph
automaton conformity
automnesia
automorphic perception
autonarcosis
autonomasia
autonomic
a. activity
a. activity-reactivity
a. affective law
a. apparatus
a. arousal
a. arousal disorder
a. ataxia
a. balance
a. conditioning
a. conversion reaction
a. denervation
a. disorganization
a. dysfunction
a. dysnomia
a. dysreactivity
a. dysreflexia
a. dysregulation
a. epilepsy
a. function
a. hyperactivity
a. hyperarousal
a. hyperreflexia
a. hyperventilation
a. imbalance
a. instability
a. motor pool
a. nerve
a. nervous system (ANS)
a. neurogenic bladder
a. neuropathy
a. reactivity
a. response
a. seizure
a. sensation
a. side effect
a. sympathomimetic drug

autonomotropic
autonomous
a. depression
a. ego function
a. functional component
a. psychotherapy
a. stage
a. superego

autonomy
bodily a.
a. of ego
functional a.
loss of a.
a. loss
a. of motives
patient a.
perseverative functional a.

autonomy-heteronomy
autopagnosia
autopathography
autopathy
autophagia, autophagy
autophagic
autophilia
autophonia
autophonomania
autoplastic
a. adaptation
a. change
a. symptom

autoplasty
autopsy
brain a.
psychological a.
a. study

autopsychic
a. delusion
a. disorientation
a. orientation

autopsychorhythmia
autopsychosis
autopsychotherapy
autopsy-negative death
autopunition
autoreceptor
autoscopic
a. hallucination
a. phenomenon
a. psychosis
a. syndrome

autosensitize
autosexing
autosexualism
autosexuality
autosmia

NOTES

autosomal
a. aberration
a. abnormality
a. anomaly
a. dominant
a. dominant gene
a. dominant inheritance
a. dominant pattern
a. recessive
a. trisomy
autosomatognosis
autosomatognostic
autosome
autosuggestibility
autosuggestion
autosymbolism
autosynnoia
autotelic
autotherapy
autotomia
autotopagnosia
autotoxic
autotrophic nutrition
autozygous
auxiliary
a. ego
a. organ
a. solution
a. therapist
auxoaction
auxotox
availability
absolute systemic a.
a. of weapon
avalanche
law of a.
avarice
avatar
avenge
avenue of administration
aver
average
a. conditioning
a. evoked response technique
a. student
averse to risk
aversion
a. conditioning
a. depression
occasional sexual a.
a. reaction
a. response
risk a.
school a.
sexual a.
a. therapy
aversion-covert conditioning
aversive
a. behavior
a. conditioning
a. control
a. drive
a. early environment
a. incentive
a. racism
a. smoking procedure
a. stimulus
a. therapy
a. training
avert
aviation medicine
aviator's
a. disease
a. effort syndrome
a. neurasthenia
avid
avidity
avocation
avoidance
anticipatory a. (AA)
a. behavior
a. category
a. cluster
cognitive a.
a. conditioning
conflict a.
conscious a.
contact a.
emotional a.
a. and escape learning
a. of exposure
eye contact a.
a. of feelings
a. gradient
harm a. (HA)
incubation of a.
master of a.
a. measure
a. of others (AO)
outside activity a.
pain a.
passive a.
a. pattern
phobic a.
a. response
a. score
social situation a.
a. speaking
a. of speech disfluency
stimulus a.
a. style
a. symptom
a. syndrome
a. therapy
a. of thoughts
a. training
withdrawal a.
avoidance-avoidance conflict

avoidant
a. attachment
a. disorder of adolescence
a. disorder of childhood
a. feature
a. neurotic personality disorder
a. personality
a. personality disorder (APD)
a. style
a. symptom
avoidant-attached behavior
avolition apathy
avow, avouch
avulsion
AWA
away without authorization
awake
a., alert, and oriented (AAO)
a. state
awakening
early morning a.
frequent nightly a.
nighttime a.
repeated nighttime a.
tiredness upon a.
aware
keenly a.
awareness
behavior a.
body a.
closed a.
conscious a.
contingency a.
a. defect
a. deficit
emotional a.
environmental a.
heightened a.
interoceptive a.
lack of interoceptive a.
lapse of a.
leisure a.
mutual pretense a.
open a.
phonemic a.
postural a.
reality a.
sensory a. (SA)
spiritual a.
a. of spirituality
state of heightened a.
subconscious a.
suspected a.
a. threshold
a. training model
away
blow a.
carry a.
explain a.
fall a.
tear a.
turn a.
a. without authorization (AWA)
awestruck
awkwardness
social a.
AWOL
absent without leave
awry
axes (*pl. of* axis)
axial
a. amnesia
a. gradient
a. hyperkinesis
a. neuritis
a. section
axilla, pl. **axillae**
coitus in a.
axiodrama
axiology
axis, pl. **axes**
defensive functioning a.
a. function
a. I, II conceptualization
a. I, II disorder
a. I, II interview
a. I, II item
a. I–IV diagnosis
5-axis system
axolysis
axonal idiocy
axonapraxia
axonometer
axonopathy
axonotmesis
axon terminal
ayahuasca
azacyclonol hydrochloride
azaloxan
azaperone
azaspirodecanedione
Azorean disease
azospermia
Aztec idiocy

NOTES

BA
blood alcohol
bone age
baah-ji
babble
phonetic b.
babbling
nonreduplicated b.
reduplicated b.
social b.
babel
babied
Babinski sign
baby-boom generation
baby-bust generation
babysitter
bacchanal
bacchant
bachelor
B. of Medical Science
B. of Social Work (BSW)
bachelorette
back
b. down
hang b.
laid b.
snap b.
b. talk
turn b.
backache
psychogenic b.
backbeat
backbite
backbone
background
cultural b.
ethnic b.
b. factor
family b.
b. interference
b. masking
b. music
b. noise
psychotherapeutic b.
regional b.
religious b.
sociocultural b.
sociodemographic b.
socioeconomic b.
backhanded
backing to velars
backlash
backpedal
backseat
backslide
backstab
backstabber
back-to-back
backward
b. association
b. coarticulation
b. conditioning
b. visual masking
backward-making technique
backwards
digit span b.
reading b.
bad
b. actor
b. blood
b. conduct discharge (BCD)
b. dream
b. karma
b. me
b. object
b. self
b. trip
badinage
BADLs
basic activities of daily living
badmouth
bad-people fear
BADS
behavioral assessment of dysexecutive syndrome
baffle
baggage
emotional b.
bagger
bagman
Bahaı
bahnung
bah tschi
bail
skip b.
bailout behavior
BAL
blood alcohol level
British anti-Lewisite
balance
acid-base b.
alternate binaural loudness b. (ABLB)
alternate monaural loudness b. (AMLB)
autonomic b.
b. control
core body b.
dynamic ambulatory b.
dynamic standing b.

balance *(continued)*
electrolyte b.
energy b.
family structural b.
fluid b.
homeostatic b.
impaired b.
inhibition-action b.
measure of b.
b. mechanism
mood b.
off b.
sitting b.
spatial b.
standing b.
structural b.
b. theory
water b.
balanced
b. diet
b. lifestyle
b. placebo
balanus
balbuties
balderdash
bald-faced lie
baleful
balefulness
Balint syndrome
balk
balky
ball
eight b.
b. of fire
b. up
ballast
isomeric b.
baller
ballet
b. technique
b. therapy
ballism
ballismus
ballistic movement
ballistics
ballistomania
ballooned neuron
balneology
balneotherapeutic
balneotherapy
banal
band
b. frequency
b. spectrum
vocal b.
Band-Aid
B.-A. medicine
B.-A. phase
bandlike headache
band-pass filter
bandwagon effect
bandy about
bane
baneful
banewort
bang
banging
head b.
sleep-related head b.
bangungot
banish
banisterine
bank
electronic data b.
patient data b.
practitioner data b.
bankrupt
bankruptcy
banter
Banting diet
BAQ
brain age quotient
baquet
baragnosis
Barbados Association of Psychiatrists
barbaralalia
barbarian
barbaric
barbarism
barbarity
barbarize
barbarous
barbed-wire
b.-w. disease
b.-w. psychosis
Barbidonna No. 2
barbital
sodium b.
barbital dependent (BD)
barbituism
barbiturate-facilitated interview
barbiturate-induced
b.-i. coma
b.-i. death
Bardet-Biedl syndrome
baresthesia
baresthesiometer
bargain
plea b.
bargaining
bariatrics
barking
BARN
body awareness resource network
Barnes global score
Barnum effect
barognosis
baroreflex sensitivity

barotrauma
barotropism
barracoon
barrage
barren
barrenness
inner b.
barrier
architectural b.
b. to care
communication b.
cultural b.
employment b.
incest b.
b. to intervention
language b.
protective b.
b. response
social b.
transportation b.
barrier-free environment
barrio
bart
baryesthesia
baryglossia
barylalia
baryphonia, baryphony
barythymia
BAS
behavioral activation system
bas
de haut en b.
basal
b. diet
b. fluency
b. ganglia-cingulate gyrus-frontal lobe loop
b. mental age
b. metabolic rate (BMR)
b. metabolism
b. narcosis
b. pitch
b. reader approach
b. resistance level
b. temperature
basalis
nucleus b.
base
b. component
ether b.
b. impulse
b. rate
b. rule
b. structure
b. word
baseborn
basedowian insanity
baseline (BL)
b. assessment
behavioral b.
b. cognitive functioning
b. measure
b. mental status
b. monitoring
b. performance
b. rating
b. scan
b. severity
b. symptom
b. visit
baseline-to-endpoint change
basement
b. chemist
b. laboratory
bases (*pl. of* basis)
bash
bashing
gay b.
basic
b. activities of daily living (BADLs)
b. anxiety
b. brain mechanism
b. brain pathway
b. conflict
b. diet
b. impairment
b. methadone service
b. mistake
b. mistrust
b. personality
b. personality type
b. reproductive number
b. rest-activity cycle (BRAC)
b. rule
b. skill
b. skill area
b. trust
basigenous
basilect
basilic
basing
basis, pl. **bases**
biologic b.
compassionate use b.
empirical b.

NOTES

basis *(continued)*
genetic b.
heritable b.
outpatient b.
pathophysiologic b.
physiologic b.
presumptive b.
psychological b.
basophilia
Cushing b.
pituitary b.
basophilism
bastard
bastardize
Bastian aphasia
bastion
bathing
resistance to b.
bathmotropic
negatively b.
positively b.
bathos
bathroom privilege
bathyanesthesia
bathyesthesia
bathyhyperesthesia
bathyhypesthesia
bathypnea
battacca
battalion
batter
battered
b. baby
b. child
b. child syndrome (BCS)
b. parent
b. spouse
b. spouse syndrome
b. wife
b. woman syndrome (BWS)
b. women's shelter
battering behavior
battery
achievement b.
aggravated b.
assault and b.
battle
abandoned during b.
b. exposure
b. fatigue
b. neurosis
b. psychoneurosis
B. sign
battlefront
battleground
Battley sedative
bawd
bawdy, bawdry
Bayesian technique
Bayle disease
Bayley behavior record
Baylorfast diet
BC
behavior control
birth control
BCD
bad conduct discharge
BCP
birth control pill
BCR
behavior control room
BCS
battered child syndrome
BCW
biologic and chemical warfare
BD
barbital dependent
barbiturate dependence
birth date
BDAC
Bureau of Drug Abuse Control
BDD
body dysmorphic disorder
bdelygmia
BDID
bystander dominates initial dominant
BDL
below detectable level
BDSM
bondage and sadomasochism
bead
worry b.'s
BEAM
brain electrical activity mapping
bearable
Beard disease
bearer
bearing
grudge b.
bearish
beast fetishism
beastly
beaten
being b.
beat generation
beatific vision
beatify
beating
beau
ideal b.
b. monde
beauteous
becalm
Beck
B. cognitive triad of depression
B. view of depressive disorder
becloud
beclouded dementia

bed
- b. crisis
- out of b. (OOB)
- b. partner

bedazzle
bedevil
bedfast
bedizen
bedlam
bedraggled
bedrest
bedridden
bedtime
bedwetter
bedwetting
befall
befitting
befool
befriend
befuddle
beggar
- emotional b.

beggary
begrudge
beguile
behavior
- aberrant b.
- abnormal illness b.
- abnormal motor b.
- abusive dating b.
- acceptable b.
- accepted b.
- accident b.
- accident-prone b.
- achievement b.
- acting-out b.
- activity and b.
- acute psychotic aggressive b.
- adaptive b.
- addictive b.
- adient b.
- adjust repetitive b.
- adolescent antisocial b.
- adolescent sexual b.
- adult self-harm b.
- age-appropriate b.
- age-inappropriate knowledge of sexual b.
- age-level b.
- aggressive objectionable b.
- aggressive psychotic b.
- agitated b.
- agnostic b.
- aimless b.
- alcohol consumption b.
- alcohol-related b.
- alexithymic b.
- b. alteration
- alternating b.
- alternative b.
- altruistic b.
- ambient b.
- amotivated b.
- b. analysis
- anarchic b.
- anger b.
- angry b.
- anomalous sexual b.
- anorexic b.
- antagonistic b.
- anticipatory and struggle b.
- antisocial b.
- anxiety-like b.
- apologetic b.
- apopathetic b.
- appetitive b.
- appropriate b.
- apraxic b.
- aroused state of disturbed b.
- arrogant b.
- assaultive b.
- assertive b.
- b. assessment
- attachment b.
- attacking b.
- attending b.
- attention-seeking b.
- atypical b.
- autistic b.
- autoaggressive b.
- autoerotic b.
- automatic b.
- aversive b.
- avoidance b.
- avoidant-attached b.
- b. awareness
- bailout b.
- battering b.
- binge-eating b.
- binge-purge b.
- bisexual b.
- bizarre b.
- borderline b.
- bulimic b.
- bullying b.
- catastrophic b.

NOTES

behavior *(continued)*
catatonic b.
ceremonial b.
b. chain
change in b.
characteristic b.
b. characteristic
child antisocial b.
childhood crossgender b.
childish b.
childlike b.
b. choice
chronic illness b.
clinging b.
clinical b.
clinically relevant b.
coercive b.
cognitive b.
collateral b.
collective b.
compelled b.
compensatory b.
competitive b.
complex motor b.
compulsive drug-taking b.
compulsive masturbatory b.
compulsive sexual b.
concealing b.
condescending b.
consensual sexual b.
consistent b.
consumer b.
contact b.
b. contract
contractual b.
b. control (BC)
b. control room (BCR)
cooperative b.
coping b.
copulatory b.
coronary-prone b.
counterphobic b.
countertransference b.
courtship b.
covert b.
criminal b.
criterion b.
cross-dressing b.
cross-gender b.
crowd b.
cuddling b.
b. cue
culturally appropriate avoidant b.
culturally condoned b.
culturally sanctioned b.
cunning and hiding b.
cyclothymic-depressive b.
dangerous b.
defensive b.
defiant b.
b. deficit
delinquent b.
delusional b.
demanding b.
dementia-related b.
dependent b.
desirable b.
desired b.
destructive b.
b. determinant
deviant political b.
deviant religious b.
differential reinforcement of other b. (DRO)
direct self-destructive b. (DSDB)
discordant b.
discriminatory b.
disinhibited violent b.
disobedient b.
b. disorder
b. disorder of childhood
disorganized attachment b.
disoriented attachment b.
b. disruption
disruptive b.
distracting spouse b.
disturbed eating b.
disturbing b.
dominant-subordinate b.
Don Juan b.
drinking b.
drive b.
driven motor b.
drug-addictive b.
drug-related HIV risk b.
drug risk b.
drug-seeking b.
drug-taking b.
drug use b.
drunk b.
b. dynamic
dysarthric b.
dysfunctional b.
dysrhythmic aggressive b.
dyssocial b.
eating b.
eccentric b.
ecstatic b.
ego-dystonic b.
ego-syntonic impulsive b.
elicited b.
embracing b.
emitted b.
empathic b.
employment-related b.
enabling b.
enraged b.
entry b.

envious b.
erotic b.
erratic b.
escape b.
ethical b.
ethnic relational b. (ERB)
evasive b.
excessive gambling b.
excitable b.
excited b.
exhibitionistic b.
experimental analysis of b.
explicit b.
exploitative-manipulative b.
exploratory b.
explosive aggressive b.
externalizing b.
extraindividual b.
extramarital b.
face-saving b.
failure to sustain consistent work b.
feeding b.
felony b.
fidgeting b.
b. field
finger-biting b.
fire-setting b.
flamboyant b.
flirtatious b.
b. fluctuation
following b.
food-related b.
forgotten b.
freezing b.
future suicidal b.
gambling b.
gang b.
b. genetics
goal-directed b.
grooming b.
grossly disorganized b.
group b.
hair-pulling b.
hallucinatory b.
haughty b.
head-banging b.
health b.
healthy adolescent b.
helping b.
help-seeking b.
heterosexual b.
hiding b.
high-risk drug b.
high-risk sexual b.
HIV risk b.
homicidal b.
homoerotic b.
homosexual b.
hostile b.
hunting b.
hyperactive b.
hyperactive impulsive b.
hyperenergetic b.
hyperoral b.
hypomanic b.
hysterical b.
idiosyncratic b.
illegal b.
illness b.
imitative b.
immediacy b.
implicit b.
impulsive b.
inappropriate social b.
inattentive b.
incestuous b.
incoherent b.
incompatible b.
inconsiderate b.
indirect life-threatening b.
indirect self-destructive b. (ISDB)
infantile b.
ingratiating b.
initiation of goal-directed b.
innate b.
instinctive b.
intense sexual b.
interictal b.
intermittent explosive b.
interpersonal b.
intimidating b.
intolerable b.
intrinsic b.
intrusive b.
invaluable b.
invariable b.
involuntary b.
irrational b.
irresponsible work b.
isolative b.
iterative b.
kinesic b.
kissing b.
kleptomanic b.
knowledge, attitude, b. (KAB)

B

NOTES

behavior *(continued)*
b. language
language b.
lawful b.
leadership b.
learned dysfunctional b.
life-threatening b. (LTB)
lifetime b.
limit-testing b.
locality-specific pattern of aberrant b.
localization of b.
loving b.
maladaptive illness b.
maladaptive pattern of b.
malevolent b.
malingering b.
management of assaultive b. (MAB)
managing b.
manipulative b.
b. mapping
masochistic b.
mass b.
masturbation b.
maternal b.
mating b.
maze b.
meddlesome b.
medication-taking b.
mercurial b.
b. method
mischievous b.
mob b.
modeled b.
b. modification
b. modification program
b. modification therapy
molar b.
molecular b.
moral b.
motor b.
multiple target b.'s
mystifying b.
needle-related HIV risk b.
negative b.
negativistic b.
nodal b.
nonaggressive objectionable b.
noncompliant b.
nonparaphilic compulsive sexual b.
nonproductive b.
nonverbal b.
nonviolent b.
normative b.
nuisance b.
obedient b.
objectionable b.
objective b.
obsessive b.
obsessive-compulsive b.
odd b.
oedipal b.
on-task b.
operant b.
operative b.
oppositional b.
oral b.
orderly b.
out-of-control b.
overt b.
pacing b.
pain b.
paranoid b.
paraphiliac b.
parasuicidal b.
parental b.
passive b.
passive-aggressive b.
past b.
paternal b.
pathologic b.
b. pattern
pattern of antisocial b.
pattern of repetitive b.
peculiar b.
pedophilic b.
perceptual-motor b.
perplexing b.
petting b.
phobic avoidance b.
phobic avoidant b.
physically aggressive b.
pleasure-oriented b.
positive attention b. (PAB)
premeditated violent b.
pressured b.
previous suicide b.
primary b.
b. problem
problematic sexual b.
promiscuous sexual b.
prosocial b.
provocative b.
psychomotor b.
psychotic aggressive b.
psychotic disruptive b.
punishing spouse b.
purging b.
purposeful b.
rage b.
b. rating
rational-emotive b.
b. reaction
real-life b.
reckless b.
b. record
b. reflex

regressive b.
rehabilitation b.
b. rehearsal
relational b.
relationship b.
religious b.
REM sleep b.
repertoire of aggressive b.
repetitious b.
repetitive checking b.
repetitive exploratory b.
repetitive pattern of b.
repressive b.
respondent b.
responsible sexual b.
restless b.
restricted b.
restricting b.
restrictive b.
b. reversal
reward-associated b.
risk-taking b.
risky sexual b.
ritual b.
ritualistic b.
b. role
sadistic b.
b. sampling
seductive b.
self-damaging b.
self-defeating b.
self-destructive b.
self-dramatizing b.
self-harming b.
self-injurious b. (SIB)
self-mutilative b.
self-punishing b.
self-stimulatory b.
sensorimotor b.
b. setting
sex-related HIV risk b.
sex-role b.
sexually arousing b.
sexually inappropriate b.
sexually seductive b.
sexual predation b.
b. shaping
sickness b.
sissy b.
sleepwalking b.
smoking b.
socially acceptable b.
socially unacceptable b.
socially undesirable b.
social phobic-like b.
social stereotypical b.
sociopathic b.
solicitous spouse b.
spatial b.
b. specimen recording
speech and language b.
b., speech, and other syndromes
spiritual b.
splitting b.
stalking b.
standard b.
stereotyped b.
stereotypical b.
stimulation-bound b. (SBB)
structural analysis of social b.
struggle b.
subliminal b.
submissive b.
substance-bound b.
substance-seeking b.
substituting b.
sucking b.
suicidal b.
suicide b.
sundowning b.
superstitious b.
suspicious b.
b. system
talking back b.
target b.
teenage smoking b.
temperamental b.
terrorism b.
b. therapy
therapy-relevant b.
B. Therapy and Research Society (BTRS)
threatening b.
tic b.
tic-like b.
tomboy b.
tool-using b.
trancelike b.
transference b.
troubling b.
b. type
type A, B b.
typical b.
tyrannical b.
unacceptable b.
uncharacteristic b.

NOTES

behavior *(continued)*
uncued b.
undersocialized conduct b.
unethical b.
unexpected b.
uninhibited b.
unlawful b.
unnatural motor b.
unpurposeful b.
unsafe sexual b.
unstable b.
unusual b.
usual b.
utilization b.
variable b.
variety of sexual b.'s
verbal b.
violating b.
violent criminal b.
voluntary b.
voyeuristic sexual b.
water-seeking b.
weird b.
b. while driving
wild b.
withdrawn b.
wrist-cutting b.

behavioral
b. abnormality
b. activation system (BAS)
b. addiction
b. approach
b. assessment of dysexecutive syndrome (BADS)
b. assessment measure
b. attribute
b. avoidance test for OCD
b. baseline
b. change
b. characteristics progression
b. conditioning
b. consistency
b. contingency
b. contract
b. couples group therapy
b. criterion
b. desensitization
b. development
b. deviancy profile
b. difference
b. disorder
b. disorganization in schizophrenia
b. disturbance
b. dyscontrol
b. dysfunction
b. dysfunction symptom
b. effect
b. emergency
b. endocrinology
b. expression
b. facilitation
b. feature
b. flexibility
b. function
b. genetics
b. health
b. health hotline
b. immunogen
b. inactivity
b. inhibition
b. inhibition deficit
b. inhibition system (BIS)
b. input
b. intervention
b. management
b. manifestation
b. marital therapy (BMT)
b. masking
b. medicine
b. memory
b. metamorphosis
b. model
b. modeling
b. monitoring
b. neuroanatomy
b. neurobiology
b. neurochemistry
b. neurology
b. neuroscience
b. objective
b. observation
b. observation audiometry (BOA)
b. oscillation
b. outburst
b. pathogen
b. perspective
b. plan
b. prosthesis
b. psychiatry
b. psychology
b. psychotherapy
b. reaction brain syndrome
b. reciprocity
b. rehearsal
b. repertoire
b. research
b. research orientation
b. science
b. semantics
b. sensitization
b. set of disturbances
b. stability
b. support
b. technique
b. teratogenicity
b. theory
b. theory of rumination
b. toxicity

b. trajectory
b. transgression
b. treatment
b. variability
behavior-altering substance
behavior-constraint theory
behaviorism
eclectic b.
operant b.
radical b.
b. school of psychology
Tolman purposive b.
behaviorist
behavioristic psychology
behavior-oriented assessment
behead
behest
behoove
Behr
B. disorder
B. syndrome
being
b. abused
b. abusive
b. beaten
b. bullied
b. cognition
b. dirty
higher b.
b. locked in
b. stared at
supreme b.
b. tormented
b. value
belabor
beleaguer
bel esprit
belie
belief
b. about identity
accepted b.
ageist b.
bizarre b.
Christian b.
coping b.
core b.
cultural b.
culture-bound b.
delusional b.
deviant b.
dominant delusional b.
dysfunctional core b.
erroneous b.
exaggerated b.
false b.
fear-related b.
firmly held b.
fixed b.
formed b.
fully organized b.
b. in God
inner b.
internal world of b.
b. in life after death
loss of b.
odd b.
paranoid delusional b.
persecutory b.
personal b.
religious b.
shared delusional b.
survival b.
sustained b.
b. system of self-help
traditional b.
true b.
unreasonable b.
unshakable b.
believable
believe
make b.
belittle
belittling
continued b.
belladonna
b. alkaloid
b. and opium
bell-and-pad technique
belle
bellicose manner
belligerence
belligerent tone
bell-shaped curve
bellwether
belonging
sense of b.
beloved
below-average
b.-a. mental function
b.-a. student
below detectable level (BDL)
belt
black b.
b. mark
bemegride
bemidone

NOTES

bemoan
bemuse
benactyzine hydrochloride
benchmark
bench warrant
bending
rule b.
benedict
benefactor
beneficence
beneficent
beneficial
b. effect
socially b.
benefit
b. of clergy
cognitive b.
coordination of b.'s
disability b.
economic b.
employee b.
nonspecific b.
benevolence
benevolent
benighted
benign
b. essential tremor
b. exertional headache
b. habit
b. psychopathy
b. stupor
b. tetanus
benignant
Benson-Geschwind classification of aphasia
bentazepam
benthamism
Benton word generation task
bent posture
ben trovato
benumb
Benylin
benzene
benzoate
benzoctamine
benzodiazepine
short-acting b.
benzodiazepine-GABA-receptor complex
benzoylmethylecgonine
BEP
brain evoked potential
berate
berdache
berdachism
bereave
bereavement
b. in children
complicated b.
conjugal b.
b. disorder
feigned b.
b. group therapy
b. support group
symptom of b.
traumatic b.
uncomplicated b.
unresolved b.
bereavement-related
b.-r. depression
b.-r. major depressive episode
b.-r. mood disorder
bereft
bergsonian
bergsonism
beriberi
wet b.
berserk
beseech
beset
beshrew
beside the point
besiege
besmirch
besot
best
b. interest of child
b. interest standard
bestial
bestialis
mixoscopia b.
bestiality
bestir
besylate
beta
b. adrenergic antagonist
b. adrenergic-blocking agent
b. adrenergic-blocking drug
b. adrenergic medication
b. adrenergic medication-induced postural tremor
b. adrenergic receptor
b. alcoholism
b. amyloid peptide
b. amyloid protein
b. arc
b. blocker
b. cell
b. endorphin
b. error
b. hydroxylase
b. hypothesis
b. index
b. level
b. movement
b. noradrenergic antagonist
b. pattern
b. rhythm
b. stimulant

b. subunit
b. wave
b. weight
betacism
betaine
chloral b.
betel nut
bęte noire
bethel
betide
betise
betray
betrayal
sense of b.
b. trauma
betrothal
betterment
better off
betting
off-track b.
parimutuel b.
sports b.
between-group variance
beverage
alcoholic b.
social b.
bewail
bewilder
bewildered
bewilderment
bewitch
bewitchery
bewitchingly
bewitchment
Bezold-Brucke phenomenon
Bhakti
bhang
Bianchi syndrome
bias
b. against elderly
age b.
clinical b.
clinician b.
computerized assessment of response b.
b. crime
emotional b.
ethnic b.
evaluator b.
exotic b.
experimental b.
experimenter b.
expression of b.
free recall b.
gender b.
healthcare b.
hostile attributional b.
information processing b.
memory b.
negativistic b.
on-the-job b.
racial b.
selection b.
societal b.
bias-accidental
AIHQ hostility b.-a.
bias-ambiguous
AIHQ hostility b.-a.
biased
bias-intentional
AIHQ hostility b.-i.
BIB
brought in by
biblicism
bibliokleptomania
bibliolatry
bibliomania
bibliophile
bibliotherapeutic strategy
bibliotherapy
Bibring view of depressive disorder
bibulous
bicircadian rhythm
bicker
Bickerstaff migraine
biconditional
BICROS
bilateral contralateral routing of signals
bicultural
bide
bidialectalism
bidirectional selection study
biduous
Bidwell ghost
Bielschowsky idiocy
biennis
Oenothera b.
bifrontal headache
bifunctional
bifurcation
Big
B. Brothers of America
B. Sisters of America
bigamist
bigamous
bigamy

NOTES

bigorexia
bigot
bigoted
bigotry
bilabial
bilateral
b. abductor paralysis
b. adductor paralysis
b. anterior capsule deep brain stimulation for OCD
b. contralateral routing of signals (BICROS)
b. ECT
b. hermaphroditism
b. myoclonic seizure
b. regions
b. speech
b. synchrony
b. transfer
bilaterally symmetric inkblot design
biliary dyskinesia
bilineal family
bilingual
bilingualism
active b.
bilious headache
bilirachia
bilirubin encephalopathy
bill
b. of goods
b. of health
b. of indictment
b. of particulars
b. of rights
billingsgate
biloba
Ginkgo b.
biloquialism
bimanual
bimodal distribution
binary principle
binaural shift
bind
b. analysis date
double b.
b. over
binding
benzodiazepine receptor b.
libido b.
nonspecific b.
b. site
Binet age
binge
alcohol b.
b. buyer
cocaine b.
b. drinker
b. drinking
drug b.
b. eater
eating b.
b. eating and purging
b. episode
b. gambler
b. and purge
b. shopping
b. spender
binge-eating
b.-e. behavior
b.-e. disorder
b.-e. pattern
bingeing, binging
binge-purge behavior
binocular
b. perception
b. vision
binomial distribution
Binswanger
B. dementia
B. disease
B. encephalopathy
bioactive
bioanalysis
bioassay
bioavailability
absolute b.
biobehavioral
b. mechanism
b. shift
biocatalyst
bioccipital headache
biochemical
b. activity
b. exposure
b. imbalance
b. information
b. pathway
b. phenotypic marker
b. study
b. tracer
biochemorphology
biocidal
biocide
bioclimatology
biocompatible
biocybernetic
biocycle
biodata
biodynamic
bioelectric potential
bioelement
bioenergetic
b. psychotherapy
b. therapy
bioengineering
bioequivalence
bioequivalent
bioethics

biofeedback
b. application
b. computer
electrodermal response b.
electroencephalogram b.
electromyography b.
EMG b.
galvanic skin response b.
b. meter
b. method
temperature b.
b. theory
b. tone
b. training
bioflavonoid
biogenesis
biogenetic mental law
biogenic
b. amine
b. amine hypothesis
b. amine neurotransmitter
b. psychosis
biogenous
biogram
biographical
b. data
b. memory
b. method
biography
reactional b.
biohazard
biokinetic
biolinguistic language theory
biologic, biological
b. act
b. age
b. basis
b. causation
b. change associated with aging
b. and chemical warfare (BCW)
b. child
b. clock
b. consideration
b. control
b. correlate
b. data
b. determinant
b. determinism
b. diathesis
b. drive
b. dysfunction
b. dysfunction symptom
b. dysregulation
b. evidence
b. father
b. foundation
b. intelligence
b. intervention
b. issue
b. marker
b. maturity
b. measure
b. mother
b. parent
b. pathogenesis
b. predisposition
b. process
b. psychiatrist
b. psychiatry
b. reductionism
b. research
b. research orientation
b. rhythm
b. risk factor
b. root of addiction
b. sex
b. sibling
b. sign depression
b. status
b. stress
b. substrate
b. taxonomy
b. theory
b. therapy
b. time
b. training
b. viewpoint
b. warfare
b. weapon
b. window on CNS function
biologism
biology
b. of affective disease
communication in behavioral b. (CBB)
b. of deceit
developmental b.
bioluminescence
biolytic
biomathematic
biome
biomechanic
biomedical
b. engineering
b. informatics (BMI)
b. model

NOTES

biomedical *(continued)*
b. monitoring system (BMS)
b. therapy
biomedicine
biometric result
biometry
bion
bionergy
bionic
bionomy
biophilia
biophysical
b. life change
b. study
b. system
biophysics
biopotential
biopsy
biopsychic
biopsychology
biopsychosocial
b. history
b. model
b. paradigm
b. stability
b. variable
biopterin
bioreversible
biorhythm
bioscience
bioscopy
biosis
biosocial
b. determinism
b. integration
b. theory
biosphere
biostatic
biostatistic
biosynthesis
biosystematic
Biot
B. breathing
B. respiration
biotaxis
biotechnology
biotelemetry
bioterrorism
exposure to b.
fear of b.
bioterrorist attack
biotic potential
biotoxication
biotoxicology
biotoxin
biotransformation
biotrepy
biotype
biotypology
biovular twins
biowarfare
bioweapon
biparental
biphasic symptom
bipolar
b. I, II
b. affective disorder
b. affective psychosis
b. cell
b. depression
b. diathesis
b. I disorder, most recent episode mixed
b. I disorder, most recent episode unspecified
b. I disorder, single manic episode
b. I-IV disorder
b. illness (BPI)
b. neuron
b. patient
b. self
b. spectrum
b. spectrum disorder
b. type, mixed
bipolar-type
b.-t. currently depressed
b.-t. schizoaffective disorder
bipotentiality
biracial
bird of passage
birth
b. brain trauma organic psychosis
b. cohort
complete b.
b. complication
b. control (BC)
b. control pill (BCP)
b. control pill contraception
b. control regimen
cross b.
b. cry
b. date (BD)
b. defect
b. family
b. father
b. injury
live b.
b. of malformed fetus
b. mother
multiple b.'s
b. name
b. order
premature b.
b. rate
season of b.
b. trauma
b. weight
year of b. (YOB)

birthmark
birthplace
birthright
BIS
  behavioral inhibition system
bisensory method
bisexual (AC/DC)
  b. behavior
  closet b.
  b. confusion
  b. libido
  b. orientation
  b. pedophilia
  b. relationship
bisexuality
  theory of constitutional b.
bitartrate
  dihydrocodeinone b.
bitemporal hypoperfusion
biter
  nail b.
biting
  b. attack
  lip b.
  b. mania
  nail b.
  b. stage
bitter
  b. end
  b. humor
  obsessively b.
bitter-ender
bitterness
bittersweet
bivariate
bizarre
  b. answer
  b. behavior
  b. belief
  b. delusion
  b. gesture
  b. idea
  b. language
  b. posture
  b. posturing
  b. repetitive mannerism
  b. speech
  b. thought content
  b. thought process
  b. variant
bizarrerie
BL
  baseline
black
  b. art
  b. belt
  b. and blue
  b. book
  b. box warning
  b. death
  b. diet
  b. eye
  b. hand
  b. magic
  b. mass
  b. patch psychosis
  b. patch syndrome
black-and-white thinking
blackball
blackguard
blacking out
blacklist
blackmail
  emotional b.
black-market medication
blackout
  alcoholic b.
  b. threshold
bladder
  autonomic neurogenic b.
  b. continence
  b. control
  nervous b.
  neurogenic b.
  pseudoneurogenic b.
  reflex neurogenic b.
  stammering of b.
  b. training
  uninhibited neurogenic b.
blame
  assign b.
  externalize b.
  place b.
  b. psychology
blameless
blame-placing communication pattern
blameworthy
bland
  b. affect
  b. diet
blandish
blank
  b. hallucination
  interest b.
  b. screen
  b. stare

NOTES

blasé
blaspheme
blasphemous thought
blasphemy
blatant
blather
blatherskite
blatter
bleak
blear
bleary-eyed
bleat
bleeding of undetermined origin (BUO)
blemish
mouth b.
blended family
blending
auditory b.
sound b.
blepharedema
blepharoplegia
blepharospasm, blepharospasmus
Bleuler diagnostic system
bleulerian type 2
blight
blind
b. alley
b. analysis
color b.
b. date
double b.
b. drunk
b. faith
b. headache
b. matching technique
b. spot
b. study
b. trust
blindism
blindness
amnesic color b.
cerebral b.
concussion b.
conversion b.
cortical psychic b.
developmental word b.
functional b.
hysterical b.
legal b.
letter b.
mind b.
music b.
note b.
object b.
psychic b.
sign b.
smell b.
soul b.
taste b.
text b.
transient b.
word b.
blink
eye b.
b. reflex
b. response
bliss
absolute b.
blithe
blithely ignored need
blithesome
bloat
bloated
bloc
en b.
block
affect b.
alpha b.
b. anesthesia
b. design
genetic b.
mental b.
methadone b.
monolithic adult b.
b. sampling
blockade
audible speech b.
central cholinergic b.
D_2 b.
emotional b.
muscarine b.
muscarinic receptor b.
narcotic b.
nicotinic receptor b.
reuptake b.
silent speech b.
thought b.
blockage
blocked
b. memory
b. speech
blocker
beta b.
blocking
b. activity
b. agent
alpha b.
emotional b.
evidence of b.
b. evidence
b. procedure
thought b.
Blocq disease
blood
b. alcohol (BA)
b. alcohol concentration (BAC)
b. alcohol content
b. alcohol level (BAL)

bad b.
b. brotherhood
b. component
b. count
b. crossmatch
b. drug screen
b. dyscrasia
b. flow change
full b.
b. group
b. injection injury
occult b.
b. oxygenation level dependent (BOLD)
b. oxygenation level dependent MRI
b. oxygen depletion
b. poisoning
b. pressure
b. psychogenic disorder
b. screen for drug test
b. smear
b. sugar
b. transfusion
b. type
b. urea nitrogen (BUN)
b. volume

bloodless decerebration

bloodletting
surreptitious b.

bloodline

bloodshed

bloodshot

bloodstain

bloodstream

bloomer

Blos developmental model

blow
b. away
death b.
lethal b.
b. over

blow-by-blow

blowhard

blue
baby b.'s
black and b.
code b.
b. edema
maternity b.'s
out of the b.
paternity b.'s
postpartum b.'s
b. velvet syndrome

blue-blooded

blue-collar
b.-c. crime
b.-c. worker

blue-nose

bluff

blunder

blunted
b. affect
b. emotional expression
b. mood
b. response

blunting
affective b.
emotional b.

blurred vision

blurring of vision

blurry

blushing

bluster

BMI
biomedical informatics
body mass index

BMR
basal metabolic rate

BMS
biomedical monitoring system

BMT
behavioral marital therapy

BO
body odor

B&O
belladonna and opium

BOA
behavioral observation audiometry

board
b. certified psychiatrist
conversation b.
direct selection communication b.
b. eligible psychiatrist
encoding communication b.
gender identity b.
institutional review b.
Ouija b.
room and b.
scanning communication b.
sounding b.

board-and-care
b.-a.-c. facility
b.-a.-c. home

NOTES

boarder
phantom b.
boarding home
boarding-out system
boast
boasting
bobbing
head b.
ocular b.
bodement
bodhisattva
bodily
b. autonomy
b. disease
b. illusion
b. movement
b. sensation
b. symptom
body
b. alienation
b. appearance
astral b.
b. awareness
b. awareness resource network (BARN)
b. boundary
b. buffer zone
b. build
b. cathexis
b. composition
b. concept-exploration maneuver
b. conceptualization disturbance
b. contact-exploration maneuver
dementia with Lewy b.'s (DLB)
b. dipping
b. dissatisfaction
b. dysgnosia
b. dysmorphia
b. dysmorphic defect
b. dysmorphic disorder (BDD)
b. dysmorphic disorder in adolescence
b. dysphoria
b. dystonia
b. ego
b. ego concept
b. ego damage
emaciated b.
fat b.
b. fat
feeling of being detached from one's b.
b. fluid
foreign b.
b. functioning
b. gesture
hitting own b.
b. ideal
b. identity
b. image
b. image agnosia
b. image distortion
b. image hallucination
immune b.
intraneuronal argentophilic Pick inclusion b.
b. language
b. mass index (BMI)
b. mechanics
b. memory
b. modification
b. modification ritual
b. monitor
b. movement
muscular b.
b. narcissism
obese b.
b. odor (BO)
b. orifice
b. percept
perception localized within b.
b. piercing
pineal b.
b. position
b. posture
b. protest
b. rocking
b. schema
b. shape
b. size
b. snatching
b. surface area
b. swaying
b. therapy
b. tic
b. type
b. water
b. weight
Winkler b.
body-image
b.-i. disturbance
b.-i. recall
body-mind dichotomy
body-related obsessive-like symptom
boggle
bogus
boisterous
aggressively b.
Bolam principle
bolasterone
BOLD
blood oxygenation level dependent
BOLD MRI
bold-faced
Bolivian Society of Psychiatry
bolster
bolus

bomb
homemade pipe b.
bombard
bombarding
bombast
bombed
bombesin
bombing
bona fide
bond
affectional b.
attachment b.
disruption of affective b.'s
emotional b.
father-child b.
high-energy b.
incapacity to sustain social b.'s
male b.
mother-child b.
pair b.
parent-child b.
parent-offspring b.
partner b.
sibling b.
bondage
b. and discipline
physical b.
b. and sadomasochism (BDSM)
sensory b.
bonding
affiliation b.
human-pet b.
b. in infancy
mother-infant b.
pair b.
parent-infant b.
bondsman
bone
b. age (BA)
b. conduction deafness
magic b.
parietal skull b.
pointing of b.
b. pointing
b. sensibility
Bonferroni adjustment
bonhomie
Bonn early recognition study
Bonnet syndrome
Bonnevie-Ullrich syndrome
Bonnier syndrome
book
black b.
closed b.
bookish
boomer
baby b.
boomlet
baby b.
boorish
boot camp
bordello
border
Doctors Without B.'s
borderline
b. behavior
b. composite description
b. diagnosis prototype
b. dull
b. intellectual functioning
b. mental retardation
b. neurotic personality disorder
b. pathology
b. patient
b. personality
b. personality disorder (BPD)
b. personality disorder with histrionic feature
b. personality organization
b. personality style
b. psychosis
b. psychosis of childhood
b. range
b. schizophrenia (BS)
b. state
b. subfactor
boredom
feeling of b.
Borjeson-Forssman-Lehmann syndrome
borne
born worrier
Bosnian
B. army veteran
B. refugee
bossy
Boston University Model of Psychiatric Rehabilitation
bothersome
bottomless
bottom-up approach
bouffée délirante
bouleversement
boulimia (*var. of* bulimia)

NOTES

bound
culturally b.
out of b.'s
b. panic attack
situationally b.
upper b.
boundary, pl. **boundaries**
analytic b.
body b.
b. case
clear boundaries
b. crossing
diagnostic b.
ego b.
b. enforcement
external b.
boundaries and gender
group b.
I b.
b. issue
language b.
loss of ego b.
normalizing b.
b. phenomenon
boundaries in postanalytic supervision
posttermination b.
b. problem
boundaries in psychoanalysis
b. respect
role b.
subsystem b.
b. violation
whole brain b.
boundless energy
bourgeois
bourgeoisie
bout of insomnia
bovarism
bovine spongiform encephalopathy
bowel
b. control
b. incontinence
irritable b.
reactive b.
stress-induced reactive b.
b. training
Bowen model
Bower model of mood-congruent memory
Bowlby
B. developmental model
B. theory of attachment
B. theory of depression
box
Goodman lock b.
obstruction b.
Skinner b.
boxer's
b. dementia
b. encephalopathy
boyfriend
former b.
BPD
borderline personality disorder
BPI
bipolar illness
BPRS
Brief Psychiatric Rating Scale
BPRS anxiety-depression score
BPRS total score
BPRS withdrawal/retardation score
BPRS-E
Brief Psychiatric Rating Scale-Expanded
BPRS-E affect factor
BPRS-E anergia factor
BPRS-E disorganization factor
BPRS-E immediate memory index
BPRS-E thought disturbance factor
BRAC
basic rest-activity cycle
bracer
brachybasia
brachymorph
bradycardia
bradycinesia (*var. of* bradykinesia)
bradyesthesia
bradyglossia
bradykinesia, bradycinesia
functional b.
bradykinetic syndrome
bradykinin
bradylalia
bradylexia
bradylogia
bradyphagia
bradyphasia
bradyphemia
bradyphrasia
bradyphrenia
bradypnea
bradypragia
bradypsychia
bradyrhythmia
bradyspermatism
bradyteleokinesis
brag
braggart
brahmanism
braid-cutting
braidism
braille
brain
b. abnormality
b. abscess
b. ache
b. activation

b. age quotient (BAQ)
archaic b.
architecture of b.
b. area
b. assault
b. atrophy
b. autopsy
b. blood flow
b. cell damage
b. cicatrix
b. circuitry
compression of b.
b. concussion
concussion of b.
b. congestion
contrecoup injury of b.
b. control
b. contusion
b. convulsion
coup injury of b.
b. damage language disorder
b. death
b. degeneration
b. depressant
b. development
b. differentiation
b. dimorphism
b. disease
b. disease organic psychosis
b. dopamine
b. dopaminergic pathway
b. dopaminergic system
b. dysfunction
b. dysmorphology
b. edema
electrical activity of b.
b. electrical activity mapping (BEAM)
electric stimulation of b. (ESB)
b. evoked potential (BEP)
evolution of b.
b. fog
b. function
b. functional failure
b. function disruption
b. functioning
b. glucose metabolism
b. illness
b. imaging
b. imaging method
b. imaging study
b. infection organic psychosis
b. injury
b. involvement
b. lactate
b. location
b. mapping
b. metabolic effect
b. metabolic mechanism
b. model
b. murmur
b. opioid activity
b. pathology
phencyclidine mixed organic b.
b. potential study
prefrontal cortex of b.
b. process
b. psychoorganic syndrome
b. region
b. research
b. response
b. seizure
somatosensory cortex of right hemisphere of b.
b. space
b. spectrin
b. SPECT scan
split b.
b. splitting
b. stimulation
b. structure
b. structure study
b. substrate
b. swelling
b. trauma
b. trauma organic psychosis
ventromedial prefrontal cortex of b.
b. volume
water on b.
b. wave
b. wave activity
b. wave complex
b. wave cycle
b. weight

brain-behavior relationship

brain-derived
b.-d. HVA concentration
b.-d. neurotrophic factor gene

BrainMap
Couples B.

brainstem
b. auditory evoked potential
b. auditory evoked response
b. control
b. disease
b. displacement

NOTES

brainstem *(continued)*
b. dysfunction
b. function
b. reticular formation
b. sign
brainstorm
BRAINSTRIP semiautomated brain extraction tool
brain-to-plasma ratio
brainwash
brainwashing
branching
b. steps in therapy
b. tree diagram
Brasdor method
bravado
Bravais-jacksonian epilepsy
bravery
bravura
Brawner
B. decision
United States vs. B.
breach
confidentiality b.
b. of confidentiality
b. of security
security b.
breadwinner
loss of b.
break
acute psychotic b.
ascending pitch b.
major b.
psychotic b.
b. shock
b. state
b. with reality
breakaway phenomenon
breakdown
analytical b.
nervous b.
breaker
rule b.
breaking of family ties
breakoff phenomenon
breakthrough
depressive b.
b. tearfulness
breakup
breast
b. augmentation
b. complex
b. envy
b. implant
b. phantom phenomenon
breastfeeding
breath
alcohol on b. (AOB)
b. analyzer
b. control play
odor of solvent on b.
shortness of b. (SOB)
b. stream
b. work
breathe
breathholding spell
breathing
apneustic b.
Biot b.
Cheyne-Stokes b.
controlled b.
crescendo-decrescendo b.
daytime mouth b.
diaphragmatic b.
b. disorder
opposition b.
b. retraining
sleep-disordered b. (SDB)
b. technique
b. tic
breathing-related sleep disorder
breathy voice
bredouillement
Brenner theory of depression
Bretazenil
bride
war b.
bridge
crossing a b.
brief
b. delusional experience
b. depressive reaction
b. dynamic psychotherapy
b. episode
b. group therapy
b. posttraumatic stress disorder
B. Psychiatric Rating Scale (BPRS)
B. Psychiatric Rating Scale-Expanded (BPRS-E)
b. psychotic disorder
b. psychotic reaction
b. pulse bilateral ECT
b. pulse unilateral ECT
b. pulse waveform
b. reactive dissociative disorder
b. reactive psychosis
b. reactive psychosis with marked stressors
b. situational depression
b. stimulus technique
b. stimulus therapy (BST)
Brieger cachexia
Briggs law
brightening
mood b.
brightness
b. adaptation
b. constancy

b. contrast
b. discrimination
b. threshold

bright normal range

bring to closure

Briquet
B. ataxia
B. disease
B. disorder
B. syndrome

brisk reflex

Brissaud
B. disease
B. infantilism
B. syndrome

Brissaud-Marie syndrome

Brissaud-Sicard syndrome

Bristowe syndrome

British
B. anti-Lewisite (BAL)
B. Journal of Psychiatry
B. Manual of the Classification of Occupations

broad
b. affect
b. heritability

broadcasting
delusion of thought b.
thought b.

Broca
B. amnesia
B. aphasia
B. area
B. center

Brodie disease

Brodmann
B. area 6
B. area 7
B. area 9
B. area 24
B. area 32
B. area 41
B. area 43
B. area 44
B. area 46
B. area 47/11

brofoxine

broken
b. engagement
b. heart
b. home
b. promise

bromatherapy

bromatology

bromatotherapy

bromide
ammonium b.
decamethonium b.
b. hallucinosis
b. intoxication
b. poisoning

bromine compound

bromism, brominism

bromisovalum

bromoiodism

bromomania

bromperidol

bronchial
b. asthma
b. respiration

bronchodilator

bronchogenic

bronchospasm

brood

brooding
b. compulsion
obsessional b.
b. personality
spells of doubting and b.

brother complex

brotherhood
blood b.

brotherliness

brotizolam

brought in by (BIB)

brow
furrowed b.

brownian
b. motion
b. movement

Brown School Behavioral Health System

Brown-Sequard syndrome

brucine

bruise

bruising
b. of undetermined origin (BUO)
unexplained b.

brujeria

Bruns ataxia

Brushfield-Wyatt disease

brusque

brutal discipline

brutality

brute pride

NOTES

bruxism
sleep b.
sleep-related b.
SSRI-induced b.
bruxomania
BS
borderline schizophrenia
BST
brief stimulus therapy
BSW
Bachelor of Social Work
BTRS
Behavior Therapy and Research Society
bubo
venereal b.
buccal
b. intercourse
b. onanism
b. speech
buccarum
morsicatio b.
buccinator muscle
buckthorn polyneuropathy
Bucladin-S Softab
Buddhism
Zen B.
Buddhist
B. healing
B. religion
B. treatment
budgeting
functional b.
buffalo neck
buffoonery
b. psychosis
b. syndrome
bufotenin
bug
cocaine b.
buggery
build
body b.
index of body b. (IB)
building
b. fear
b. restriction
team b.
bulb
auditory b.
jugular b.
bulbocapnine
bulesis
bulimia, boulimia
b. nervosa
b. nervosa, nonpurging type
b. nervosa, purging type
purging-type b.
bulimic
b. behavior
b. episode
b. purge
bulimic-anorexic spectrum
bulimorexia
bulletin
Psychopharmacology B.
bullied
being b.
bully
bullying
b. behavior
continued b.
b. culture
b. experience
repeated b.
b. target
bum
skid-row b.
bump
goose b.'s
BUN
blood urea nitrogen
Bunney-Hamburg
B.-H. global psychosis rating
B.-H. nurse rating
BUO
bleeding of undetermined origin
bruising of undetermined origin
buoyancy
high-spirited b.
buprenorphine
burden
caregiver b.
family b.
b. interview
psychological b.
screen for caregiver b.
bureaucrat
Bureau of Drug Abuse Control (BDAC)
burial
proper b.
buried alive
burn
cigarette b.
napalm b.
B. and Rand theory
burned-out
b.-o. anergic schizophrenia
b.-o. schizophrenic
burning
b. oneself
b. pain
b. rubber
burnout
caretaker b.
parent b.
professional b.
b. syndrome

burr
Burton theory of depression
Burundanga intoxication
business readjustment
buster
baby b.
butanediol
butane-sniffing dependence
butaperazine
butethal
butoctamide
butterfly coil
button
mescal b.
panic b.
butyrolactone
gamma b. (GBL)
butyrophenone agent
butyrophenone-based neuroleptic drug
buyer
binge b.
buying
compulsive b.
b. spree
buzz
b. group
b. session
buzzing sensation
buzzword
BWS
battered woman syndrome
by
brought in by (BIB)
by-idea
bypass
gastric b.
byproduct
bystander dominates initial dominant (BDID)

NOTES

CA
chronologic age
Cocaine Anonymous
CA4-1
area CA4-1
caapi
cabal
cabin fever
cable graft
CABS
chronic alcoholic brain syndrome
cacation
cacesthesia
cache
cachectic infantilism
cachexia
Brieger c.
c. hypophysiopriva
pituitary c.
cachinnation
cacodemonomania
cacoethes
cacogenesis
cacogenic
cacogeusia
cacography
cacolalia
cacophonous
cacophony
cacophoria
cacoplastic
cacosmia
cacothenic
cacotrophy
cactus
peyote c.
cacuminal
cadaver
cadaverous
cadence
cadent
caducity
caelotherapy
cafard
caffeinated substance
caffeine-abstinent subject
caffeine-containing drug
caffeine-induced
c.-i. anxiety
c.-i. anxiety disorder
c.-i. contracture
c.-i. sleep disorder
c.-i. vasoconstriction
caffeine-intolerant individual
caffeine-related
c.-r. disorder
c.-r. sequela
caffeine-restricted diet
caffeine-sensitive individual
caffeinism
cage
population c.
Cain
C. complex
raise C.
Cairns stupor
cajole
calami
lapsus c.
calamus scriptorius
calcarine sulcus
calcium
acamprosate c.
calcium signaling
calculate
ability to abstract and c.
calculation
calendar c.
c. skill
calculus, pl. **calculi**
cerebral c.
Caldwell high speed magnetic stimulator
calefacient
calendar
c. age
c. calculation
life history c.
caliber
.22-c. handgun
.38-c. handgun
.44-c. handgun
calibrate
calibrated loop
calibration
California drug-endangered children's unit
calipers
calisthenics
call
c. girl
obscene phone c.
caller
obscene telephone c.
callomania
callosal
c. area
c. disconnection syndrome

C

callosal *(continued)*
c. disconnection syndrome aphasia
c. sulcus
callous
calmative
calming effect
calmodulin
calm wakefulness state
caloric
c. intake
c. stimulation test for vestibular function
calorie
calorifacient
calorigenic action
calumny
CAM
complementary and alternative medicine
camaraderie
camazepam
Cambodian refugee
Cameron
Rouse vs C.
camouflage
cAMP
cyclic adenosine monophosphate
cAMP response element (CRE)
cAMP response element binding protein
camp
boot c.
concentration c.
day c.
death c.
labor c.
refugee c.
camptocormia, camptocormy
camptospasm
Canadian Academy of Child Psychiatry
canal
anal c.
anterior vertical c.
auditory c.
central c.
craniopharyngeal c.
intramedullary c.
medullary c.
canalization
canard
Canavan
C. disease
C. sclerosis
cancerophobe
cancer reaction
candid
candidate gene strategy
canine
c. hysteria
c. spasm
caninus
risus c.
spasmus c.
canities
canker
cannabidiol
cannabin
cannabinoid
cross-reacting c.'s
cannabinol
cannabis
c. abuse
c. delusional disorder
c. dependence
c. intoxication
c. intoxication delirium
c. intoxication-related disorder
c. intoxication with perceptual disturbance
c. organic mental disorder
c. psychosis
C. sativa
C. sativa
c. use disorder
cannabis-induced
c.-i. anxiety
c.-i. anxiety disorder
c.-i. delirium disorder
c.-i. drowsiness
c.-i. euphoria
c.-i. mental change
c.-i. psychotic disorder with delusions
c.-i. psychotic disorder with hallucinations
cannabism
cannabis-related
c.-r. disorder
c.-r. disorder, NOS
cannibalism
cannibalistic
c. fantasy
c. fixation
Cannon-Bard
C.-B. theory
C.-B. theory of emotion
Cannon theory
canny
canonical correlation
cant
cantankerous
Cantelli sign
cantharis, pl. **cantharides**
CAP
carotid Amytal procedure
CAPA
child and adolescent psychiatric assessment

capability
cognitive c.
metabolic c.
capable
capacitance
capacity
adaptive c.
channel c.
code c.
c. code
cognitive c.
contractual c.
diminished c.
dissociative c.
empathic c.
functional c. (FC)
functional residual c. (FRC)
hedonic c.
hypnotic c.
c. for independent living
intellectual c.
intrinsic c.
legal c.
c. to love
measured c.
mental c.
metacognitive c.
nonverbal intellectual c.
orgasmic c.
oxygen-carrying c.
paranormal c.
physical c.
potential intellectual c.
psychological c.
self-regulatory c.
self-soothing c.
speaking c.
testamentary c.
volitional c.
caper
Capgras
C. delusion
C. phenomenon
C. syndrome
capistratus
capita (*pl. of* caput)
capital
c. offense
c. sin
capitalize
capitis (*gen. of* caput)
capitium
capping technique
caprice
capricious
Caps
Nytol Quick C.
capsule
drug-containing c.
external c.
gauze-wrapped glass c.
capsulothalamic syndrome
CAPTA
Child Abuse Prevention and Treatment Act
captation
captious
captivate
captivation
captive
indoctrination while c.
captivus
penis c.
captodiamine
capture
capuride
caput, gen. **capitis**, pl. **capita**
dolor capitis
per capita
c. succedaneum
carbamate
carbamylcholine chloride
carbinol
carbohydrate
c. craving
c. metabolism
carbon
c. dioxide (CO_2)
c. dioxide intoxication
c. dioxide poisoning
c. dioxide therapy
c. disulfide exposure
c. disulfide intoxication
c. monoxide
c. monoxide exposure
c. monoxide intoxication
c. monoxide poisoning
c. tetrachloride
carbonate
carbonic anhydrase inhibitor
carbonyl modification
carcinogen
card
daily report c.
diary c.
c. game gambling

NOTES

card *(continued)*
mother c.
c. playing
Rorschach c.
c. stacking
tarot c.
cardiac
c. arrest
c. arrhythmia
c. disorder
c. neurosis
c. psychosis
c. reaction
c. rhythm
c. symptom
cardinal
c. ocular movement
c. sign
c. sin
c. symptom
c. trait
c. virtue
cardiomyopathy
alcoholic c.
cardioneurosis
cardiophrenia
cardiopulmonary
c. arrest
c. resuscitation (CPR)
cardiopulmonary-obesity syndrome
cardiospasm
psychogenic c.
cardiotoxic
cardiovascular
c. neurosis
c. psychogenic disorder
c. seizure
card-sorting function
care
acute stabilization inpatient c.
adequate c.
adoption from foster c.
adoptive c.
ambulatory c.
ancillary c.
barrier to c.
child psychiatric c.
classification of level of c.
clinical c.
community c.
community mental health c. (CMHC)
comprehensive c.
compulsory c.
continuing c.
continuity of c.
continuum of c.
crisis residential c.
custodial c.
elder c.
eligibility for c.
end-of-life c.
enhanced standard c.
c. ethics
excessive need for c.
extended c.
family c.
foster c. (FC)
grossly pathogenic c.
health c.
home c.
hospice c.
inappropriate dependent c.
individual c.
inpatient c.
institutional c.
level of c.
long-term c.
managed c.
c. management for chronic addiction (CMCA)
medical c.
mental health c.
need for c.
obesity c.
online mental health c.
optimal c.
c. organization
outpatient c.
palliative c.
parental c.
pastoral c.
paternal c.
pathogenic c.
pathologic c.
pattern of c.
personal c.
primary c.
c. and protection proceeding
psychiatric c.
psychosocial residential c.
resistance to c.
routine clinical c.
secondary c.
c. seeker
skilled nursing c. (SNC)
specialized foster c.
standard of c.
tender loving c. (TLC)
tertiary c.
career
c. change
c. choice
c. conference
c. counseling
c. counselor
c. decision-making
c. development

c. evaluation
c. planning
c. planning program (CPP)
c. workshop
carefree
careful observation
caregiver
adoptive c.
c. burden
coping in c.'s
c. depression
c. distress
c. education
family c.
home c.
intimate attachment to c.
primary c.
c. stress
caregiving
enhance daily c.
careless dressing
caress
caretaker
c. assault
c. burnout
primary c.
caretaking role
careworn
cargo culture
Caribbean
caricature
carinatum syndrome
caring
expression of c.
quality of c.
carnal knowledge
carnosine
carotic
carotid
c. Amytal procedure (CAP)
c. sinus reflex death
carping
carpipramine
carpopedal
c. contraction
c. spasm
carrier
insurance c.
trait c.
Carroll-Klein model of bipolar disorder
carrot-and-stick approach
carry
c.'s a gun
c. away
c. off
c. on
c. through
carrying a weapon
caruncula, pl. **carunculae**
CAS
child assessment schedule
casanthranol
cascade
pathophysiologic c.
case
abuse c. (AC)
basket c.
boundary c.
c. control experimental study design
c. control study
Dora c.
c. ethics
false-negative c.
c. fatality rate
c. finding
c. formulation
high-profile c.
c. history
c. history study
incident c.
index c.
c. index
juvenile justice c.
c. method
c. mix
parole violation c.
c. in point
polysymptomatic c.
c. register
c. report
Schreber c.
self-reported c.
Tarasoff c.
test c.
textbook c.
typical-onset c.
caseload
casework
social c.
caseworker
CASI
casino gambling
cassina leaf
caste
castigate

C

NOTES

cast on
castrate
castration
c. anxiety
chemical c.
c. complex
emotional c.
c. fear
female c.
male c.
CASTT
child abuse-specific treatment of trauma
casual sex
casualty
combat c.
casuistic
casuistry
CAT
cognitive analytic therapy
computed axial tomography
CAT scan
catabasia
catabolic force
catabolism
catabolite
cataclysmic headache
catagenesis
catalepsy
epidemic c.
schizophrenic c.
cataleptic somnambulism
cataleptiform
cataleptoid
catalexia
catalogia
catalogue
explanatory model interview c.
catalyst
catalytic agent
catamenia
catamite
catamnesis
catamnestic
cataphasia
cataphora
cataphoric
cataphrenia
cataplasia
cataplectic
cataplexy, cataplexis
c. episode
catastrophe theory
catastrophic
c. ancataplexy syndrome
c. anxiety
c. behavior
c. effect
c. event
c. expectation
c. illness
c. reaction
c. response
c. schizophrenia
c. stress
catathymia
catathymic
c. amnesia
c. crisis
catatonia
deadly c.
depressive c.
excited c.
lethal c.
maniac c.
c. mitis
periodic c.
c. protracta
psychotic c.
recurrent c.
schizophrenic c.
Stauder lethal c.
stuporous c.
treatment-refractory c.
catatonic
c. behavior
c. cerebral paralysis
c. dementia
c. disorder
c. disorder due to general medical condition
c. excitation
c. excitement
c. feature
c. mutism
c. negativism
c. patient
c. posturing
c. presentation
c. rigidity
c. schizophrenia
c. state
c. stupor
c. symptom
c. syndrome
catatonic-type schizophrenia
catatonoid attitude
catatony
catchment area
cat-cry syndrome
catecholamine
c. hypophysis
c. neurotransmitter
peripheral c.
c. receptor
catecholamine-induced
c.-i. change
c.-i. thermogenesis
catechol-*O*-methyltransferase (COMT)

categorical
c. approach
c. attitude
c. change
c. classification
c. definition
c. imperative
c. model
c. personality disorder diagnosis
c. perspective
c. system
c. thinking
c. thought
categorization
symbolic c.
symptom c.
categorizing people
category
arousal c.
avoidance c.
diagnostic c.
disorder c.
dysphoric c.
early-onset c.
histrionic diagnostic c.
late-onset c.
c. mistake
NOS c.
reexperiencing c.
c. retrieval task
schizotypal c.
semantic c.
somatic c.
syntactic c.
catelectrotonus
catenating
catenation
catharsis
activity c.
community c.
conversational c.
emotional c.
psychodramatic c.
cathartic
c. abuse
c. event
c. method
cathectic discharge
catheresis
catheterization
diagnostic cardiac c.
cathexis
affective c.
body c.
ego c.
fantasy c.
libidinal c.
object c.
oral-sadistic c.
positive c.
word c.
cathinone
Catholic religion
CATIE-SZ
clinical antipsychotic trials of intervention effectiveness-schizophrenia
catnip
catochus
cat's eye syndrome (CES)
Caucasian
caudate
c. nucleus overactivity in OCD
c. tissue
caumesthesia
causa
causal
c. association
c. factor
c. indication
c. link
c. mechanism
c. possibility
c. relationship
c. texture
causal-attributional theory
causalgia
causalis
indicatio c.
causality
circular c.
direct c.
linear c.
phenomenistic c.
presumed c.
psychic c.
reverse c.
causation
biologic c.
organismic c.
causative
c. agent
c. mechanism
c. stress
cause
contextual c.
efficient c.

NOTES

cause *(continued)*
c. efficient
c. of identification
neurobiological c.
psychological c.
reversible c.
substance-related c.
cause-effect relationship
caustic
c. ingestion
c. remark
caution
cautious
CAVD
completion, arithmetic problems, vocabulary, and following directions
caveat
Caverject
cavort
CBASP
cognitive-behavioral analysis system of psychotherapy
CBB
communication in behavioral biology
CBC
child behavior characteristic
CBF
cerebral blood flow
CBGT
cognitive-behavioral group therapy
CBR
chemical, bacteriological, and radiological
CBRNE
chemical, biological, radiological, nuclear, and explosive
CBS
chronic brain syndrome
CBT
cognitive-behavioral therapy
cognitive behavior therapy
CBW
chemical and biological warfare
CC
chief complaint
CCD
charge-coupled device
CCS
concentration camp syndrome
CCTV
closed-circuit television
CD
character disorder
combination drug
communication disorder
conduct disorder
copying drawing
current diagnosis
Cd
color denial
CDC
chemical dependency counselor
CDD
certificate of disability for discharge
cease
ceaseless pacing
cecocentral scotoma
CEI
character education inquiry
ceiling
c. age
c. effect
celibacy vow
celibate
cell
alpha c.
c. assembly
beta c.
bipolar c.
detention c.
c. differentiation
jail c.
locked c.
lymphoblastoid c.
c. nucleus
padded c.
pallidal c.
photoreceptor c.
Pick c.
reactive c.
somatic c.
wandering c.
white blood c.
cellular
c. immunity factor
c. immunologic response
c. store
cellulotoxic
celsi
alopecia c.
Celsus alopecia
cement
cenesthesia, coenesthesia
cenesthesic, cenesthetic
cenesthopathic schizophrenia
cenotrope
censor
freudian c.
psychic c.
censorship
dream c.
censure
peer c.
census
juvenile residential facilities c.
c. tract

center
- academic medical c.
- acoustic c.
- addiction c.
- adult diagnostic and treatment c.
- appetitive c.
- association c.
- c. of attention
- Broca c.
- communal residential c.
- community mental health c. (CMHC)
- cortical c.
- counseling c.
- crisis c.
- daycare c.
- day reporting c.
- day treatment c. (DTC)
- Defense Manpower Data C.
- developmental evaluation c. (DEC)
- C.'s for Disease Control and Prevention
- drug information c. (DIC)
- ego c.
- guidance c.
- higher brain c.
- language c.
- c. median
- medical c.
- C. for Mental Health Services (CMHS)
- methadone c.
- motor cortical c.
- nonpublic residential treatment c.
- pleasure c.
- psychocortical c.
- public residential treatment c.
- rape crisis c.
- reflex c.
- regulatory c.
- residential treatment c. (RTC)
- satiety c.
- speech intention c.
- speech monitoring c.
- C. for Stress and Anxiety Disorders
- C. for Substance Abuse Treatment (CSAT)
- suicide prevention c.
- visual c.
- Wernicke c.
- word c.
- work-release c.

centered
- child c.
- community c.
- group c.

centering

center-surround response

centimorgan (cM)

central
- c. alexia
- c. anesthesia
- c. aphasia
- c. canal
- c. cholinergic blockade
- c. conflict
- c. convulsion
- c. deafness
- c. dysautonomia
- C. European subtype
- c. excitatory state
- c. executive component
- c. fissure
- c. force
- c. gray matter (CGM)
- c. gray matter region
- c. inhibition
- c. language disorder (CLD)
- c. language imbalance
- c. limit theorem
- c. masking
- c. motive state
- c. nervous system (CNS)
- c. neuritis
- c. neurogenic hyperventilation
- c. pain
- c. paralysis
- c. processing dysfunction
- c. reflex time
- c. role
- c. scotoma
- c. seizure
- c. sensory deficit
- c. sensory loss
- c. sleep apnea
- c. sulcus
- c. tegmental nucleus
- c. tendency
- c. tendency measure
- c. theme
- c. timing process
- c. trait
- c. transactional core
- c. vision

centralism

NOTES

C

centralist psychology
centrality
centraphose
centration
Centre
Early Psychosis Prevention and Intervention C.
centrencephalic
c. epilepsy
c. seizure
centripetal
centrokinesia
centrokinetic
centromere
centrophenoxine
cephalalgia, cephalgia
histaminic c.
orgasmic c.
cephalea attonita
cephaledema
cephalemia
cephalgia (*var. of* cephalalgia)
cephalic
c. aura
c. index
c. seizure
c. tetanus
cephalitis
cephalodynia
cephalogenesis
cephalometric analysis
cephalometry
cephalomotor
cephalopathy
ceptor
chemical c.
contact c.
distance c.
CER
conditioned emotional response
cercle
arc de c.
cerea
flexibilitas c.
c. flexibilitas
cerebellar
c. activation
c. ataxia
c. cortex
c. gait
c. hypoperfusion
c. metabolism
c. nucleus
c. pathway
c. region
c. rigidity
c. seizure
c. sign
c. speech
c. tremor
cerebral
c. activity
c. agraphia
c. anoxia
c. asymmetry
c. atrophy
c. blindness
c. blood flow (CBF)
c. calculus
c. compression
c. compromise
c. contusion
c. convulsion
c. cortex
c. cortical function
c. death
c. decompression
c. decortication
c. depressant
c. disorder
c. disorganization
c. dominance
c. dynamic imaging
c. dysfunction
c. dysplasia
c. eclipse
c. edema
c. electrotherapy (CET)
c. fissure
c. glucose metabolic-type organic psychosis
c. glucose metabolism
c. hemisphere
c. hemodynamic variation
c. hyperesthesia
c. hyperplasia
c. hypoplasia
c. hypoxia
c. impairment
c. infarct
c. infection
c. injection
c. integration
c. irritation
c. localization
c. location
c. malaria
c. mapping of apraxia
c. neurosyphilis
c. outflow tremor
c. oxygen consumption
c. pacemaker
c. perfusion pressure (CPP)
c. porosis
c. potential
c. region
c. seizure

c. sign
c. syphilis
c. tetanus
c. thumb
c. trauma
c. voxel
cerebrate posturing
cerebration
unconscious c.
cerebri
commotio c.
lacuna c.
cerebrocranial defect
cerebropathia
cerebropsychosis
cerebrospinal
c. convulsion
c. fluid (CSF)
c. index
c. pressure
c. seizure
c. system
cerebrotonia
cerebrovascular disease organic psychosis
ceremonial behavior
ceremonious
ceremony
collaring c.
secret c.
CERS
Crisis Evaluation Referral Service
certainty
certifiable
certificate
dependent adult c.
detention c.
c. of disability for discharge (CDD)
c. of incompetency
c. of need
certification
certified
c. addiction disease specialist
c. social worker (CSW)
certify
ceruleus
locus c.
cervicodynia
CES
cat's eye syndrome
cessation
caffeine c.
cocaine c.
gambling c.
habit c.
smoking c.
CET
cerebral electrotherapy
C factor
CFS
chronic fatigue syndrome
CGI-BP
clinical global impression-bipolar
CGM
central gray matter
CGPP
comparative guidance and placement program
CHADD
children and adults with attention deficit disorder
children and adults with attention deficit/hyperactivity disorder
chain
c. analysis
behavior c.
c. reflex
c. reproduction
c. smoker
chained reinforcement
chaining response
chair
tranquilizer c.
challenge
diagnostic c.
ethical c.
hostile c.
c. strategy
chamber
echo c.
gas c.
Chamorro
CHAMPUS
Civilian Health and Medical Program of the Uniformed Service
chance
c. action
c. difference
c. error
last c.
c. medley
c. response parameter
c. variation
chancre
hard c.

NOTES

chancre *(continued)*
mixed c.
monorecidive c.
soft c.
sporotrichositic c.
true c.
tularemic c.
chancroid
chancrous
change
c. abilitator
abulic mental c.
adolescent sexual c.
age-appropriate cognitive c.
age-inappropriate cognitive c.
c. agent
agent of c.
age-related brain c.
age-related genomic c.
age-related pharmacokinetic c.
analogic c.
anatomic brain c.
c. in appetite
appetite c.
c. of attitude
autoplastic c.
baseline-to-endpoint c.
c. in behavior
behavioral c.
biophysical life c.
blood flow c.
cannabis-induced mental c.
career c.
catecholamine-induced c.
categorical c.
chronic c.
circumscribed c.
cognitive c.
compulsive c.
cultural c.
culture c.
c. in demeanor
dietary c.
digital c.
disease-related c.
c. in energy
environmental c.
global c.
c. in health
c. of heart
hyperintensity c.
intrapsychic c.
job c.
language c.
c. in libido
life c.
c. of life
life-cycle c.
lifestyle c.
c. in living arrangement
major life c.
maladaptive behavioral c.
maladaptive psychological c.
maturational c.
medication c.
mental status c.
c. in mentation
metabolic c.
methylphenidate-induced c.
moment-to-moment mood c.
mood c.
negative c.
neurochemical c.
newly emergent categorical c.
nutritional c.
c. of pace
pathologic c.
personality c.
c. in personality characteristic
pharmacodynamic c.
pharmacokinetic c.
physical c.
c. point
positive attitude c.
postural c.
psychological c.
psychomotor c.
psychophysiological c.
reflex c.
sense of bodily c.
sex c.
sleep c.
c. in sleep pattern
c. in sociability
socioeconomic life c.
stigma c.
stoichiometric c.
structural c.
subjective mood c.
sustainability of c.
c. of topic
toxemia-related personality c.
transitional c.
treatment c.
trophic c.
unpredictable mood c.
white matter c.
changeable versus constant
changed body image
changeover
changeup
changing
c. clothes
c. emotion
c. environment
c. needs
c. sleep-wake pattern

channel
acid-sensing ion c.
c. capacity
communication c.
c. of communication
chant
chaos
organizational c.
c. theory
chaotic environment
chaplain
hospital c.
military c.
character
acquired c.
anal c.
anal-aggressive c.
c. analysis
c. armor
c. assassination
c. attack
authoritarian c.
Cloninger psychobiological model of temperament and c.
compulsive c.
c. defect
c. defense
c. deficit
dependent c.
depressive c.
c. development
c. dimension
c. disorder (CD)
c. displacement
dominant c.
c. education inquiry (CEI)
epileptic c.
erotic c.
exploitative c.
c. flaw
genital c.
histrionic c.
hoarding c.
hysterical c.
c. impulse disorder
impulsive c.
in c.
masochistic c.
narcissistic c.
national c.
c. neurosis
obsessional c.
oral c.
oral-aggressive c.
oral-passive c.
oral-receptive c.
out of c.
paranoiac c.
c. pathology
phallic c.
phallic-narcissistic c.
phobic c.
receptive c.
c. resistance
sex-conditioned c.
sex-limited c.
sex-linked c.
c. spectrum disorder
c. structure
c. trait
c. type
c. witness
characteristic
aberrant parental c.
c. age
association c.
c. association
c. behavior
behavior c.
change in personality c.
child behavior c. (CBC)
clang association c.
clinical c.
comorbid c.
consumer c.
core c.
culturally specific c.
demand c.
demographic c.
dominant c.
electrical c.
environment c.
c. feature
c. manifestation
neuropsychologic c.
objective trauma c.
overrepresented c.
c. paraphiliac focus
parental environment c.
c. pattern
c. pattern of affectivity
c. pattern of motivation
c. pattern of thought
perceived trauma c.
performance c.
personality c.

NOTES

characteristic *(continued)*
phenomenological c.
predictive c.
presenting c.
primary sex c.
psychological c.
psychometric performance c.
receiver operating c. (ROC)
secondary sex c.
sex c.
c. sign
signal-noise c.
subjective sleep c.
temperamental c.
temporal c.
trait c.
trauma c.
unique c.
c. withdrawal syndrome
characterization wit
characterological
c. depression
c. disorder
characterology
charas
Charcot
C. disease
C. grand hysteria
C. triad
C. vertigo
charge-coupled device (CCD)
charisma
charismatic
c. group
c. personality
c. religious experience
charlatan
charlatanry
Charles Bonnet syndrome
Charlson comorbidity score
charm
superficial c.
Charpentier law
chart
astrology c.
autobiographical life c.
Dartmouth COOP functioning c.
expectancy c.
mood c.
pediatric growth c.
progress c.
chary
chase
idea c.
chaser
ambulance c.
chaste tree
chastise
chastisement
chastity
chatterbox effect
checkerboard pattern
checking
c. compulsion
mirror c.
c. and touching rituals
checklist
aberrant behavior c.
c. approach
checkup
drinkers' c.
cheeking medication
cheerful
cheerfulness
forced c.
sudden c.
unnatural c.
cheerless
cheilophagia
cheirognostic, chirognostic
cheirokinesthesia, chirokinesthesia
cheirokinesthetic
cheirology
chelating agent
chelation therapy
chemical
c., bacteriological, and radiological (CBR)
c., biological, and radiological
c., biological, radiological, nuclear, and explosive (CBRNE)
c., radiological, and biological
c., radiological, and biological warfare
c. of use and abuse
chemical-mechanical transduction
cheminosis
chemist
basement c.
chemistry
clinical c.
mental c.
psychiatric c.
chemopsychiatry
chemoreceptor trigger zone
chemoreflex
chemoresistance
chemosensitive
chemosensory
chemotherapy
chemotropism
cheromania
chest
c. discomfort
c. pain
c. pulse
c. restraint
c. voice

chewing
c. automatism
c. method
c. and spitting
chewing-speech relationship
Cheyne-Stokes
C.-S. aspiration
C.-S. breathing
C.-S. psychosis
C.-S. respiration
CHI
closed head injury
chi
tai c.
chiaroscuro
chide
chief complaint (CC)
child
abandoned c.
c. abandonment
C. Abuse Prevention and Treatment Act (CAPTA)
c. abuse-specific treatment of trauma (CASTT)
c. abuse syndrome
c. and adolescent fear and anxiety treatment program
c. and adolescent psychiatric assessment (CAPA)
c. and adolescent psychiatry
adopted c.
c. advocate
c. of alcoholic (COA)
c. analysis
antisocial c.
c. antisocial behavior
c. assessment schedule (CAS)
atypical c.
autistic c.
battered c.
c. behavior characteristic (CBC)
best interest of c.
biologic c.
c. centered
conduct-disordered c.
c. counselor
c. custody
c. development clinic
c. development specialist
difficult c.
easy c.
c. endangerment
exceptional c.
c. fixation
foster c.
gifted c.
c. group therapy
c. guidance
c. guidance clinic
c. guidance therapy
C. Health and Development Study
homeless c.
c. homicide
c. inpatient service
c. inpatient unit
c. language development
latchkey c.
love c.
malnourished c.
c. maltreatment
manic c.
c. mental health professional
c. mental health service
mentally retarded c.
misbehaving c.
c. molestation
c. molestation allegation
c. molester
neglect of c.
c. neglect
neglected c.
normal c.
obese c.
c. outpatient service
c. physical abuse
c. pornography
c. posttraumatic stress reaction index
prepubertal c.
preschool c.
problem c.
c. prodigy
c. psychiatric care
c. psychiatrist
c. psychiatry (CHP, CP)
c. psychologist
c. psychology (CP)
c. psychopathology
c. psychopharmacology
c. psychosis
c. psychotherapy
c. rearing
scatter c.
school-age c.
c. sexual abuse
sexual abuse of c.

NOTES

child *(continued)*
c. sexual abuser
c. sexual assault
sexually abused c.
c. snatcher
c. support
traumatized c.
troubled c.
unruly c.
unwanted c.
violent c.
vulnerable c.
C. Welfare League of America (CWLA)
childbearing age
childbirth
c. amnesia
c. organic psychosis
psychosis in c.
childcare
c. aide
c. facility
c. worker
child-focused
childhood
abuse in c.
adjustment reaction of c.
c. adversity
anxiety disorder of c.
c. anxiety disorder
c. aphasia
c. autism
avoidant disorder of c.
behavior disorder of c.
c. bipolar disorder
borderline psychosis of c.
c. crossgender behavior
dementia-aphonia syndrome of c.
developmental experimentation in c.
c. developmental stage
c. disease
c. disintegrative disorder
disorder of c.
early c.
emotional disturbance of c.
c. encephalopathy
c. environment
c. experience
c. fear
fearfulness disorder of c.
c. figure
gender identity disorder of c.
happy c.
hyperkinetic reaction of c.
hyperkinetic syndrome of c.
identity disorder of c.
introverted disorder of c.
c. loss of parent
c. loss of sibling
c. maltreatment
c. maltreatment history self-report
c. memory
c. mistreatment history
c. motivation
c. obsessive-compulsive disorder
c. onset
oppositional disorder of c.
overanxious disorder of c.
problem of c.
c. psychosexual identity disorder
c. psychosis
psychosis of c.
reaction of c.
reactive attachment disorder of infancy or early c.
relationship problem of c.
schizoid disorder of c.
c. schizophrenia
schizophrenic syndrome of c.
second c.
sensitivity reaction of c.
c. separation anxiety
separation anxiety disorder of c.
c. sexual abuse
shyness disorder of c.
c. social dysfunction
social withdrawal of c.
c. stressor
symbiotic psychosis of c.
c. Tourette syndrome
c. tradition
transient tic disorder of c.
c. trauma
withdrawal reaction of c.
c. years
childhood-onset
c.-o. depression
c.-o. insomnia
c.-o. obsessive-compulsive disorder
c.-o. pervasive developmental disorder
c.-o. phobia
c.-o. psychosis
c.-o. schizophrenia
c.-o. Tourette syndrome
childish
c. behavior
c. emotion
childlike
c. behavior
c. innocence
c. mannerism
c. silliness
child-parent
c.-p. concordance
c.-p. fixation
child-penis wish
child-placement counseling

child-raising period
childrearing
maternal c.
paternal c.
children
c. and adults with attention deficit disorder (CHADD)
c. and adults with attention deficit/hyperactivity disorder (CHADD)
aid to dependent c. (ADC)
American Association of Psychiatric Services for C. (AAPSC)
amnesia in c.
c. at risk
autistic-spectrum c.
bereavement in c.
emotional maltreatment of c.
exploitation of c.
feral c.
gender identity disorder in c.
halfway c.
identity-disordered c.
kleptomania in c.
latchkey c.
latency-age c.
prepubertal c.
relaxation training in c.
suicide in c.
taxonomy of problematic social situations for c.
c. of transsexual parent
troubled c.
children's
c. development of moral thought
C. Health Care Act of 2000
C. Health Study (CHS)
c. language processes
C. Protective Services (CPS)
Chilean refugee
chill
nervous c.
c. out
chill-out room
chilophagia
chimeric
c. stimulant
c. stimulation
China syndrome
Chinese
C. classification of mental disorders
C. ginseng
C. medicine
chin jerk
chirobrachialgia
chirognostic (*var. of* cheirognostic)
chirokinesthesia (*var. of* cheirokinesthesia)
chirospasm
chlamydia, pl. **chlamydiae**
chlamydial
chlamydiosis
chloral
c. alcoholate
c. betaine
c. derivative
chloralism
chloride
amyl c.
carbamylcholine c.
c. channel flux assay
diphenylaminearsine c.
mercuric c.
chlormezanone
chloroform
chlorohydrocarbon dependence
chlorprothixene
choice
behavior c.
career c.
drug of c.
forced c.
laxative of c. (LOC)
narcissistic object c.
object c.
occupational c.
odd word c.
c. point
c. reaction
stimulant c.
symptom-based drug c.
treatment c.
vocational c.
choke hold
choking
c. feeling
c. game
cholecystokinin
choleric type
cholesteryl ester transfer protein
choline
cholinergic
c. activity
c. approach

NOTES

cholinergic *(continued)*
c. neuron
c. receptor
c. side effect
c. synapse
c. therapy
c. tract
c. transmission
cholinomimetic
choo-choo phenomenon
choose
freedom to c.
chorea
automatic c.
chronic progressive c.
conversion c.
dancing c.
electric c.
fibrillary c.
habit c.
hysterical c.
juvenile c.
laryngeal c.
c. major
methodical c.
mimetic c.
c. minor
c. nutans
procursive c.
rhythmic c.
c. rotatoria
saltatory c.
senile c.
tetanoid c.
choreal
choreic
c. ataxia
c. insanity
c. movement
choreicus
status c.
choreiform
c. movement
c. syndrome
choreoathetosis
choreoid
choreophrasia
CHP
child psychiatry
chrematomania
Christian
C. belief
C. religion
Christianity
chroma
chromaffinoma
chromaffinopathy
chromatic
c. audition
c. color
c. contrast
c. dimming
c. flicker
c. response
chromaticity
chromatid
chromatin
c. negative
c. positive
sex c.
chromatinolysis
chromatography
chromatolytic
chromatopsia
chromesthesia
chromium picolinate
chromolysis
chromosomal
c. aberration
c. abnormality
c. locus
c. translocation
chromosome
c. 4, 13, 18, 21
accessory c.
acrocentric c.
fragile X c.
c. number
sex c.
c. 13, 18, 21 trisomy
c. 21-trisomy syndrome
X c.
Y c.
chromotherapy
chromotrichia
chromotrichial
chromotropic
chronaxia, chronaxy
chronic
adjustment disorder, c.
c. administration
c. African sleeping sickness
c. alcohol abuse
c. alcoholic brain syndrome (CABS)
c. alcoholic delirium
c. alcoholic mania
c. alcoholism
c. amnesia
c. anorexia nervosa
c. antidepressant inhibition
c. anxiety
c. brain syndrome (CBS)
c. change
c. cocaine user
c. course
c. deficit state
c. delusional state

c. depressive personality
c. disability
c. disease score
c. distrust
c. drinker
c. drug abuse
c. drunkenness
c. dysthymia
c. ethanol exposure
c. ethanol user
c. factitious illness
c. familial polyneuritis
c. fatigue
c. fatigue syndrome (CFS)
c. feeling of emptiness
c. headache
c. hyperventilation syndrome
c. hypomanic personality
c. illness behavior
c. insomnia
c. integrative deficit
c. intoxication
c. lead poisoning
c. major depression
c. melancholia
c. mental distress
c. mental illness
c. motor tic
c. motor tic disorder
c. neurologic disease-associated dementia
c. neuropsychologic disorder
c. pain
pain disorder, c.
c. paranoid psychosis
c. paranoid reaction
c. paranoid schizophrenic reaction (CPSR)
c. pattern
c. pessimism
c. phase of stable sleep difficulty
c. posttraumatic neurosis
c. posttraumatic stress disorder
c. progressive chorea
c. psychosocial turbulence
c. psychotic illness
c. response
c. schizophrenia
c. sleep disturbance
c. spasm tic
c. state of anger
c. stress
c. stressor
c. stress reaction
c. suspiciousness
c. tissue damage
c. toxic effect
c. type
c. undifferentiated
c. undifferentiated schizophrenia
c. undifferentiated schizophrenic reaction
c. use
c. vertigo
c. wasting disease

chronically
c. depressed patient
c. disabling pattern
c. mentally ill

chronicity
(Hymovich) C. Impact and Coping Instrument (CICI)
c. of symptoms

chronobiological disorder
chronobiology
chronognosis
chronograph
chronologic age (CA)
chronological
c. drinking record
c. order
c. relationship

chronology of symptoms
chronometry
mental c.

chronotaraxis
chronotherapy
CHS
Children's Health Study

chum period
CI
coefficient of intelligence
confidence interval

cibi
fastidium c.

CIC
crisis intervention clinic

cicatrices (*pl. of* cicatrix)
cicatricial alopecia
cicatrisata
alopecia c.

cicatrix, pl. **cicatrices**
brain c.

CICI
(Hymovich) Chronicity Impact and Coping Instrument

NOTES

CIDI
composite international diagnostic interview
cigarette burn
ciliary neurotrophic factor
cilium, pl. **cilia**
cinanesthesia (*var. of* kinanesthesia)
cinchonism
cinclisis
Cinderella
C. complex
C. syndrome
cingula (*pl. of* cingulum)
cingulate
anterior c.
c. cortex
c. gyrus overactivity in OCD
posterior c.
c. response
c. sulcus
c. tissue
cingulectomy
cingulotomy
cingulum, pl. **cingula**
cinq
folie á c.
cintriamide
CIP
comprehensive identification process
critical illness polyneuropathy
circadian
c. clock
c. clock gene
c. hormone
c. marker
c. pacemaker mechanism
c. phase of sleep
c. quotient (CQ)
c. realignment
c. rhythm
c. rhythm sleep disorder
c. rhythm sleep disorder, delayed sleep phase
c. rhythm sleep disorder, shift work
c. system
c. timing
c. variation
circannual rhythm
circaseptan rhythm
circle
Papez c.
vicious c.
circuit
attentional c.
convergence c.
cortex c.
divergence c.
dysfunctional neural c.
error detection c.
frontosubcortical brain c.
limbic c.
neuroanatomic c.
neuronal c.
Papez c.
reverberating c.
traditional limbic c.
worry c.
circuitry
amygdala-fear c.
brain c.
dysfunctional c.
c. of emotion
frontal-cerebellar-thalamic c.
limbic c.
normal c.
reciprocal c.
reward c.
striatofrontal c.
circulaire
folie c.
circular
c. causality
c. dementia
c. insanity
c. pattern response
c. psychosis
c. questioning
c. reaction
c. thinking
circulating leptin level
circulatory psychosis
circumambulate
circumcision
female c.
male c.
circumfix morpheme
circumlocution
circumplex
multifacet c.
c. of premorbid personality types
circumscribed
c. amnesia
c. change
c. craniomalacia
c. delusion
c. edema
c. pyocephalus
c. region
circumscripta
alopecia c.
circumscription
monosymptomatic c.
circumspect
circumstance
abnormal c.
altered life c.
clinical c.

distressing c.
extenuating c.
frightening c.
inappropriate c.
other specified family c.
real-life c.
circumstantial
c. evidence
c. information
c. migraine headache
c. speech
c. thought process
circumstantiality
CIRP
cooperative institutional research program
cirrhosis
alcoholic c. (AC)
Laennec c.
liver c.
syphilitic c.
toxic c.
cirrhotic liver
9-*cis* retinoic acid receptor (RXR)
cisternal puncture
cisterna magna
cisvestism
cite
Citelli syndrome
citizen
law-abiding c.
naturalized c.
senior c.
citizenship
original c.
citrate
sildenafil c.
civil
c. commitment
c. commitment procedure
c. conflict
c. disobedience
c. marriage
c. rights
c. rights violation
civilian
c. catastrophe reaction
C. Health and Medical Program of the Uniformed Service (CHAMPUS)
c. sexual assault
c. trauma
civilization
CJD
Creutzfeldt-Jakob disease
cladiosic
claim review
clairaudience
clairsentience
clairvoyance
clairvoyant dream
clammy skin
clamor
clan
clandestine
clang association characteristic
clanging
clannish
clansman
clarification
clarify
clarity
diagnostic c.
phonetic c.
clash
paradigm c.
personality c.
clasp-knife
c.-k. effect
c.-k. phenomenon
c.-k. response
c.-k. rigidity
c.-k. spasticity
class
closed c.
c. conscious
diagnostic c.
c. discrimination
elite c.
c. inclusion
c. interval
c. limit
middle c.
parental socioeconomic c.
c. size
skip c.
social c.
socioeconomic c.
c. word
classic
c. apraxia
c. euphoric mania
c. migraine
c. psychoanalysis
classical
c. analysis

NOTES

classical *(continued)*
c. conditioning
c. depression
c. migraine headache
c. paranoia
c. psychoanalytical theory
classification
alcoholic c.
categorical c.
c. of depression
dichotomous c.
DSM-IV-R c.
empirical c.
Kendell c.
c. of level of care
c. method
multiaxial c.
neo-kraepelian c.
Newcastle c.
Paykel c.
c. system
classism
classless
classroom
Claude
C. hyperkinesis sign
C. syndrome
clausa
rhinolalia c.
clause
disturbance between c.'s
disturbance within c.'s
claustra (*pl. of* claustrum)
claustral complex
claustrophobic
claustrum, pl. **claustra**
clavus hystericus
clawing attack
clay eater
clay-modeling
c.-m. equipment
c.-m. therapy
CLD
central language disorder
cleanliness of clothing
cleansing
virgin c.
clear
c. boundaries
c. and convincing evidence
c. rules and consequences
c. sensorium
c. thinking
c. twilight state
clearance
dopamine c.
clearcut
c. attachment
c. schizophrenia
clearheaded
clearheadedness
clearinghouse
privacy c.
self-help c.
clearly demarcated relationship
clearsighted
clearsightedness
cleft palate speech
clemency
clench
clenched teeth
clenching
fist c.
Clerambault erotomania syndrome
Clerambault-Kandinsky complex
clergy
benefit of c.
cleric
clerical
c. perception (Q)
c. response
cleverness factor
cliché
client-centered
c.-c. approach
c.-c. psychotherapy
c.-c. therapy
climacteric, climacterium
c. age
c. insanity
c. melancholia
c. neurosis
c. paranoid psychosis
c. paranoid reaction
c. paranoid state
c. paraphrenia
c. psychoneurosis
climate
emotional c.
group c.
climax
normal libido, coitus, and c. (NLC&C)
sexual c.
climber
social c.
climbing
clinging
c. behavior
c. dependence
clingy housewife
clinic
affective disorders c. (ADC)
chemical dependence c.
child development c.
child guidance c.
community-based c.
crisis intervention c. (CIC)

guidance c.
mental health c. (MHC)
mental hygiene c.
outpatient c.
pain c.
c. patient
c. patient population
research c.
satellite c.
sex c.
supportive medication c.

clinical
c. analysis
c. anecdote
c. antipsychotic trial of intervention effectiveness-schizophrenia (CATIE-SZ)
c. approach
c. armamentarium
c. behavior
c. bias
c. care
c. case discussion
c. characteristic
c. chemistry
c. circumstance
c. comparison
c. comparison study
c. conceptualization
c. condition
c. correlate
c. counseling
c. course
c. data
c. decision-making
c. depression
c. description
c. diagnosis
c. diagnostic practice
c. difference
c. effect
c. efficacy
c. encounter
c. equivalent
c. evaluation
c. example
c. experience
c. facilitated intervention
c. feature
c. finding
c. formulation
c. global impression-bipolar (CGI-BP)
c. global impression severity and improvement score
c. grouping
c. heterogeneity
c. history
c. immunology
c. implication
c. importance
c. impression
c. improvement
c. inference
c. intervention program
c. interview
c. judgment
c. laboratory
c. management
c. manifestation
c. material
c. medicine
c. method
c. monitoring
c. monitoring technique
c. need
c. neuropsychology
c. neuroscientist
c. observation
c. outcome
c. performance score (CPS)
c. perspective
c. phenomenology
c. phenomenon
c. phenotype
c. picture
c. population
c. poverty
c. poverty syndrome
c. practice setting
c. prediction
c. presentation
c. procedure
c. profile
c. progression
c. psychiatrist
c. psychiatry
c. psychobiology
c. psychologist
c. psychology
c. psychopharmacology
c. purpose
c. reasoning
c. record review
c. relevance
c. resemblance

NOTES

clinical *(continued)*
c. response
c. responsibility
c. sequela
c. sign
c. situation
c. social worker
c. sociology
c. stability
c. status
c. subtype
c. symptom
c. teaching
c. theory
c. thinking
c. training
c. trial
c. understanding
c. use
c. validity
c. variable
c. visit
clinically
c. adverse sequela
c. recommended dose
c. relevant behavior
c. significant
c. significant anxiety
c. significant distress
c. significant impairment
clinician
c. bias
evaluating c.
c. observation
psychiatric c.
psychodynamic c.
c. rating
clinician-client relationship
clinician-consultant
clinician-observer
clinician-rated cognitive symptom
clinicopathologic
clinimetrics
clinodactyly
clipped speech
clipping
peak c.
clitoral
c. erection
c. hood
c. stimulation
clitoridis
erector c.
glans c.
clitoris, pl. **clitorides**
clitorism
clitoromania
cloacal theory
cloaca therapy
clock
biologic c.
circadian c.
c. drawing
clominorex
clone
clonic
c. convulsion
c. movement
c. seizure
c. spasm
clonicity
clonic-tonic-clonic seizure
Cloninger psychobiological model of temperament and character
clonism
clonospasm
clonus
ankle c.
subsultus c.
toe c.
wrist c.
clopenthixol
clophenoxate
clorazepic acid
close
c. clinical monitoring
c. observation
c. observation protocol
c. watch restriction
closed
c. adoption
c. anesthesia
c. awareness
c. book
c. class
c. group
c. head injury (CHI)
c. head trauma
c. horizon
c. juncture
c. place
closed-circuit television (CCTV)
closed-ended
c.-e. query
c.-e. question
closed-loop feedback system
close-knit
c.-k. community
c.-k. family
closemouthed
closeness
closesightedness
closet
c. alcoholic
c. bisexual
c. drinker
c. homosexual
out of c.

closure
auditory c.
bring to c.
law of c.
perceptual c.
c. principle
c. process
visual c.
clothes
changing c.
plucking at c.
pulling of c.
clothing
adaptive c.
cleanliness of c.
condition of c.
inappropriate c.
odor of solvent on c.
tattered c.
clotiazepam
cloud
up in c.'s
clouded
c. sensorium
c. state
c. state epilepsy
cloudiness
sensorium c.
clouding
c. of consciousness
mental c.
cloudy sensorium
cloverleaf skull syndrome
clownery
clowning
provocative c.
clownish gait
clownism
cloxazolam
CLS
confused language syndrome
club
c. drug
social c.
clucking
nervous c.
c. sound
tongue c.
clue
diagnostic c.
clumsiness
motor c.
c. syndrome
clumsy
c. child syndrome
c. gesture
Clunis inquiry forensic psychiatry
cluster
c. A, B, C disorder
c. A, B personality disorder
c. analysis
anxious-fearful c.
c. approach
avoidance c.
c. B trait
c. C, D symptoms
c. characteristics in personality disorder
confidence c.
diagnostic c.
dissociative symptom c.
dramatic emotional c.
DSM c.'s
eccentric A c.
emotional B c.
fearful C c.
c. headache
inner battery c.
c. marriage
c. migraine
odd eccentric c.
problem behavior c.
c. reduction
c. of resources
situation c.
c. of situations
suicide c.
c. suicide
c. of symptoms
clustering
c. criterion
familial c.
semantic c.
clutter
hoarding and c.
cluttering
Clytemnestra complex
cM
centimorgan
CMA
conflict management appraisal
CMCA
care management for chronic addiction
CME
continuing medical education

NOTES

CMHC
community mental health care
community mental health center
CMHS
Center for Mental Health Services
CMV
cytomegalovirus
CNS
central nervous system
CNS depressant
CNS disease group
CNS stimulant
CNS syphilis
CNS trauma
CNT
could not test
current night terror
CNV
conative negative variation
contingent negative variation
CO_2
carbon dioxide
CO_2 inhalation
COA
child of alcoholic
coach
coactivation
coactive strategy
coaddiction
coalcoholic
coalcoholism
coalesce
coalescence
coalition
confusingly fluid c.
coarctated personality
coarse tremor
coarticulation
anticipatory c.
backward c.
coast memory
cobalamin deficiency
cocaethylene assay
Cocaine Anonymous (CA)
cocaine-dependent
c.-d. baby
c.-d. individual
cocaine-free
c.-f. urine sample
c.-f. urine screen
cocaine-heroin combination
cocaine-induced
c.-i. anxiety
c.-i. dopamine stimulation
c.-i. psychotic disorder
c.-i. psychotic disorder with delusions
c.-i. psychotic disorder with hallucinations
c.-i. sexual dysfunction
cocaine-related
c.-r. disorder
c.-r. disorder, NOS
c.-r. response
c.-r. stroke
cocainism
cocainization
cocainize
cocainomania
CocAnon
cockalorum
cockamamy
cocky
coconsciousness
coconscious personality
coconut sound
cocooning
CODA
Codependents Anonymous
coddle
code
c. blue
capacity c.
c. capacity
c. of ethics
genetic c.
ICD-9 c.
imagery c.
model penal c.
moral c.
penal c.
professional c.
psychiatric CPT c.
c. of silence
substitution accuracy c.
substitution efficiency c.
V c.
Z c.
codependence
codependency disorder
codependent
C.'s Anonymous (CODA)
c. personality
codification
coding
codominance
coefficient
alienation c.
c. alpha
alpha c.
alternate form reliability c.
association c.
comparable forms reliability c.
concordance c.
confidence c.
contingency c.

c. of correlation
correlation c.
equivalence c.
familiar correlation c.
high alpha c.
c. of inbreeding
c. of intelligence (CI)
kappa c.
low alpha c.
odd-even method reliability c.
reliability c.
scoring c.
split-half reliability c.
test-retest reliability c.
validity c.
c. of variation (CV)

coenesthesia (*var. of* cenesthesia)
coenesthetic schizophrenia
coerce
coerced treatment
coercion
c. program
sexual c.

coercive
c. behavior
c. communication
c. legal action
c. persuasion
c. philosophy
c. treatment

coeundi
impotentia c.

coeur
cri de c.

coexcitation
coexist
coexistence
dysfunctional c.
c. of neurotransmitter
peaceful c.

coexistent culture
coexisting
c. disorder
c. psychopathology

coffee consumption
COGA
Collaborative Study on the Genetics of Alcoholism

cogent
cogitate
cognate confusion
cognition
affect, behavior, c. (ABCs)
altered c.
being c.
constriction of c.
c. disorder
dysfunctional c.
empiric c.
frontal-based c.
neurologic c.
paranormal c.
social c.
theory of c.

cognitive
c. ability
c. analytic therapy (CAT)
c. antecedent
c. appraisal approach
c. approach to dreaming and repression
c. assessment
c. avoidance
c. awareness level
c. behavior
c. behavior therapy (CBT)
c. benefit
c. capability
c. capacity
c. change
c. conditioning
c. control
c. coping
c. decline
c. decrement
c. defect
c. deficiency
c. deficit
c. derailment
c. deterioration
c. development
c. development stage
c. disability
c. disorder
c. disorganization
c. disruption
c. dissonance
c. dissonance theory
c. distancing
c. distortion
c. disturbance
c. domain
c. dysfunction
c. dysmetria
c. element
c. enhancement therapy

NOTES

C

cognitive *(continued)*
c. enhancer
c. fatigue
c. flexibility
c. function
c. functioning
c. generation of affect
c. growth
c. impairment
c. impairment of depression
c. impairment level
c. improvement
c. interpretation
c. learning theory
c. loss
c. map
c. mapping
c. maturation
c. maturity
c. measure
c. mechanism
c. mediation
c. method
c. model
c. model of depression
c. need
c. neuropsychology
c. neuroscience
c. nonability
c. pathology
c. performance
c. personality trait
c. process
c. processing
c. psychodynamics
c. psychology
c. psychotherapy
c. rehabilitation
c. rehearsal
c. remediation
c. remediation therapy
c. research orientation
c. reserve
c. response prevention
c. restitution
c. restructuring
c. risk factor
c. ritual
c. route
c. schema
c. science
c. score
c. self-hypnosis training
c. self-reinforcement
c. slippage
c. state
c. status
c. stimulation
c. strategy
c. structure
c. style
c. subsystem
c. symptom
c. task
c. technique
c. tendency
c. testing
c. theory of depression
c. theory of learning
c. trajectory
c. triad
c. variable
c. violence

cognitive-behavioral
c.-b. analysis system of psychotherapy (CBASP)
c.-b. approach
c.-b. coping skills training group
c.-b. factor
c.-b. group therapy (CBGT)
c.-b. intervention
c.-b. psychotherapy
c.-b. technique
c.-b. therapy (CBT)
c.-b. treatment

cognitive-linguistic treatment

cognitively
c. elicited emotion
c. intact

cognitive-perceptual disturbance

cognitive-physiological therapy

cognitivist

cognizance

cognizant

cogwheel
c. phenomenon
c. rigidity

cohabitant

cohabitation

Cohen
C. syndrome
C. view of depressive disorder

coherence

coherent
c. negative picture-caption pair
c. positive picture-caption pair
c. stream of thought

cohesion
community c.
figural c.
group c.
law of c.

cohesive
c. device
c. family
c. image

cohesiveness
level of c.
c. level
cohoba snuff
cohort
birth c.
c. effect
c. experimental design
c. study
coil
butterfly c.
induction c.
coin
c. new phrase
c. new slang term
c. new word
c. rubbing
coinage
word c.
coincidence direction
coital
c. headache
c. orgasm
c. position
coition
coitus
c. analis
c. in ano
c. in axilla
c. condomatus
c. inter femora
c. interruptus
c. à la vache
oral c.
c. prolongatus
psychogenic painful c.
c. representation
c. reservatus
c. saxonus
c. a tergo
cold
c. acclimation
c. comfort
c. effect
c. effector
emotionally c.
c. exposure
c. fear
c. intolerance
c. mottled insensate leg
paradoxical c.
c. sensitivity
c. shoulder
c. spot
cold-blooded
coldhearted
coldness
emotional c.
cold-pack treatment
cold-sensitive neuron
colicky
colinearity
collaborate
collaboration
collaborative
c. empiricism
c. relationship
C. Study on the Genetics of Alcoholism (COGA)
c. therapy
c. treatment process
collapse delirium
collapsing anchor
collaring ceremony
collateral
c. behavior
c. information
c. source
collecting mania
collection
data c.
information c.
statistics c.
collective
c. behavior
c. ego
c. experience
c. hypnotization
c. hysteria
c. monologue
c. neurosis
c. psychosis
c. representation
c. suicide
c. transference
c. unconscious
collectivist culture
college
c. degree
c. graduate
invisible c.
c. student
Collet-Sicard syndrome
colligation
colloquial

NOTES

collusion
colony
Gheel c.
color
achromatic c.
c. agnosia
c. amblyopia
c. anomia
c. blind
chromatic c.
c. constancy
c. contrast
c. denial (Cd)
c. discrimination
c. in dream
flash of c.
flight of c.
gang c.'s
c. hearing
c. mixture
c. perception
c. preference
primary c.
c. response
c. taste
c. theory
c. therapy
c. weakness
c. zone
Colorado symptom index
Columbia suicide history form
Columbine High School shooting
columella, pl. **columellae**
column
cortical c.
ocular dominance c.
coma
alcoholic c.
apoplectic c.
barbiturate-induced c.
diabetic c.
hepatic c.
irreversible c.
Kussmaul c.
metabolic c.
c. therapy
thyrotoxic c.
trance c.
c. vigil
comatose patient
combat
armed c.
c. casualty
c. exhaustion
c. fatigue
c. fear
c. flashback
hors de c.
c. hysteria
military c.
c. neurosis
c. reaction
single c.
c. stress
c. stress disorder
c. stress exposure
c. tension
c. trauma
c. veteran
combative
c. patient
c. posture
c. stance
combat-related trauma
combination
aspirin c.
cocaine-heroin c.
c. drug (CD)
c. drug dependence
frequency c.
c. headache
law of c.
orthogonal c.
paradoxical c.
c. strategy
c. therapy
combinative thinking
combined
c. anesthesia
c. factor
c. predictive power
c. sclerosis
c. system disease
c. therapy
c. transcortical aphasia
combined-type
c.-t. attention deficit hyperactivity disorder
c.-t. personality disorder
comfort
cold c.
contact c.
c. dream
emotional c.
c. food
c. level
comic relief
comitial mal
command
c. auditory hallucination
c. automatism
embedded c.
c. hallucination
c. law
negative c.
c. negativism
2-step c.

c. style commitment
written c.
comme il faut
comment
condescending c.
derogatory c.
discriminatory c.
obscene sexual c.
threatening c.
value-laden c.
commentary
running c.
sexual c.
commenting
voice c.
commiserate
Commission
National Nuclear Energy C.
C. on Psychotherapy by Psychiatrists
commissural aphasia
commit
commitment
civil c.
command style c.
conscious c.
criminal c.
ideological c.
institutional c.
involuntary civil c.
involuntary outpatient c.
laws of c.
legal c.
long-term c.
observation c.
c. period
c. procedure
religious c.
sense of c.
short-term c.
temporary c.
voluntary c.
committed
legally c.
committee
C. on Family Violence and Sexual Abuse
C. on Standards and Survey Procedures
utilization review c.
common
c. central process
c. experience
c. goal
c. law marriage
c. migraine
c. migraine headache
c. precipitant exposure
c. sense
c. sense psychiatry
c. sense therapy
c. shared feature
c. theme
c. trait
commonality
commonplace
commotio
c. cerebri
c. spinalis
communality
communal residential center
commune
communicable
c. disease
c. hysteria
communicated insanity
communicating
c. empathy
c. epilepsy
communication
c. ability
augmentative c.
c. barrier
c. in behavioral biology (CBB)
c. channel
channel of c.
coercive c.
consummatory c.
c. deviance
c. disorder (CD)
email c.
emotional c.
enhance c.
c. ethics
exaggeration of language and c.
facilitated c.
facilitation of c.
fragmented c.
c. function
gestural c.
hesitant c.
human c.
illogical c.
impaired effective c.
c. impairment
indexical c.

C

NOTES

communication *(continued)*
inhibited c.
irreverent c.
language and c.
c. magic
manual c.
c. network
nonverbal c.
nonvocal c.
oral c.
paradoxical c.
pathologic c.
c. pattern
personal c.
persuasive c.
physician-patient c.
privileged c.
c. problem
problem-solving c.
qualitative impairment in c.
reciprocal c.
scale for assessment of thought, language, and c.
secure c.
signed c.
c. in sign language
c. skill
c. skills assessment
c. skills training
social c.
c. theory
therapeutic c.
c. therapy
c. tool
total c.
unaided augmentative c.
c. unit
vague c.
vehicle for c.
verbal c.
visual c. (VC, VIC)
c. with adolescent
written c.
communication/cognition treatment
communicative
c. competence
c. comprehension
c. disorder
c. function
c. interaction
c. skill
communicatively impaired
communicology
communion principle
communiquée
folie c.
community
c. action group
alternative lifestyle c.
c. assessment
c. care
c. catharsis
c. centered
close-knit c.
c. cohesion
c. connectedness
c. diagnosis
c. divorce
c. effort
elite c.
c. feeling
c. functioning
gay c.
homosexual c.
impoverished c.
inner city c.
integrated c.
c. integration
c. intervention
mental health c.
c. mental health
c. mental health care (CMHC)
c. mental health center (CMHC)
C. Mental Health Construction Act of 1963
middle-class c.
minority c.
c. need
Oneida c.
online support c.
c. outreach program
c. placement
c. population
c. psychiatry
c. psychiatry program (CPP)
c. psychology
c. reinforcement approach
c. reintegration
religious c.
c. resource
c. responsibility
c. role
c. safety
segregated c.
senior citizen c.
sense of c.
c. service
c. setting
singles c.
c. spirit
c. study
suburban c.
c. support
c. support system
therapeutic c. (TC)
c. treatment and reintegration program

c. violence
working c.
community-based
c.-b. clinic
c.-b. intervention
c.-b. mental health treatment
c.-b. psychiatric program
community-institutional relations
community-residing patient
comorbid
c. alcohol dependence
c. anxiety disorder
c. Axis II diagnosis
c. characteristic
c. cluster B personality disorder
c. condition
c. depressive disorder
c. mental disorder
c. mood disorder
c. past alcoholism
c. psychiatric diagnosis
c. psychiatric disorder
c. psychiatric illness
c. psychopathology
c. schizophrenia and PTSD
c. substance abuse
c. tic
comorbidity
age-related c.
anxiety c.
anxiety-mood c.
medical c.
multiple anxiety c.'s
psychiatric c.
somatopsychiatric c.
substantial c.
compacta
companion
imaginary c.
phobic c.
companionate marriage
companionship
animal c.
human c.
imaginary c.
company
NDCHealth health information service c.
comparable
c. finding
c. forms reliability coefficient
c. worth
comparative
c. efficacy
c. guidance and placement program (CGPP)
c. judgment
c. medicine
c. psychiatry
c. psychology
c. research
c. scanning
comparison
clinical c.
c. condition
factor c.
gender c.
positive c.
post hoc c.
c. region
systematic c.
compartment
synaptic c.
compartmentalize
compassion
compassionate
c. feeling
c. marriage
c. use basis
compatibility
compatible
compelled behavior
compelling evidence
compensate
compensated work therapy
compensation
c. defense mechanism
c. neurosis
c. neurotic disorder
c. psychoneurosis
c. schizophrenia
synaptic c.
compensatory
c. behavior
c. education
c. fantasy
c. mechanism
c. mood swing
c. movement
c. technique
c. trait
compete
competence
apparent c.
assessment of c.

NOTES

competence *(continued)*
communicative c.
cultural c.
facade of c.
juvenile c.
c. knowledge
measure of c.
mental c.
c. motivation
presumption of c.
social c.
competency
c. assessment
assessment of basic c. (ABC)
high degree of c.
legal criteria for c.
low threshold of c.
maternal c.
mental c.
paternal c.
c. standard
competency-based
c.-b. examination
c.-b. instruction
competent
c. decision
c. decision-making
mentally c.
c., optimal relational functioning
c. relationship
c. to stand trial
competing theories of motivation
competition
competitive
c. behavior
c. employment
c. motives
complacence
complacent attitude
complain
complainant-listener relationship
complainer
help-rejecting c.
complaint
chief c. (CC)
frequent physical c.'s
habitual c.'s
hypochondriacal c.
nuisance c.
pain c.
primary c.
repetitive c.'s
sleep c.
somatic c.
subjective insomnia c.
unexplained pain c.
unfounded c.
vague c.
complemental air
complementarity of interaction
complementary
c. and alternative medicine (CAM)
c. instinct
c. role
complement symptom-focused assessment
complete
c. amnesia
c. aphasia
c. birth
c. cross-dressing
c. delusion
c. genital primacy
c. learning method
c. mother
c. Oedipus complex
c. substrate
c. treatment plan
completed suicide
completion
c., arithmetic problems, vocabulary, and following directions (CAVD)
picture c. (PC)
sentence c.
stem c.
suicide c.
task c.
treatment c.
complex
c. absence
active castration c.
AIDS dementia c. (ADC)
AIDS-related c. (ARC)
c. aspect of fear conditioning
authority c.
benzodiazepine-GABA-receptor c.
brain wave c.
breast c.
brother c.
Cain c.
castration c.
Cinderella c.
claustral c.
Clerambault-Kandinsky c.
Clytemnestra c.
c. cognitive function
complete Oedipus c.
culture c.
c. delusion
Diana c.
c. disease
disorganized symptom c.
dorsal vagus c.
ego c.
Electra c.
c. equivalence
Eshmun c.
father c.
femininity c.

c. finger routine
Friedmann c.
function c.
GABA receptor c.
c. genetic disorder
God c.
grandfather c.
Griselda c.
c. hallucination
c. hand routine
heir of Oedipus c.
hippocampal c.
homosexual c.
hypersexual c.
I c.
c. of ideas
inferiority c.
inferior orbitofrontal c.
inverted Oedipus c.
Jocasta c.
K c.
kernel c.
Lear c.
c. learning process
Madonna c.
Madonna-prostitute c.
martyr c.
Medea c.
messiah c.
mother c.
Mother Superior c.
c. motor behavior
c. motor tic
negative Oedipus c.
c. noise
obscenity-purity c.
oedipal c.
Oedipus c.
organ inferiority c.
c. partial epilepsy
c. partial seizure (CPS)
particular c.
passive castration c.
persecution c.
Phaedra c.
c. phenomenon
Pierre Robin c.
Polycrates c.
posttraumatic stress disorder c.
c. precipitated epilepsy
c. psychological construct
c. psychological trait
c. PTSD
Quasimodo c.
c. readiness
c. relationship
c. segregation analysis
c. sentence
small penis c.
c. social interaction
spike-and-wave c.
superiority c.
symptom c.
c. tone
c. type
c. vocal tic
c. whole body movement

complexion

complexity
diagnostic c.
environmental c.
etiological c.
human c.
syntactic c.
c. of torture

compliance
c. masking covert resistance
motor c.
overt c.
patient c.
privacy c.
c. rate
social c.
strategic c.
sustained c.
c. therapy
treatment c.

compliant

complicate

complicated
c. bereavement
c. grief disorder
c. migraine headache
c. relationship

complication
c. of adolescence
adverse neurologic c.
birth c.
drug-induced medical c.
pregnancy and birth c.
psychiatric c.
psychosocial c.

complicity

complimentary

comply
failure to c.

NOTES

component
adrenomedullary c.
articulatory loop c.
autonomous functional c.
base c.
blood c.
central executive c.
cross-sectional c.
functional c.
general c.
genetic c.
heritable c.
inotropic c.
masochistic c.
moral c.
physiologic c.
prominent phobic anxiety c.
slave system c.
sudomotor c.
thermogenic c.
true c.
vasomotor c.
3-component theory
composed
composite
c. index
c. international diagnostic interview (CIDI)
narcissistic c.
c. person
c. personality
c. personality description
c. score
total battery c.
composition
body c.
group c.
mixed-sex group c.
same-sex group c.
sociodemographic c.
compos mentis
composure
compound
active c.
antidepressant c.
antipsychotic c.
arsenic c.
bromine c.
c. medicine
primary active c.
comprehend
comprehension
auditory c.
communicative c.
c. deficit
language c.
passage c.
c. span
comprehensive
c. assessment
c. care
C. Crime Control Act of 1984
c. distancing
C. Drug Abuse Prevention and Control Act of 1970
c. evaluation
c. examination
c. identification process (CIP)
c. review
c. service
c. solution
c. therapeutic approach
c. treatment
c. treatment planning
comprehensiveness
compression
c. anesthesia
c. of brain
cerebral c.
c. paralysis
compromise
cerebral c.
c. distortion
c. formation
compromised
c. function
medically c.
severely c.
compulsion
antisocial c.
brooding c.
checking c.
counting c.
eating c.
c. neurosis
c. psychoneurosis
repetition c.
c. score
sexual c.
tapping c.
thinking c.
uncontrollable c.
unreasonable c.
compulsion-obsession
compulsive
c. act
c. action
c. buying
c. change
c. character
c. computer game playing
c. defense
c. disturbance
c. drawing
c. drinker
c. drug administration
c. drug-taking behavior

c. eater
c. exercise
c. exercising
c. fixation on unobtainable partner
c. gambler
c. gambling
c. habit
c. hoarding
c. idea
c. insanity
c. laughter
c. loser theory
c. magic
c. mania
c. masturbation
c. masturbatory behavior
c. neurosis
c. neurotic personality disorder
c. orderliness
c. personality
c. psychasthenia
c. psychogenic disorder
c. psychogenic tic
c. psychoneurotic reaction
c. quality
c. repetition
c. restraint
c. ritual
c. severity
c. sex
c. sexual behavior
c. spasm and tic
c. stealing
c. substance use
c. suicide
c. swearing
c. swearing syndrome
c. symptom
c. thought
c. water drinking
c. writing

compulsivity
National Council on Sexual Addiction and C. (NCSAC)

compulsivity-impulsivity dimension

compulsory care

compurgation

computation
symbolic c.

computational process

computed axial tomography (CAT)

computer
c. addict
c. addiction
biofeedback c.
c. file
c. game
c. geek
c. hacker
c. security

computer-aided therapy

computer-assisted
c.-a. review
c.-a. speech device

computer-guided therapy

computerized
c. assessment of response bias
c. tomography scan

COMT
catechol-*O*-methyltransferase
COMT Val$^{108/158}$ Met genotype

con
ability to c.

CONAMORE
Conflict and Management of Relationships study

conarium

conation

conative
c. appetitive striving
c. negative variation (CNV)

conatus

concatenation

concavity

conceal

concealed handgun

concealing behavior

conceit

conceivable

conceive

concentrate
inability to c.

concentrating
difficulty c.
trouble c.

concentration
approximate lethal c. (ALC)
attention and c.
blood alcohol c. (BAC)
brain-derived HVA c.
c. camp
c. camp syndrome (CCS)
decreased c.
c. deficit
c. difficulty
c. disturbance

NOTES

concentration *(continued)*
impaired c.
information memory c. (IMC)
c. method
minimum effective c. (MEC)
peak methadone c.
plasma R-methadone c.
time of maximum c.
concentration-related problem
concept
abstract c.
body ego c.
c. of brain function
c. of cardinal numbers
concrete c.
conjunctive c.
critical band c.
cultural c.
feces-child-penis c.
folk diagnostic c.
c. formation
grandiose c.
humanistic c.
key c.
c. learning
lexica c.
mall treatment c.
medicine c.
mental c.
object c.
permanence c.
psychoanalytic c.
psychodynamic c.
self-derogatory c.
self-role c.
c. of spiritual coping
c. of spiritual healing
traditional psychoanalytic c.
Western diagnostic c.
c. of will
Zanarini c.
concept-driven perception
conception
hallucination of c.
imperative c.
conceptual
c. ability
c. disorder
c. disorganization
c. disturbance
c. endeavor
c. learning
c. limitation
c. nervous system
c. planning
c. problem
c. quotient (CQ)
c. reasoning
c. skill
c. tempo
c. thinking
conceptualization
abstract c.
axis I, II c.
clinical c.
conceptualized
conceptualizing
concern
abandonment c.
dispassionate c.
eating c.
ethical c.
interpersonal c.
malevolent c.
physical c.
psychological c.
sense of c.
sexual c.
shape c.
social c.
spiritual c.
unconscious c.
ventilate c.
weight c.
concernment
conciliate
concomitant
concordance
child-parent c.
c. coefficient
parent-youth c.
c. rate
twin c.
concordant result
concrete
c. abstractive ability
c. attitude
c. concept
c. image
c. intelligence
c. operation
c. operational development
c. operational stage
c. operation period
c. operation stage
c. picture
c. representation
c. thinking
c. thought process
concreteness
concretistic thinking
concretization
active c.
concretizing attitude
concubinage
concubine
concubitus
concupiscence

concurrent
c. alcohol and substance abuse
c. personality disorder
c. psychiatric diagnosis
c. psychiatric problems
c. reinforcement
c. review
c. therapy
c. validity
concussion
c. amnesia
c. blindness
brain c.
c. of brain
c. syndrome
condemn
condemnation
condensation
condescend
condescending
c. attitude
c. behavior
c. comment
c. evaluation
c. manner
c. speech
c. tone of voice
condescension
condition
abnormal pathologic c.
activating c.
active general medical c.
adverse working c.'s
atmospheric c.
autism-like c.
catatonic disorder due to general medical c.
clinical c.
c. of clothing
comorbid c.
comparison c.
congenital intersex c.
delirium due to general medical c.
deplorable living c.'s
deplorable working c.'s
desperate financial c.
developmental c.
drug-free c.
emergency psychiatric c.
emotional c.
etiological neurological c.
experimental c.
fatigue c.
general medical c. (GMC)
haloperidol c.
heterogeneous c.
illumination c.
insomnia-type sleep disorder due to general medical c.
intersex c.
life-threatening c.
material home c.
medical c.
mental disorder due to general medical c.
mood disorder due to general medical c.
necessary c.
neurologic c.
neuropsychiatric c.
noise c.
c. not attributable to mental disorder
organic psychotic c.
paranoid c.
parole c.
c. of parole
pathologic c.
persistent emotional c.
personality change due to general medical c.
physical intersex c.
preexisting c.
proband c.
prodromal c.
psychiatric c.
psychological factor affecting medical c. (PFAMC)
psychological factor affecting a mental c.
psychologic factor affecting physical c.
psychosis due to physical c.
psychotic disorder due to general medical c.
respondent c.
school handicap c.
sexual dysfunction due to general medical c.
sexually transmitted c. (STC)
sleep disorder due to general medical c.
stimulation c.
subcortical c.
test c.

C

NOTES

condition *(continued)*
treatment c.
underlying c.
conditional
c. arousal
c. discharge
c. probability
conditioned
c. avoidance response
c. cue
c. drug response
c. emotional response (CER)
c. escape response
c. fear association
c. inhibition
c. place preference (CPP)
c. reflex (CR)
c. reflex therapy
c. reinforcer
c. stimulation
c. stimulus (CS)
c. suppression
c. withdrawal
conditioning
approximation c.
assertive c.
autonomic c.
average c.
aversion c.
aversion-covert c.
aversive c.
avoidance c.
backward c.
behavioral c.
classical c.
cognitive c.
complex aspect of fear c.
counter c.
cross c.
decorticate c.
escape c.
esprit de corps c.
exteroceptive c.
eyelid c.
false c.
fear c.
female c.
higher order c.
instrumental c.
interoceptive c.
negative c.
operant c.
pavlovian c.
place c.
primary reward c.
respondent c.
secondary reward c.
second-order c.
simple aspect of fear c.
skinnerian c.
taste aversive c.
c. therapy
trace c.
vicarious c.
condom
condomatus
coitus c.
condonation
condone
conducive
conduct
adjustment disorder with disturbance of c.
consistent pattern of c.
c. disorder (CD)
disorderly c.
c. disturbance
c. disturbance adjustment disorder
c. disturbance adjustment reaction
moral c.
pattern of c.
persistent pattern of c.
c. problem
solitary aggressive-type c.
conduct-disordered child
conduction
air c.
c. aphasia
c. deafness
c. delay
electronic c.
ephaptic c.
excitation and c.
motor nerve c.
nerve c.
saltatory c.
conductor
conduit
confabulans
paraphrenia c.
confabulate
confabulated
c. detail response (dD)
c. whole response (DWR)
confabulation
conference
career c.
family c. (FC)
confession
c. of guilt
patient c.
confessor
father c.
mother c.
confidante
confide
confidence
c. artist

c. cluster
c. coefficient
diagnostic c.
c. interval (CI)
lack of c.
c. level
level of c.

confidential
c. documentation
c. interview
c. record

confidentiality
c. breach
breach of c.
c. issue

confident status

configuration
personality c.
word c.

configurative culture

confinement
c. effect
c. fear
home c.
prison c.
solitary c.

confirmation

conflict
approach-approach c.
approach-avoidance c.
c. avoidance
avoidance-avoidance c.
basic c.
central c.
civil c.
culture c.
emotional c.
escalating c.
ethical c.
extrapsychic c.
family c.
horizontal c.
increased interpersonal c.
inferred c.
infrequent interpersonal c.
inner c.
c. of interest
internal c.
interpersonal c.
intolerable inner c.
intrafamilial c.
intrapersonal c.
intrapsychic c.
c. level
level of c.
c. management
c. management appraisal (CMA)
C. and Management of Relationships study (CONAMORE)
marital c.
c. of meaning
c. mediation
moral c.
oedipal c.
parent-child c.
partner c.
psychiatric c.
psychodynamic c.
religious c.
c. resolution
c. resolution skill
c. resolution strategy
resolve c.
role c.
roommate c.
significant c.
soldier in armed c.
unconscious c.
unresolved c.
vertical c.
c.'s with peers

conflicted feeling

conflict-free
c.-f. area
c.-f. function
c.-f. sphere

conflicting
c. emotion
c. feelings
c. message
c. motives

conflictual
c. home environment
c. relationship
c. situation

confluence method

conform
failure to c.

conformance
functional c.

conformity
automaton c.
conventional role c.
morality of conventional role c.
social c.

confounding factor

NOTES

confront
confrontation
direct c.
premature c.
reality c.
simple c.
c. stage
supportive c.
confrontational experience
confrontative
confrontive coping
confucianism
confused
c. delusion
c. language syndrome (CLS)
c. speech
confusingly fluid coalition
confusion
acute c.
c. assessment method diagnostic algorithm
authority c.
bisexual c.
cognate c.
episodic c.
feeling of c.
gender identity c.
identity vs role c.
mental c.
nocturnal c.
personal identity c.
postictal c.
psychogenic c.
reactive c.
c. reactive psychosis
right-left c.
role c.
time c.
c. of values
confusional
c. arousal
c. arousal from sleep
c. episode
c. excitement
c. insanity
c. migraine headache
c. psychotic reaction
c. schizophreniform psychosis
c. state presenile dementia
c. twilight state
confusional-arousal disorder
congener
congenial
congenital
c. adrenal hyperplasia
c. atonic pseudoparalysis
c. defect
c. facial diplegia
c. intersex condition
c. neurosyphilis
c. paramyotonia
c. spastic paraplegia
c. sutural alopecia
c. syphilitic paralytic dementia
congenitalis
alopecia c.
congestion
brain c.
congruence
congruent
c. affect
mood c.
conjoined
c. nerve roots
c. twins
conjoint
c. counseling
c. interview
c. synapses
c. therapy
conjugal
c. bereavement
c. consequence of promiscuity
c. paranoia
c. psychosis
c. tension
c. visit
c. visitation
conjugate
c. gaze
c. paralysis
conjunction
illusory c.
conjunctival injection
conjunctive
c. concept
c. reinforcement
conjure
connate
connatural
connectedness
community c.
emotional c.
family c.
impaired c.
social c.
connection
interneuronal c.
neuroanatomic c.
reciprocal c.
social c.
therapeutic c.
connotation
consanguineous marriage
consanguinity
conscience
authoritarian c.

humanistic c.
troubled c.
conscientiousness
conscious
c. avoidance
c. awareness
class c.
c. commitment
c. deceit
c. decision
c. feigning
c. guidance
c. level
c. memory
c. perception
c. process
c. resistance
c. simulation
c. state
consciously
c. accessible process
c. inaccessible process
consciousness
active mode of c.
altered level of c.
altered state of c. (ASC)
clouding of c.
cosmic c.
crowd c.
crude c.
declining c.
depression of c.
discrimination c.
disintegration of c.
c. disturbance
c. disturbance stress reaction
double c.
effect of trauma on c.
episodic change of c.
expanded c.
c. expansion
field of c.
fluctuating level of c.
fringe of c.
group c.
head c.
higher level of c.
higher state of c.
impaired c.
impairment of c.
level of c. (LOC)
loss of c. (LOC)
marginal c.
mystical state of c.
parasomniac c.
passive mode of c.
perceptual c.
post September 11 c.
c. raising
reduced level of c.
social c.
state of c. (SOC)
stream of c.
subliminal c.
threshold of c.
time c.
unitary c.
consecutive insanity
consensual
c. action
c. gaze
c. reaction
c. reflex
c. sex
c. sexual behavior
c. understanding
c. validation
consensually
consent
age of c.
c. form
informed c.
mutal c.
valid c.
Willowbrook c.
written informed c.
consenting
c. adult
c. partner
c. patient
consequence
c. of action
c. association
clear rules and c.'s
c. of decision
destructive social c.
fatal c.
harmful c.
health-related c.
interpersonal c.
legal c.
long-term c.
negative life c.
neurobehavioral c.
painful c.
personal c.'s

NOTES

consequence *(continued)*
psychiatric c.
psychological c.
serious c.
short-term c.
social c.
c.'s of war
consequent
consequentialism
consequentialist ethics
conservation
conservatism
politicoeconomic c. (PEC)
conservative
c. cutoff score
c. management
c. medication
c. treatment
conservator
conservatorship
considerable external support
considerate
consideration
biologic c.
developmental c.
treatment c.
considered thought
consistency
behavioral c.
internal c.
moral c.
perceptual c.
c. principle
consistent
c. behavior
c. delivery
c. irresponsibility
c. mood
c. pattern of conduct
c. relationship
c. response
consociate
consolation dream
console
consolidated sleep
consolidation
memory c.
conspicuous consumption
conspiratorial
conspire
constancy
brightness c.
color c.
emotional object c.
extrinsic c.
intrinsic c.
law of c.
libidinal object c.
location c.
object c.
perceptual c.
c. phenomenon
constant
c. anger
changeable versus c.
Heinis c.
relaxation c.
c. routine
c. worry
constantium
constellation
family c.
c. of grief
self-pitying c.
c. of signs and symptoms
consternation
constipation
psychogenic c.
constitution
epileptic psychopathic c.
hyperadrenal c.
posttraumatic psychopathic c.
psychopathic c.
constitutional
c. bisexuality theory
c. depression
c. depressive disposition
c. disease
c. factor
c. insanity
c. manic disposition
c. medicine
c. psychology
c. psychopathic inferiority
c. psychopathic state (CPS)
c. psychosis
c. type
constrain
constraint
morality of c.
c. of movement
c. of thought
thought c.
constraint-induced therapy
constrict
constricted
c. activity
c. affect
emotionally c.
c. pupil
constriction
affective c.
c. of cognition
emotional c.
pupillary c.
c. of thought
construct
complex psychological c.

core c.
multidimensional c.
personal c.
psychological c.
c. validity

construction
c. ability
c. apraxia
exocentric c.
hierarchy c.
phrase c. (PC)
social c.
visual field c.

constructional
c. apraxia
c. dyspraxia

constructive
c. aggression
c. approach
c. criticism
c. discipline
c. feedback
c. memory
c. support

consult
psychiatric c.

consultant
juvenile court c.
medical c.
prescribing c.

consultation
agency-centered c.
crisis c.
forensic c.
patient-oriented c.
psychiatric c.
c. psychiatry
psychopharmacology c.
social service c.

consultation-liaison
c.-l. psychiatry
c.-l. service

consultative relationship

consulting
c. psychiatrist
c. psychologist
c. room
c. staff

consumer
c. behavior
c. characteristic
c. education
c. psychology
c. research

consuming
time c.

consummate

consummatory
c. act
c. communication
c. reward

consumption
abnormal calorie c.
abnormal food c.
alcohol c.
caffeine c.
cerebral oxygen c.
coffee c.
conspicuous c.
daily caffeine c.
daily cigarette c.
drug c.
nervous c.
parental alcohol c.
regular caffeine c.

contact
absent eye c.
c. avoidance
c. behavior
c. ceptor
c. comfort
continuity of c.
eye c.
fixed eye c.
frequency of c. (FOC)
genital sexual c.
orogenital c.
poor eye c.
sexual c.
social c.
unwanted sexual c.
warm c.
c. with reality

contagion
emergency c.
psychic c.

containment
emotional c.

contaminated needle

contamination
fear of c.
c. fear
c. obsession
purposeful c.

contemplate

NOTES

contemplation
contemplative
contemporary
c. approach
c. practice
contemptible
contempt for others
contemptuous
contendere
nolo c.
content
c. addressability
c. analysis
bizarre thought c.
blood alcohol c.
c. of delusion
dream c.
grandiose c.
c. of hallucination
language c.
latent c.
manifest c.
mood, orientation, judgment, affect, c. (MOJAC)
paucity of speech c.
positive speech c.
poverty of c.
c. psychology
self-derogatory c.
speech c.
c. of thought
thought c.
c. thought disorder
unusual thought c.
c. validity
contention
contentious
contentiousness
contentment
context
cultural c.
historical c.
c. processing
c. reframing
social c.
space c.
spatial-temporal c.
taken out of c.
time c.
contextual
c. association
c. cause
c. control
c. cue
c. influence
c. therapy
contextualism
contiguity
c. aphasia
c. disorder
law of c.
spatial c.
temporal c.
contiguous voxel
continence
bladder c.
fecal c.
urinary c.
continent
contingency
c. awareness
behavioral c.
c. coefficient
c. contract
c. learning
c. management
c. model
c. reinforcement
contingent
c. negative variation (CNV)
c. punishment
continua (*pl. of* continuum)
continuance
continuation
depression c.
c. therapy
c. treatment
continued
c. abuse
c. belittling
c. bullying
c. stay review (CSR)
continuing
c. care
c. medical education (CME)
c. petit mal seizures
continuity
c. of attachment
c. of care
c. of contact
sense of c.
sleep c.
worse sleep c.
continuous
c. amnesia
c. antipsychotic drug treatment
c. antipsychotic medication
c. approach
c. bath treatment
c. cognitive testing
c. course
c. daytime drowsiness
c. epilepsy
c. group
c. growth
c. infusion
c. maintenance medication
c. narcosis

c. observation
c. panel
c. performance task-accuracy (CPT-ACC)
c. performance task-efficiency (CPT-EFF)
c. reinforcement
c. reinforcement schedule
c. sleep
c. sleep therapy
c. tremor
c. variable

continuum, pl. **continuums, continua**
c. of care
epilepsia corticalis continua
epilepsia partialis continua
hypothetical c.
introversion-extroversion c.
c. theory

contort

contraception
birth control pill c.
rhythm method of c.
withdrawal method of c.

contraceptive
c. device
oral c.
postcoital c.
c. practice

contract
c. against self-harm
c. against suicide
behavior c.
behavioral c.
contingency c.
employment c.
evaluation c.
c. evaluation
formal c.
formalized c.
group c.
homicide-suicide protection c.
individualized c.
informal c.
interactional c.
legal c.
marriage c.
c. negotiation
patient c.
c. review
c. for safety
sweetheart c.
therapeutic c.
c. therapy

contraction
carpopedal c.
lead pipe c.
rhythmic c.
tetanic c. (Te)

contraction-relaxation

contractual
c. agreement
c. alliance
c. arrangement
c. behavior
c. capacity
c. psychiatry
c. psychotherapy

contracture
caffeine-induced c.
functional c.
organic c.

contradict

contradiction

contradictory
c. data
c. information

contrafissura

contraindication
medical c.
medication c.

contralateral
c. hemiplegia
c. neglect syndrome
c. parietal lobe dysfunction
c. parietal lobes
c. reflex
c. sign

contrariness

contrary

contrasexual component of psyche

contrast
brightness c.
chromatic c.
color c.
cultural c.
c. effect
law of c.
maximal c.
c. sensitivity

contrastimulus

contrastive
c. analysis
c. distribution
c. stress

NOTES

contravolitional
contrecoup injury of brain
contrectation
contretemps
contributing role
contribution
extracellular c.
intracellular c.
therapeutic c.
contributor
contributory
c. element
c. negligence
contrite
contrition
contrive
control
c. analysis
appetite c.
attentional c.
automatic gain c.
automatic volume c.
aversive c.
balance c.
behavior c. (BC)
biologic c.
birth c. (BC)
bladder c.
bowel c.
brain c.
brainstem c.
Bureau of Drug Abuse C. (BDAC)
cognitive c.
contextual c.
crowd c.
degree of c.
delusion of c.
c. delusion
c. device
diminished c.
disorder of impulse c.
distribution of c.
ego c.
excitatory c.
executive c.
experimental c.
external force c.
external locus of c.
c. feedback
feedback c.
feeling of c.
c. frustration
c. group
gun c.
handgun c.
idiodynamic c.
image c.
immediate c.
impaired impulse c.
impulse c.
in c.
inadequate impulse c.
inhibitory c.
inner c.
internal-external c.
internal locus of c.
interpersonal c.
island of c.
lack of c.
learned autonomic c.
locus of c. (LOC)
locus of c.-chance (LOC-C)
locus of c.-external (LOC-E)
locus of c.-internal (LOC-I)
losing c.
loss of c.
mental c.
mind c.
multidimensional health locus and c.
National Center for Injury Prevention and C.
need to c.
neurologic c.
out of c. (OOC)
outside c.
pain c.
parental c.
personal locus of c. (PLC)
c. picture-caption pair
poor impulse c.
c. preoccupation
psychooptical reflex c.
rate c.
reflex c.
rigid c.
secret c.
self-control pain c.
sense of c.
social c.
sociopolitical locus of c. (SLC)
sphincter c.
stimulus c.
superego c.
superstitious c.
swing phase c.
synergic c.
taking c.
thought c.
tonic inhibitor c.
vestibuloequilibratory c.
voluntary c.
weak ego c.
worry c.
yoked c.
controllability attribution
controlled
c. analgesic

c. anger
c. association
c. attention
c. breathing
delusion of being c.
c. drinking
c. emotion
c. environment
c. exposure
c. medication trial
c. sampling
c. substance
C. Substances Act (CSA)

controlling
c. external entities
c. external spirit
c. identity
c. parent
c. personality

controversial diagnosis

contumacious

contumacy

contumely

contusion
brain c.
cerebral c.
scalp c.
wind c.

convalescence

convalescent dream

convenience
c. dream
c. gambling
marriage of c.

conventional
c. antipsychotic drug
c. antipsychotic medication
c. dopamine receptor-blocking antipsychotic
c. factor analysis
c. neuroleptic
c. neuroleptic agent
c. neuroleptic drug
c. neuroleptic treatment
c. pharmacotherapy
c. role conformity
c. sign

converge

convergence circuit

convergent
c. and divergent validity
c. thinking

conversation
c. board
meaningful c.

conversational
c. catharsis
c. skill
c. voice

converse

conversing
voice c.

conversion
c. anesthesia
c. aphonia
c. ataxia
c. blindness
c. chorea
c. defense mechanism
c. disorder
c. disorder, mixed type
c. disorder, motor type
c. disorder, seizure type
c. disorder, sensory type
c. disorder with mixed presentation
c. disorder with motor symptoms or deficits
c. disorder with seizure or convulsion
c. disorder with sensory symptom or deficits
c. of emotion
c. hysteria
c. hysteria neurosis
c. hysteria psychoneurosis
metabolic c.
c. paralysis
c. phenomenon
c. psychoneurotic reaction
c. seizure
c. sensory charge
c. symptom
tonic-clonic c.
c. unconsciousness
unconsciousness c.

conversion-type
c.-t. hysterical neurosis
c.-t. neurotic hysterical disorder

convert

convexobasia

convicted sex offender

conviction
delusional c.
felony c.
inferred delusional c.

NOTES

conviction *(continued)*
misdemeanor c.
religious c.
convince
convolute
convolution
convulsant threshold
convulsion
apoplectiform c.
brain c.
central c.
cerebral c.
cerebrospinal c.
clonic c.
conversion disorder with seizure or c.
coordinate c.
drug-induced c.
epileptic c.
epileptiform c.
essential c.
hysterical c.
immediate posttraumatic c.
infantile c.
jacksonian c.
local c.
mimic c.
myoclonic c.
paroxysmal c.
psychogenic c.
psychomotor c.
puerperal c.
reflex c.
repetitive c.
salaam c.
spasmodic c.
spontaneous c.
static c.
tetanic c.
tonic c.
toxic c.
uncinate c.
uremic c.
convulsive
c. disorder
c. equivalent
c. melancholia
c. reflex
c. seizure
c. shock therapy
c. state
c. status epilepticus
c. therapy
c. tic
co-occur
co-occurrence of depression
co-occurring
c.-o. addictive disorder
c.-o. association
c.-o. mental disorder
cookbook
c. diagnosis
c. fashion
cookie theft picture
cool-headed
cooling
c. of affect
c. off
cooperate
cooperation
morality of c.
cooperative
c. behavior
c. education
c. institutional research program (CIRP)
c. motives
c. psychotherapy
c. reward structure
c. therapy
c. training
c. urban house
cooperativity
criterion of c.
level of c.
Cooper method
coordinate
c. convulsion
c. seizure
coordinated
c. epilepsy
c. reflex
coordination
c. of benefits
decreased c.
c. developmental delay disorder
eye-hand c.
fine motor c.
fluid c.
maze c.
motor c.
subaverage motor c.
visuomotor c.
coordinatus
spasmus c.
coparental divorce
COPE
coping operations preference enquiry
COPE computer software program for depression therapy
co-pharmacy
cophica
alalia c.
coping
c. ability
active c.
adaptive c.

c. behavior
c. belief
c. in caregivers
cognitive c.
concept of spiritual c.
confrontive c.
c. deficit
detached c.
emotion-focused c.
ideational style of c.
maladaptive c.
c. mechanism
c. operations preference enquiry (COPE)
proactive c.
problem-focused c.
rational cognitive c.
resource for c.
c. response
c. skill
c. strategy
c. style
c. tendency
c. trait
c. with aging
c. with bipolar prodromes schedule

copper poisoning
coprolagnia
coprolalia
multiple tics with c.
tic convulsive with c.
coprolalomania
coprology
coprophagia, coprophagy
coprophagous
coprophemia disorder
coprophil, coprophilic
coprophilia
coprophrasia
copropraxia
copulate
copulation
copulatory behavior
copy
copycat
c. crime
c. suicide
copying
c. drawing (CD)
c. mania
coquetting
flirting and c.
cordial
cordiality
core
c. belief
c. body balance
c. body temperature
central transactional c.
c. characteristic
c. cognitive disturbance
c. conflictual relationship theme
c. consensual understanding
c. construct
c. mindfulness skill
c. pain
c. problem
c. temperature fluctuation
c. values
Cornelia de Lange syndrome
3-cornered therapy
corollary discharge
coronal
c. orientation
c. plane
c. section
coronary
coronary-prone behavior
corpora (*pl. of* corpus)
corporal
c. agnosia
c. punishment
corporate
c. crime
c. criminal
c. fraud
c. hierarchy
c. icon
corpse
corpulence
corpulent
corpus, pl. **corpora**
c. arenacea
c. callosum syndrome
habeas c.
corpora quadrigemina
c. striatum
correction
age c.
medical record c.
correctional
c. facility
c. psychiatry
c. psychology
c. transfer (CT)
correctitude

NOTES

corrective
- c. emotional experience
- c. feedback
- c. technique
- c. therapist
- c. therapy (CT)

correlate
- anatomic c.
- biologic c.
- clinical c.
- differential c.
- psychophysiologic c.

correlation
- canonical c.
- coefficient of c.
- c. coefficient
- familial c.
- intraclass c.
- item-total c.
- c. method
- multiple c.'s
- negative c.
- partial c.
- positive c.
- potential c.
- product-moment c.
- rank c.
- rank-difference c.
- c. ratio
- c. redundancy
- c. study

correlational method

correlative
- objective c.

correspondence
- cross c.
- email c.
- encrypted c.
- point-for-point c.
- secure c.

corrigible

corroborate

corroborating dream

corrode

corrosion

corrosive

corrupt

corruptible

cortex, pl. **cortices**
- allocortical c.
- association c.
- cerebellar c.
- cerebral c.
- cingulate c.
- c. circuit
- deep c.
- dorsolateral prefrontal c.
- entorhinal c.
- extrinsic c.
- frontal c. (FC)
- inferior prefrontal c.
- inferior temporal c. (ITC)
- language-associated c.
- lateral orbitofrontal c.
- medial frontal c.
- medial orbitofrontal c.
- medial prefrontal c.
- mesial prefrontal c.
- motor c.
- occipital c.
- occipitotemporal c.
- orbital prefrontal c.
- orbitofrontal c.
- parietal c.
- periamygdaloid c.
- prefrontal c.
- primary auditory c.
- primary sensory c.
- rostral medial prefrontal c.
- sensory c.
- sulcal prefrontal c.
- supramarginal/angular c.
- temporal c.
- ventromedial c.
- visual association c.

cortical
- c. activity
- c. alexia
- c. amnesia
- c. aphasia
- c. apraxia
- c. area
- c. center
- c. column
- c. deafness
- c. dementia
- c. epilepsy
- c. evoked potential
- c. evoked response
- c. function
- c. gray matter
- c. input
- c. lateralization
- c. mapping
- c. metabolism
- c. network
- c. pathology
- c. psychic blindness
- c. region
- c. sensibility
- c. sensory loss
- c. structure
- c. testing
- c. thumb position
- c. volume
- c. zone

corticalization

cortical-subcortical network activity

cortices (*pl. of* cortex)
corticis
corticoadrenal insufficiency
corticobasal degeneration
corticoid therapy
corticotropin-releasing
c.-r. factor
c.-r. hormone
cortin
cortisol
plasma c.
c. secretion
coruscation
corybantism
cosmetic
c. issue
c. reconstruction
cosmic
c. consciousness
c. identification
c. sensitivity
cosmology
cost
maximum allowable c. (MAC)
treatment c.
Costa-McCrae factor
cost-benefit analysis
cost-reward
c.-r. analysis
c.-r. model
Cotard syndrome
co-therapy
cotinine
cottage plan
Cotunnius disease
couch
analytic c.
cough
habit c.
psychogenic c.
could not test (CNT)
coulomb
Council on Psychiatric Services
counsel
counseling
abuse c.
adolescent c.
alcohol c.
career c.
c. center
child-placement c.
clinical c.
conjoint c.
crisis c.
divorce c.
drug c.
eclectic c.
educational c.
exercise c.
extended c.
family c.
followup c.
genetic c.
group c.
individual c.
Internet c.
c. interview
c. ladder
marital c.
marriage c.
mental health c.
online c.
parent-child conflict c.
pastoral c.
placement c.
practical c.
premarital c.
c. process
c. psychologist
c. psychology
reevaluation c.
reinforcement c.
relapse prevention c.
c. relationship
risk-reduction c.
c. service
sex c.
telephone c.
traditional c.
vocational c.
Web c.
counselor
career c.
chemical dependency c. (CDC)
child c.
couples c.
disability c.
drug c.
family c.
genetic c.
grief c.
group c.
guidance c.
individual c.
industrial rehabilitation c.
legal c.

NOTES

counselor *(continued)*
licensed professional c. (LPC)
marital c.
marriage c.
mental health c.
pastoral c.
personal c.
professional c.
rehabilitation c.
school c.
spiritual c.
substance abuse c.
youth c.
counselor-centered therapy
count
blood c.
radioactive c.
countenance
counter
c. conditioning
over the c. (OTC)
under the c.
counteracting impulsivity
counteraction
counteraggression
counterargue
counterattack
counterbalance
counterbalancing
countercompulsion
counterconditioning
counterconformity
countercriticism
counterculture
counterego
counteridentification
counterinfluence
counterintuitive
counterinvestment
counterirritant
counterphobic
c. attitude
c. behavior
countershock
countertransference
c. behavior
c. experience
c. neurosis
countertransferential reaction
counterwill
counter-wish dream
counting
c. compulsion
c. money tremor
c. obsession
coup injury of brain
couple
C.'s BrainMap
c.'s counselor
c.'s group therapy
c. member
c.'s sex therapy
c. skills group
c.'s therapy
coupling
courage
Dutch c.
lack of c.
courageous
courant
au c.
course
atypical c.
chronic c.
clinical c.
continuous c.
deteriorating c.
developmental c.
episodic c.
fluctuating c.
global c.
c. of illness
c. of illness measure
life c.
longitudinal c.
long-term c.
perilous c.
planned c.
rapid-cycling c.
recurrent c.
c. specifier
tempestuous c.
temporal c.
c. of treatment
court
appeals c.
c. custody
c. of domestic relations
family c.
c. of honor
juvenile c.
c. of law
mental health c.
c. order
ruling of c.
supreme c.
traffic c.
trial c.
court-appointed
c.-a. guardian
c.-a. psychiatrist
courteous
court-mandated
c.-m. evaluation
c.-m. treatment
court-ordered involuntary outpatient treatment
court-related problem

courtroom psychology
courtship behavior
couth
couvade
covariance
analysis of c. (ANCOVA)
covariate
coven
member of c.
covenant
crapulous c.
covenantee
covenanter
covert
c. anxiety
c. behavior
c. feeling
c. hostility
c. message
c. modeling
c. narcissism
c. observation
c. reinforcement
c. resentment
c. resistance
c. response
c. self-esteem
c. sensitization
c. visuospatial attention
coverture
covetous
coward
Cox regression analysis
cozen
cozenage
CP
child psychiatry
child psychology
CPP
career planning program
cerebral perfusion pressure
community psychiatry program
conditioned place preference
cranial perfusion pressure
CPR
cardiopulmonary resuscitation
CPS
Children's Protective Services
clinical performance score
complex partial seizure
constitutional psychopathic state
cumulative probability of success
CPSR
chronic paranoid schizophrenic reaction
CPT-ACC
continuous performance task-accuracy
CPT-EFF
continuous performance task-efficiency
CQ
circadian quotient
conceptual quotient
CR
conditioned reflex
crack
sexual favor for c.
crackling
parchment c.
craft
c. neurosis
c. palsy
crafty
cramp
accessory c.
menstrual c.
miner's c.
musician's c.
occupational c.
pianist's c.
piano player's c.
seamstress' c.
shaving c.
stoker's c.
tailor's c.
Wernicke c.
crania (*pl. of* cranium)
cranial
c. anomaly
c. nerve
c. nerve abnormality
c. perfusion pressure (CPP)
craniognomy
craniology
Gall c.
craniomalacia
circumscribed c.
craniopharyngeal canal
craniosinus fistula
craniostenosis
cranium, pl. **crania**
crapuleux
délire c.
crapulous covenant
crash
depressive c.
crass

NOTES

crassitude
crave
craven
craving
alcohol c.
carbohydrate c.
cocaine c.
cue-elicited c.
cue-induced c.
decreased c.
drug c.
food c.
c. management
nicotine c.
c. reducer
strong c.
withdrawal-based c.
craving-related urge
craze
crazy
CRE
cAMP response element
creative
c. imagination
c. outlet
c. self
c. talent
c. thinking
creativeness
creativity
credence
credibility
scientific c.
witness c.
credible
credit card abuse
credulous
creed
creeping-crawling sensation
creeping palsy
crepuscular
crescendo-decrescendo breathing
crescendo sleep
cresomania
crestfallen
cretin
cretinism
cretinistic
cretinoid idiocy
cretinous
Creutzfeldt-Jakob
C.-J. disease (CJD)
C.-J. syndrome
cri
c. de coeur
c. du chat syndrome
crib death
criblé
état c.
cribrosus
status c.
Crigler-Najjar
C.-N. disease
C.-N. syndrome, type 1 and 2
crime
accessory to c.
c. against humanity
bias c.
blue-collar c.
C. Control Act of 1984
copycat c.
corporate c.
c. á deux
drug-related c.
hate c.
heinous c.
high-profile c.
multiple personality c.
nonviolent c.
c. of passion
sex c.
United Nations Office on Drugs and C.
c. victim
c. of violence
violent c.
witness to c.
criminal
c. abortion
c. activity
adolescent c.
c. anthropology
c. behavior
c. commitment
corporate c.
c. degeneracy
habitual c.
high-profile c.
c. history
c. hygiene
c. insanity
c. intent
c. irresponsibility
c. justice patient
c. justice system
juvenile c.
c. offender
c. past
c. population
c. profile
c. psychiatry
c. psychology
c. record
report c.
c. response
c. responsibility
c. responsibility assessment

c. sexual act
c. sexual psychopath (CSP)
criminalistics
criminality
criminally insane
criminology
cripple
emotional c.
social c.
crisis, pl. **crises**
accidental c.
acute situational c.
c. of adolescence
adolescent c.
bed c.
catathymic c.
c. center
c. consultation
c. counseling
custody c.
c. effect
emotional c.
C. Evaluation Referral Service (CERS)
existential c.
financial c.
c. group
c. hotline
hypertensive c.
identity c.
in c.
interpersonal c.
c. intervention
c. intervention clinic (CIC)
c. intervention group psychotherapy
c. intervention technique
laryngeal c.
life c.
magnetic c.
c. management
c. management strategy
maturational c.
mesmeric c.
midlife c.
neurotoxicant-related cholinergic c.
normative c.
occupational c.
oculogyric c.
oral c.
c. period
postencephalitic oculogyric c.
precipitating c.
psychogenic oculogyric c.
psychosexual identity c.
rapprochement c.
c. residential care
c. resolution
c. situation
situational c.
c. stabilization
suicidal c.
tabetic c.
c. team
teens in c.
c. theory
therapeutic c.
c. therapy
unanticipated c.
urban c.
widowhood c.
criteria-defined borderline personality disorder
criterion, pl. **criteria**
C. A, A2, B, C, D, E, F
abuse c.
admission c.
c. of associativity
autism criteria
c. behavior
behavioral c.
clustering c.
c. of cooperativity
c. data
death criteria
dependence c.
depression c.
diagnostic criteria
c. dimension
DSM-IV axis II c.
equivalent criteria
equivalent intoxication c.
equivalent withdrawal c.
c. evaluation
exclusion criteria
field-tested c.
full symptom criteria
c. group
impairment c.
c. level
level-of-care c.
lifetime depression c.
method of defining criteria
patient placement c.
a priori c.
psychiatric c.
relevant diagnostic c.

NOTES

criterion *(continued)*
restrictive c.
Schooler-Kane criteria
c. of specificity
statutory criteria
symptom criteria
theta c.
Thorndike-Lorge criteria
c. validity
c. variable
von Knorring c.
withdrawal criteria
criterion-related validity
critical
c. age
c. analysis
c. band concept
c. flicker frequency
c. illness polyneuropathy (CIP)
c. incident technique
c. judgment
c. parent
c. period
c. point
c. ratio
c. region
c. review
c. score
c. submodality
c. thinking
c. value
criticism
ability to take c.
constructive c.
destructive c.
fear of c.
implied c.
objective c.
overt c.
parental c.
peer c.
professional c.
subjective c.
criticize
criticus
status c.
critique
age c.
crochet
main en c.
crocodile tears
Cronbach alpha
crooked
cross
c. adaptation
c. addiction
c. birth
c. conditioning
c. correspondence
c. dependence
c. modal fluency
cross-aggregation
crossbones
skull and c.
crossbreed
cross-correlation mechanism
cross-cultural
c.-c. adaptation
c.-c. difference
c.-c. homogeneity
c.-c. psychiatry
c.-c. testing
cross-culture
c.-c. approach
c.-c. issue
c.-c. psychiatry
cross-dependence
cross-dressing
c.-d. behavior
complete c.-d.
forced c.-d.
motivation for c.-d.
partial c.-d.
crossed
c. adductor jerk
c. anesthesia
c. dominance
c. eyes
c. hemianesthesia
c. hemiplegia
c. knee jerk
c. laterality
c. paralysis
c. phrenic phenomenon
cross-fostering
cross-gender
c.-g. behavior
forced c.-g.
c.-g. identification
c.-g. interest
crossing
boundary c.
c. a bridge
cross-linkage theory
cross-match
blood c.
cross-modality perception
crossover
c. mirroring
c. study
cross-reacting cannabinoids
cross-sectional
c.-s. area (CSA)
c.-s. assessment
c.-s. component
c.-s. data
c.-s. definition
c.-s. evaluation

c.-s. experimental study design
c.-s. method
c.-s. observation
c.-s. prevalence
c.-s. research
c.-s. snapshot
c.-s. study
cross-sex role
cross-taper
cross-tolerance
cross-training
cross-validation
Crouzon syndrome
crowd
c. behavior
c. consciousness
c. control
c. fear
milling c.
crowded place
Crown crisp experiential index
crucial
crucifixion attitude
crucify
crude
c. consciousness
c. opium
cruel
c. impulse
c. punishment
cruelty to animals
cruising
crural ataxia
crus, pl. **crura**
crusade
crush
c. in adolescence
c. syndrome
crust
upper c.
crusty
cry
birth c.
epileptic c.
c. for help
hue and c.
inability to c.
c. reflex
cryalgesia
cryanesthesia
cryesthesia
crying
c. attack
c. cat syndrome
excessive c.
frequent c.
inappropriate c.
c. jag
pathologic c.
c. spell
uncontrollable c.
crymodynia
cryomania
cryoprobe
cryospasm
cryosurgery
cryptanamnesia
cryptesthesia
cryptic
c. depression
c. message
cryptogenic
c. epilepsy
c. epileptic syndrome
c. seizure
c. symbolism
cryptomnesia
cryptorchidism
cryptotia
crystalize
crystalline powder
crystallization
symptom c.
crystallized
c. ability
c. grandiose delusion
c. intelligence
CS
conditioned stimulus
CSA
Controlled Substances Act
cross-sectional area
CSAT
Center for Substance Abuse Treatment
CSF
cerebrospinal fluid
CSP
criminal sexual psychopath
CSR
continued stay review
CSSA
cocaine symptom severity assessment
CSW
certified social worker

NOTES

CT
correctional transfer
corrective therapy
Cuban glossary of psychiatry
cuckold
cuddling behavior
cuddly
cue
accessing c.
anxiety-provoking c.
audiovisual c.
auditory distance c.
behavior c.
cocaine c.
conditioned c.
contextual c.
drug-related c.
c. effect
environmental c.
c. exposure
exposure to biowarfare c.
external c.
eye accessing c.
gambling c.
innocuous environmental c.
internal c.
interoceptive c.
kinesthetic c.
learning c.
c. management
minimal c.
nonverbal c.
obliviousness to social c.'s
orientation c.
perceptual c.
phase c.
c. reduction
response-produced c.
semantic c.
sensory c.
social c.
specific sensory c.
trauma c.
verbal c.
visual c.
cued
c. panic attack
c. speech
cue-elicited craving
cue-induced
c.-i. craving
c.-i. subjective effect
cueing
cuirass
analgesic c.
tabetic c.
culpability
culpable
cult
homophobic c.
c. indoctrination syndrome
killer c.
c. member
personality c.
religious c.
satanic c.
cultural
c. absolutism
c. adaptability
c. adjustment
c. adjustment following migration
c. anthropology
c. area
c. assessment
c. assimilation
c. assumption
c. attitude
c. background
c. barrier
c. belief
c. change
c. competence
c. concept
c. context
c. contrast
c. deprivation
c. determinism
c. difference
c. disadvantage
c. discrimination
c. diversity
c. element
c. experience
c. factor
c. formulation
c. frame of reference
c. healer
c. identity
c. influence
c. inventory
c. item
c. lag
c. norm
c. parallelism
c. phenomenon
c. poison
c. process
c. psychiatry
c. reference group
c. relativism
c. role
c. roots
c. sensitivity
c. shock
c. stereotype
c. subgroup
c. taboo

c. testing
c. theme
c. tradition
c. training
c. transmission
c. value
c. variation
cultural-familial mental retardation
culturally
c. appropriate
c. appropriate avoidant behavior
c. bound
c. condoned behavior
c. deprived
c. different
c. diverse population
c. parallel
c. sanctioned
c. sanctioned behavior
c. sanctioned experience
c. sanctioned response
c. sanctioned symptom
c. specific characteristic
c. unsanctioned
c. unsanctioned response
culture
adolescent c.
c. and alcoholism
bullying c.
cargo c.
c. change
coexistent c.
collectivist c.
c. complex
configurative c.
c. conflict
diagnosing organizational c.
dominant c.
drug c.
hip-hop c.
hippie c.
host c.
indigenous family c.
industrialized c.
c. norm
c. of origin
phallocentric c.
pop c.
popular c.
school c.
sexual c.
c. shock
c. trait
youth c.
culture-bound
c.-b. belief
c.-b. syndrome
culture-related feature
culture-specific
c.-s. feature
c.-s. intervention
c.-s. syndrome
cumulative
c. dose
c. drug action
c. effect
c. incidence rate
c. medication reduction
c. probability of success (CPS)
c. record
c. response
c. response curve
c. stressors
c. trauma disorder
cunnilingus
cunning and hiding behavior
curandero, curanderismo
curare
curarization-induced flaccidity
curativa
indicatio c.
cure
faith c.
c. rate
talking c.
transference c.
work c.
curfew
curiosity
sexual c.
curiosum eroticum
curled-into-fetal-position posture
current
action c.
alternating c. (AC)
alternating current and/or direct c. (AC/DC)
c. cognitive status
c. defense level
demarcation c.
c. depression
c. diagnosis (CD)
c. episode duration
c. of injury
c. night terror (CNT)

NOTES

current *(continued)*
c. psychotic episode
c. suicide attempt
c. tic
curse
Ondine c.
cursing magic
cursiva
epilepsia c.
cursive epilepsy
curtailed sleep
curve
bell-shaped c.
cumulative response c.
developmental c.
distribution c.
dose-response c.
frequency c.
gaussian c.
learning c.
logistic c.
luetic c.
nonlinear developmental c.
normal c.
paretic c.
probability c.
response c.
Cushing
C. basophilia
C. disease
C. response
cuss
custodial
c. care
c. parent
custody
child c.
court c.
c. crisis
c. dispute
c. issue
joint c.
parental c.
c. quotient
c. relinquishment
single c.
split c.
transfer of c.
c. transfer
custom
dietary c.
eating c.
expression of c.'s
foreign c.
cut
visual field c.
cutaneous
c. anesthesia
c. experience
c. hyperalgesia
c. psychogenic disorder
c. reaction
cutoff score
cutting
c. oneself
self-inflicted hair c.
self-inflicted skin c.
wrist c.
CV
coefficient of variation
CWLA
Child Welfare League of America
cyamemazine
cyanosis
cyanotic syndrome of Scheid
cyberchondria
cybercrime
cybermedicine
cybernetic
c. theory
c. theory of aging
cyberporn
cyberpsych
cybersex addiction
cyberstalker
cyberstalking
c. law
c. victim
cybertherapy
cyclandelate
cyclazocine
cycle
aberrant c.
basic rest-activity c. (BRAC)
brain wave c.
desire phase of sexual response c.
duration duty c.
estrous c.
excitement phase of sexual response c.
fusion-defusion c.
genesial c.
gonadal c.
introjective-projective c.
c. length
life c.
menstrual c.
non-24-hour sleep-wake c.
orgasmic phase of sexual response c.
perceptual c.
phase shift of sleep-wake c.
resolution phase of sexual response c.
sexual response c.
short c.
sleep c.

sleep-wake c.
vicious c.
cycler
rapid c.
cycles-per-second tremor
cyclic
c. abulia
c. adenosine monophosphate (cAMP)
c. depression
c. ether
c. headache
c. history
c. illness
c. insanity
c. medication
c. mood disorder
c. mood swing
c. psychiatric disorder
c. schizophrenia
c. vomiting
c. vomiting syndrome
cyclical
c. depression
c. pattern of symptoms
c. psychogenic vomiting
cycling
mania with rapid c.
mood disorder with rapid c.
rapid c.
cyclohexyl nitrite
cycloid
c. personality
c. psychosis
cyclooxygenase-2
cyclophrenia
cycloplegia
cyclothymia
cyclothymic, cyclothymiac
c. personality
c. personality disorder
cyclothymic-depressive behavior
Cymbalta
cynanthropy
cynical humor
cynicism
cynic spasm
cynomania
cynorexia
cyophoria
cypenamine
cyprodenate
cyproheptadine
cyproximide
cytoarchitectural organization
cytochrome
c. P-450 2D6 gene
c. P-450 2E1
c. P-450 metabolic enzyme
c. P-450 metabolism
c. P450 system
cytogenetic
cytogenic
cytomegalovirus (CMV)
cytoplasm
cytosine

NOTES

D4
receptor D4
D_2
D_2 blockade
D_2 occupancy
DA
developmental age
dabbler
d'accoucheur
main d.
DaCosta syndrome
d'action
folie d.
dactylophasia
dactylospasm
dad
deadbeat d.
daft
daily
d. caffeine consumption
d. cigarette consumption
d. dose
d. living
d. living aid
d. living skill
d. record of severity of problems (DRSP)
d. report card
d. symptom rating
Dale law
dally
DAMA
discharged against medical advice
damage
alcoholic liver d.
amygdala d.
body ego d.
brain cell d.
chronic tissue d.
diencephalic d.
DNA d.
drug-related brain d.
extent of d.
hippocampal d.
intrinsic d.
liver d.
minimal brain d.
neuronal d.
property d.
dammed-up
d.-u. emotion
d.-u. feeling
d.-u. libido
damming up
damn
damnable
damnify
damning
dampen
damping effect
dampness
dance
d. education
Saint John's d.
shadow d.
St. Vitus d.
d. therapy
dancing
d. chorea
d. disease
d. eye
d. mania
d. spasm
danger
acute d.
focus of anticipated d.
future d.
immediate d.
life-threatening d.
long-term d.
d. to others
perceived d.
physical d.
poor awareness of d.
d. to self
d. situation
underestimating d.
danger-laden schema vulnerability
dangerous
d. activity
d. behavior
d. behavior reaction
d. coping strategy
d. delusion
d. drug
d. image
d. to oneself
d. to others
d. patient
sexually d.
d. situation
d. stunt
dangerousness
perception of d.
prediction of d.
Dantrium
dantrolene sodium
DARE
drug abuse resistance education
dare

daredevil
dark
d. adaptation
d. environment
d. mood
darkening vision
darkness
D/ART
Depression: Awareness, Recognition, and Treatment
Dartmouth COOP functioning chart
darwinian reflex
darwinism
neural d.
social d.
Dasein analysis
dashing
dastard
DAT
dementia of Alzheimer type
data
anecdotal d.
biographical d.
biologic d.
clinical d.
d. collection
contradictory d.
criterion d.
cross-sectional d.
empirical d.
epidemiological d.
evaluability-assessment d.
field d.
followup d.
functional imaging d.
historical d.
identifying d.
laboratory d.
longitudinal expert evaluation using all available d. (LEAD)
long-term d.
mental d.
narrative d.
normative d.
nutriceutical d.
paucity of d.
pedigree d.
personal followup d.
postmortem d.
psychiatric d.
Q d.
quantitative d.
d. reanalysis strategy
reanalyzed d.
self-report d.
d. set
d. snooping
supporting d.
survey d.
d. tampering
Database
Total Army Injury and Health Outcomes D.
date
anniversary d.
bind analysis d.
birth d. (BD)
blind d.
personnel d.
d. rape
d. rape drug
d. stamp
dating
d. bar
d. experience
d. life
d. relationship
d. violence
daughter language
daunt
dauntless
dawdle
DAWN
Drug Abuse Warning Network
dawn
day
d. camp
drinks per drinking d.
drug-free d.
d. fatigue
d.'s of heavy drinking
d. hospital
d. one
packs per d. (PPD)
d. reporting center
d. residue
d. school
d. trading
d. treatment center (DTC)
d. treatment program
d. treatment unit
daycare
d. center
d. program
d. residential treatment
daydream
hero d.
suffering hero d.
daydreaming
daylight
daymare
3-day schizophrenia
daytime
d. drowsiness
d. dysfunction
d. fatigue
d. hallucination

d. mouth breathing
d. sedation
d. sleep episode
d. sleep hangover
d. somnolence

day-to-day
d.-t.-d. function
d.-t.-d. stress

Daytrana transdermal patch

daze

dazzle

db
decibel

DBT
dialectical behavior therapy

DD
dysthymic disorder

Dd
unusual detail response

dD
confabulated detail response

DDAVP tablet

DDNOS
dissociative disorder, NOS

DDS
disability determination service

Dds
detail response to small white space

DdW
detail response elaborating whole

de
de Clerambault syndrome
de facto
de haut en bas
de Lange syndrome
de lunatico inquirendo
de novo mechanism

DEA
Drug Enforcement Administration

DEA#
Drug Enforcement Administration number

dead
desire to be d.
d. end
d. hand
identification with d.
playing d.
d. room

deadbeat
d. dad
d. mom

deadhead

deadline

deadlock

deadly
d. catatonia
d. nightshade
d. nightshade poisoning
d. sin

deadness
emotional d.

deadpan

deaf

deaf-blind

deafferentation

deaf-mute

deafness
acoustic trauma d.
air conduction d.
bone conduction d.
central d.
conduction d.
cortical d.
developmental word d.
exposure d.
functional d.
high-frequency d.
hysterical d.
midbrain d.
music d.
nerve d.
occupational d.
organic d.
perceptive d.
prelingual d.
psychic d.
psychogenic d.
selective d.
temporary d.
tone d.
word d.

deaf signer

dealer
dope d.
drug d.

dealing

Dear John letter

death
accidental d.
actual or threatened d.
adolescent attitude toward d.
d. anxiety
apoptotic cell d.
apparent d.
attended d.

NOTES

death *(continued)*
attitude to d.
autoerotic d.
autopsy-negative d.
barbiturate-induced d.
belief in life after d.
black d.
d. blow
brain d.
d. camp
carotid sinus reflex d.
cerebral d.
d. of close friend
crib d.
d. criteria
desire for d.
d. domain
drug overdose d.
d. and dying
excitotoxic d.
exhaustion d.
expectation of d.
expected d.
exposure to d.
d. feigning
fetal d.
functional d.
hastened d.
hypoxyphilia-caused d.
impending d.
inhalant-related d.
d. instinct
intentional d.
d. by lethal injection
d. mask
necrotic cell d.
nerve cell d.
d. neurosis
parental d.
pervasive desire for d.
premature d.
d. preoccupation
preoccupation with d.
d. rate
d. rattle
reaction to d.
d. of relative
d. row
d. of self
d. sentence
serious desire for d.
sniffing d.
spousal loss through d.
d. of spouse
sudden d.
suffering d.
survivor of d.
d. theme
thoughts of d.
d. threat
threat of d.
threatened d.
time of d.
timely d.
d. trance
d. trap
traumatic d.
d. trend
unattended d.
unintentional d.
untimely d.
violent d.
voodoo d.
d. warrant
d. wish

deathbed

deathblow

deathwatch

debacle

debase

debate

debauchee

debauchery

debilitate

debilitating
d. anxiety
d. dysphoric symptom
d. illness
d. mental disorder

debility
nervous d.

debonair, debonaire

debriefing
psychological d.

debris
word d.

debt
gambling d.

debug

debunk

DEC
developmental evaluation center

decadent

decamethonium bromide

decanoate
Prolixin d.

decay
memory d.
reflex d.
d. theory
tooth d.

deceit
biology of d.
conscious d.
determinant of d.
facial d.
technological detection of d.
d. tendency

deceitfulness
deceitful style
deceivable
deceive
intention to d.
deceleration injury
decency
decent
decenter
decentralization
decentration
deception
effect of d.
d. style
decerebrate
d. plasticity
d. posture
d. rigidity
decerebration
bloodless d.
decerebrize
decibel (db)
decimate
decinormal
decision
Brawner d.
competent d.
conscious d.
consequence of d.
Durham d.
Gault d.
impulsive lifestyle d.
informed d.
legal d.
limiting d.
moral d.
Parham d.
philosophical d.
d. support
d. support system
Tarasoff d.
d. theory
treatment d.
d. tree
unilateral d.
decision-maker
executive d.-m.
decision-making
career d.-m.
clinical d.-m.
competent d.-m.
destructive d.-m.
end-of-life d.-m.
ineffective d.-m.
d.-m. organizer
d.-m. process
rash d.-m.
real-life d.-m.
d.-m. skill
decisive
declaim
declaration
dying d.
declarative
d. emotional memory processing
d. memory
d. memory process
declare
declass
declassify
decline
d. in academic functioning
age-related d.
age-related cognitive d.
cognitive d.
functional d.
postpubertal social d.
precipitous cognitive d.
d. rate
declining consciousness
decode
decoding skill
decompensation
acute d.
d. ego
frequent d.
full psychotic d.
impending d.
psychotic d.
severe d.
decompensative neurosis
decomposition
d. in dreams
ego d.
d. of ego
d. of movement
decompress
decompression
cerebral d.
internal d.
d. operation
orbital d.
d. sickness
suboccipital d.
subtemporal d.
trigeminal d.

NOTES

D

deconditioning
decontaminate
decoration scruple
decorticate
d. conditioning
d. posturing
decortication
cerebral d.
reversible d.
decorum
decreased
d. arm swing
d. brain weight
d. concentration
d. coordination
d. craving
d. interest
d. interest in activity
d. job satisfaction
d. libido
d. memory
d. motivation
d. need for sleep
d. respiratory rate
d. work performance
decree
divorce d.
decrement
cognitive d.
work d.
decremental procedure
decrepitude
decriminalize
decrudescence
decry
decussation
pyramidal d.
DED
depressive executive dysfunction
dedifferentiation
dedolation
deduction
deductive reasoning
deefferentation
deem
de-emphasize
deep
d. brain stimulation for mood disorder
d. cortex
d. depression
d. inner resource
d. place
d. sensibility
d. side
d. sleep
d. structure
d. tendon reflex (DTR)
d. trance
d. trance identification
d. white matter
d. white matter hyperintensity
d. white matter pathology
d. white matter region
deeply buried anger
deep-pressure sensitivity
deep-rooted
deep-seated
de-erotize
de-escalate
deescalation technique
deface
defalcate
defamation
defatigation
defaulter
drug d.
defeat
defeatist attitude
defecate
defecation reflex
defect
alcohol-related birth d. (ARBD)
awareness d.
birth d.
body dysmorphic d.
cerebrocranial d.
character d.
cognitive d.
congenital d.
developmental d.
exaggerated d.
excessive concern for d.'s
field d.
genetic d.
high-grade d.
imagined body d.
imagined physical appearance d.
learning d.
memory d.
mental d.
metabolic d.
neurologic d.
organic d.
perceptual d.
physical d.
polytrophic d.
d. preoccupation
preoccupation with d.
retention d.
sensory d.
slight d.
teratologic d.
d. theorist
visual field d.
visuoperceptive d.
defected eye

defective
mentally d.
defeminization
defend
defense
d. attitude
attitude d.
character d.
compulsive d.
ego d.
heat d.
d. hysteria
hysterical character d.
hysteroid d.
immature d.
insanity d.
d. interpretation
lack of mature d.
d. level
masochistic character d.
mature d.
d. mechanism
normal heat d.
d. organization
perceptual d.
d. psychoneurosis
d. reaction
d. reflex
screen d.
stormed d.
d. strategy
defensible space
defensive
d. adultomorphic stance
d. behavior
d. dysregulation
d. emotion
d. functioning axis
d. process
d. reaction
defensiveness
psychological d.
defer diagnosis
deference
reciprocal d.
deferential attitude
deferred
d. diagnosis
diagnosis or condition d. on axis I, II
d. obedience
d. reaction
d. shock
defiance
oppositional d.
defiant
d. behavior
d. rage
stubbornly d.
deficiency
autoimmune d.
cobalamin d.
cognitive d.
environmental d.
familial d.
folate d.
hereditary d.
immune d.
literacy d.
d. love
mental d.
moral d.
d. motivation
d. motive
niacin d.
nicotinic acid d.
nutritional d.
orgasmic d.
oxygen d.
secondary mental d.
thiamine d.
vitamin B, B12 d.
deficiens
ejaculatio d.
orgasmus d.
deficient
d. affective experience
mentally d. (MD)
d. sense of reality
d. sexual desire
deficit
attention d.
awareness d.
behavior d.
behavioral inhibition d.
central sensory d.
character d.
chronic integrative d.
cognitive d.
comprehension d.
concentration d.
conversion disorder with motor symptoms or d.'s
conversion disorder with sensory symptom or d.'s
coping d.

D

NOTES

deficit *(continued)*
emotional memory d.
executive function d.
expressive language d.
gaze d.
global cognitive d.
gross motor d.
gross neurologic d.
gross sensory d.
immediate memory d.
information processing d.
intellectual function d.
interpersonal relationship d.
ipsilateral d.
language d.
memory function d.
mental d.
motor d.
multiple cognitive d.'s
neural d.
neurocognitive d.
neurolinguistic d.
parietotemporal perfusion d.
perception d.
perceptual d.
perseveration d.
pixelated parietotemporal perfusion d.
presynaptic functional d.
primary motor d.
d. reversal
d. schizophrenia
self-care d.
sensory d.
serotonergic d.
sleep d.
social relations d.
social skills d.
speech-motor d.
d. symptom
temporal integration d.
verbal d.
vigilance d.
visual perceptual d.

defile
define
definite
definition
categorical d.
cross-sectional d.
diagnostic d.
operational d.

definitive treatment
deflate
deflated narcissism
deflected eye
deflection
defloration scruple
deflower
deformation
morphological d.
d. of self

deformation-based morphometry
deformity
defraud
deft
defuse
defusion
defy
degeneracy
criminal d.
d. theory

degenerate
degeneration
alcohol-related cerebellar d.
ascending d.
brain d.
corticobasal d.
descending d.
focal d.
orthograde d.
progressive hepatolenticular d.
d. psychosis
reaction of d. (RD)
retrograde d.
secondary d.
senile d.

degenerative
d. disorder
d. encephalopathy
d. insanity
d. primary dementia
d. psychosis
d. status

degenerativus
status d.

degradation
degrade
degrading ritual
degree
d. of amnesia
college d.
d. of control
d. of dependence
d. of disability
d. of freedom
d. of hopelessness
d. of impairment
d. of pain
third d.

degustation
dehumanization
dehumanize
dehumanizing
dehydration
d. reaction
voluntary d.

dehypnotize

deictic
deify
deign
deindividuation
deinstitutionalization
deinstitutionalize
deism
deity
inflated relationship to d.
spectral relationship to d.
deixis
person d.
place d.
time d.
déjà
d. entendu
d. éprouvé
d. fait
d. pense
d. raconté
d. vécu
d. voulu
d. vu
d. vu phenomenon
dejected mood
dejection
delahara
delate
delay
conduction d.
developmental language d.
ejaculatory d.
global d.
inhibition of d.
language d.
orgasm d.
patient d.
phase d.
specific d.
delayed
d. auditory feedback
d. development
d. discharge
d. ejaculation
d. gratification
d. grief
d. language
d. memory
d. orgasm
d. postanoxic encephalopathy
d. posttraumatic stress disorder
d. reaction
d. reaction experiment
d. recall
d. recall index
d. rectifier
d. reflex
d. reinforcement
d. response
d. reward
d. sensation
d. shock
d. sleep phase
d. sleep-phase syndrome
d. speech
d. therapy
d. toilet training
delayed-phase preference
delectation
deleterious mutation
deletion
thought d.
deliberate
d. feigning
d. fire setting
d. infliction of pain
d. self-harm (DSH)
d. therapy
deliberation
ethical d.
legal d.
medical d.
delicate self-cutting
delicto
Delilah syndrome
delimitation
delineate
delineation
delineator
delinquency
adaptive d.
d. in adolescence
adolescent neurotic d.
geriatric d.
group d.
juvenile d.
neurotic d.
recovery from d.
socialized d.
delinquent
d. adolescent
d. behavior
juvenile d.
nonviolent d.
predatory d.

D

NOTES

delinquent *(continued)*
violent d.
d. youth
deliquium
délirante
bouffée d.
délire
d. aigu
d. ambitieux
d. chronique à évolution systematique
d. crapuleux
d. d'embleé
d. de negation
d. de toucher
d. doublé
d. oneirique
d. terminal
d. tremblant
deliria (*pl. of* delirium)
deliriant
delirifacient
delirio
sine d.
deliriosa
schizophrenia d.
delirious
d. mania
d. patient
d. reaction
d. shock
d. transient organic psychosis
delirium, pl. **deliria**
abstinence d.
active d.
acute alcoholic d.
alcoholic d.
d. alcoholicum
alcohol-induced d.
alcohol withdrawal d.
amphetamine d.
anticholinergic d.
anxiolytic d.
anxious d.
asthenic d.
cannabis intoxication d.
chronic alcoholic d.
cocaine intoxication d.
collapse d.
digitalis-induced d.
drug-induced d.
d. due to general medical condition
d. due to multiple etiologies
d. ebriosorum
d. epilepticum
exhaustion d.
febrile d.
d. ferox
focused d.
frank d.
full-blown d.
grandiose d.
grave d.
hallucinogen intoxication d.
history of d.
hypnotic d.
hypoglycemic d.
hysterical d.
d. hystericum
inhalant-induced d.
inhalant intoxication d.
intoxication d.
lingual d.
low d.
macromaniacal d.
manic d.
marijuana d.
medication-induced d.
melancholia with d.
micromaniacal d.
microptic d.
d. mussitans
muttering d.
d. of negation
occupational d.
oneiric d.
opioid-induced d.
opioid intoxication d.
organic d.
panic d.
partial d.
d. of persecution
phencyclidine intoxication d.
posttraumatic d.
d. in presenile dementia
psychasthenic d.
psychoactive substance d.
puerperal d.
rhyming d.
secondary d.
sedative d.
senile d.
d. in senile dementia
d. state drug psychosis
steroid-induced d.
subacute d.
substance-induced d.
substance withdrawal d.
superimposed d.
sympathomimetic d.
d. symptom interview
thyroid d.
toxic d.
d. transient organic psychosis
trauma-induced d.
traumatic d.
d. tremens (DT, DTs)

d. tremens alcoholic psychosis
unfocused d.
d. unit
vascular dementia with d.
withdrawal d.

delirium-like state
delirium-related mental disorder
Delis-Kaplan executive function system (DKEFS)
deliteralization
delitescence
delivery

consistent d.
method of d.

delta

d. activity
d. alcoholism
d. index
d. level
d. opiate receptor
d. rhythm
d. sleep-inducing peptide
d. wave

delta-wave sleep
delude
delusion

affect-laden d.
alcohol-induced psychotic disorder with d.'s
allopsychic d.
amphetamine-induced psychotic disorder with d.'s
anxiolytic-induced psychotic disorder with d.'s
autochthonous d.
autopsychic d.
d. of being controlled
bizarre d.
cannabis-induced psychotic disorder with d.'s
Capgras d.
circumscribed d.
cocaine d.
cocaine-induced psychotic disorder with d.'s
complete d.
complex d.
confused d.
content of d.
d. of control
control d.
crystallized grandiose d.
dangerous d.
depressive d.
disorganized d.
d. of doubles
dysmorphic d.
d. of emotional passivity
encapsulated d.
erotic d.
erotomanic d.
established d.
expansion d.
expansive d.
expressive d.
first-rank symptom of d.
fixed d.
fleeting d.
fragmentary d.
global bizarre d.
d. of grandeur
grandiose d.
hallucinogen-induced psychotic disorder with d.'s
hopelessness d.
hypnotic-induced psychotic disorder with d.'s
d. of ill health
induced psychotic disorder with d.'s
infestation d.
d. of infidelity
d. of influence
inhalant-induced psychotic disorder with d.'s
insane d.
interpretation d.
isolated d.
jealous d.
jealous-type d.
jealousy d.
Mignon d.
mild d.
d. of mind reading
d. of misidentification
mixed-type d.
mood-congruent d.
mood-incongruent d.
multiple d.'s
negation d.
d. of negation
negative d.
nihilistic d.
nonbizarre d.
nonsystematized d.
object of d.

NOTES

delusion *(continued)*
observation d.
organic d.
d. of orientation
Othello d.
paranoid d.
d. of parasitosis
partial d.
passivity d.
pejorative d.
persecution d.
d. of persecution
persecutory d.
persistent d.
phencyclidine-induced psychotic disorder with d.'s
poorly systematized d.
d. of poverty
d. of power
primordial d.
psychotic disorder with d.'s
reference d.
referential d.
reformist d.
religious d.
d. in schizophrenia
schneiderian d.
sedative-induced psychotic disorder with d.'s
d. of self-accusation
sexual d.
simple d.
d. of sin
d. of sinfulness
somatic d.
d. of somatic passivity
d. stupor
substance-induced psychotic disorder with d.'s
d. symptom
systematized d.
systemic d.
d. of thought broadcasting
thought broadcasting d.
thought insertion d.
d. of thought insertion
d. of thought withdrawal
unspecified-type d.
unsystematized d.
vascular dementia with d.'s
d. of wealth
well-formed d.
well-systemized d.

delusional
d. anxiety
d. behavior
d. belief
d. belief in intimacy
d. conviction
d. depression
d. equivalent
d. experience
d. feature
floridly d.
d. ideation
d. insanity
d. intensity
d. jealousy
d. loving
d. misidentification syndrome
d. network
d. paranoid disorder
d. percept
d. projection
d. proportion
d. subtype
d. syndrome drug psychosis
d. system
d. thinking
d. thought
d. thought passivity
d. thought pattern
d. transient organic psychosis
d. transient organic syndrome

delusion-like
d.-l. idea
d.-l. preoccupation

delusive

delve

demagogue

demand
attentional d.
d. characteristic
external d.
functional d.
internal d.
job d.
role d.
sexual d.
d. of society
unreasonable d.

demanding
d. behavior
d. interaction
d. in nature
d. temperament

demarcated relationship

demarcation
d. current
d. potential
d. in sensory testing

demarche

demasculinization

d'embleé
délire d.

demean

demeanor
change in d.
mild eccentricity in d.
demented patient
dementia
acute primary d.
advanced d.
d. and aging
alcohol-associated d.
alcoholic d.
alcohol-induced d.
alcoholism associated with d.
alcohol persisting d.
Alzheimer d.
Alzheimer-like senile d. (ALSD)
d. of Alzheimer type (DAT)
d. of Alzheimer type, with early onset
d. of Alzheimer type, with late onset
anxiolytic-induced persisting d.
apoplectic d.
d. apoplectica
d. associated with alcoholism
Association for Frontotemporal D.
atrophic d.
beclouded d.
Binswanger d.
boxer's d.
catatonic d.
chronic neurologic disease-associated d.
circular d.
confusional state presenile d.
congenital syphilitic paralytic d.
cortical d.
degenerative primary d.
delirium in presenile d.
delirium in senile d.
depressed-type presenile d.
depression in d.
depression-associated d.
developmental d.
dialysis d.
diffuse Lewy body d.
driveling d.
drug-induced d.
d. due to brain injury
d. due to Creutzfeldt-Jakob disease
d. due to head trauma
early phase of d.
endocrine disease-associated d.
endstage d.
d. in epilepsy
epileptic d.
d. evaluation
exhaustion senile d.
familial d.
frontal lobe d.
frontosubcortical d.
frontotemporal d.
global d.
hallucinatory d.
hebephrenic d.
Heller d.
higher d.
HIV d.
HIV-1-associated d.
HIV-based d.
HIV-induced d.
hypnotic-induced persisting d.
impairment of d.
induced persisting d.
infantile d.
d. infantilis
infectious disease-associated d.
inflammatory disease-associated d.
inhalant-induced d.
irreversible d.
juvenile paralytic d.
lacunar d.
language disorder in d.
medication-induced d.
mixed d.
multiinfarct d.
d. myoclonica
neurosyphilis-associated d.
nondegenerative nonvascular d.
old-age d.
organ failure-associated d.
organic d.
paralytic d.
d. paralytica
d. paralytica juvenilis (DPJ)
paranoid d.
d. paranoides
d. paranoides gravis
d. paranoides mitis
paranoid-type arteriosclerotic d.
paranoid-type presenile d.
paranoid-type senile d.
paraphrenic d.
d. paratonia progressiva
paretic d.
Parkinson disease with d. (PDD)
d. patient

NOTES

dementia *(continued)*
persisting d.
d. phase
Pick disease d.
polyarteritis nodosa d.
postanoxic d.
postfebrile d.
postoperative d.
posttraumatic d.
d. praecocissima
d. praecox
preexisting d.
presenile d.
d. presenilis
primary degenerative d. (PDD)
primary senile d.
d. process
d. prodrome
profound d.
d. progression
progressive d.
psychoactive substance d.
psychobiological process of d.
puerperal d.
d. pugilistica
rapidly progressive d.
relative d.
remitting d.
repeated infarct d.
reversible d.
schizophrenic d.
secondary d.
sedative-, hypnotic-, or anxiolytic-induced persisting d.
sedative-induced persisting d.
d. sejunctiva
semantic d.
senile d.
severe d.
d. severity
simple depressive d.
simple senile d.
socialized d.
solvent d.
d. stage
static d.
subcortical d.
substance-abuse persisting d.
substance-induced persisting d.
superimposed d.
d. syndrome
d. syndrome of depression
syphilitic paralytic d.
syphilitic progressive d.
tabetic-form paralytic d.
tardive d.
terminal d.
thalamic d.
toluene d.
toxic d.
transitional Lewy body d.
transmissible virus d. (TVD)
traumatic d.
uncomplicated arteriosclerotic d.
uncomplicated presenile d.
uncomplicated senile d.
vascular d.
vitamin deficiency-associated d.
Wernicke d.
white matter d.
Wilson disease d.
d. with Lewy bodies (DLB)

dementia-aphonia
d.-a. syndrome
d.-a. syndrome of childhood

dementia-related
d.-r. behavior
d.-r. mental disorder
d.-r. psychiatric syndrome

dementia-state drug psychosis

dementing
d. illness
d. process

demerit

demigod

demimonde

demise
untimely d.

demissio animi

Demiurge

democratic leadership pattern

demographic
d. characteristic
d. feature
d. risk factor
d. variable

demography
dynamic d.
static d.

demolish

demon

demoniac

demonic possession

demonolatry

demonology

demonomania

démonomaniaque
folie d.

demonstrable

demonstrate

demonstration

demonstrator

demoralization
personal d.

demoralize

demorphinization

demote

demotivate

demulcent
demure
demutization
demyelinating disorder
demystify
den
denarcotize
denegation
denervate
denervation
autonomic d.
law of d.
d. level
deneutralization
deniable
denial
d. of anergy
color d. (Cd)
d. defense mechanism
d. of external reality
parental d.
psychodynamic d.
psychotic d.
reality d.
d. of responsibility
denied grief
denigrate
denigrated self-esteem
denigration
denizen
denomination
religious d.
denotation
denote
denounce
dense
d. scotoma
d. sensory loss
densitometry
density
frontal lobe neuronal d.
inside d.
outside d.
population d.
dental
d. amalgam
d. anxiety
d. enamel erosion
d. jurisprudence
d. patient reaction
dentata
vagina d.
denuding
hair d.
denunciation
denutrition
Denver developmental screening test II
deny
deodoratum
deodorized opium
deontological ethics
deontologic theory
deontologism
deontologist
deontology
deoppilant
deorality
deoxyribonucleic acid (DNA)
Depade
department
emergency d. (ED)
D. of Health and Human Services (DHHS)
D. of Mental Health (DMH)
psychiatric emergency d.
depatterning
dependence, dependency
absinthe d.
additional drug d.
aerosol spray d.
affective d.
airplane glue d.
alcohol d.
amphetamine d.
anxiolytic d.
barbiturate d. (BD)
benzodiazepine d.
butane-sniffing d.
caffeine d.
cannabis d.
chemical d.
chlorohydrocarbon d.
clinging d.
cocaine d.
codeine d.
combination drug d.
comorbid alcohol d.
d. criterion
cross d.
degree of d.
diet drug d.
d. disorder
drug d.
emotional d.
ethanol d.

NOTES

dependence *(continued)*
ether d.
excessive d.
field d.
full d.
hallucinogen d.
hallucinogenic drug d.
hypnotic d.
increased d.
inhalant d.
instrumental d.
interpersonal d.
laxative d.
lighter fluid d.
long-term d.
LSD d.
marijuana d.
methadone d.
methamphetamine d.
morbid d.
morning glory seed d.
morphine d.
narcotic drug d.
nicotine d.
nitrous oxide d.
d. on therapy
opioid d.
oral d.
passive d.
peyote d.
pharmacology of abuse and d.
phencyclidine d.
physical d.
physiologic d.
polysubstance d.
pornography d.
prescription drug d.
propoxyphene d.
psilocybin d.
psychedelic agent d.
psychic d.
psychoactive substance d.
psychostimulant d.
psychotomimetic agent d.
reward d. (RD)
sedative d.
social d.
solvent d.
soporific drug d.
state d.
substance abuse and d.
d. syndrome
synthetic drug d.
synthetic heroin d.
d. tendency
tetrahydrocannabinol d.
THC d.
therapeutic dose d.
tobacco d.
d. trait
tranquilizer drug d.
unmet d.
unspecified substance d.
volatile solvent d.

dependence-independence
field d.-i.

dependent
d. adult certificate
alcohol d.
d. behavior
blood oxygenation level d. (BOLD)
d. character
dose d.
d. edema
d. feature
d. neurotic personality disorder
d. passive personality disorder
d. patient role
d. personality
d. relationship
trait d.
d. variable

dependent-protective relationship

depersonalization
d. episode
d. experience
d. neurosis
d. neurotic disorder
neurotic state with d.
d. psychoneurosis
d. psychoneurotic reaction
recurrent d.
d. syndrome

depersonalize

depersonalized image

depict

deplete

depleted emotion

depletion
blood oxygen d.
metabolic volume d.

deplorable
d. living conditions
d. working conditions

deploy

depolarization

depolarizing muscle relaxant

deportment

depose

deposit
intracytoplasmic protein d.

deposition

depot
d. antipsychotic
d. antipsychotic preparation
fat d.
d. form
d. medication

d. medication injection
d. medication injection therapy
Piportil D.
depot-administered antipsychotic drug
depravation
depraved
depravity
deprecate
deprecatory
depreciate
depreciated subsystem
deprementia
depressant
brain d.
cerebral d.
CNS d.
motor d.
depressed
d. affect
d. bipolar affective psychosis
bipolar-type currently d.
depressive-type currently d.
d. mania
d. manic state
d. mood
d. mood adjustment disorder
d. mood adjustment reaction
d. mood episode
d. mood theme
d. new mother
d. patient
d. preschooler
d. presentation
d. reflex
schizoaffective disorder, d.
d. schizoaffective schizophrenia
d. suicide victim
d. tone
d. type
depressed-type presenile dementia
depression
Abraham theory of d.
acute anxiety d.
acute situational d.
adjustment d.
adolescent d.
adult major d.
agitated d.
akinetic d.
alcohol-induced d.
anaclitic d.
anancastic d.
anergic d.
anxiety d.
anxious somatic d.
arteriosclerotic d.
atypical d.
autogenous d.
autonomous d.
aversion d.
D.: Awareness, Recognition, and Treatment (D/ART)
Beck cognitive triad of d.
bereavement-related d.
biologic sign d.
bipolar d.
Bowlby theory of d.
Brenner theory of d.
brief situational d.
Burton theory of d.
caregiver d.
characterological d.
childhood-onset d.
chronic major d.
classical d.
classification of d.
clinical d.
cognitive impairment of d.
cognitive model of d.
cognitive theory of d.
d. of consciousness
constitutional d.
d. continuation
co-occurrence of d.
d. criterion
cryptic d.
current d.
cyclic d.
cyclical d.
deep d.
delusional d.
d. in dementia
dementia syndrome of d.
depression sine d. (DSD)
double d.
drug-induced d.
drug-resistant d.
d. during pregnancy
dysthymia with major d.
dysthymia without major d.
elevated mood followed by d.
Endicott substitution criteria for d.
endogenomorphic d.
endogenous d.
d. in epilepsy
Esquirol theory of d.

NOTES

D

depression *(continued)*
exaggerated d.
exogenous d.
d. factor
feeling of d.
first episode of d. (FED)
Freud theory of d.
future d.
gamble to escape from d.
geriatric d.
d. history
holiday d.
homeopathy and d.
hopelessness and d.
hypersomnia associated with d.
hypersomnic d.
hyposomnia associated with d.
hysterical delirium d.
ictal d.
insomnia associated with d.
intense d.
interictal d.
involutional d.
Klein theory of d.
Kohut theory of d.
Kraepelin theory of d.
late-life d.
level of d.
light treatment for winter d.
long-term recurrent d.
major d.
manic d.
manifestation of d.
marked d.
masked d.
maternal d.
Maudsley theory of d.
melancholic d.
menopausal d.
mental d.
Meyer theory of d.
mild d.
moderate to severe d.
monopolar d.
myxedema d.
nervous d.
neurotic d.
d. neurotic disorder
nonbipolar major d.
nonmajor d.
nonpsychotic unipolar d.
nonreactive d.
nuclear d.
overt sign of d.
overwhelming d.
paradoxical d.
paralyzing d.
d. period
physiogenetic d.
postdivorce d.
post dormital d.
posthysterectomy d.
postictal d.
postinfection d.
postnatal d. (PND)
postoperative d.
postpartum d. (PPD)
postpsychotic d.
postschizophrenic d.
poststroke d.
post-TIA d.
prevention and treatment of d. (PTD)
prolonged situational d.
propensity for d.
psychogenic d.
psychoneurotic d.
psychotic d. (PD)
reactive clinical d.
reactive psychotic d.
recurrent psychotic d.
refractory d.
resistant d.
respiratory d.
retarded d.
reversible cognitive impairment of d.
rhythmopathy and d.
d. risk
ruminative d.
d. score
secondary d.
self-blaming d.
self-reported d.
Seligman theory of d.
senile d.
severe d.
d. severity
sign d.
simple affective d.
single-episode psychotic d.
situational d.
sleep and d.
sleeplessness associated with d.
somatic treatment for d.
somatized d.
somatizing clinical d.
d. spectrum disease
sporadic d.
spreading d.
stupor and d.
stuporous d.
subjective d.
subsyndromal d.
d. subtype
d. symptom
symptomatic d.
syndromic d.

d. treatment
treatment-refractory d.
treatment-resistant d. (TRD)
underlying d.
unipolar chronic d.
unipolar major d.
unipolar recurrent d.
unspecified d.
vascular d.
winter d.
withdrawal-related d.
d. with psychotic feature

depression-associated dementia

depressione
depressio sine d.

depression-hyperglycemia relationship

depression-induced cognitive impairment

depression-related
d.-r. hypersomnia
d.-r. mental disorder
d.-r. psychiatric syndrome

depressio sine depressione

depressive
d. auditory hallucination
d. breakthrough
d. catatonia
d. character
d. character structure
d. crash
d. delusion
d. disease
d. disorder, NOS
d. episode
d. equivalent
d. executive dysfunction (DED)
d. experience
d. mixed state
d. neurosis
d. olfactory hallucination
d. personality
d. phase
d. position
d. pseudodementia
d. psychoneurotic reaction
d. psychotic reaction
d. rumination
d. situational reaction
d. spectrum disorder (DSD)
d. stupor
d. symptom
d. symptomatology
d. symptom level
d. syndrome
d. transient organic psychosis
d. turmoil
d. visual hallucination

depressive-dysphoric personality disorder

depressive-type
d.-t. currently depressed
d.-t. nonorganic psychosis
d.-t. psychoneurosis
d.-t. psychoorganic syndrome

depressor

deprivation
activity d.
cultural d.
early parental d.
emotional d.
environmental d.
food d.
masked d.
maternal d.
oxygen d.
paternal d.
perceptual d.
psychological d.
psychosocial d.
role d.
sensory d.
severe environmental d.
sleep d.
social d.
d. syndrome
thought d.
water d.

deprived
culturally d.
d. early life
educationally d.

depth
analysis in d.
d.'s of despair
d. of mood
d. perception
d. psychology
d. recording
d. of sleep
d. therapy

derailment
actual d.
cognitive d.
frequent d.
d. in schizophrenia
speech d.
thought d.
d. of volition

NOTES

deranged
mentally d.
d. neural development
derangement
mental d.
metabolic d.
derealization
dereflection
dereism
dereistic thinking
derelict
skid-row d.
dereliction
deride
derision
derivation
derivative
alcohol d.
chloral d.
ergot d.
indole d.
thioxanthene d.
dermatitis, pl. **dermatitides**
factitial d.
psychogenic d.
self-induced factitial d.
dermatoglyphic
dermatoneurosis
dermatothlasia
dermoneurosis
derogate
derogatory
d. comment
d. remark
d. word
dervish
De Sanctis-Cacchione syndrome
desanimania
descendant
descending
d. degeneration
d. dyscontrol
d. neuritis
d. technique
descent
identity by d.
description
borderline composite d.
clinical d.
composite personality d.
DSM-IV d.
graphic d.
hallucination d.
histrionic composite d.
narrative d.
psychological d.
Q-Sort d.
schizoid composite d.
supervisory behavior d. (SBD)
SWAP-200 d.
textual d.
descriptive
d. approach
d. detail
d. feature
d. psychiatry
d. statistic
d. validity
descriptor score
descry
desecrate
desegregate
desensitization
behavioral d.
eye movement d.
imaginal d.
phobic d.
psychological d.
reciprocal inhibition and d.
systematic d.
systemic d.
desensitize
Desert Storm veteran
deserted place
deserter
desertion
d. anxiety
maternal d.
paternal d.
deserved
d. punishment
d. punishment theme
desexualize
desiccant
desiccate
desiccation
desiderate
design
A/B/A d.
bilaterally symmetric inkblot d.
block d.
case control experimental study d.
cohort experimental d.
cross-sectional experimental study d.
environmental d.
equipment d.
Equipoise Stratified D.
experimental d.
factorial d.
geometric d.
independent group experimental study d.
interdisciplinary environmental d.
job d.
longitudinal experimental study d.
memory for d. (MFD)
mixed d.

multiple baseline d.
naturalistic d.
prospective experimental study d.
quasi-experimental d.
randomized group d.
retrospective experimental study d.
study d.
time-series d.

designate

designer
d. drug
d. hallucinogen
d. label

desirability
low social d.
social d.

desirable behavior

desire
absent sexual d.
active d.
d. to be dead
d. to be thin
d. for death
deficient sexual d.
d. to die
disorder of d.
disturbance in sexual d.
drug d.
hyperactive sexual d.
hypoactive sexual d.
impaired sexual d.
incestuous d.
increased sexual d.
d. to inflict harm
inhibited sexual d.
d. to instill fear
intense d.
irrational d.
d. level
low sexual d.
morbid d.
d. for personal gain
d. phase of sexual response cycle
reduced sexual d.
d. for revenge
sexual d.
situational hypoactive sexual d.
d. state
stated d.

desired
d. behavior
d. effect

desire-for-death rating

desirous

desist

desmethylimipramine

desmethylmirtazapine

desmodynia

DESNOS
disorders of extreme stress, not otherwise specified

desolate

desomorphine

despair
depths of d.
ego integrity versus d.
existential d.
feeling of d.
integrity vs d.

despeciation

desperate financial condition

desperation
feeling of d.

despicable

despise

despondency

despondent

destiny
manifest d.

destitute

destruction
property d.
d. of property

destructive
d. aggression
d. behavior
d. criticism
d. decision-making
d. drive
d. family relationship pattern
d. instinct
d. obedience
d. relationship
d. social consequence
d. tendency

destructiveness
withdrawal d.

destrudo

desultoriness

desultory

desynchronization
event-related d. (ERD)

desynchronized discharge pattern

desynchronous

detached
d. coping

NOTES

detached *(continued)*
emotionally d.
d. manner
detachment
emotional d.
feeling of d.
d. from social relationship
pattern of d.
sense of d.
social d.
somnolent d.
detail
descriptive d.
minimization of emotional d.
preoccupation with d.
d. response elaborating whole (DdW)
d. response to small white space (Dds)
detailed
d. dream
d. history
detectability threshold
detection
d. of adolescent killer
arousal d.
lie d.
signal d.
d. threshold
detector
lie d.
detention (detn)
d. cell
d. certificate
d. facility
d. home
deter
deteriorated
d. affective disorder
d. bipolar disorder
deteriorating
d. course
d. function
deterioration
age-related d.
alcoholic d.
appearance d.
cognitive d.
d. effect
emotional d.
d. epilepsy
epileptic d.
functional d.
global d.
grooming d.
habit d.
hygiene d.
d. index (DI)
intellectual d.
irradiation-induced mental d.
language function d.
manners d.
memory d.
mental d.
mood d.
motivation d.
personality d.
posttraumatic d.
d. process
progressive d.
prominent d.
psychopathologic d.
d. quotient
radiation-induced mental d.
reaction-type d.
senile d.
significant d.
simple d.
social skills d.
status d.
stepwise d.
uniformly progressive d.
determinant
behavior d.
biologic d.
d. of deceit
dominant d.
dream d.
environmental d.
interpersonal environmental d.
psychological d.
determination
forensic d.
legal d.
sex d.
determining quality
determinism
biologic d.
biosocial d.
cultural d.
linguistic d.
psychic d.
reciprocal d.
deterrence
deterrent
d. to suicide
d. therapy
detest
detestable
detn
detention
detoxicate
detoxification
alcohol d.
methadone d.
previous d.
d. program

protracted d.
social d.
detoxified alcoholic
detoxify
detract
detractor
d'etre
raison d.
detriment
detrimental
detumescence
deuteropathy
deux
á d.
crime á d.
egoisme à d.
folie á d.
DEV
deviant
deviation
devaluation
devalue
devastate
devastating effect
develop
failure to d.
developed
poorly d.
developing psychotic disorganization
development
abnormal d.
adolescent moral d.
adult d.
anal stage psychosexual d.
arrested d.
atypical d.
behavioral d.
brain d.
career d.
character d.
child language d.
cognitive d.
concrete operational d.
delayed d.
deranged neural d.
deviant pathway of d.
disturbance of intellectual d.
ego d.
egocentric stage of d.
emotional d.
expressive language d.
fetal d.
formal operational d.
gender identity psychosexual d.
impaired d.
intellectual d.
kohlbergian theory of moral reasoning d.
language d.
latency period psychosexual d.
late speech d.
learning d.
level of d.
libidinal d.
lifespan d.
McLean study of adult d.
mental d.
moral d.
motor d.
neurobiology of early childhood d.
normal childhood d.
optimal d.
oral stage psychosexual d.
personal d.
personality d.
pervasive impairment of d.
phallic stage psychosexual d.
postnatal d.
preoperational d.
d. profile
d. program
d. psychobiology
psychomotor d.
psychosexual d.
psychosocial d.
receptive language d.
retarded d.
scale to assess narrative d.
sensorimotor d.
sexual d.
slow rate of language d.
social d.
standards d.
subsequent d.
task of emotional d. (TED)
developmental
d. age (DA)
d. agraphia
d. aphasia
d. apraxia
d. arithmetic disorder
d. articulation disorder
d. assessment
d. biology
d. condition
d. consideration

NOTES

developmental *(continued)*
d. coordination disorder
d. course
d. curve
d. defect
d. dementia
d. disability
d. disorder associated with hyperkinesis
d. domain
d. dyslexia
d. dysphasia
d. effect
d. evaluation center (DEC)
d. experience
d. experimentation in childhood
d. expressive writing disorder
d. heterogeneity
d. history
d. hyperactivity
d. idiocy
d. imbalance
d. impact
d. influence
d. landmark
d. language delay
d. language disorder
d. learning problem (DLP)
d. level
d. lines
d. milestone
d. moodiness
d. pattern
d. period
d. perspective
d. phase
d. process
d. psychology
d. reading disorder
d. retardation
d. roots
d. schedule
d. screening
d. skill
d. stage
d. task
d. theory
d. trajectory
d. word blindness
d. word deafness

developmental-behavioral pediatrics

developmentally
d. appropriate self-stimulatory behaviors in the young
d. cumulative alcoholism
d. disabled
d. inappropriate social relatedness
d. limited alcoholism

developmental-vulnerability model

deviance
communication d.
personality d.
psychiatric d.
psychopathic d.
role d.
secondary d.
sexual d.
social d.

deviant (DEV)
d. arousal
d. attitude
d. belief
d. language
d. pathway of development
d. political behavior
psychopathic d. (PD)
d. religious behavior
sexual d.

deviation (DEV)
ego d.
d. from physiological norm
mean d.
personality d.
population standard d.
primary sexual d.
quartile d. (q)
d. quotient
response d.
sample standard d.
sexual d.
skew d.
standard d. (SD)
statistical d.

device
Actigraph d.
adaptive d.
charge-coupled d. (CCD)
cohesive d.
computer-assisted speech d.
contraceptive d.
control d.
inanimate learning d.
interrupter d.
language acquisition d. (LAD)
manipulative d.
prosthetic d.
safety d.

devil's
d. advocate
d. pact

devil worship

devil-may-care attitude

deviltry

devious manner

devitalize

devoid

devoir

devolution

devolutive
devolve
devotion
devour
devout
religiously d.
devoutly spiritual
dewy-eyed
dexamphetamine
dexterity
fine motor d.
manual d.
dextral
dextrality
dextrality-sinistrality
dextromanual
dextropedal
dextropropoxyphene
dextrosinistral
DHHS
Department of Health and Human Services
DI
deterioration index
drug information
drug interaction
diabetes
d. mellitus
d. self-care
d. self-management
type 1, 2 d.
diabetic
d. coma
insulin-dependent d.
d. ketoacidosis (DKA)
diablerie
diabolepsy
diabolic
diabolism
diacetylmorphine
diachorema
diachoresis
diachronic study
diacrisis
diacritic
diadochokinesis
diagnosable
diagnosed
newly d.
diagnosing organizational culture
diagnosis, pl. **diagnoses (DX, Dx)**
admitting d. (AD)
alcohol-related d.
alternative d.
anxiety d.
assessment and d.
axis I–IV d.
categorical personality disorder d.
clinical d.
community d.
comorbid Axis II d.
comorbid psychiatric d.
concurrent psychiatric d.
d. or condition deferred on axis I, II
controversial d.
cookbook d.
current d. (CD)
defer d.
deferred d.
differential d.
dimensional d.
direct d.
discharge d.
DSM d.
dual d.
entering d. (ED)
equivalent d.
d. by exclusion
d. ex juvantibus
false-negative d.
false-positive d.
final d.
folk d.
geriatric d.
ICD-10 psychiatric d.
incorrect d.
laboratory d.
Latin American guide for psychiatric d.
missed d.
narcissistic d.
negative d.
pathologic d.
pendulum of d.
personality disorder d.
primary d.
principal d.
proband d.
provisional d.
provocative d.
psychiatric d.
reliable d.
schizophrenic d.
schizophreniform d.
secondary d.

NOTES

D

diagnosis *(continued)*
serum d.
single d.
social d.
structural d.
tentative d.
unclear d.
unrelated d.
valid d.
wastebasket d.
Western d.
working d.
diagnosis-related group
diagnostic
d. algorithm
d. ambiguity
d. anesthesia
d. aspect
d. assessment
d. boundary
d. cardiac catheterization
d. category
d. challenge
d. clarity
d. class
d. clue
d. cluster
d. complexity
d. confidence
d. criteria
d. definition
d. feature
d. group
d. importance
d. impression
d. interview
d. judgment
d. laboratory
d. manual
d. measure
d. method
d. noise
d. orphan
d. overshadowing
d. procedure
d. process
d. profile
d. prototype
D. and Statistical Manual of Mental Disorders (DSM)
D. and Statistical Manual of Mental Disorders, Fourth Edition (DSM-IV)
D. and Statistical Manual of Mental Disorders, Fourth Edition, Revised (DSM-IV-R)
D. and Statistical Manual of Mental Disorders, Fourth Edition, Text Revision (DSM-IV-TR)
d. subgroup
d. subtype
d. teaching
d. template
d. therapy
d. truth telling
d. use of hypnosis
diagnostician
diagnostics
diagram
branching tree d.
scatter d.
dialectic
dialectical
d. behavior theory
d. behavior therapy (DBT)
d. dilemma
dialing
random digital d. (RDD)
dialogue
offensive chat-room d.
dialysis
d. dementia
d. encephalopathy syndrome
diametrically opposed
diamorphine
Diana complex
dianoetic
diaphemetric
diaphoresis
diaphragm
diaphragmatic breathing
diarrhea
nocturnal d.
psychogenic d.
diary
d. card
personal d.
sleep d.
symptom d.
diasostic
diathesis
asthenic d.
biologic d.
bipolar d.
neuropathic d.
panic d.
psychopathic d.
spasmodic d.
stress-driven d.
d. stress paradigm
diathesis-stress theory of schizophrenia
diatribe
dibenzepin
dibenzothiazepine
DIC
drug information center
dice game
dichloralphenazone

dichlorotetrafluoroethane
dichotic
d. listening paradigm
d. listening task
d. message
dichotomization of score
dichotomize
dichotomous
d. classification
d. thinking
dichotomy
body-mind d.
present-absent d.
dichromatic
dichromatopsia
dictatorial
diction
dictum
dicyclic
DID
dissociative identity disorder
didactic
d. analysis
d. group psychotherapy
dido
die
desire to d.
wish to d.
diehard personality
diencephalic
d. damage
d. epilepsy
d. seizure
d. stupor
diencephalon, pl. **diencephala**
diestrus
gestational d.
lactational d.
diet
absolute d.
ADA d.
adequate d.
American Diabetes Association d.
aspartame-restricted d.
balanced d.
Banting d.
basal d.
basic d.
Baylorfast d.
black d.
bland d.
caffeine-restricted d.
dietetic d.
d. drug
d. drug abuse
d. drug dependence
elemental d.
elimination d.
fad d.
Feingold d.
high-calorie d.
high-fat d.
high-fiber d.
high-protein d.
improper d.
isocaloric d.
Jenny Craig d.
ketogenic d.
lactoovovegetarian d.
lactovegetarian d.
light d.
limited d.
liquid d.
low-calorie d.
low-carbohydrate d.
low-fat d.
low-salt d.
low-tyramine d.
macrobiotic d.
d. management
Nutri/System d.
Optifast d.
optimal d.
ovovegetarian d.
Pritikin d.
recommended d.
reduced-sodium d.
regular d.
restricted d.
salt-free d.
soft d.
South Beach d.
Spartan d.
subsistence d.
d. treatment
unrestricted d.
vegan vegetarian d.
vegetarian d.
Weight Watchers d.
dietary
d. amenorrhea
d. change
d. chaos syndrome
d. custom
d. excess
d. habit

NOTES

dietary *(continued)*
d. modification
d. restraint
d. restriction
d. state
d. supplement
d. theory
d. toxin
diet-controlled
dietetic diet
diethylamide
lysergic acid d. (LSD)
diethylmalonylurea
dieting
d. technique
unwise d.
dietitian
difference
behavioral d.
chance d.
clinical d.
cross-cultural d.
cultural d.
dose-related d.
ethnic d.
functional d.
gender d.
gender-based mental health d.'s
genetic d.
gray-white matter d.
group d.
hormonal d.
individual d.'s
just noticeable d. (JND)
d. limen
metabolic d.
morphological d.
nonsignificant d.
pharmacological d.
phase d.
qualitative d.
religious d.
significant d.
standard error of d.
true d.
different
culturally d.
differentia
differential
d. beneficial effect
d. correlate
d. diagnosis
d. diagnostic technique
d. equation
d. extinction
d. function
d. increase
d. interaction
d. prevalence
d. reinforcement
d. reinforcement of other behavior (DRO)
d. relaxation
d. response
semantic d.
threshold d.
d. threshold
differentiate
differentiation
brain d.
cell d.
regional d.
sex d.
sexual d.
difficult
d. child
d. to manage
d. to subdue
difficulty
academic d.
acculturation d.
d. in changing response set
chronic phase of stable sleep d.
d. concentrating
concentration d.
d. controlling anger
d. describing feelings
emotional d.
emotional and behavioral d.'s (EBD)
gambling-related d.
d. identifying feelings
interpersonal d.
item d.
language d.
learning d.
d. level
life d.
memory d.
moderate d.
multiple life d.'s
practical d.
protracted d.
school d.
sensory d.
specific reading d. (SRD)
speech d.
spelling d.
stable sleep d.
sublimation d.
d. swallowing
tactile sensory d.
d. waking up
d. with thought
word-finding d.
diffidence
diffident

diffuse
d. affect
d. anxiety
d. axonal injury
d. brain atrophy
d. brain dysfunction
d. encephalopathy
d. function
d. Lewy body dementia
d. phoneme
d. sclerosis
d. slowing of EEG
diffused reflex
diffusion
identity vs role d.
d. respiration
role d.
D. Tensor Imaging (DTI)
diffusional state
digamy
digestible
digestive
d. epilepsy
d. psychogenic disorder
digit
d. recall
d. span (DS)
d. span backwards
d. stamp
d. symbol (DS)
d. symbol substitution
digital change
digitalgia paresthetica
digitalis-induced delirium
digit-symbol
d.-s. coding task
d.-s. and incidental memory
dignify
dignitary
dignity
digraph
digress
digressed speech
digressive
dihybrid
dihydrochloride
dihydrocodeine
dihydrocodeinone bitartrate
dihydromorphine
dihydromorphone
DIL
drug information log
Dilantin
D. Infatabs
D. Kapseals
Dilantin-125
dilate
dilated pupil
dilation
papillary d.
dilatory nature
dildo
dilemma
dialectical d.
ethical d.
legal d.
moral d.
need-fear d.
organic-functional d.
diligence
diligent
dilly-dally
dilution
transference d.
dimension
abstract versus representational d.
character d.
compulsivity-impulsivity d.
criterion d.
disorganization d.
group d.
hyperactivity-impulsivity d.
inattention d.
job d.
micropsychotic d.
negative symptom d.
personality d.
positive symptom d.
sensory d.
spiritual d.
symptom d.
dimensional
d. approach
d. diagnosis
d. model
d. rating
d. setting
d. system
1-dimensional
2-dimensional
2-d. electrophoresis
2-d. proton echo-planar spectroscopic imaging
3-dimensional
dimensionality

NOTES

dimethoxyamphetamine
2,5-dimethoxy-4-methylamphetamine (DOB)
dimethyltryptamine (DMT)
diminish
diminished
d. capacity
d. control
d. effect
d. emotional expression
d. libido
d. pleasure in everyday activities
d. reality testing
d. recall
d. reflex
d. response to pain
d. responsibility
d. responsiveness
d. sensation
d. sexual interest
d. social interest
diminution
d. of affect
d. of thought
diminutive
dimming
chromatic d.
dimorphic
sexually d.
dimorphism
brain d.
sexual d.
DIMS
disorders of initiating and maintaining sleep
ding-dong theory
dinomania
diode
Dionysian attitude
diotic
d. listening
d. message
dioxide
carbon d. (CO_2)
dioxyamphetamine
diphasic
diphenylaminearsine chloride
diphenylchlorarsine
diphosphate
diplacusis dysharmonica
diplegia
ataxic d.
congenital facial d.
facial d.
infantile d.
masticatory d.
spastic d.
diplegic idiocy
diploid
diploma
high school d.
d. in psychological medicine (DPM)
diplomacy
diplomatic
diplomyelia
diplopia
dipole tracing (DT)
dipping
body d.
dippoldism
dipropyltryptamine (DPT)
dipsesis
dipsetic
dipsomania
dipsosis
DIR
disturbed interpersonal relationship
direct
d. association
d. causality
d. causative pathophysiological mechanism
d. confrontation
d. diagnosis
d. genetic influence
d. genital stimulation
d. image
d. interview
d. motor system
d. observation
d. physiological effect
d. question
d. selection communication board
d. self-destructive behavior (DSDB)
d. suggestion under hypnosis (DSUH)
d. tension indicator
d. thermogenic effect
d. threat
d. threat to life
d. treatment
directed
d. group therapy
inner d.
other d.
d. thinking
tradition d.
d. violent fantasy
direction
coincidence d.
completion, arithmetic problems, vocabulary, and following d.'s (CAVD)
d. prognosis
psychotic d.
spiritual d.
directionality

directive
advance d.
genetic d.
proxy d.
d. psychotherapy
directness
direful situation
dire straits
dirigation
dirt
d. eater
d. eating
dirtiness
feeling of d.
dirty
being d.
d. needle
d. pool
quick and d.
d. urine
d. words
disability
abstracting d.
associated d.
d. benefit
chronic d.
cognitive d.
d. counselor
degree of d.
d. determination service (DDS)
developmental d.
drawing d.
early retirement with d. (ERD)
emotional d.
functional d.
general language d.
d. insurance
language d.
learning d. (LD)
d. level
long-term d. (LTD)
manifested d.
memory d.
mental d.
mild d.
mobility d.
motor d.
observable d.
output d.
overall d.
partial permanent d.
perceptual d.
perceptual-motor d.
permanent d.
posttraumatic chronic d.
progressive d.
psychiatric d.
reading d.
residual d.
d. risk factor
sequencing d.
service-connected d. (SCD)
severe d.
social role d.
specific learning d.
specific reading d.
speech d.
temporary d.
total d.
work d.
disability-adjusted life years
disabled
developmentally d.
emotionally disturbed/learning d. (ED/LD)
learning d.
mentally d.
partially d.
psychiatrically d.
temporarily d.
totally d.
d. by war
disabling
d. anxiety
d. headache
d. mental illness
d. psychiatric symptom
socially d.
d. stress
d. worry
disadvantage
cultural d.
economic d.
educational d.
symptomatic d.
disaggregation
disappointment
romantic d.
disapproval
social d.
disapproving voice
disarming
disarray
disassimilation
disassociate
disassociation (*var. of* dissociation)

NOTES

D

disaster
man-made d.
natural d.
d. psychiatry
d. situation
d. stressor
technological d.
d. trauma
d. victim
d. work
d. worker
disaster-related
d.-r. avoidant symptom
d.-r. intrusive symptom
disastrous
disavowal level
disavows responsibility
disband
disbelief
discern
discernible
discharge
affective d.
anxiety d.
bad conduct d. (BCD)
cathectic d.
certificate of disability for d. (CDD)
conditional d.
corollary d.
delayed d.
d. diagnosis
dishonorable d.
early d.
epileptiform d.
exercise-induced sympathetic d.
honorable d.
intensity, severity, and d. (ISD)
interference pattern of d.
involuntary d.
medical d.
d. pattern
premature d.
rate of recovery at d.
sympathetic d.
discharged against medical advice (DAMA)
dischronation
disciplinarian
disciplinary
d. action
d. infraction
d. problem
d. segregation
discipline
bondage and d.
brutal d.
constructive d.
excessive d.
formal d.
harsh d.
inadequate d.
inconsistent parental d.
mental d.
physical d.
disciplined lifestyle
disclaim
disclose
disclosure
emotional d.
same-sex d.
truth d.
discombobulate
discomfiture
discomfort
chest d.
emotional d.
gender role persistent d.
d. level
persistent d.
physical d.
threshold of d. (TD)
d. threshold
d. with emotion
d. with gender role
discommodity
discompose
disconcert
disconnected
d. idea
d. thought
disconnection
d. apraxia
d. hypothesis
social d.
d. syndrome
d. thought disorder
d. with reality
disconnect speech
disconsolate
discontent
discontented
discontinuance
discontinuation
drug d.
SSRI d.
d. syndrome
discontinuity
discord
marital d.
discordance
d. of movement
d. of voice
discordant
d. behavior
d. facial expression
discountenance
discourage

discourse
spontaneous narrative d.
discourteous
discredit
discreet
discrete
d. behavioral state
d. emotional response
d. period
d. symptom
discretion
discriminant
d. analysis
d. stimulus
d. validity
discrimination
age d.
auditory d.
brightness d.
class d.
color d.
d. consciousness
cultural d.
ethnic d.
form d.
gender d.
index of d.
d. learning
loss d.
minority d.
pattern d.
pitch d.
racial d.
reverse d.
right-left d.
score d.
sensory d.
sexual d.
training d.
visual d.
weight d.
discriminative stimulus
discriminator
discriminatory
d. behavior
d. comment
discursive
discussion
clinical case d.
heated d.
leaderless group d. (LGD)
open d.
philosophical d.
discutient
disdain
disease
Acosta d.
d. adaptation
affective d.
alcoholic liver d. (ALD)
altitude d.
Alzheimer d. (AD)
Andes d.
association d.
aviator's d.
Azorean d.
barbed-wire d.
Bayle d.
Beard d.
Binswanger d.
biology of affective d.
Blocq d.
bodily d.
brain d.
brainstem d.
Briquet d.
Brissaud d.
Brodie d.
Brushfield-Wyatt d.
Canavan d.
Charcot d.
childhood d.
chronic wasting d.
combined system d.
communicable d.
complex d.
constitutional d.
Cotunnius d.
Creutzfeldt-Jakob d. (CJD)
Crigler-Najjar d.
Cushing d.
dancing d.
dementia due to Creutzfeldt-Jakob d.
depression spectrum d.
depressive d.
disturbance associated with organic mental d.
drug d.
dynamic d.
emotional d.
endstage liver d.
d. etiology
d. exacerbation
exposure to d.
familial pure depressive d. (FPDD)

NOTES

disease *(continued)*
fatigue d.
feared d.
flight into d.
d. frequency
Friedreich d.
Fuerstner d.
functional d.
Gairdner d.
Gaucher d.
genetic d.
genetotrophic d.
heart d.
hepatolenticular d.
human prion d.
Iceland d.
infantile Gaucher d.
International Classification of D.'s, Clinical Modification, Ed. 9 (ICD-9CM)
International Classification of D.'s, Ed. 9 (ICD-9)
International Classification of D.'s, Ed. 10 (ICD-10)
Janet d.
juvenile nonneuropathic Niemann-Pick d.
Kempf d.
kinky-hair d.
Korsakoff d.
Kraepelin d.
Kraepelin-Morel d.
laughing d.
Lewy body variant of Alzheimer d.
life-threatening d.
liver d.
longitudinal exploration of psychosocial factors in sickle cell d.
long-term d.
Lyme d.
maple sugar syrup urine d.
Marateaux-Lamy d.
Marchiafava-Bignami d.
mental d.
Neftel d.
nervous d.
neurodegenerative d.
occupational d.
organic brain d. (OBD)
d. prevention
prion d.
d. process
progressive d.
psychiatric d.
psychotic d.
pure depressive d.
rectal d.
Saint Dymphna d.
Saint Martin d.
Saint Mathurin d.
Sander d.
Sanfilippo d.
Seitelberger d.
self-induced d.
self-perpetuated d.
self-rated impact of d.
Selter d.
d. severity
sexually transmitted d. (STD)
skin d.
social d.
sporadic depressive d. (SDD)
Steele-Richardson-Olszewski d.
suspected d.
d. theme
d. trigger
venereal d. (VD)
von Hippel-Lindau d.
Werdnig-Hoffmann d.
Wernicke d.
Westphal d.
white matter d.
Wilson hepatolenticular degeneration d.
Winkelman d.

disease-related
d.-r. change
d.-r. fatigue

disembody

disenchant

disenfranchise

disengage

disengagement

disentangle

disequilibrium
linkage d.
neurochemical d.

disesteem

disfavor

disfigure

disfigurement
facial d.

disfluency
avoidance of speech d.
d. dyskinesia
speech d.

disgrace

disgruntle

disguise

disguised wish fulfillment

disgust
feeling of d.
image eliciting d.

dishabille

disharmonious state of mind

disharmony
affective d.
marital d.
dishearten
disheveled
d. appearance
d. patient
dishonest simulation of symptoms
dishonesty
professional d.
dishonor
dishonorable discharge
disillusion
disingenuous
disinhibited
d. sexual impulse
d. type of passive developmental disorder
d. violent behavior
disinhibition
anxiolytic d.
emotional d.
initial d.
motor d.
disinhibitory psychopathology
disintegrate
disintegration
d. anxiety
d. of consciousness
personality d.
disintegrative
d. childhood psychosis
d. disorder
disinter
disinterest in eating
disjunction
disk-over-water apparatus
disloyal
disloyalty
feeling of d.
dismal
dismantle
dismay
dismember
dismiss
disobedience
civil d.
disobedient behavior
disobey
disoblige
disodium
disomy
uniparental d.

disorder
abnormal involuntary movement d. (AIMD)
Abraham view of depressive d.
academic skills d.
academic underachievement d.
acquired sexual d.
acute neuropsychologic d.
acute paranoid d.
acute stress d. (ASD)
addictive d.
adjustment interface d.
adjustment reaction conduct d.
adolescent-onset conduct d.
adrenal d.
adult depressive d.
adult-life psychosexual identity d.
d. of affect
affective bipolar d.
affective determined d.
affective neurotic personality d.
affective spectrum d.
aggressive-type undersocialized conduct d.
agoraphobia without history of panic d.
alcohol anxiety d.
alcohol-dependent sleep d.
alcoholic amnestic d.
alcoholic organic mental d.
alcohol-induced psychotic d.
alcohol intoxication-related d.
alcohol mood d.
alcohol-related use d., NOS
alcohol sleep d.
alcohol use d.
allergic psychogenic d.
alpha methyldopa-induced mood d.
alternating bipolar d.
alternative criterion B for dysthymic d.
amitriptyline-induced mood d.
amnestic d.
amphetamine delusional d.
amphetamine-induced psychotic d.
amphetamine-related d.
amphetamine use d.
antisocial personality d. (APD, ASPD)
anxiety adjustment d.
anxiety-avoiding personality d.
anxiety due to physical d.
anxiety psychogenic d.

NOTES

disorder *(continued)*
anxiety-related mental d.
anxiety state neurotic d.
anxiolytic amnestic d.
anxiolytic substance-use d.
anxiolytic use d.
apathetic-type personality d.
aphasia d.
appetite psychogenic d.
apraxic d.
arithmetic developmental delay d.
arousal d.
arteriosclerotic brain d.
articulation developmental delay d.
artificial d.
Asperger d.
associated d.
asthenic personality d.
attachment d.
attachment-separation d.
attention d.
attention deficit d. (ADD)
attention deficit and disruptive behavior d. (AD-DBD)
attention deficit hyperactivity d. (ADHD)
attention deficit hyperactivity d.-predominantly inattentive (ADHD-PI)
atypical affective d.
atypical anxiety d.
atypical bipolar d.
atypical conduct d.
atypical dissociative d.
atypical eating d.
atypical gender identity d.
atypical impulse control d.
atypical mixed or other personality d.
atypical paranoid d.
atypical pervasive developmental d.
atypical somatoform d.
atypical specific developmental d.
atypical stereotyped movement d.
atypical tic d.
auditory perceptual d.
autism spectrum d.
autistic d.
autoimmune obsessive-compulsive tic d.
autonomic arousal d.
avoidant neurotic personality d.
avoidant personality d. (APD)
axis I, II d.
Beck view of depressive d.
behavior d.
behavioral d.
Behr d.
bereavement d.
bereavement-related mood d.
Bibring view of depressive d.
binge-eating d.
bipolar affective d.
bipolar I-IV d.
bipolar spectrum d.
bipolar-type schizoaffective d.
blood psychogenic d.
body dysmorphic d. (BDD)
borderline neurotic personality d.
borderline personality d. (BPD)
brain damage language d.
breathing d.
breathing-related sleep d.
brief posttraumatic stress d.
brief psychotic d.
brief reactive dissociative d.
Briquet d.
caffeine-induced anxiety d.
caffeine-induced sleep d.
caffeine-related d.
caffeine use d.
cannabis delusional d.
cannabis-induced anxiety d.
cannabis-induced delirium d.
cannabis intoxication-related d.
cannabis organic mental d.
cannabis-related d.
cannabis-related d., NOS
cannabis use d.
cardiac d.
cardiovascular psychogenic d.
Carroll-Klein model of bipolar d.
catatonic d.
d. category
Center for Stress and Anxiety D.'s
central language d. (CLD)
cerebral d.
character d. (CD)
character impulse d.
characterological d.
character spectrum d.
d. of childhood
childhood anxiety d.
childhood bipolar d.
childhood disintegrative d.
childhood obsessive-compulsive d.
childhood-onset obsessive-compulsive d.
childhood-onset pervasive developmental d.
childhood psychosexual identity d.
children and adults with attention deficit d. (CHADD)
children and adults with attention deficit/hyperactivity d. (CHADD)
Chinese classification of mental d.'s
chronic motor tic d.

chronic neuropsychologic d.
chronic posttraumatic stress d.
chronobiological d.
circadian rhythm sleep d.
cluster A, B, C d.
cluster A, B personality d.
cluster characteristics in personality d.
cocaine anxiety d.
cocaine delusional d.
cocaine-induced psychotic d.
cocaine intoxication-related d.
cocaine mood d.
cocaine-related d.
cocaine-related d., NOS
cocaine sleep d.
cocaine use d.
codependency d.
coexisting d.
cognition d.
cognitive d.
Cohen view of depressive d.
combat stress d.
combined-type attention deficit hyperactivity d.
combined-type personality d.
communication d. (CD)
communicative d.
comorbid anxiety d.
comorbid cluster B personality d.
comorbid depressive d.
comorbid mental d.
comorbid mood d.
comorbid psychiatric d.
compensation neurotic d.
complex genetic d.
complicated grief d.
compulsive neurotic personality d.
compulsive psychogenic d.
conceptual d.
concurrent personality d.
condition not attributable to mental d.
conduct d. (CD)
conduct disturbance adjustment d.
confusional-arousal d.
content thought d.
contiguity d.
conversion d.
conversion-type neurotic hysterical d.
convulsive d.
co-occurring addictive d.
co-occurring mental d.
coordination developmental delay d.
coprophemia d.
criteria-defined borderline personality d.
cumulative trauma d.
cutaneous psychogenic d.
cyclic mood d.
cyclic psychiatric d.
cyclothymic personality d.
debilitating mental d.
deep brain stimulation for mood d.
degenerative d.
delayed posttraumatic stress d.
delirium-related mental d.
delusional paranoid d.
dementia-related mental d.
demyelinating d.
dependence d.
dependent neurotic personality d.
dependent passive personality d.
depersonalization neurotic d.
depressed mood adjustment d.
depression neurotic d.
depression-related mental d.
depressive-dysphoric personality d.
depressive d., NOS
depressive spectrum d. (DSD)
d. of desire
deteriorated affective d.
deteriorated bipolar d.
developmental arithmetic d.
developmental articulation d.
developmental coordination d.
developmental expressive writing d.
developmental language d.
developmental reading d.
Diagnostic and Statistical Manual of Mental D.'s (DSM)
digestive psychogenic d.
disconnection thought d.
disinhibited type of passive developmental d.
disintegrative d.
disorganized-type schizophrenic d.
displacement d.
disruptive behavior d.
dissociative identity d. (DID)
dissociative d., NOS (DDNOS)
dissociative trance d.
dissociative-type neurotic hysterical d.
dream anxiety d.

NOTES

disorder *(continued)*
drug dependence d.
drug-induced mental d.
drug-related d.
d. due to combined factors
dyscontrol d.
dysmorphic somatoform d.
dysphoric personality d.
dyspneic psychogenic d.
dyssocial personality d.
dysthymic d. (DD)
dysthymic neurotic d.
early childhood behavioral d.
early trauma hypothesis of autistic d.
eating d.
eating d.'s, NOS (EDNOS)
ejaculation d.
electroconvulsive therapy-induced mood d.
elimination d.
emaciation d.
emancipation d.
emancipatory d.
emotional d. (ED)
emotional disturbance adjustment d.
emotional dyscontrol d.
emotional instability personality d.
emotionally based d.
emotionally unstable character d. (EUCD)
d. of empathy
endocrine psychogenic d.
endogenous affective d.
environmental sleep d.
epileptic d.
epileptoid personality d.
episodic affective d.
episodic behavior d.
erectile arousal d.
erotomanic d.
erotomanic-type delusional d.
esophagus psychogenic d.
evidence of dissociation d.
d. of excessive sleepiness
d. of excessive somnolence (DOES)
experimental d.
explosive neurotic personality d.
expressive language development d.
expressive writing development d.
extractive d.
extrapyramidal d.
d.'s of extreme stress, not otherwise specified (DESNOS)
eye psychogenic d.
factitious d., combined type
factitious dissociative identity d.
factitious interface d.
factitious d., physical type
factitious d., psychological type
factitious-type neurotic hysteric d.
false role d.
familial bipolar mood d.
familial hormonal d.
familial pediatric bipolar d.
fantasy and dissociative d.
feeding and eating d.
feeding psychogenic d.
female hypoactive sexual desire d.
female orgasmic d.
female sexual arousal d.
fluency d.
food intake d.
formal thought d.
French classification for child and adolescent mental d.'s
Freud view of depressive d.
frontal perceptual d.
functional psychogenic d.
functional voice d.
gait d.
gambling d.
gastric psychogenic d.
gastroesophageal reflux d. (GERD)
gastrointestinal functional psychogenic d.
gender identity d. (GID)
generalized anxiety d. (GAD)
genetic d.
genitourinary psychogenic d.
geriatric depressive d.
grandiose-type delusional d.
grandiose-type paranoid d.
group-type conduct d.
habit d.
hallucinogen affective d.
hallucinogen delusional d.
hallucinogen-induced delirium and anxiety d.
hallucinogen persisting perception d.
hallucinogen-related d., NOS
hallucinogen use d.
Hartnup d.
heart psychogenic d.
hereditary d.
heterogenous d.
histrionic neurotic personality d.
homosexual conflict d.
hospital-treated mental d.
Hyogo Institute for Aging Brain and Cognitive D.'s
hyperactive impulse attention deficit d.
hyperactivity d.
hyperkinetic conduct d.
hyperkinetic impulse d.
hypersomnia d.

hypersomnia-type sleep d.
hypersomnolence d.
hyperthymic personality d.
hypnosis and dissociative d.
hypnotic-dependent sleep d.
hypnotic-induced d.
hypnotic use d.
hypoactive sexual desire d.
hypochondriacal psychogenic d.
hypochondriasis neurotic d.
hypomanic d.
hypothermic d.
hypothymic personality d.
hysteria neurotic d.
hysterical gait d.
hysterical movement d.
hysterical personality d.
hysterical psychogenic d.
hysterical psychomotor d.
iatrogenic d.
identity d.
imitative dissociative identity d.
immature personality d.
impulse control d. (ICD)
d. of impulse control
impulse control conduct d.
inadequate personality d.
inattentive-type attention deficit hyperactivity d.
induced anxiety d.
induced delusional d.
induced mood d.
induced paranoid d.
induced persisting amnestic d.
induced psychotic d.
induced sleep d.
d. of infancy, childhood, or adolescence
inhalant-induced d.
inhalant-related d.
inhalant use d.
d. inheritability
inhibited-type reactive attachment d. of infancy or early childhood
d.'s of initiating and maintaining sleep (DIMS)
insomnia related to another mental d.
insomnia-type substance-induced sleep d.
intelligence d.
intermittent explosive d.
international classification of sleep d.'s
Internet addiction d.
intersensory d.
intersexual d.
intestinal psychogenic d.
intracranial d.
introverted personality d.
intrusive sexual d.
isolated explosive d.
Jacobson view of depressive d.
jealous-type delusional d.
jealous-type paranoid d.
jet lag sleep d.
joint psychogenic d.
Klein view of depressive d.
labile personality d.
labyrinthine d.
language developmental delay d.
language and speech d.
late luteal phase dysphoric d.
later reading d.
learning development d.
learning psychogenic d.
less pervasive d.
lifelong personality d.
lifetime anxiety d.
light therapy-induced mood d.
limbic system d.
limb psychogenic d.
low back pain psychogenic d.
low-grade thought d.
lymphatic psychogenic d.
major affective d.
major depressive d. (MDD)
major mood d.
major psychiatric d.
male erectile d.
male hypoactive sexual desire d.
male orgasmic d.
malingered dissociative identity d.
malingering d.
manic bipolar d.
manic-depressive d.
marijuana delusional d.
masochistic personality d.
mathematics d.
medication-induced d.
memory d.
menstrual psychogenic d.
mental psychoneurotic d.
mental subnormality d.
metabolic d.

NOTES

disorder *(continued)*
micturition psychogenic d.
mild neurocognitive d.
minor depressive d.
mixed anxiety depression d. (MADD)
mixed developmental delay d.
mixed mood d.
mixed personality d.
mixed psychoneurotic d.
mixed receptive-expressive language d.
mixed specific developmental d.
mixed-type delusional d.
monoplegic psychogenic d.
mood-cyclic d.
mood spectrum d.
moral deficiency personality d.
motility d.
motor psychogenic d.
motor skills d.
motor tic d.
motor-verbal tic d.
motor-vocal tic d.
movement d.
multiple-personality d. (MPD)
muscle psychogenic d.
musculoskeletal psychogenic d.
narcissistic neurotic personality d.
narcissistic personality d. (NPD)
negativistic personality d.
neurasthenia neurotic d.
neurocirculatory psychogenic d.
neurocognitive d.
neurodevelopmental d.
neuroleptic-induced acute movement d.
neuroleptic treatment of childhood conduct d.
neurologic d.
neuropsychiatric movement d.
neuropsychologic d.
neuropsychological d.
neurotic hysteric d.
neurotic mental d.
neurotic personality d.
nicotine-induced d.
nicotine organic brain d.
nicotine-related d., NOS
nicotine use d.
nightmare d.
nocturnal fragmentation d.
nocturnal sleep-related eating d.
nonaggressive-type undersocialized conduct d.
nonfearful panic d.
nonorganic steep d.
nonpsychotic mental d.
nonpsychotic psychiatric d.
nonstress-induced personality d.
nonsubstance-induced mental d.
non-tic-related obsessive-compulsive d.
nontranssexual cross-gender d.
no trauma personality d.
nutritional deficiency d.
obsessional personality d.
obsessive-compulsive d. (OCD)
obsessive-compulsive neurotic d.
obsessive-compulsive personality d. (OCPD)
obsessive personality d.
obsessive psychogenic d.
occupational neurotic d.
occupational psychogenic d.
OCD spectrum d.
operational checklist for psychotic d.'s
opioid-induced psychotic d.
opioid use d.
oppositional d.
oppositional defiant d. (ODD)
oppression artifact d.
organic anxiety d.
organic brain d. (OBD)
organic delusional d.
organic mental d. (OMD)
organic mood d.
organic personality d.
organic psychiatric d.
orgasmic d.
orientation d.
other type personality d.
overanxious d.
overconscientious personality d.
overreactive d.
over-the-counter drug-related d.
pain d.
panic d. (PD)
paralytic psychosomatic d.
paranoid neurotic personality d.
paranoid-schizotypal personality d.
paranoid-type schizophrenic d.
paraphiliac coercive d.
parasomnia-type substance-induced sleep d.
passive-aggressive neurotic personality d.
past lifetime d.
pathologic gambling d. (PGD)
pathologic grooming d.
PCP-induced anxiety d.
PCP-related d., NOS
pediatric bipolar d. (PBPD)
perception d.
perceptual d.
periluteal phase dysphoric d.
periodic limb movement d.

permissive hypothesis of affective d.
persecutory delusional d.
persecutory-type delusional d.
persecutory-type paranoid d.
persistent vegetative state d.
persisting perception d.
personality d. (PD)
personality change d.
personality neurotic d.
pervasive anger d.
pervasive developmental d. (PDD)
pervasive disinhibited type developmental d.
phencyclidine delusional d.
phencyclidine-induced d.
phencyclidine-related d.
phencyclidine use d.
phobic neurotic d.
phobic psychogenic d.
phonological d.
physical comorbid d.
physical psychogenic d.
pica d.
polysubstance-related d.
polysubstance use d.
positive thought d.
possession trance d.
postconcussion d.
posthallucinogen perception d.
postpsychotic depressive d.
posttraumatic dissociative d.
posttraumatic personality d.
posttraumatic stress d. (PTSD)
preexisting mental d.
preexisting seizure d.
premenstrual dysphoric d. (PMDD)
prescription drug-related d.
presenile mental d.
primary affective d. (PAD)
primary anxiety d.
primary behavior d.
primary care evaluation of mental d. (PRIME-MD)
primary mood d.
primary psychiatric d.
primary sleep d.
primary thought d.
processing d.
prolonged posttraumatic stress d.
pruritic psychosomatic d.
pseudosocial personality d.
psychiatric comorbid d.
psychiatric system interface d.
psychic d.
psychoactive substance abuse d.
psychoactive substance-induced organic mental d.
psychoactive substance use d. (PSUD)
psychoaffective d. (PAD)
psychogenic learning d.
psychogenic limb d.
psychogenic motor d.
psychogenic muscle d.
psychogenic musculoskeletal d.
psychogenic neurocirculatory d.
psychogenic obsessional d.
psychogenic pain d.
psychogenic phobic d.
psychogenic respiratory d.
psychogenic rheumatic d.
psychogenic sexual d.
psychogenic skin d.
psychogenic sleep d.
psychogenic stomach d.
psychomotor d.
psychoneurotic mental d.
psychophysiologic d.
psychosexual gender identity d.
psychosomatic paralytic d.
psychosomatic pruritic d.
psychosomatic skin d.
psychotic d., NOS
psychotic presenile d.
pyromania d.
Rado view of depressive d.
rapid cycling bipolar d.
reactive attachment d.
reading developmental delay d.
receptive language d.
rectal psychogenic d.
recurrent brief depressive d.
recurrent mood d.
Reitan rules to assess learning d.
related sleep d.
REM behavior d. (RBD)
REM sleep behavior d.
REM sleep-related d.
repetitive impulse d.
residual-type schizophrenic d.
resistant mood d.
resonance d.
respiratory impairment sleep d.
respiratory psychogenic d.
retardation developmental delay d.

NOTES

disorder *(continued)*
Rett d.
rheumatic psychogenic d.
rhythmic movement d.
rumination d.
sadistic personality d.
sadomasochistic personality d.
Sandler view of depressive d.
schizoaffective d.
schizoid neurotic personality d.
schizoid-schizotypal personality d. (SSPD)
schizophrenia spectrum d.
schizophrenic d.
schizophreniform d.
schizotypal personality d.
seasonal affective d. (SAD)
seasonal mood d.
secondary mood d.
secondary sleep d.
sedative-, hypnotic-, or anxiolytic-induced anxiety d.
sedative-induced d.
sedative use d.
seductive personality d.
self-defeating personality d.
self-perceived cognitive d.
Seligman view of depressive d.
semantic pragmatic d.
semantogenic d.
senile psychotic mental d.
separation anxiety d. (SAD)
sexual arousal d.
sexual aversion d.
sexual desire d.
sexual deviance d.
sexual deviation neurotic d.
sexual and gender identity d.
sexual pain d.
sexual psychogenic d.
sham d.
shamanistic thought d.
shared paranoid d.
shared psychotic d.
shift work-related sleep d.
shyness d.
simple deteriorative d.
situational-type female orgasmic d.
situational-type female sexual arousal d.
skin psychogenic d.
sleep-associated movement d.
sleep behavior d.
sleep psychogenic d.
sleep starts d.
sleeptalking d.
sleep terror d.
sleep-wake schedule d.
sleep-wake transition d.
sleepwalking d.
social anxiety d.
socialized conduct d.
sociopathic personality d. (SPD)
solitary aggressive-type conduct d.
somatic paranoid d.
somatization neurotic d.
somatizing d.
somatoform interface d.
somatoform pain d. (SPD)
somatopsychic d.
specific developmental d. (SDD)
spectrum d.
speech developmental delay d.
speech and language d.
spoken language d.
stereotyped movement d.
stereotypic movement d. (SMD)
stereotypy and habit d.
steroid-induced mood d.
stimulant-dependent sleep d.
stress d.
stress-induced personality d.
stress-related d.
subaffective d.
substance abuse d.
substance dependence d.
substance-induced organic mental d.
substance-induced psychotic d.
substance-related d.
substance use d. (SUD)
substitution d.
subsyndromal thought d.
sympathomimetic delusional d.
tactile-perceptual d.
taxonomy of anger d.
temporal-perceptual d.
temporary personality d.
The Systematic Treatment Enhancement Program for Bipolar D.
thinking d.
thought d.
thyroid d.
tic d.
tic-related obsessive-compulsive d.
time and rhythm d.
tobacco use d.
Tourette d.
toxic d.
trance-possession d.
transient situational personality d.
transient tic d.
trauma spectrum d.
unaggressive conduct d.
underachievement d.
undersocialized d.
undifferentiated attention-deficit d.
undifferentiated somatoform d.

undifferentiated-type conduct d.
undifferentiated-type schizophrenic d.
unhappiness and misery d.
unipolar d.
unitary d.
unknown substance-induced mood d.
unsocialized aggressive d.
unspecified mental d.
violent conduct d.
Virginia Adult Twin Study of Psychiatric and Substance Use D.'s
visceral d.
visuospatial d.
vocal, chronic motor, or tic d.
voice d.
walking d.
well-delineated psychiatric d.
withdrawal d.
withdrawal-related mood d.
writing d.
d. of written expression

disordered
d. mentally
d. mental status
d. personality function
d. relating
d. thinking

disorderly
d. conduct
drunk and d.

disorganization
autonomic d.
cerebral d.
cognitive d.
conceptual d.
developing psychotic d.
d. dimension
d. dimension of positive schizophrenic symptoms
linguistic d.
mental d.
psychotic d.
spatial d.
d. syndrome
thought d.

disorganized
d. attachment behavior
d. delusion
d. factor
d. factor in schizophrenia
d. form of attachment
d. schizophrenia
d. speech
d. speech assessment
d. speech in schizophrenia
d. state
d. subtype
d. symptom complex
d. thinking
d. thought process

disorganized-type
d.-t. schizophrenia
d.-t. schizophrenic disorder

disorient

disorientation
auditory d.
autopsychic d.
graphic d.
posttraumatic d.
right-left d.
spatial d.
speech d.
thought d.
time d.
topographical d.
visuospatial d.

disoriented
d. attachment behavior
d. form of attachment
d. patient

disown

disparage

disparaging remark

disparity
phase d.
vision d.

dispassionate concern

dispel

dispensation

disperse

dispersion
response d.

dispirited

displaceability of libido

displaced
d. child syndrome
d. person

displacement
activity d.
affect d.
brainstem d.
character d.
d. defense mechanism

NOTES

D

displacement *(continued)*
d. disorder
dream d.
geographic d.
guilt d.
retroactive d.
d. substitute
symbolic d.
d. wit
display
affect d.
emotional d.
facial d.
temper d.
displease
displeasure
disposition
constitutional depressive d.
constitutional manic d.
personal d.
placid d.
polymorphous perverse d.
d. system
volatile d.
dispositional coping style
dispraise
disproportion
disproportionate impairment
disprove
disputatious
dispute
custody d.
disputing
disqualify
disquiet
disquietude
patient d.
disregard
pervasive pattern of d.
d. for rules
disreputable
disrepute
disrespect
act of d.
disrespectful treatment
disrobing
inappropriate d.
public d.
disrupt
disrupted
d., dysfunctional relational functioning
d. parenting
d. relationship
d. sleep organization
disruption
d. of affective bonds
behavior d.
brain function d.
cognitive d.
family d.
level of d.
marital d.
d. of normal activity
sleep d.
d. of thought process
disruptive
d. behavior
d. behavior disorder
d. emotion
d. family functioning
d. impact
d. psychotic patient
d. verbal threat
dissatisfaction
body d.
marital d.
perceived life d.
dissectible cognitive operation
dissemble
disseminata
alopecia d.
disseminate
dissemination
evaluation d.
dissension
dissent
disservice
dissidence
dissident
dissimilar
dissimilation rule
dissimulation
dissimulator
dissipate
dissipation
heat d.
dissociable
dissociate
dissociated
d. learning
d. sensory loss
d. state
dissociate-dysmnesic substitution reaction
dissociation, disassociation
adult d.
d. defense mechanism
double d.
d. of learning
d. level
d. measure
nonpathological d.
pathological d.
peritraumatic d.
psychological d.
semantic d.
d. sensibility
sensory d.

sleep d.
somatoform d.
d. syndrome
visual-kinetic d.

dissociative
d. amnesia
d. anesthesia
d. anesthetic
d. capacity
d. disorder, NOS (DDNOS)
d. experience
d. flashback episode
d. fugue
d. hysteria
d. hysteria psychoneurosis
d. identity disorder (DID)
d. paranoia
d. patient
d. phenomenon
d. psychoneurosis
d. psychoneurotic reaction
d. response
d. state
d. symptom
d. symptom cluster
d. tendency
d. trance
d. trance disorder

dissociative-type
d.-t. hysterical neurosis
d.-t. neurotic hysteria
d.-t. neurotic hysterical disorder

dissolute

dissolution

dissonance
cognitive d.

dissonant

dissuade

dissuasive

distal distinctive feature analysis

distance
d. ceptor
emotional d.
functional d.
optimal interpersonal d.
d. perception
professional d.
d. receptor
social d.
sociometric d.

distancing
cognitive d.
comprehensive d.

distant
emotionally d.

distasteful

distension

distinct
d. depressed presentation
d. dysphoric presentation
d. euphoric presentation

distinction
primary-secondary d.

distinctive feature analysis

distingue

distinguish

distort

distorted
d. body image
d. communication in schizophrenia
d. grief
d. ideas of reference
d. inferential thinking
d. language in schizophrenia
d. perception
d. perception of reality

distortion
apperceptive d.
auditory d.
body image d.
cognitive d.
compromise d.
ego d.
figure-ground d.
inferential behavioral monitoring d.
d. of inferential behavioral monitoring
inferential perception d.
d. of inferential thinking
d. of interpretation
intrapsychic d.
language and communication d.
memory d.
metonymic d.
nonlinear d.
paratactic d.
parataxic d.
perceptual d.
psychological d.
psychotic d.
reality d.
sensorium d.
social avoidance and d.
spatial d.
subjective d.
time d.

NOTES

distortion *(continued)*
transient d.
visual d.
visuospatial d.
distract
easy to d.
distracted easily
distractibility
easy d.
distractible speech
distracting
d. spouse behavior
d. stimuli
distraction
pleasurable d.
distraught
d. former lover
d. former partner
d. spouse
distress
abdominal d.
acute d.
caregiver d.
chronic mental d.
clinically significant d.
elevated psychological d.
emotional d.
event-related d.
general psychological d.
global index of d.
intense psychological d.
intrapsychic d.
d. level
menopausal d.
mental d.
obvious d.
physical symptom d.
posttraumatic d.
present d.
psychic d.
psychological d.
separation d.
sexual orientation d.
social avoidance and d. (SAD)
spiritual d.
subjective d.
d. tolerance
d. tolerance skill
unconscious d.
distressed personality
distressing
d. circumstance
d. dream
d. thought
distributed
d. effort
d. memory
d. processing
distribution
bimodal d.
binomial d.
contrastive d.
d. of control
d. curve
fixed d.
frequency d.
gaussian d.
illicit drug d.
noncontrastive d.
normal d.
Poisson d.
d. of power
regional d.
d. of responsibility
skew d.
unequal d.
distributive
d. analysis
d. analysis and synthesis
district
red-light d.
distrust
chronic d.
interpersonal d.
malevolent d.
pervasive d.
distrustful
disturbance
acid-base d.
activity and attention d.
acute situational d.
adjustment reaction d.
affective d.
amphetamine intoxication with perceptual d.
analyzing new information d.
anxiety d.
aphasic d.
appetite d.
assimilating information d.
d. associated with conversion phenomenon
d. associated with organic mental disease
d. of attention
attentional d.
behavioral d.
d. of behavioral activation
behavioral set of d.'s
d. between clauses
body conceptualization d.
body-image d.
cannabis intoxication with perceptual d.
chronic sleep d.
cocaine intoxication with perceptual d.

cognitive d.
cognitive-perceptual d.
compulsive d.
concentration d.
conceptual d.
conduct d.
consciousness d.
d. in content of thought
core cognitive d.
domestic d.
eating d.
electrolyte d.
emotional d.
executive functioning d.
explosive d.
fluctuating mood d.
fluency d.
fluid d.
d. in form of thinking
frequency d.
functioning d.
gait d.
gastrointestinal d.
habit d.
high-level perceptual d.
hyperkinetic d.
identity d.
infancy and early childhood d.
d. of intellectual development
intermittent explosive d.
isolated explosive d.
language d.
learning new information d.
level of d.
linguistic d.
memory d.
d. of memory
menstrual d.
mental d.
metabolic d.
mild sleep d.
mood d.
motor skill d.
occipital metabolic d.
oculomotor d.
perception d.
perceptual d.
d. in perceptual motor ability
personality pattern d.
personality trait d.
phencyclidine intoxication with perceptual d.
physical d.
planning d.
posttraumatic d.
predominant mood d.
psychiatric d.
psychic d.
psychographic d.
psychological d.
psychomotor d.
psychotic d.
rate of fluency d.
reasoning d.
recalling new information d.
d. of recognition
sensory d.
d. in sexual desire
sexual orientation d.
significant sleep d.
situational d.
sleep continuity d.
socialized d.
social relatedness d.
sociopathic personality d. (SPD)
speech d.
speed of information processing d.
SSRI-induced sexual d.
stress-related d.
d. in suggestibility
superego d.
thought d.
transient emotional d.
transient situational d.
undersocialized socialized d.
visual field d.
will d.
d. of the will
d. within clauses
word-finding ability d.

disturbed

d. adolescent
d. attachment relationship
d. eating behavior
emotionally d. (ED)
d. home environment
d. interpersonal relationship (DIR)
d. orientation
d. person
d. personality
d. sense of self
d. sleep
d. sleep pattern
d. social relatedness
d. ward

NOTES

disturbing
d. behavior
d. experience
d. feeling
d. thought
disturb the peace
disunite
disunity
disuse principle
disutility
disvalue
dither
diuretic misuse
diurnal
d. enuresis
d. epilepsy
d. mood variation
diurnus
pavor d.
divagate
divagation
diverge
divergence circuit
divergent
d. production
d. thinking
diverging trend
diverse
d. group
d. medicinal application
d. need
diversion
diversional therapy
diversionary
d. activity
d. tactic
diversity
cultural d.
group d.
sensitivity to d.
diversive exploration
divest
divided attention
divination
diving reflex
division
divisive
divorce
community d.
coparental d.
d. counseling
d. decree
economic d.
emotional consequences of d.
legal d.
overt behavior consequence of d.
parental d.
psychic d.
d. rate
d. status
stressful d.
d. therapy
divorcee
divulge
divulsion
dixyrazine
dizygotic twins
dizziness
dizzy spell
DKA
diabetic ketoacidosis
olanzapine-associated DKA
DKEFS
Delis-Kaplan executive function system
DLB
dementia with Lewy bodies
DLP
developmental learning problem
DMH
Department of Mental Health
DMT
dimethyltryptamine
DNA
deoxyribonucleic acid
DNA damage
genomic DNA
DNA transcription factor
DNR
do not resuscitate
do
do not resuscitate (DNR)
tae kwon do
DOB
2,5-dimethoxy-4-methylamphetamine
d'Ocagne nomogram
docile
docility
docket
doctor-patient relationship
Doctors Without Borders
doctrine
dualistic d.
Flourens d.
neuron d.
parental right d.
documentation
confidential d.
doddering
dodger
doer
DOES
disorder of excessive somnolence
dog
guide d.
d. track gambling
dog-eat-dog attitude
dogged
dogma

dogmatic
do-gooder
doing
 learning by d.
doldrums
doleful
Dole-Nyswauder program
doll's
 d. eye reaction
 d. eye reflex
 d. eye sign
dolor capitis
dolore
dolorific
dolorimetry
dolorogenic zone
dolorology
dolorosa
 analgesia d.
 anesthesia d.
 facies d.
dolorous
domain
 adaptive skill d.
 cognitive d.
 death d.
 developmental d.
 d. of functioning
 neuropsychologic d.
 outcome d.
 spiritual d.
dome
 double d.
domestic
 d. aggression
 d. disturbance
 d. environment
 d. fight
 d. medicine
 d. partner abuse
 d. quarrel
 d. violence (DV)
domesticated pride
domicile
domiciliary care home
dominance
 cerebral d.
 crossed d.
 eye d.
 feeling of d.
 d. hierarchy
 lateral d.
 left hemisphere d.
 manual d.
 mixed cerebral d.
 right hemisphere d.
 social d.
 territorial d.
 theory of social d.
 time d.
 X-linked d.
dominant
 d. association
 autosomal d.
 bystander dominates initial d. (BDID)
 d. character
 d. characteristic
 d. culture
 d. delusional belief
 d. determinant
 d. feature
 d. gene
 d. genotype
 d. hand
 d. hemisphere
 d. hemisphere parietal area
 d. hemisphere temporal area
 d. idea
 d. language
 d. laterality
 left-hand d.
 d. mentality
 mixed-foot d.
 d. person
 d. personality
 right-hand d.
 d. spouse
 d. trait
 d. waking frequency
dominantly inherited
dominant-subordinate behavior
dominate
domination
 sexual d.
 d. and submission
dominatrix
domineering
Don
 D. Juan
 D. Juan behavior
 D. Juan dress
 D. Juanism
 D. Juan syndrome
 D. Juan type
 D. Quixote

D

NOTES

Donaldson
O'Connor vs D.
donation
organ d.
donna
prima d.
do-not-care attitude
do-nothing
doom
feeling of d.
impending d.
sense of impending d.
doomsayer
doomsday
door
revolving d.
d. slamming
door-in-the-face effect
dopaminergic
d. antagonist
d. drug
d. effect
d. hyperactivity
d. inhibition
d. medication-induced postural tremor
d. modulation
d. pathway
d. stimulant
d. synapse
d. system
d. tone
d. tract
dope dealer
Doppelganger phenomenon
Doppler shift
Dora case
doramania
Dorian love
d'orient
mal d.
dormant
dormido
sangue d.
dormifacient
dormitory
doromania
dorsal
d. anterior cingulate region
d. column stimulation
d. gray matter
d. limbic region
d. neocortical region
d. raphe nucleus
d. reflex
d. vagus complex
dorsolateral
d. pathway
d. prefrontal cortex
dosage
equivalent d.
medication d.
neuroleptic d.
total neuroleptic d.
dose
anticholinergic d.
clinically recommended d.
cumulative d.
daily d.
d. dependent
effective d.
d. escalation
full d.
improper d.
lethal d. (LD)
lithium d.
low d.
maintenance d.
marginally therapeutic d.
maximum permissible d.
maximum recommended human d. (MRHD)
measured d.
minimum d.
missed d.
modal d.
neuroleptic d.
optimum d.
oral d.
permissible d.
priming d.
d. range
recommended d.
d. reduction
d. reduction method
sequential d.
standard d.
steady-state d.
subtherapeutic d.
therapeutic d.
d. titration
tolerance d.
toxic d.
dose-dependent
d.-d. effect
d.-d. seizure
dose-reduction strategy
dose-related difference
dose-response
d.-r. curve
d.-r. relation
d.-r. relationship
dosimetric medicine
dosing
energy d.
fixed d.
flexible neuroleptic d.

neuroleptic d.
set-by-age d.

dotage

dote

dot-probe task

double

d. agentry
d. assimilation
d. bind
d. bind theory of schizophrenia
d. blind
d. consciousness
delusion of d.'s
d. depression
d. dissociation
d. dome
d. entendre
d. hemiplegia
illusion of d.'s
d. insanity
d. meaning
d. orientation
d. personality
d. simultaneous stimulation (DSS)
d. standard
subjective d.'s
d. superego
d. take
d. taper
d. vision

doublé

délire d.

double-agentry

double-blind

d.-b. drug study
d.-b. experiment
d.-b. study
d.-b. theory

double-cross

double-dealing

double-edged

double-faced

double-masked experiment

double-point threshold

doublespeak

doublethink

doubling

doubly

doubt

irrational d.
d. of loyalty
morbid d.
obsessive d.
d.'s of trustworthiness

doubtful

doubting

d. insanity
d. mania
d. spell

douce

mort d.

doughty

dour

doute

folie du d.
maladie du d.

douze

folie á d.

dowdy

down

back d.
dress d.
d. from overdose
gunned d.
let d.
simmer d.
slap d.
stare d.
take d.
talk d.
tear d.
ups and d.'s
wear d.
weigh d.

down-and-out

downbeat nystagmus

downcast gaze

downfall

downgrade

downhearted

downhill

downplay

down-regulated

downright

downsizing

down-the-line

down-to-earth

downtrodden

downturned corners of the mouth

downward

d. drift
d. drift hypothesis

DPJ

dementia paralytica juvenilis

NOTES

DPM
diploma in psychological medicine
DPP
dropout prediction and prevention
DPT
dipropyltryptamine
dr
unusual rare detail response
drab
DRADA
Depression and Related Affective Disorders Association
draft
Dragons
Dungeons and D.
dramatic
d. affect
d. behavioral swing
d. emotional cluster
emotionally d.
d. interpersonal relationship
d. interpersonal style
d. play
d. speech
verbally d.
dramatism
dramatization
dramatize
DRAMS
drug risk analysis message system
drapetomania
drastic
drawback
drawing
d. ability
automatic d.
clock d.
compulsive d.
copying d. (CD)
d. disability
mirror d.
spontaneous d.
d. task
drawl
drawn laughter
DRD4
D. Exon II polymorphism
D. gene
dread
feeling of d.
d. of insanity
talion d.
dreaded situation
dream
anxiety d.
d. anxiety attack
d. anxiety disorder
artificial d.
d. association
bad d.
d. censorship
clairvoyant d.
color in d.
comfort d.
consolation d.
d. content
convalescent d.
convenience d.
corroborating d.
counter-wish d.
decomposition in d.'s
detailed d.
d. determinant
d. displacement
distressing d.
dream within a d.
d. ego
d. embarrassment
erotic d.
examination d.
exhibition d.
d. experience
d. exploration
Freud theory of d.'s
frightening d.
frustration d.
d. function
d. illusion
d. induction
d. interpretation
made-to-order d.
manifest d.
masochistic wish d.
d. pain
paired d.'s
parallel d.
perennial d.
pipe d.
prophetic d.
punishment d.
d. recall
reconstruction d.
recurrent distressing d.
recurring d.
d. regression
d. screen
secondary elaboration of d.
Sisyphus d.
speech in d.
d. state
d. stimulus
d. symbolism
telepathic d.
terror d.
d. time
unpleasant d.
d. up
veridical d.

vivid d.
wet d.
wish d.
d. work
d. world

dreamer

dreaming
amnesia for sleep and d.

dreamland

dreamless sleep

dreamlike
d. hallucination
d. state

dream-work

dreamy state

dreary

D_4-receptor antagonist

dredge

dress
Don Juan d.
d. down

dressing
d. apraxia
careless d.
inappropriate d.
unusual d.

Drexel Tour of London

drift
downward d.
genetic d.
d. hypothesis
observer d.

drifter

drink
malternative d.
mixed d.
d.'s per drinking day

drinker
binge d.
chronic d.
closet d.
compulsive d.
evening d.
incurable problem d. (IPD)
jag d.
periodic d.
problem d. (PD)
repeated heavy d.
social d.
weekend d.

drinkers' checkup

drinking
aftereffect of d.
air d.
alcohol d.
d. behavior
binge d.
compulsive water d.
controlled d.
days of heavy d.
d. days per week
dyssocial d.
early-onset d.
escape d.
d. history
inveterate d.
jag d.
light d.
morning d.
nonproblematic d.
occupational d.
paroxysmal d.
periodic d.
problem d.
recreational d.
social d.
somatopathic d.
state marker of heavy d.
volitional d.
water d.
weekend d.

drive
absent d.
achievement d.
acquired d.
activity d.
affectional d.
affiliation d.
aggressive d.
appetitive d.
aversive d.
d. behavior
biologic d.
destructive d.
ego d.
elimination d.
erotic d.
exploration d.
exploratory d.
fear d.
hedonic d.
homonomy d.
hunger d.
innate d.
instinctual d.
internal d.

NOTES

drive *(continued)*
kinetic d.
learned d.
libidinal d.
manipulative d.
maternal d.
obstruction d.
paternal d.
physiologic d.
physiologic d.
primary d.
primitive d.
d. reduction
d. reduction theory
repressed instinctual d.
secondary d.
sex d.
stimulus d. (Sd)
subjective d.
thermal d.
thirst d.
drive-by shooting
drivel
driveling dementia
driven
d. motor behavior
treatment d.
drivenness
driver
drunk d.
slave d.
driving
behavior while d.
erratic d.
photic d.
reckless d.
d. under influence (DUI)
d. while intoxicated (DWI)
DRO
differential reinforcement of other behavior
droit
droll
dromolepsy
dromomania
drone
droning speech
drool
drooping eyelid
drop
d. attack
foot d.
knockout d.'s
toe d.
wrist d.
dropout
d. prediction and prevention (DPP)
d. rate
school d.
treatment d.
drowsiness
cannabis-induced d.
continuous daytime d.
daytime d.
incapacitating d.
pathologic d.
drowsy
DRSP
daily record of severity of problems
drub
drubbing
drudge
drudgery
drug
d. abreaction
abreactive d.
d. absorption
d. abstinence
d. abuse
abuse of nonprescribed d.
d. abuser
d. abuse rehabilitation program
d. abuse resistance education (DARE)
D. Abuse Warning Network (DAWN)
d. action
d. addict
d. addiction
addictive potential of d.
add-on d.
d. administration
d. allergy
alpha adrenergic-blocking d.
alpha adrenergic-stimulating d.
antagonist d.
antianxiety d.
anticholinergic d.
anticonvulsant d.
antidepressant d.
antiepileptic d.
antipsychotic d.
antiseizure d.
anxiolytic d.
d. assay
ataractic d.
atypical antipsychotic d.
d. augmentation
autonomic sympathomimetic d.
beta adrenergic-blocking d.
d. binge
butyrophenone-based neuroleptic d.
caffeine-containing d.
club d.
combination d. (CD)
d. concentration variability
d. consumption

conventional antipsychotic d.
conventional neuroleptic d.
d. counseling
d. counselor
d. court program
d. craving
d. culture
dangerous d.
date rape d.
d. dealer
d. defaulter
d. dependence
d. dependence disorder
depot-administered antipsychotic d.
designer d.
d. desire
diet d.
d. discontinuation
d. disease
dopaminergic d.
d. effect
d. efficacy
D. Enforcement Administration (DEA)
D. Enforcement Administration number (DEA#)
experimental d.
d. family
gateway d.
d. habit
d. half-life
hallucinatory d.
hallucinogenic d.
heterocyclic antidepressant d.
high-dose d.
d. holiday
d. hunger
hypnotic d.
hypnotic-sedative d.
illegal d.
illicit psychoactive d.
d. information (DI)
d. information center (DIC)
d. information log (DIL)
d. ingestion
inhalation of d.
injectable d.
d. insanity
d. interaction (DI)
d. intervention
d. intolerance
d. intoxication
intravenous d.
investigational new d. (IND)
legal d.
d. level
maintenance d.
d. maintenance treatment
d. management
mind-altering d.
mood-altering d.
mood-elevating d.
mood-stabilizing d.
narcotic agonist d.
narcotic antagonist d.
narcotic-blocking d.
neuroleptic d.
new-generation antipsychotic d.
nonprescription d.
nonpsychotropic d.
noradrenergic d.
nosotropic d.
novel antipsychotic d.
orphan d.
d. overdose
d. overdose death
d. paraphernalia
parasympathomimetic d.
parenteral d.
d. possession
d. preparation
prescription d.
psychoactive d.
psychodysleptic d.
psychogenic d.
d. psychosis
d. psychosis hallucinatory state
psychostimulant d.
psychotherapeutic d.
psychotomimetic d.
psychotropic d. (PTD)
rave d.
recreational d.
d. regimen
d. reinforcement
d. related
d. response rate
d. risk analysis message system (DRAMS)
d. risk behavior
schedule d.
d. screen
second-generation antipsychotic d.
sedative d.
sedative-hypnotic d.

NOTES

drug *(continued)*
self-administration of psychoactive d. (SAPD)
d. smoke
d. snorting
street d.
d. supply
sympathomimetic d.
d. tapering
tertiary amine tricyclic antidepressant d.
d. tetanus
d. theft
d. therapy
d. tolerance
d. toxicity
d. trading
d. traffic
d. trafficking
d. transporter
tricyclic d.
tricyclic antidepressant d. (TCAD)
d. trip
unaltered d.
d. under investigation
d. use behavior
d. use forecasting (DUF)
d. use history
d. user
d. use review (DUR)
war on d.'s
d. washout
d. withdrawal
d. withdrawal seizure
d. withdrawal syndrome
wonder d.

drug-addictive behavior

drug-associated
d.-a. mortality
d.-a. weight gain

drug-containing capsule

drug-dependent
d.-d. individual
d.-d. insomnia

drug-drug interaction

drug-facilitated
d.-f. interview
d.-f. rape
d.-f. robbery
d.-f. sexual assault

drug-free
d.-f. condition
d.-f. day
d.-f. employee
d.-f. patient
d.-f. period
d.-f. program

drug-fueled music marathon

drug-induced
d.-i. agitation
d.-i. agranulocytosis
d.-i. confusional state
d.-i. convulsion
d.-i. delirium
d.-i. dementia
d.-i. depression
d.-i. dystonia
d.-i. encephalopathy
d.-i. floating sensation
d.-i. hallucination
d.-i. hallucinatory state
d.-i. hallucinosis
d.-i. high
d.-i. mania
d.-i. medical complication
d.-i. mental disorder
d.-i. negative symptom
d.-i. paranoid state
d.-i. psychosis
D.-I. Rape Prevention and Punishment Act
d.-i. seizure
d.-i. semihypnotic state
d.-i. sexual dysfunction
d.-i. syndrome
d.-i. treatment

drug-injecting equipment

drug-like desire state

drugmaker

drug-negative urine

drug-related
d.-r. brain damage
d.-r. crime
d.-r. cue
d.-r. disorder
d.-r. HIV risk behavior
d.-r. incarceration
d.-r. insomnia
d.-r. sexual side effect
d.-r. violence

drug-resistant depression

drug-responsive treatment

drug-seeking behavior

drug-specific intervention

drug-taking behavior

drug-using
d.-u. man
d.-u. woman

drum up

drunk
d. behavior
blind d.
d. and disorderly
d. driver
dry d.
legally d.

drunkard

drunken
drunkenness
acute d.
alcoholic d.
chronic d.
ether d.
maudlin d.
pathologic d.
public d.
simple alcoholic d.
sleep d.
sleeping d.
dry
d. drunk
d. leprosy
d. mouth
d. orgasm
d. out
d. up
DS
digit span
digit symbol
DSD
depression sine depression
depressive spectrum disorder
DSDB
direct self-destructive behavior
DSH
deliberate self-harm
DSM
Diagnostic and Statistical Manual of Mental Disorders
DSM clusters
DSM diagnosis
DSM disorder overlap
DSM-IV
Diagnostic and Statistical Manual of Mental Disorders, Fourth Edition
DSM-IV axis II criterion
DSM-IV description
DSM-IV-R
Diagnostic and Statistical Manual of Mental Disorders, Fourth Edition, Revised
DSM-IV-R classification
DSM-IV-TR
Diagnostic and Statistical Manual of Mental Disorders, Fourth Edition, Text Revision
DSM-IV-TR diagnostic grouping
DSS
double simultaneous stimulation
DSUH
direct suggestion under hypnosis
DT
delirium tremens
dipole tracing
duration tetany
DTC
day treatment center
DTI
Diffusion Tensor Imaging
DTR
deep tendon reflex
DTs
delirium tremens
dual
d. addictions
d. ambivalence
d. diagnosis
d. diagnosis patient
d. diagnosis program
d. leadership
d. mechanism of action
d. personality
d. purpose
d. relationship
d. reuptake inhibitor
d. transference therapy
dual-arousal model
dual-instinct theory
dualism
mind-body d.
psychic d.
dualistic doctrine
dual-process theory
dual-sex therapy
dub
dubiety
dubious
dubitable
Dubois method
Dubowitz syndrome
dud
duel
duende
due process
DUF
drug use forecasting
DUF program
DUI
driving under influence
dulcify
dull
d. affect

NOTES

dull *(continued)*
borderline d.
d. normal range
dullard
dullness
emotional d.
dumbfound
dumbness
word d.
dumbstruck
Dunedin Multidisciplinary Health and Development Study
Dungeons and Dragons
Dunnett-Hsu procedure
dupe
duplex transmission
duplicate
duplication
d. of ego
d. phenomenon
duplicative reaction
duplicity
DUR
drug use review
durable
d. power of attorney
d. power of attorney for healthcare
duration
current episode d.
d. of drug action
d. duty cycle
emergency dyscontrol d.
minimum d.
d. of mood
short sleep d.
sleep d.
d. tetany (DT)
treatment d.
d. of treatment
duress
episodic dyscontrol d.
Durham
D. decision
D. rule
Durkheim theory of suicide
dusky
Dutch courage
duteous
dutiful
duty
fiduciary d.
line of d.
neglect of d.
omission of d.
d. to warn
DV
domestic violence
dwarfism
psychosocial d.
DWI
driving while intoxicated
DWR
confabulated whole response
DX, Dx
diagnosis
dyad
mother-child d.
parent-child d.
parent-youth d.
sister-sister d.
social d.
dyadic
d. level
d. parent-child interaction coding system
d. psychotherapy
d. session
d. symbiosis
dybbuk
dying
adolescent attitude toward d.
death and d.
d. declaration
fear of d.
stages of death and d.
dynamic
adaptation d.
d. ambulatory balance
d. aphasia
attachment d.
behavior d.
d. demography
d. disease
d. equilibrium
family d.'s
d. formulation
group d.'s
hemispheric d.
infantile d.'s
intermediate hemispheric d.
lateral hemispheric d.
medial hemispheric d.
narcissistic d.
personality d.'s
d. personality
d. physical activity
power d.
d. principle
prominent narcissistic d.
d. psychiatry
d. psychology
d. psychotherapy
d. range
d. reasoning
religious d.
d. standing balance
temporal d.
d. variable

dynamica
alopecia d.
dynamism
lust d.
mental d.
dynamo
dynorphin
dysacusis
dysanagnosia
dysantigraphia
dysaphia
dysaphic
dysarthria
ataxic d.
dysarthric
d. behavior
d. speech
dysarthrosis
dysautonomia
central d.
familial d.
peripheral d.
dysautonomic
d. feature
d. illness
dysbasia, dysbasis
d. lordotica progressiva
dysbulia, dysboulia
dysbulic
dyscalculia
dyschezia
dyschronism
dyscoimesis
dyscontrol
affective d.
behavioral d.
descending d.
d. disorder
emergency d.
emotional d.
episodic d.
impulsive d.
instinctual d.
organic d.
seizure d.
temper d.
dyscrasia
blood d.
dyseneia
dysequilibrium state
dyserethism
dysergastic reaction
dysergia
dysesthesia
dysesthetic
dysexecutive syndrome
dysfunction
academic d.
acquired sexual d.
adult social d.
alcohol-induced sexual d.
amphetamine-induced sexual d.
anorectal physiological d.
antipsychotic-associated sexual d.
anxiolytic-induced sexual d.
arousal d.
attentional d.
atypical psychosexual d.
autonomic d.
behavioral d.
biologic d.
brain d.
brainstem d.
central processing d.
cerebral d.
childhood social d.
cocaine-induced sexual d.
cognitive d.
contralateral parietal lobe d.
daytime d.
depressive executive d. (DED)
diffuse brain d.
drug-induced sexual d.
educational d.
ejaculatory d.
emotional d.
endothelial d.
erectile d.
executive system d.
focal lateralized d.
frontal lobe d.
frontocortical d.
functional dyspareunia psychosexual d.
functional vaginismus psychosexual d.
generalized sexual d.
hemispherical d.
higher cerebral d. (HCD)
higher cortical d.
household d.
hypnotic-induced sexual d.
hypothalamic d.
hypothalamic-pituitary axis d.
immunologic d.
induced sexual d.

NOTES

dysfunction *(continued)*
inhibited female orgasm psychosexual d.
inhibited male orgasm psychosexual d.
inhibited sexual desire psychosexual d.
inhibited sexual excitement psychosexual d.
interpersonal d.
language d.
lateralized d.
lifelong sexual d.
lobar d.
lobe d.
male erectile d.
maternal d.
midbrain d.
minimal brain d. (MBD)
neurodevelopmental d.
neurologic d.
occupational d.
opioid-induced sexual d.
organic brain d.
orgasm d.
orgasmic d.
parental d.
parietal lobe d.
perceived maternal d.
perceived parental d.
perceptual motor d.
personality d.
posttraumatic cortical d.
premature ejaculation psychosexual d.
primary orgasmic d.
psychological d.
psychosexual d.
refractory erectile d.
school d.
secondary erectile d.
secondary orgasmic d.
self-care d.
sensory integration d. (SID)
severe diffuse brain d.
sexual d.
situational orgasmic d.
situational sexual d.
sleep d.
social d.
speech d.
SSRI-induced erectile d.
striatofrontal d.
substance-induced sexual d.
sympathetic d.
work d.

dysfunctional
d. alliance
d. behavior
d. circuitry
d. coexistence
d. cognition
d. core belief
d. dopamine system
d. family
d. family factor
d. family style
d. father
d. home life
d. mother
d. neural circuit
d. personality style
d. relational functioning
d. relationship
socially d.
d. thought record

dysgenesis
gonadal d.

dysgenic

dysgenitalism

dysgeusia

dysgnosia
auditory-verbal d.
body d.
number d.
visual letter d.
visual number d.

dysgonesis

dysgrammatism

dysgraphia

dysgraphicus
status d.

dysharmonica
diplacusis d.

dysidentity

dysjunction
personal d.

dyskinesia
biliary d.
disfluency d.
extrapyramidal d.
medication-induced tardive d.
neuroleptic-induced tardive d.
orofacial d.
paroxysmal d.
spontaneous d.
tardive d.
withdrawal d.

dyskinetic movement

dyskoimesis

dyslalia

dyslexia
acquired d.
developmental d.

dyslexic

dyslogia

dyslogistic

dysmaturation
social d.
dysmegalopsia
dysmenorrhea
psychogenic d.
dysmentia
neuroleptic-induced d.
tardive d.
dysmetria
cognitive d.
dysmetric hand movement
dysmetropsia
dysmimia
dysmnesia
dysmnesic
d. psychosis
d. syndrome
dysmorphia
body d.
muscle d.
dysmorphic
d. delusion
d. somatoform disorder
dysmorphism
muscle d.
dysmorphogenesis
dysmorphology
brain d.
dysmorphomania
dysmorphopsia
dysmyelination
dysmyotonia
dysnomia
autonomic d.
dysnystaxis
dysorexia
dysorthographia
dysorthography
dysosmia
dysostosis multiplex
dyspallia
dyspareunia
female d.
functional d.
generalized-type d.
lifelong-type d.
male d.
psychogenic d.
situational-type d.
dyspepsia
psychogenic d.
dysperception
metabolic d.
dysphagia
d. globosa
d. nervosa
dysphasia
developmental d.
expressive d.
receptive d.
Wernicke d.
dysphemia
dysphonia
adductor spasmodic d.
hyperkinetic d.
spasmodic d.
spastic d.
d. spastica
ventricular d.
dysphoretic
dysphoria
body d.
gender d.
hysteroid d.
intense episodic d.
d. nervosa
neuroleptic-induced d.
omnipresent d.
postcoital d.
premenstrual d.
dysphoriant
dysphoric
d. affect
d. category
d. character structure
d. mania
d. manic state
d. mood
d. patient
d. personality disorder
d. presentation
d. Q factor
d. response
d. subfactor
d. subjective experience
dysphrasia
dysphrenia
dysphylaxia
dysplasia
cerebral d.
septooptic d.
dysplastic constitutional type
dyspnea response
dyspneic psychogenic disorder
dysponderal amenorrhea
dysponesis

NOTES

dyspragia
dyspraxia
constructional d.
speech d.
spelling d.
d. syndrome
dyspraxic movement
dysprosody
dysraphic
dysraphicus
status d.
dysreactivity
autonomic d.
dysreflexia
autonomic d.
dysregulate
dysregulated
d. neurotransmission
d. stress response
dysregulation
affective d.
anger d.
autonomic d.
biologic d.
defensive d.
emotional d.
endocrine d.
level of defensive d.
limbic d.
prefrontal cortical activity d.
dysrhythmic
d. aggressive behavior
d. movement
d. speech
dyssocial
d. behavior
d. drinking
d. personality
d. personality disorder
d. reaction
dyssomnia
jet lag-type d.
shift work-type d.
sleep phase d.
unspecified-type d.
dysspondylism
dysstasia
dyssymbiosis
dyssymbolia
dyssynergia
d. cerebellaris myoclonica
d. cerebellaris progressiva
dystaxia
dysteleology
dysthymia
chronic d.
primary d.
subaffective d.
d. with major depression
d. without major depression
dysthymic
d. adjustment reaction
d. disorder (DD)
d. neurotic disorder
dystonia
acute d.
body d.
drug-induced d.
focal d.
idiopathic d.
mandibular d.
neuroleptic-induced acute d.
nocturnal paroxysmal d.
paroxysmal d.
psychogenic d.
substance-induced d.
tardive d.
torsion d.
withdrawal d.
dystonic
d. movement
d. posturing
d. reaction
d. tremor
dystopia
dystrophia adiposogenitalis
dystrophin
dystropy
dysuria
psychic d.
psychogenic d.

E
E trisomy
2E1
cytochrome P-450 2E1
e4/e4 genotype
EA
educational age
eagerness
ear
glue e.
listening with third e.
e. pulling
third e.
wet behind e.'s
early
e. abuse
e. adulthood
e. aggression
e. childhood
e. childhood behavioral disorder
e. childhood identifiable antecedent
e. component waveform
E. Developmental Stages of Psychopathology Study
e. discharge
e. environment
e. experience
e. full remission
e. genital primacy
e. infantile autism
e. interventionist
e. latency potential
e. life stressor
e. manic agitation
e. medical trauma
e. morning awakening
e. parental deprivation
e. and periodic screening, diagnosis, and treatment (EPSDT)
e. pharmacological intervention
e. phase of dementia
e. posttraumatic epilepsy
e. predictor
e. Psychosis Prevention and Intervention Centre
e. psychotherapeutic intervention
e. relationship
e. retirement with disability (ERD)
e. separation
e. speech impairment
e. stage in adolescence
e. trauma hypothesis of autistic disorder
e. traumatic epilepsy
e. treatment
e. warning sign
early-onset
e.-o. alcoholism
e.-o. category
e.-o. drinking
e.-o. mental illness
e.-o. schizophrenia
Early Psychosis Prevention and Intervention Centre
earner
wage e.
earth
e. eater
e. eating
earthy
ease
e. of fatigue
ill at e.
easily
distracted e.
e. disturbed sleep
e. influenced
e. provoked
Eastern
E. Psychiatric Research Association
E. religion
E. subtype
easy
e. child
e. to distract
e. distractibility
e. fatigue
free and e.
e. mark
e. virtue
easygoing
eat
refusal to e.
eater
binge e.
clay e.
compulsive e.
dirt e.
earth e.
emotional e.
erratic e.
finicky e.
picky e.
starch e.
eating
e. aid
e. attitude
e. behavior
e. binge

E

eating *(continued)*
e. compulsion
e. concern
e. custom
dirt e.
disinterest in e.
e. disorder
e. disorder examination (EDE)
e. disorder investigation (EDI)
e. disorders, NOS (EDNOS)
e. disturbance
earth e.
e. fear
e. habit
e. hair
e. and purging
social e.
starch e.
e. symptom
e. without satiation
eavesdropper
EBD
emotional and behavioral difficulties
EBM
evidence-based medicine
Ebonics
ebriety
ebriose
ebriosorum
delirium e.
ebrious
ebullience
ebullient
ebullition
EBV
Epstein-Barr virus
ECA
epidemiological catchment area
ECA study
eccentric
e. A cluster
e. behavior
e. paranoia
e. personality
e. projection
e. thinking
eccentricity
ecchordosis physaliformis
ecclesiasticism
ecdemiomania
ecdemonomania
ecdysiasm
ecdysist
ecgonine
echelon
higher e.
echeosis
echinacea
echo, pl. **echoes**
e. chamber
e. de la pensée
e. phenomenon
e. principle
e. reaction
e. sign
e. speech
thought e.
echoacousia
echoencephalography
echoes (*pl. of* echo)
echographia
echoic memory
echoing
thought e.
echokinesis, echokinesia
echolalia
immediate e.
mitigated e.
unmitigated e.
echolalus
echolocation
echomatism
echomimia
echomotism
echopathy
echophenomena
echophotony
echophrasia
echopraxia, echopraxis
eclaircissement
eclamptic symptom
éclat
eclectic
e. behaviorism
e. counseling
e. theoretical orientation
eclecticism
eclipse
cerebral e.
mental e.
ECM
external chemical messenger
ecmnesia
ecocide
ecofreak
ecogenetic
ecological
e. perception
e. psychiatry
e. study
e. system model
e. validity
ecologic framework
ecology
human e.
social e.
ecomania

economic
e. advantage
e. approach
e. benefit
e. disadvantage
e. divorce
e. principle
e. viewpoint
ecopharmacology
ecopsychiatry
ecopsychology
ECOScales
e-counseling
ecphorize
ECS
electrocerebral silence
electroconvulsive shock
epileptic confusional state
ECST
electroconvulsive shock therapy
electroconvulsive shock treatment
ecstasy
religious e.
ecstasy-associated malignant hyperthermia
ecstatic
e. behavior
e. pain
e. trance
ECT
electroconvulsive therapy
electroshock therapy
ECT administration
bilateral ECT
brief pulse bilateral ECT
brief pulse unilateral ECT
involuntary ECT
sine wave unilateral ECT
suprathreshold ECT
unilateral brief pulse ECT
unilateral nondominant-hemisphere ECT
unilateral sine wave ECT
ectoderm
ectodermogenic neurosyphilis
ectomorph
ectomorphic constitutional type
ectopic ACTH syndrome
ectoplasm
ectype
ecumenic
ecumenicist
eczema
psychogenic e.
ED
emergency department
emotional disorder
emotionally disturbed
entering diagnosis
EDE
eating disorder examination
edema
blue e.
brain e.
cerebral e.
circumscribed e.
dependent e.
hunger e.
nutritional e.
pitting e.
toxic e.
edetate
edge
e. artifact
on e.
edgy
EDI
eating disorder investigation
edict
Edinburgh
Edinger-Westphal nucleus
ED/LD
emotionally disturbed/learning disabled
EDNOS
eating disorders, not otherwise specified
EDR
electrodermal response
EDS
excessive daytime sleepiness
educable mentally retarded (EMR)
educated
poorly e.
education
advanced e.
caregiver e.
compensatory e.
consumer e.
continuing medical e. (CME)
cooperative e.
dance e.
drug abuse resistance e. (DARE)
environmental e.
formal e.
high-quality e.
level of e.

NOTES

education *(continued)*
e. level
low e.
mean years of e.
online e.
parental e.
patient e.
physical e.
postgraduate e.
progressive e.
psychiatric e.
e. quotient (EQ)
sex e.
special e.
undergraduate e.
vocational rehabilitation and e. (VR&E)

educational
e. acceleration
e. achievement
e. age (EA)
e. attainment
e. counseling
e. disadvantage
e. dysfunction
e. functioning
e. history
e. information
e. intervention
e. level
e. measurement
e. opportunity
e. program
e. psychology
e. psychotherapy
e. quotient (EQ)
e. setting
e. situation
e. stressor
e. therapist
e. treatment
e. value

educationally
e. deprived
e. mentally handicapped (EMH)
e. subnormal (ESN)

educational-socialization model

education-focused session

educative intervention

educe

eduction

edulcorate

Edwards syndrome

EE
expressed emotion

EEG
electroencephalogram
electroencephalograph
electroencephalography
EEG activation
EEG activity measurement
diffuse slowing of EEG
nonspecific abnormality on EEG
phase lag on EEG
phase spike on EEG
sleep-deprived EEG
sleep spindle on EEG
EEG tracing
waking EEG

eerie

Efavirenz

effect
adverse drug e.
adverse medication e.
adverse negative immunosuppressive e.
age e.
air pressure e.
alerting e.
antiadrenergic e.
antiaggressive e.
anticholinergic e.
anticonvulsant e.
antihistaminergic e.
antiimpulse e.
antimuscarinic e.
antipsychotic e.
antiserotonergic e.
anxiolytic e.
aspirin e.
assimilation e.
asymmetry and order e.
atmosphere e.
audience e.
autokinetic e.
autonomic side e.
bandwagon e.
Barnum e.
behavioral e.
beneficial e.
brain metabolic e.
calming e.
catastrophic e.
ceiling e.
chatterbox e.
cholinergic side e.
chronic toxic e.
clasp-knife e.
clinical e.
cocktail party e.
cohort e.
cold e.
confinement e.
contrast e.
crisis e.
cue e.
cue-induced subjective e.
cumulative e.

damping e.
e. of deception
desired e.
deterioration e.
devastating e.
developmental e.
differential beneficial e.
diminished e.
direct physiological e.
direct thermogenic e.
door-in-the-face e.
dopaminergic e.
dose-dependent e.
drug e.
drug-related sexual side e.
empathogenic e.
enhanced e.
enlightenment e.
environmental e.
ether e.
euphoric e.
euphorigenic e.
expectancy e.
experimenter-expectancy e.
extrapyramidal medication side e.
fetal alcohol e. (FAE)
first-pass e.
genetic e.
Glick e.
e. gradient
Halloween e.
hallucinogen toxic e.
halo e.
hangover e.
harmful side e.
Hawthorn e.
head shadow e.
hedonic psychoactive e.
humidity e.
hypermetabolic e.
iatrogenic e.
idiosyncratic side e.
immunosuppressive e.
impaired recovery e.
inhibitory e.
interaction e.
interactive e.
interviewer e.
intolerable side e.
isolation e.
kindling e.
late-emerging medical side e.
law of e.
e. law
less than maximal e.
limbic e.
limited e.
long hot summer e.
long-lasting drug e.
long-term e.
loss of e.
main e.
maximal e.
measurement e.
mediating e.
medical e.
medication side e.
Mellanby e.
mere-exposure e.
metabolic e.
misinformation e.
modified Stroop e.
movement disorder e.
Mozart e.
muscle-relaxing e.
negative immunosuppressive e.
neurotropic e.
nonsignificant protective e.
nonspecific e.
noradrenergic e.
off e.
on e.
Orbeli e.
partial reinforcement e. (PRE)
passing stranger e.
peak behavioral e.
peripheral sympathomimetic e.
personal e.'s
physiologic e.
placebo e.
positive e.
potential adverse e.
practice e.
primary e.
protective e.
psychiatric e.
psychoactive e.
psychodynamic e.
psychological e.
psychostimulant e.
psychotropic e.
putative e.
Pygmalion e.
rebound e.
reinforcing e.
rewarding e.

NOTES

effect *(continued)*
secondary e.
secure base e.
sedative e.
serotonergic side e.
sexual side e.
short-lasting drug e.
side e.
e. size
specific e.
SSRI-induced sexual side e.
stimulant e.
stimulation-related adverse e.
e.'s of stress
Stroop e.
subjective e.
suggestibility e.
sundowner e.
sympathomimetic e.
temperature e.
therapeutic e.
thermogenic e.
Thorndike law of e.
toxic side e.
Transylvania e.
e. of trauma
e. of trauma on consciousness
treatment e.
treatment-emergent extrapyramidal side e.
tricyclic e.
undifferentiated e.
unintended e.
untoward cholinergic e.
Vulpian e.
Wever-Bray e.
wind e.
withdrawal e.
Zeigarnik e.

effective
e. action
e. dose
e. ego
e. habit strength
e. level
e. masking
occupationally e.
e. reaction potential
socially e.
e. stimulus
e. technique
e. treatment

effectiveness
long-term e.
treatment e.

effectiveness-schizophrenia
clinical antipsychotic trials of intervention e.-s. (CATIE-SZ)

effector
cold e.
heat e.
e. operation
warm e.

effectual

effeminate homosexual

effemination

efferent
e. feedback
e. motor aphasia
e. nerve
e. relation

effervesce

effervescent

effete

Effexor

efficacious

efficacy
clinical e.
comparative e.
drug e.
lack of e.
relational e.
therapeutic e.

efficiency
good sleep e.
habitual sleep e.
index of forecasting e.
masking e.
neural e.
REM sleep e.
sleep e.

efficient
cause e.
e. cause

effigy

effort
e. after meaning
community e.
distributed e.
e. level
e. syndrome

effort-reward imbalance

effort-shape technique

effrontery

effulgence

effusive

EFT
extended family therapy

egalitarianism

egersis

ego
e. alien
alter e.
alternative alter e.
e. analysis
e. anxiety
autonomy of e.

auxiliary e.
body e.
e. boundary
e. boundary loss
e. cathexis
e. center
collective e.
e. complex
e. control
e. coping skill
decompensation e.
decomposition of e.
e. decomposition
e. defense
e. defense mechanism
e. development
e. deviation
e. distortion
dream e.
e. drive
duplication of e.
effective e.
e. eroticism
escape from e.
extinction of e.
e. formation
fragmentation of e.
e. function
e. ideal
e. identity
e. instinct
e. integration
e. integrity
e. integrity versus despair
e. involvement
e. libido
loss of boundaries of e.
e. maximization
mental e.
e. model
motor control of e.
e. narcissism
negation of e.
e. neurosis
e. nucleus
oral e.
perception e.
pleasure e.
preschizophrenic e.
e. proper
e. psychology
e. psychotherapy
purified pleasure e.
reality life of e.
reasonable e.
e. resistance
e. restriction
e. retrenchment
safety of e.
split in e.
e. splitting
stability of e.
e. state
e. strength (ES)
e. stress
e. structure
e. subject
e. substance
e. suffering
supportive e.
surface e.
e. transcendence
e. trip
weak e.
e. weakness

egocentric
e. language
e. speech
e. stage of development
e. thinking
e. thought process

egocentricity

ego-dystonic
e.-d. behavior
e.-d. homosexuality
e.-d. intrusion
e.-d. obsession
e.-d. orientation
e.-d. promiscuity
e.-d. pseudohallucination

egoism
alter e.

egoisme à deux

egoity

egomania

ego-oriented individual therapy

ego-state therapy

ego-syntonia

ego-syntonic
e.-s. gambling urge
e.-s. impulsive behavior

egotism

egotistical

egotistic suicide

egotropic

egregious

NOTES

egress
Egyptian Psychiatric Association
EH
emotional handicap
E&H
environment and heredity
Ehret syndrome
Eichhorst neuritis
eidetic
e. ability
e. image
e. imagery
e. personification
e. type
eidolon
eidoptometry
eight
e. ball
Section E.
e. stages of man
eighth-month anxiety
EIO
exploratory insight-oriented psychotherapy
Eisenlohr syndrome
either-or
e.-o. situation
e.-o. thinking
ejaculate
inability to e.
ejaculatio
e. deficiens
e. praecox
e. retardata
ejaculation
delayed e.
e. disorder
e. failure
female e.
immediate e.
e. physiology
premature e.
primary retarded e.
e. reflux
retarded e.
retrograde e.
secondary retarded e.
ejaculatory
e. delay
e. dysfunction
e. impotence
e. incompetence
e. pain
e. reflex
Ekbom syndrome
ekistic
EL
elopement
elaborate dream sequence
elaboration
secondary e.
symbolic e.
élan vital
elasticity
elated
e. affect
e. mood
elation
elder
e. abuse
e. adult neglect
e. care
E. Justice Act
e. maltreatment
elderly
acute care of e. (ACE)
bias against e.
e. depressed patient
psychiatric disorders in e.
psychosis in e.
e. suicide
eldest
eldritch
elective
e. abortion
e. admission
e. anorexia
e. mutism
e. mutism adjustment
e. mutism adjustment reaction
e. sterility
e. therapy
Electra complex
electric
e. anesthesia
e. aura
e. chorea
e. field
e. irritability
e. shock therapy
e. shock treatment
e. skin shock
e. sleep
e. stimulation of brain (ESB)
e. wine
electrical
e. activity of brain
e. characteristic
e. current brain trauma organic psychosis
e. habituation
e. intracranial stimulation
e. potential
e. shock
e. synapse
e. transcranial stimulation (ETS)
e. vibrator

electricity
feeling of e.
electrify
electroanalgesia
electroanalysis
electroanesthesia
electrobasograph
electrocerebral silence (ECS)
electrocoma
electrocontractility
electroconvulsive
e. shock (ECS)
e. shock therapy (ECST)
e. shock treatment (ECST)
e. therapy (ECT)
e. therapy-induced mood disorder
electrocortical activity
electrocorticogram
electrocorticography
electrode
e. placement
reference e.
electrodermal
e. response (EDR)
e. response biofeedback
electrodiagnosis
electrodiagnostic study
electroencephalogram (EEG)
e. biofeedback
flat e.
quantitative e. (QEEG)
electroencephalograph (EEG)
electroencephalographic
electroencephalography (EEG)
quantitative e. (QEEG)
electrokinetic
electrolyte
e. abnormality
e. balance
e. disturbance
e. imbalance
e. replacement
electromagnetic
e. hypersensitivity
e. trigger
e. wave
electromicturation
electromigratory
electromotive force (EMF)
electromyograph (EMG)
electromyography biofeedback
electron
electronarcosis (EN)
electroneurography
electronic
e. aid
e. conduction
e. data bank
e. disaster recovery plan
e. health record
e. media
e. medical record (EMR)
e. monitoring
electrooculographic activity
electroolfactogram (EOG)
electropathology
electrophoresis
2-dimensional e.
electrophrenic respiration
electrophysiology
electroplexy
electroshock (ES)
maximal e.
e. therapy (ECT, EST, est)
e. threshold (EST, est)
e. treatment (EST, est)
electroshock-induced
e.-i. psychosis
e.-i. psychotic syndrome
electrosleep therapy
electrospectrography
electrostimulation
electrostriatogram
electrosynthesis
electrotherapeutic
e. sleep
e. sleep therapy
electrotherapist
electrotherapy
cerebral e. (CET)
transcerebral e. (TCET)
electrotonus
electrovibratory massage
element
cAMP response e. (CRE)
cognitive e.
contributory e.
cultural e.
identical e.
thyroid response e. (TRE)
elemental
e. diet
e. mercury
elementarily
elementary
e. anxiety

NOTES

E

elementary *(continued)*
e. hallucination
e. manner
e. partial seizure
e. process
Eleutherococcus senticosus
eleutheromania
elevated
e. mood
e. mood followed by depression
e. psychological distress
e. risk
e. score
elevation
mood e.
nonfocal e.
prolactin e.
sleep e.
T-score e.
elevator
mood e.
elfin facies
elicitation
affect e.
emotion e.
elicited
e. behavior
e. imitation
eligibility for care
eliminant
elimination
e. diet
e. disorder
e. drive
e. half-life
process of e.
ELISA
enzyme-linked immunoabsorbent assay
elision
elite
e. class
e. community
Elixhauser comorbidity index
elixir
amobarbital e.
high alcoholic e.
elocution
elopement (EL)
e. ideation
e. precaution
e. protocol
e. status (ES)
eloping from home
eloquence
eloquent
ELP
estimated learning potential
Elpenor syndrome
eltoprazine
elucidation
elude
elusion
elusive
e. illness state
e. syndrome
emaciated
e. appearance
e. body
emaciation disorder
email
e. communication
e. correspondence
e. harassment
e. relationship
emanate
emanative
emancipated
e. adolescent
e. minor
emancipation
e. disorder
e. disorder of adolescence
emancipatory
e. disorder
e. striving
emasculate
emasculation
embarrass
embarrassing
embarrassment
dream e.
fear of e.
e. psychosis
embattle
embedded command
embeddedness
structural e.
embellish
embezzle
embezzlement
embezzler
embitter
emblazon
emblem
embodiment
embody
embolalia, embololalia
embolden
embolophrasia
emboloplasia
embonpoint
embracing behavior
embroil
embryopathy
rubella e.
EMDR
eye movement desensitization and reprocessing

emergence
emergency
behavioral e.
e. care facility
e. contagion
e. department (ED)
e. dyscontrol
e. dyscontrol duration
e. hospitalization
e. intervention
medical e.
e. medical technician (EMT)
e. medicine
opiate-induced e.
psychiatric e.
e. psychiatric condition
e. psychiatric first aid
e. psychiatric setting
e. psychiatry
e. psychotherapy
e. room (ER)
e. service (ES)
e. situation
spiritual e.
suicidal e.
e. theory
e. theory of emotion
e. treatment
e. unit (EU)
emergent
e. evolution
treatment e.
emetatrophia
emetocathartic
emetomania
EMF
electromotive force
EMG
electromyograph
EMG biofeedback
EMH
educationally mentally handicapped
emigrant
emigration
forced e.
eminence
eminent
emission
nocturnal e.
e. tomography scan
emitted behavior
emotiomotor
emotiomuscular
emotion
activation theory of e.
adjustment disorder with mixed disturbance of e.'s
altered e.
e. attitude
Cannon-Bard theory of e.
changing e.
childish e.
circuitry of e.
cognitively elicited e.
conflicting e.
controlled e.
conversion of e.
dammed-up e.
defensive e.
depleted e.
discomfort with e.
disruptive e.
e. elicitation
emergency theory of e.
expressed e. (EE)
expression of e.
2-factor theory of e.
gatekeeper e.
ictal e.
image eliciting neutral e.
inability to experience e.
e. induction
James-Lange theory of e.
level of expressed e.
maladaptive pattern of e.
manifestation of e.
memory by e.
monotonous e.
moral e.
natural e.
negative e.
Papez theory of e.
pervasive e.
pleasurable e.
positive e.
e. production
public display of e.
recall-generated e.
e. regulation
e. regulation training
repressed e.
retraining e.
roller coaster e.
stereotyped e.
stirred-up e.
sustained e.

NOTES

E

emotion *(continued)*
taboo e.
uncanny e.
unconscious e.
welfare e.

emotional
e. abandonment
e. abuse
e. abyss
e. activity
e. adjustment
e. age
e. agitation
e. amalgam
e. amenorrhea
e. amnesia
e. anesthesia
e. arousal
e. atmosphere
e. attainment
e. attitude
e. avoidance
e. awareness
e. baggage
e. B cluster
e. beggar
e. and behavioral difficulties (EBD)
e. bias
e. blackmail
e. blockade
e. blocking
e. blunting
e. bond
e. castration
e. catharsis
e. cause of seizure
e. climate
e. coldness
e. comfort
e. communication
e. condition
e. conflict
e. connectedness
e. consequences of divorce
e. constriction
e. containment
e. control therapy
e. cripple
e. crisis
e. deadness
e. dependence
e. deprivation
e. detachment
e. deterioration
e. development
e. difficulty
e. disability
e. disclosure
e. discomfort
e. disease
e. disinhibition
e. disorder (ED)
e. display
e. distance
e. distress
e. disturbance
e. disturbance adjustment disorder
e. disturbance adjustment reaction
e. disturbance of adolescence
e. disturbance of childhood
e. disturbance stress reaction
e. dullness
e. dyscontrol
e. dyscontrol disorder
e. dysfunction
e. dysregulation
e. eater
e. emptiness
e. engagement
e. episode
e. event
e. experience
e. facial expression
e. factor
e. fatigue
e. fatigue study
e. flatness
e. flattening
e. flavor
e. flooding
e. functioning
e. handicap (EH)
e. health
e. illness
e. immaturity
e. impairment
e. incontinence
e. information
e. information processing
e. inhibition
e. inoculation
e. input
e. insanity
e. insight
e. instability
e. instability personality disorder
e. insulation
e. investment
e. involvement
e. lability
e. learning
e. leukocytosis
e. maltreatment of children
e. manipulation
e. marker
e. material
e. maturation
e. maturity

e. mechanism
e. memory
e. memory deficit
e. memory process
e. memory processing
e. memory score
e. misery
e. modulation
e. monomania
e. need
e. neglect
e. numbing
e. numbness
e. nutriment
e. object amalgam
e. object constancy
e. overlay
e. overreaction
e. personality
e. problem
e. range
e. reactivity
e. reciprocity
e. recovery period
e. reeducation
e. reenactment
e. regulation
e. release
e. release therapy
e. repression
e. response
e. responsiveness
e. responsivity
e. salience
e. scar
e. security
e. self-disclosure
e. shading
e. significance
e. speech
e. stability
e. state
e. stimulation
e. stimulus
e. storm
e. stress
e. stress depressive psychosis
e. stress precipitating tremor
e. stress reaction
e. stroke
e. stupor
e. suffering
e. supply
e. support
e. symptom
e. tension
e. thought
e. tone
e. trajectory
e. trauma
e. turmoil
e. unresponsiveness
e. upheaval
e. upset
e. valence
e. variant
e. vulnerability
e. well-being
e. withdrawal
e. word

emotionalism

emotionality

excessive e.
labile e.
negative e.
pathologic e.
positive e.

emotionally

e. arousing information
e. based disorder
e. charged attitude
e. cold
e. constricted
e. detached
e. distant
e. disturbed (ED)
e. disturbed/learning disabled (ED/LD)
e. dramatic
e. handicapped
e. impaired
e. inhibited
e. invested
e. isolated
e. laden topic
e. loaded event memory
e. numb
e. provoking stimulus
e. salient trigger
e. sensitive
e. stable
e. taxing
e. unavailable
e. unstable
e. unstable character disorder (EUCD)

NOTES

emotionally *(continued)*
e. unstable immaturity
e. unstable immaturity reaction
e. unstable personality
e. upset
e. vulnerable
emotion-cognition interface
emotion-conduct adjustment reaction
emotion-consistent account
emotion-focused coping
emotion-laden situation
emotionless
emotion-related
e.-r. activation
e.-r. feedback stimulus
e.-r. meaning
emotiovascular
emotive
e. energy
e. imagery
e. language
e. process
e. speech
e. stimulus
e. theory
e. therapy
empacho
empathic
e. behavior
e. capacity
e. failure
e. identification
e. index
e. understanding
empathize
empathogenic effect
empathy
accurate e. (AE)
communicating e.
disorder of e.
failure to develop e.
generative e.
lack of e.
support, autonomy, fusioning, e. (SAFE)
victim e.
emphatic speech
empiric
e. cognition
e. drug treatment
e. risk
e. risk figure
empirical
e. approach
e. basis
e. classification
e. criterion keying
e. data
e. evidence
e. finding
e. formula
e. investigation
e. law
e. limitation
e. process
e. question
e. research
e. review
e. self
e. study
e. support
systematic, complete, objective, practical, e. (SCOPE)
e. validity
empirical-rational strategy
empiricism
collaborative e.
scientific e.
empiricist theory
empleomania
employ
employable
employed
gainfully e.
employee
e. benefit
drug-free e.
e. drug use
e. evaluation
semiskilled e.
employment
e. barrier
competitive e.
e. contract
e. failure
e. impairment
e. intervention
e. interview
e. problem
e. problem rating
e. profile
e. workshop
employment-related behavior
empower
empowered family
empowerment
sense of e.
empressement
emprosthotonos
emptiness
e. of affect
chronic feeling of e.
emotional e.
e. fear
feeling of e.
spiritual e.
empty
e. chair technique

e. nest
e. nest syndrome
e. organism
e. set
e. stare
e. word
empty-handed
emptying reflex
EMR
educable mentally retarded
electronic medical record
Emsam
EMT
emergency medical technician
emulate
emulation
emulous
emulsion
emylcamate
EN
electronarcosis
en
en bloc
en frenzy
en masse
en rapport
enabler
enabling behavior
enact
enactive
e. mode
e. period
enactment
enanthate
enantiodromia
enantiopathic
encapsulated delusion
encephalasthenia
encephalatrophic
encephalatrophy
encephalauxe
encephalemia
encephalic
encephalitis
herpes e.
e. lethargica
syphilitic e.
encephalitogen
encephalitogenic
encephalization
encephaloclastic
encephalopathy, encephalopathia
acute toxic e.
AIDS e.
air e.
alcoholic pancreatic e.
alcoholic pellagra e.
anoxic e. (AE)
bilirubin e.
Binswanger e.
bovine spongiform e.
boxer's e.
childhood e.
degenerative e.
delayed postanoxic e.
diffuse e.
drug-induced e.
epileptogenic e.
familial e.
hepatic e. (HE)
hyperkinetic e.
hypernatremic e.
hypertensive e.
hypoglycemic e.
hypoxic-ischemic e. (HIE)
idiopathic e.
lead e.
mercury e.
metabolic e.
neurotoxicant-related e.
painter's e.
palindromic e.
portosystemic e. (PSE)
postanoxic e.
postcontusion syndrome e.
posttraumatic e.
progressive degenerative subcortical e.
progressive traumatic e.
punch-drunk e.
recurrent e.
saturnine e.
static e.
subacute spongiform e.
subcortical arteriosclerotic e.
thiamine deficiency e. (TDE)
thyrotoxic e.
toxic e.
traumatic progressive e.
uremic e.
Wernicke e.
Wernicke-Korsakoff e.
encephalopsy
encephalopsychosis
encephalopyosis
encephalorrhagia

NOTES

encephaloscopy
encephalosis
encephalothlipsis
encephalotome
enchain
enchant
enclose
enclosed space
enclosure law
encoding
e. communication board
memory e.
e. skill
encopresis
functional e.
overflow e.
primary e.
encounter
clinical e.
forced sexual e.
gang e.
e. group
indiscriminate sexual e.
intuitive e.
marriage e.
meaningful e.
e. movement
online e.
physician-patient e.
sexual e.
stressful e.
encrypted correspondence
enculturate
enculturation
encumber
encumbrance
encyclical
end
bitter e.
dead e.
e. organ
e. point
e. product
e. spurt
e. state
e. state functioning
endangerment
child e.
endear
endeavor
conceptual e.
endemic
e. neuritis
e. paralytic vertigo
endemica
endergonic
endermic
Endicott substitution criteria for depression
ending
sympathetic nerve e.
endocrine
e. disease-associated dementia
e. dysregulation
e. function
e. obesity
e. psychogenic disorder
e. therapy
endocrine-type organic psychosis
endocrinology
behavioral e.
end-of-life
e.-o.-l. care
e.-o.-l. decision-making
e.-o.-l. issue
e.-o.-l. question
endogamy
endogenetic
endogenomorphic depression
endogenous, endogenic
e. adenosine
e. affective disorder
e. brain mechanism
e. chemical
e. circadian pacemaker
e. circadian period
e. circadian rhythm phase
e. depression
e. factor
e. negativity
e. obesity
e. opioid
e. pain
e. rhythm
e. smile
e. stimulation
e. zeitgeber
endogenously produced substance
endogeny
endomorph
endomorphic constitutional type
endomusia
endoneurium
endonuclease
restriction e.
endoperineuritis
endopredator
endoreactive mood
endorphin
beta e.
endorse
endoscopic
endosymbiosis
endothelial dysfunction
endothelium-relaxing factor
endothelium-releasing factor
endowment
genetic e.

endplate
end-pleasure
endpoint
e. CGI score
e. tremor
endstage
e. dementia
e. liver disease
endurance level
enduring
e. pattern
e. pattern of inflexibility
e. problem
enema
e. addiction
e. drug administration
nutritive e.
enemator
energetic
energy
acoustic e.
active displacement of emotive e.
e. affect
e. balance
boundless e.
change in e.
e. dosing
emotive e.
e. expenditure
increased e.
intense e.
kinetic e.
lack of e.
e. level
libidinal e.
life e.
loss of e.
low e.
mental e.
metabolic e.
e. metabolism
e. output
potential e.
psychic e.
sexual e.
e. swing
vital e.
enervate
enervation
enfold
enforced treatment
enforcement
boundary e.
engagement
broken e.
emotional e.
e. level
engender
engineering
biomedical e.
genetic e.
human e.
e. psychologist
e. psychology
social e.
English
E. as second language (ESL)
fluent E.
E. language fluency
engrafted schizophrenia
engram
e. entitlement
function e.
engraphia
engrave
engrossment
engulfment
enhance
e. communication
e. daily caregiving
e. memory
enhanced
e. effect
e. methadone maintenance treatment
e. sensitivity
e. standard care
e. standard methadone maintenance treatment program
e. standard methadone service
enhancement
enhancer
cognitive e.
enigma
enjoin
enkephalin
neuronal e.
enlargement
enlighten
enlightenment effect
enlisted man
enliven
enmesh
enmeshment
enmity
ennui
enormity

E

NOTES

enosimania
enounce
enquiry
coping operations preference e. (COPE)
enrage
enraged behavior
enrapt
enrapture
enriched environment
enrichment
environmental e.
job e.
e. program
ensconce
enserf
enslave
ensoul
ensure
entailment
entangle
entelechy
entendre
double e.
entendu
déjà e.
enteric nervous system
entering diagnosis (ED)
enterocolitis
autistic e.
enterprising
entheomania
enthlasis
enthrall
enthusiasm
enthusiastic
enthymeme
entitlement
engram e.
exaggerated sense of e.
e. program
sense of e.
entity
attribute e.
controlling external e.'s
external e.
entoderm
entomomania
entopic vision
entorhinal cortex
entourage
entrainment
entrance event
entreat
entrench
entropy
entrust
entry
e. behavior
organizational e.
enunciate
enuresis
diurnal e.
e. nocturna
primary nocturnal e.
psychogenic e.
enuretic
e. absence
e. event
envenom
enviable
envious behavior
environ
environment
aberrant parental e.
adolescent e.
adult e.
adverse psychosocial e.
aversive early e.
barrier-free e.
changing e.
chaotic e.
e. characteristic
childhood e.
conflictual home e.
controlled e.
dark e.
disturbed home e.
domestic e.
early e.
enriched e.
facilitating e.
free-access e.
ghetto e.
e. and heredity (E&H)
holding e.
home e.
hostile work e.
immediate e.
impoverished early e.
inadequate school e.
individual-specific e.
institutional e.
interdisciplinary e.
invalidating e.
litigious e.
low sensory e.
low stimulation e.
managed care e.
milieu e.
e. modification
multicultural e.
natural e.
negatively tuned rearing e.
novel e.
nurturing e.

parental e.
perception of e.
permissive e.
physical e.
planned learning e.
post-9/11 e.
quiet e.
rearing e.
respond to e.
response to e.
safe e.
secluded e.
secondary e.
secure e.
sensory e.
social e.
socially disruptive e.
stimulating e.
stressful e.
structured e.
therapeutic e.
unawareness of e.
working e.

environmental
e. adaptability
e. adjustment
e. aesthetics
e. approach
e. assessment
e. attribution
e. awareness
e. change
e. complexity
e. cue
e. deficiency
e. dependency syndrome
e. deprivation
e. design
e. determinant
e. disturbance of sleep
e. education
e. effect
e. enrichment
e. etiology
e. experimentation
e. factor
e. hazard
e. influence
e. learning theory
e. load theory
e. manipulation
e. medicine
e. modification
e. mold trait
e. neurosis
e. press
e. pressure
e. problem
e. process
e. psychologist
e. psychology
e. resistance (ER)
e. sleep disorder
e. stimulation (ES)
e. stimulus
e. stress
e. stressor
e. stress theory
e. support
e. susceptibility
e. therapy
e. toxin

environmentalism

environmentalist

environmentally
e. aesthetic
e. induced anxiety

environment-centered service

envisage

envy
breast e.
penis e.
phallus e.
vaginal e.
womb e.

enzyme
cytochrome P-450 metabolic e.
e. gene
e. induction
lipolytic e.
liver e.'s
neurotransmitter synthesizing e.
rate-limiting e.

enzyme-linked immunoabsorbent assay (ELISA)

enzyme-multiplied immunoassay

E&O
evaluation and observation

EOG
electroolfactogram

eonism

eosinopenia

EOT
externally oriented thinking

EP
evoked potential

NOTES

epena
ependyma
ependymitis
ephaptic conduction
epharmony
ephebiatrics
ephebic
ephebogenesis
ephebology
ephebophilia
ephedra
Ephedra sinica
ephedrine
ephemera
ephemeral mania
EPI
  extrapyramidal involvement
epicrisis
epicritic
  e. sensation
  e. sensibility
  e. system
epicure
epidemic
  e. catalepsy
  e. of fear
  e. germ exposure
  e. hysteria
epidemiologic
epidemiological
  e. catchment area (ECA)
  e. data
  e. research
  e. study
epidemiologist
  psychiatric e.
epidemiology
  pandemic e.
  psychiatric e.
epidurography
epigastric aura
epigenesis
epigenetic
  e. principle
  e. theory
epilation
  permanent e.
  temporary e.
epilepsy, epilepsia
  absence e.
  acousticomotor e.
  acquired e.
  activated e.
  affective e.
  akinetic e.
  alcoholic e.
  alcohol-precipitated e.
  audiogenic e.
  automatic e.
  autonomic e.
  Bravais-jacksonian e.
  centrencephalic e.
  clouded state e.
  communicating e.
  complex partial e.
  complex precipitated e.
  continuous e.
  coordinated e.
  cortical e.
  cryptogenic e.
  cursive e.
  dementia in e.
  depression in e.
  deterioration e.
  diencephalic e.
  digestive e.
  diurnal e.
  early posttraumatic e.
  early traumatic e.
  erotic e.
  essential e.
  extrapyramidal e.
  extrinsic e.
  e. fear
  focal e.
  gelastic e.
  generalized flexion e.
  generalized tonic-clonic e.
  genuine e.
  gestational e.
  grand mal e.
  hallucinatory e.
  haut mal e.
  hippocampal e.
  hysterical e.
  idiopathic e.
  impulsive petit mal e.
  inhibition e.
  inhibitory e.
  intractable grand mal e.
  Jackson e.
  jacksonian e.
  juvenile myoclonic e.
  larval e.
  larvated e.
  laryngeal e.
  latent e.
  late traumatic e.
  limbic e.
  local e.
  localization-related e.
  localized e.
  major e.
  masked e.
  matutinal e.
  minor e.
  mixed-type e.
  musicogenic e.

myoclonic astatic e.
myoclonus e.
nocturnal e.
organic e.
e. organic psychosis
parasympathetic e.
partial e.
pattern-induced e.
pattern-sensitive e.
perceptive e.
peripheral e.
petit mal e.
photic e.
photogenic e.
photosensitive e.
postanoxic e.
precipitating of e.
primary generalized e.
procursive e.
psychic e.
psychomotor e.
psychopathology of e.
psychosensory e.
reactive e.
reading e.
reflex inhibition of e.
regional e.
retropulsive e.
rolandic e.
secondary generalized e.
seizure e.
senile e.
sensorial e.
sensory-induced e.
sensory-precipitated e.
serial e.
short stare e.
situation-related e.
sleep e.
sleep-related e.
somatomotor e.
somatosensory e.
somnambulic e.
startle e.
status e.
sympathetic e.
symptomatic e.
tardy e.
temporal lobe e. (TLE)
tetanoid e.
thalamic e.
tonic e.
tornado e.
traumatic e.
true e.
twilight e.
uncinate e.
vasomotor e.
vasovagal e.
vertiginous e.
visceral e.
visual e.

epileptic
e. absence
e. aphasia
e. aura
e. automatism
e. character
e. clouded state
e. confusional state (ECS)
e. convulsion
e. cry
e. dementia
e. deterioration
e. disorder
e. equivalent
e. focus
e. fugue
e. furor
e. idiocy
e. mania
e. personality
e. psychopathic constitution
e. seizure
e. stupor
e. swindler
e. syndrome (ES)
e. transient organic psychosis
e. twilight state
e. variant
e. vertigo

epileptica
absentia e.

epilepticum
delirium e.

epilepticus
convulsive status e.
furor e.
ictus e.
nonconvulsive status e.
status e.

epileptiform
e. convulsion
e. discharge
e. neuralgia
e. seizure

NOTES

epileptogenic
e. encephalopathy
e. focus
e. stimulation
e. stimulus
e. zone
epileptoid
e. amaurosis
e. personality disorder
epiloia
epinosic gain
epiphany
moment of e.
epiphenomenalism
epiphenomenon
epiphysiopathy
episode
absence e.
acute manic e.
acute psychotic e.
acute schizophrenic e.
adult depressive e.
affective e.
aggressive e.
amnestic e.
aphonic e.
bereavement-related major depressive e.
binge e.
bipolar I disorder, single manic e.
brief e.
bulimic e.
cataplexy e.
confusional e.
current psychotic e.
daytime sleep e.
depersonalization e.
depressed mood e.
depressive e.
dissociative flashback e.
emotional e.
first psychotic e.
florid e.
flushing e.
full-blown depressive e.
full psychotic e.
future e.
gray-out e.
hypomanic e.
index e.
intoxication e.
length of e.
lifetime e.
major depressive e. (MDE)
manic-like e.
manic mood e.
micropsychotic e.
mini-psychotic e.
mixed mania e.
mixed mood e.
mood e.
nocturnal sleep e.
personal e.
prodromal e.
prolonged nocturnal sleep e.
psycholeptic e.
psychotic schizophrenic e.
purge e.
real-life emotional e.
recurrent e.
schizoaffective e.
schizophrenic e.
single e.
sleep-onset e.
sleep terror e.
substance-induced manic e.
unintentional daytime sleep e.
uninterrupted e.
unspecified mood e.
untreated e.
e. version
episodic
e. affective disorder
e. amnesia
e. behavior disorder
e. bilateral loss of muscle tone
e. body movement
e. change of consciousness
e. confusion
e. course
e. dyscontrol
e. dyscontrol duress
e. dyscontrol syndrome
e. memory
e. memory function
e. substance abuse
epistemic
epistemophilia
epistolary
epithalamus
epithet
national e.
epitonic
epitonos
epoch
wakefulness e.
epochal amnesia
EPR
evoked potential response
éprouvé
déjà e.
EPS
extrapyramidal symptom
extrapyramidal syndrome
extrapyramidal system
EPSDT
early and periodic screening, diagnosis, and treatment

epsilon
e. alcoholism
e. movement
EPSP
excitatory postsynaptic potential
Epstein-Barr
E.-B. syndrome
E.-B. virus (EBV)
EQ
educational quotient
education quotient
equable
equal-and-unequal-cases method
equal-appearing intervals method
equal employment opportunity
equality
e. law
point of subjective e. (PSE)
e. stage
subjective e.
equalization of excitation
equanimity
equate
equation
differential e.
logistic regression e.
personal e.
regression e.
equatorial phase
Equetro
equicaloric
equidominant
equilibration
equilibratory
e. ataxia
e. sense
equilibrium
dynamic e.
genetic e.
Hardy-Weinberg e.
homeostatic e.
narcissistic e.
nutritive e.
sense of e.
steady-state e.
equine gait
equipment
clay-modeling e.
e. design
drug-injecting e.
Equipoise Stratified Design
equiponderant
equipotential
equipotentiality law
equitable
equity
e. stage
e. theory
equivalence
e. coefficient
complex e.
equivalent
age e. (AEq)
arithmetic grade e.
clinical e.
convulsive e.
e. criteria
delusional e.
depressive e.
e. diagnosis
e. dosage
epileptic e.
e. form
e. form reliability
grade e.
grammatical e.
e. group
e. intoxication criterion
masturbation e.
e. method
pharmaceutical e.
psychic e.
reading grade e.
spelling grade e.
e. symptom
e. symptomatic presentation
e. withdrawal criterion
equivocal finding
equivocate
ER
emergency room
environmental resistance
evoked response
extended release
era
juvenile e.
neomyerian e.
eradicate
ERB
ethnic relational behavior
ERD
early retirement with disability
event-related desynchronization
erectile
e. arousal disorder

NOTES

erectile *(continued)*
e. disorder due to combined factors
e. disorder due to psychological factors
e. dysfunction
e. failure
e. impotence
erection
clitoral e.
penile e.
pharmacologically induced penile e. (PIPE)
psychogenic painful e.
sleep e.
erector
e. clitoridis
e. penis
eremiomania
eremite
eremophilia
erethism
e. mercurialis
sexual e.
erethismic shock
erethistic, erethitic
e. idiocy
e. idiot
erethisophrenia
ERG
existence, relatedness, and growth
ERG theory
ergasia
ergasiatry
ergasiology
ergasiomania
ergasthenia
ergastic
ergogenic aid
ergograph
ergoloid
ergomania
ergometer
ergot
e. alkaloid
e. derivative
ergotherapist
ergotherapy
ergotism
ergotropic
e. process
e. system
Erhardt seminar training
Erickson
E. developmental model
E. theory of latency
erigendi
impotentia e.
Erikson 8 stages of man
eristic
erode
erodible
erogeneity
erogenous zone
eromania
eros
erosion
dental enamel e.
e. of privacy
erotic
e. arousal
e. arousal pattern
e. asphyxiation
e. behavior
e. character
e. delusion
e. dream
e. drive
e. epilepsy
e. fantasy
e. image
e. instinct
e. language
e. obsession
e. paranoia
e. pyromania
e. seizure
e. stimulus
e. transference
e. type
e. zoophilism
erotica
eroticism, erotism
anal e.
ego e.
genital e.
lip e.
muscle e.
olfactory e.
oral e.
organ e.
paranoid e.
skin e.
temperature e.
urethral e.
eroticize
eroticized fantasy
eroticomania
eroticum
curiosum e.
érotique
monomanie e.
erotization
erotize
erotized
e. anxiety
e. hanging
erotogenesis

erotogenic
e. masochism
e. zone
erotographomania
erotolalia
erotology
erotomania
erotomaniac
erotomanic
e. delusion
e. delusional state
e. disorder
e. subtype
e. type
erotomanic-type delusional disorder
erotopath
erotopathic
erotopathy
ERP
event-related potential
exposure and response prevention
errant thought
erratic
e. absorption
e. behavior
e. driving
e. eater
e. mood
e. parenting
e. sleep
e. speech rhythm
e. thinking
erroneous
e. belief
e. impression
error
accidental e.
alpha e.
e. analysis
anomic e.
anticipatory e.
aphasic e.
attribution e.
beta e.
chance e.
e. detection circuit
experimental e.
fundamental attribution e.
genetic e.
gross medical e.
e. of measurement
measurement e.
medication e.
memory intrusion e.
motivated e.
paraphasic e.
perceptual e.
perseverative e.
probable e. (PE)
standard e.
subjective e.
time e.
trial and e.
type I, II e.
e. variance
vicarious trial and e. (VTE)
word retrieval e.
eructation
erudite
erudition
eruption
skin e.
erythromania
erythroplasia
erythroplastic lesion
ES
ego strength
electroshock
elopement status
emergency service
environmental stimulation
epileptic syndrome
experimental study
ESB
electric stimulation of brain
escalating conflict
escalation
dose e.
escapade
sexual e.
escape
e. artist
e. behavior
e. conditioning
e. drinking
e. from ego
e. from freedom
e. from reality
e. into illness
e. learning
e. mechanism
e. phenomenon
e. reaction
e. training
escape-avoidance
escapism

NOTES

escapist
eschatology
Escherich sign
eschew
eschrolalia
escort
escutcheon
ESEP
extreme somatosensory evoked potential
Eshmun complex
ESL
English as second language
ESN
educationally subnormal
esophageal
e. neurosis
e. voice
esophagus psychogenic disorder
esophoria
esoteric
ESP
extrasensory perception
extrasensory projection
especial
espial
espousal
espouse
esprit
bel e.
e. de corps conditioning
Esquirol theory of depression
essence
essential
e. alcoholism
e. anosmia
e. convulsion
e. epilepsy
e. feature
e. headache
e. hypertension
e. psychopharmacology
e. seizure
e. tremor (ET)
e. vertigo
essentialism
EST, est
electroshock therapy
electroshock threshold
electroshock treatment
established
e. delusion
e. risk
establishment
establish predictability
estate guardianship
esteem-enhancing
esteem need
esthematology
esthesia
esthesic
esthesiodic system
esthesiogenesis
esthesiogenic
esthesiography
esthesiology
esthesiomania
esthesiometer
esthesiometry
esthesiophysiology
esthesioscopy
esthesodic
esthetic (*var. of* aesthetic)
estimable
estimated
e. learning potential (ELP)
e. length of stay
estimator
estranged partner
estrangement
feeling of e.
inner e.
sense of e.
estrogen replacement therapy
estromania
estrous cycle
estrual
estrus
esurience
esurient
eszopiclone
état criblé
eternal suckling
eternity fear
eternize
e-therapy
ethereal
etherism
etherize
etheromania
ethical
e. approach
e. behavior
e. challenge
e. concern
e. conflict
e. deliberation
e. dilemma
e. highbrow
e. imperative
e. issue in adolescence
e. obligation
e. principle
e. quandary
e. reasoning
e. restraint
e. risk hypothesis
e. self
ethically permissible

ethics
achievement e.
care e.
case e.
code of e.
communication e.
consequentialist e.
deontological e.
medical e.
normative e.
professional e.
e. of psychiatric research
situation e.
situational e.
structure-based e.
e. violation
virtue e.
western e.
work e.
ethnic
e. background
e. bias
e. difference
e. discrimination
e. factor
e. group
e. hate
e. identity
e. minority
e. prejudice
e. profiling
e. reference group
e. relational behavior (ERB)
e. status
e. subgroup
ethnically diverse family
ethnicity
ethnocentrism
ethnocultural factor
ethnographic approach
ethnography
ethnology
ethnopsychiatry
ethnopsychology
ethnopsychopharmacology
ethnoracial issue in aging
ethogram
ethological
e. model of personal space
e. study
ethologist
ethology
ethopharmacology
ethos
ethyl alcohol addiction
ethylamine
ethylism
etiolate
etiological
e. agent
e. association
e. complexity
e. factor
e. heterogeneity
e. neurological condition
e. relationship
e. validity
etiologic role
etiology, pl. **etiologies**
delirium due to multiple etiologies
disease e.
environmental e.
4-factor theory of e.
general medical e.
medical e.
multifactorial e.
organic e.
presumed e.
social e.
substance-induced e.
e. theory
unclear e.
underlying organic e.
etiopathogenesis
etiopathogenic
etiopathology
etiotropic
etiquette
ETOH, EtOH
ethanol
ethyl alcohol
etomidate
etoperidone
etryptamine
ETS
electrical transcranial stimulation
etymology
EU
emergency unit
expected utility
eubiotics
eucaine
EUCD
emotionally unstable character disorder
euchromatopsy
eucodal

NOTES

E

eucrasia
eudemonia
euergasia
eugenicist
eugenics
negative e.
positive e.
eugenic sterilization law
eugenism
eugnathia
eugnosia
eukinesia
eukinetic
eulogize
eumetria
eunoia
eunuch
eunuchism
pituitary e.
eunuchoidism
female e.
eunuchoid voice
euosmia
eupeptic
euphemism
euphenics
euphonia
euphonic
euphoretic
euphoria
cannabis-induced e.
cocaine e.
event-related e.
false e.
giddy e.
indifferent e.
methamphetamine e.
postcoital e.
euphoriant
euphoric
e. affect
e. apathy
e. effect
e. experience
e. mood
e. presentation
e. speech
euphorigenic effect
euphuism
eupnea
eupraxia
Eurasian
European American
eurymorph
eurytopic
eusthenia
eusthenic
eustress
eutelegenesis
euthanasia
active e.
passive e.
slow e.
voluntary e.
euthenic
eutherapeutic
euthymia
euthymic
e. memory
e. mood
e. state
euthyroid
eutonia sclerotica
eutonic
eutrophia
evacuant
evacuation
evacuator
evade
evaluability
evaluability-assessment data
evaluating clinician
evaluation
e. of adolescent
career e.
clinical e.
comprehensive e.
condescending e.
e. contract
contract e.
court-mandated e.
criterion e.
cross-sectional e.
dementia e.
e. dissemination
employee e.
event-related potentials e.
face-to-face e.
false e.
family e.
home e.
in-house e.
e. interview
job e.
medical care e. (MCE)
mental capacity e.
multiaxial e.
multiple outcomes of raloxifene e. (MORE)
negative e.
neurologic e.
neuropsychologic e.
e. and observation (E&O)
operational e.
e. period
poor performance e.
psychiatric e.
psychoeducational e.

psychological e.
psychometric e.
psychosocial factor e.
rehabilitation e.
e. research
social e.
symptom e.
testing and e. (T&E)
e. of training
transactional e.
unbiased e.
e. utilization
vocational e.

evaluative
e. rating
e. reasoning

evaluator bias

evanescent

evangelical

evasion

evasive
e. behavior
e. tendency

evasiveness

evenhanded

evening
e. drinker
e. headache
e. primrose
e. treatment

event
acute extrapyramidal e.
adverse race-related e.
amnesia for sleep terror e.
antecedent e.
anxiety-provoking e.
catastrophic e.
cathartic e.
emotional e.
entrance e.
enuretic e.
evocation of e.
exit e.
external e.
extrapyramidal e.
genomic e.
heinous e.
horrendous e.
humiliating e.
independent e.
life e.
life-threatening e.
e. memory
milestone e.
multifactorial e.
negative life e.
neuroleptic-related e.
parasuicidal e.
past e.
personal e.
place-specific e.
positive e.
potential positive e.
precipitating e.
psychosocial e.
e. recall
e. recall score
recent life e. (RLE)
reexperienced traumatic e.
sequence of e.'s
significant life e.
sleep terror e.
stressful life e.
stressful precipitating e.
time-specific e.
totality of possible e.'s
traumatic life e.
treatment-emergent adverse e.
triggering e.

event-related
e.-r. brain potentials study
e.-r. desynchronization (ERD)
e.-r. distress
e.-r. euphoria
e.-r. potential (ERP)
e.-r. potentials evaluation
e.-r. synchronization

eventuate

eversion theory of aging

everyday
e. activities in life
e. function

EVF
ethanol volume fraction

evict

eviction
evidence e.

evidence
admissible e.
e. of amnesia
anatomic e.
anecdotal e.
biologic e.
e. of blocking
blocking e.
circumstantial e.

NOTES

evidence *(continued)*
clear and convincing e.
compelling e.
e. of dissociation disorder
empirical e.
e. eviction
incontrovertible e.
indirect e.
e. of interruption
e. of intrusion of idiosyncratic material
e. of intrusion of private material
new e.
preponderance of e.
psychiatric e.
rule of e.
supporting e.
e. of weight loss
evidence-based
e.-b. approach
e.-b. medicine (EBM)
e.-b. process
e.-b. psychiatry
evidentiary hearing
evil
e. eye
e. force
e. influence
e. manner
e. person
e. reputation
e. spirit
e. temper
e. thought
e. tyrant
evil-minded
evince
eviration
evocation of event
evoked
e. affect
e. potential (EP)
e. potential response (EPR)
e. response (ER)
e. somatosensory response
evolution
e. of brain
emergent e.
mental e.
saltatory e.
e. theory
evolutionary intervention
evolutionism
evolve
evulsion
ex
ex post facto
ex vivo
exacerbated symptom
exacerbation
e. of acting out
acute e.
disease e.
pain e.
psychotic e.
e. rate
schizophrenic e.
symptom e.
exactitude
exact science
exaggerated
e. achievement
e. belief
e. body language
e. communication in schizophrenia
e. defect
e. defect in physical appearance
e. depression
e. expression
e. fear
e. feeling
e. inferential thinking in schizophrenia
e. movement
e. negative quality
e. perception
e. positive quality
e. self-opinion
e. sense of entitlement
e. sense of importance
e. sense of self
e. startle response
exaggeration
e. of inferential behavioral monitoring
e. of language and communication
e. in wit
exaltation
reactive e.
exalted paranoia
examination, exam
e. anxiety
comprehensive e.
e. dream
eating disorder e. (EDE)
followup e.
longitudinal mental status e.
mental status e. (MSE)
neurobehavioral cognitive status e.
neurologic e.
neuropathologic e.
objective e.
peripheral e.
physical e. (PE)
psychiatric e.
psychological e.
screening e.
sexological e.

status e.
e. stupor
examiner
medical e.
trial e.
example
clinical e.
exasperate
exceptional
e. child
e. stress
exception question
Excerpta Medica
excess
dietary e.
excessive
e. acting out
e. admiration
e. alcohol intake
e. concern for defects
e. crying
e. daytime sleepiness (EDS)
e. daytime somnolence
e. dependence
e. discipline
e. drug use
e. emotionality
e. excitement
e. exercise
e. fatigue
e. food intake
e. gambling
e. gambling behavior
e. grooming
e. guilt
e. happiness
e. jewelry
e. jocularity
e. laughing
e. laxative use
e. makeup
e. motor activity
e. need
e. need for care
e. optimism
e. pride
e. responsibility
e. rigidity
e. skin scratching
e. sleep
e. social anxiety
e. spending
e. stress
e. talkativeness
e. talking
e. volubility
e. worry
e. worrying
excessively
e. impressionistic speech
e. loud speech
e. preoccupied
e. soft speech
e. upset
exchange
angry word e.
fetal-maternal e.
excipient
excitability of neuron
excitable behavior
excitant
excitation
catatonic e.
e. and conduction
equalization of e.
e. gradient
psychogenic e.
e. psychosis
e. psychotic reaction
reactive e.
subliminal e.
excitation-contraction
excitative psychosis
excitative-type nonorganic psychosis
excitatory
e. agent
e. amino acid receptor inhibitor
e. control
e. field
e. impulse
e. neurotransmitter
e. postsynaptic potential (EPSP)
e. stimulus
e. synapse
excitatory-inhibitory process
excited
e. behavior
e. catatonia
e. mood
e. schizoaffective schizophrenia
e. state
excitement
anniversary e.
catatonic e.
confusional e.
excessive e.

NOTES

E

excitement *(continued)*
hypomanic e.
inhibited sexual e. (ISE)
manic e.
mental e.
e. phase
e. phase of sexual response cycle
psychomotor e.
reactive mental e.
schizophrenic e.
sexual e.
substance-induced e.
excitement-seeking tendency
excitomotor
excitomuscular
excitonutrient
excitor
excitotoxic death
excitotoxicity
exclamation theory
exclusion
e. criteria
diagnosis by e.
exclusive
mutually e.
excogitate
excommunicate
excommunicative
excoriation
neurotic e.
psychogenic e.
excrement fear
excrescence
excretory perversion
excruciate
exculpate
excursive
excusatory
execrable
execrate
executive
e. aphasia
e. aspect
e. control
e. decision-maker
e. ego function
e. function deficit
e. functioning
e. functioning disturbance
e. function model
e. language
e. organ
e. process
e. speech
e. stress
e. subsystem
e. system dysfunction
exegesis
analytic e.
exemplar
exemplify
exencephalic
exencephalous
exencephaly, exencephalia
exercise
e. addict
e. addiction
aerobic e.
compulsive e.
e. counseling
excessive e.
holding e.
imagery e.
intellectual e.
intergroup e.
journaling e.
law of e.
mental e.
mirror e.
modeling e.
patterning e.
physical e.
e. plan
sensate focus e.
spiritual e.
therapeutic e.
e. therapy
e. treatment
verbal memory e.
exercise-induced sympathetic discharge
exerciser container
exercising
compulsive e.
exert
exertional headache
exhaustion
combat e.
e. death
e. delirium
level of e.
e. management
mental e.
nervous e.
e. paralysis
e. psychosis
e. senile dementia
stage of e.
e. stage
e. state
stuporous e.
e. syndrome
exhaustive
e. psychosis
e. stupor
exhibition
e. dream
sexual e.
e. wit

exhibitionism
e. paraphilia
shock e.
exhibitionistic behavior
exhibitionist need
exhilarant
exhilarate
exhortation
ex-husband
exigent
exile situation
existence
e. need
e., relatedness, and growth (ERG)
existential
e. analysis
e. anguish
e. anxiety
e. crisis
e. despair
e. ego function
e. living
e. neurosis
e. phenomenology
e. psychiatry
e. psychoanalysis
e. psychology
e. psychotherapy
e. school
e. vacuum
existential-humanistic
e.-h. theory
e.-h. therapy
existentialism
exit
e. event
e. interview
exocathection
exocentric construction
exocytosis
exogamy
exogenesis
exogenetic
exogenous
e. chemical
e. depression
e. factor
e. obesity
e. psychosis
e. smile
e. stimulation
e. stress
e. zeitgeber
exonerative moral reasoning
exon III
exophoria
exopsychic
exorbitance
exorcism
exorcist
exosomatic method
exotic
e. bias
e. psychosis
exoticism
expanded consciousness
expansion
consciousness e.
e. delusion
e. idea
e. mood
perceptual e.
expansiva
paraphrenia e.
expansive
e. delusion
e. idea
e. mood
e. solution
expansiveness
grandiose e.
expatiate
expectancy
e. chart
life e.
lifetime e.
outcome e.
e. theory
expectant analysis
expectation
anxious e.
apprehension e.
catastrophic e.
e. of death
failed e.
internal world of e.
e. of life
negative e.
e. neurosis
optimistic e.
realistic e.
serial linguistic e.
unrealistic e.
expected
e. death
e. frequency

NOTES

expected *(continued)*
- e. level of achievement
- e. utility (EU)
- e. weight gain

expenditure
- energy e.
- resting energy e.

experience
- accidental e.
- adverse childhood e.
- affective e.
- atypical delusional e.
- brief delusional e.
- bullying e.
- charismatic religious e.
- childhood e.
- clinical e.
- collective e.
- common e.
- confrontational e.
- corrective emotional e.
- countertransference e.
- cultural e.
- culturally sanctioned e.
- cutaneous e.
- dating e.
- deficient affective e.
- delusional e.
- depersonalization e.
- depressive e.
- developmental e.
- dissociative e.
- disturbing e.
- dream e.
- dysphoric subjective e.
- early e.
- emotional e.
- euphoric e.
- external world e.
- false sensory e.
- fantasized sexual e.
- frontline combat e.
- gambling e.
- group e.
- hallucinatory e.
- heterosexual sexual e.
- homosexual sexual e.
- horrific e.
- human therapeutic e.
- identity e.
- immediate e.
- inner e.
- intimate e.
- job-sample e.
- learning e.
- life e.
- life-changing spiritual e.
- life-threatening e.
- loss e.
- mother-child e.
- mystical e.
- narcolepsy e.
- near-death e.
- negative race-related e.
- online sexual e.
- openness to e.
- opposite sex sexual e.
- out-of-body e. (OBE)
- outside range of normal human e.
- overrepresented e.
- overwhelming childhood e.
- overwhelming intimate e.
- paradigmatic stress from life e.
- past e.
- peak e.
- perceptual e.
- personal e.
- personally saddening e.
- physical e.
- pleasure e.
- practice e.
- prisoner-of-war e.
- psychic e.
- psychologically overwhelming e.
- religious e.
- repeated painful e.'s
- same-sex sexual e.
- sensory e.
- sexual e.
- social learning e.
- spiritual possession e.
- split-off and denied e.
- stimulating e.
- stress from life e. (SFLE)
- stressful life e.
- subjective e.
- success e.
- syntaxic mode of e.
- terrifying e.
- thought transfer e.
- transient hallucinatory e.
- traumatic e.
- treatment e.
- troubling e.
- unusual perceptual e.
- e. with criminal activity

experiential
- e. factor
- e. group
- e. psychotherapy
- e. therapy

experiment
- analog e.
- delayed reaction e.
- double-blind e.
- double-masked e.
- factorial e.
- field e.

experimental
e. analysis of behavior
e. bias
e. condition
e. control
e. design
e. disorder
e. drug
e. error
e. game
e. group
e. hypothesis
e. intervention
e. marriage
e. medication
e. medicine
e. method
e. neurasthenia
e. neurosis
e. psychiatry
e. psychology
e. psychometric setting
e. realism
e. series
e. sexual activity
e. study (ES)
e. therapy
e. treatment
e. variable
experimentation
environmental e.
pharmacological e.
role e.
sexual e.
experimenter bias
experimenter-expectancy effect
expert
mental health e.
physician e.
e. system
e. testimony
e. witness
expertise
expiate
expiation
expiatory
e. punishment
e. self-punishment
explain away
explanation
alternative e.
post hoc e.
reassuring e.
explanatory model interview catalogue
expletive
use of e.'s
explicable
explicit
e. behavior
e. gesture
e. language
e. memory
e. process
e. recollection
e. rejection
e. role
e. type
explicitly religious
exploding head syndrome
exploit
exploitation
e. of children
gender e.
interpersonal e.
exploitative
e. character
e. orientation
e. personality
exploitative-manipulative behavior
exploiter
professional e.
exploiting type
exploitive
interpersonally e.
exploration
diversive e.
dream e.
e. drive
therapeutic e.
exploratory
e. behavior
e. drive
e. insight
e. insight-oriented psychotherapy (EIO)
e. therapy
explosion readiness
explosive
e. aggressive behavior
chemical, biological, radiological, nuclear, and e. (CBRNE)
e. disturbance
e. neurotic personality disorder
e. outburst
e. personality
e. psychotic state

NOTES

E

explosive *(continued)*
e. rage
e. speech
e. temper
e. therapy
explosivity
exposition attitude
expostulate
exposure
e. to abuse
aluminum e.
anthrax e.
antipsychotic medication e.
arsenic e.
atmospheric pollution e.
avoidance of e.
battle e.
biochemical e.
e. to bioterrorism
e. to biowarfare cue
carbon disulfide e.
carbon monoxide e.
chronic ethanol e.
cold e.
combat stress e.
common precipitant e.
controlled e.
cue e.
e. deafness
e. to death
e. to disease
epidemic germ e.
ethanol e.
exteroceptive e.
fetal e.
germ e.
graded e.
e. to grief
habit e.
e. to hate
e. hierarchy
e. to hostility
imaginal e.
indecent e.
interoceptive e.
lead e.
manganese e.
mercury e.
neuroleptic e.
neurotoxicant e.
nickel e.
occupational e.
e. of person
prolonged e.
e. and response prevention (ERP)
self-directed e.
smoking e.
e. to terrorist activity
e. to torture
toxic gas e.
toxic metal e.
e. to toxin
e. to trauma
e. to trigger
e. to violence
e. in vivo
war zone e.
exposure-based
e.-b. cognitive behavior therapy
e.-b. intervention
expound
expressed
e. emotion (EE)
e. motivation
expression
abrupt shift in affective e.
abstract e.
affective e.
akinesia/diminished emotional e.
appropriate facial e.
behavioral e.
e. of bias
blunted emotional e.
e. of caring
e. of customs
diminished emotional e.
discordant facial e.
disorder of written e.
e. of emotion
emotional facial e.
exaggerated e.
facial e.
e. of feelings
gene e.
e. of grief
e. of hospitality
e. of hostility
inappropriate sexual e.
involuntary emotional e.
line of e.
lines of e.
e. method
nonverbal e.
obscene e.
parenthetical e.
passivity in anger e.
pattern of e.
e. of prejudice
proapoptotic gene e.
rapid shift in affective e.
repeated shift in affective e.
restricted range of emotional e.
sexual e.
shallow e.
e. of sharing
staring facial e.
unassertive e.
unhappy facial e.

unusual facial e.
verbal e.
e. with feelings
written e.

expressionism factor

expressive
e. amimia
e. amusia
e. aphasia
e. delusion
e. dysphasia
e. function
e. gesture
e. glance
e. language
e. language deficit
e. language development
e. language development disorder
e. language quotient
e. language skill
e. movement
e. pattern
e. psychotherapy
e. therapy
e. writing development disorder

expressiveness
lack of e.

expressive-receptive aphasia

expurgate

expurgatory

ex-smoker

extemporaneous

extended
e. care
e. counseling
e. family
e. family therapy (EFT)
e. jargon paraphasia
e. pedigree
e. play
e. release (ER)
e. sick leave

extended-care
e.-c. facility
e.-c. insurance
e.-c. review

extended-stay review

extension semantics

extensor
e. plantar reflex
e. plantar response
e. rigidity
e. tetanus
e. thrust

extent
e. of abuse
e. of damage
e. prognosis

extenuating circumstance

extérieur
milieu e.

exteriorization

exteriorize

external
e. boundary
e. capsule
e. chemical messenger (ECM)
e. cue
e. demand
e. entity
e. event
e. force
e. force control
e. genitalia
e. incentive
e. incentive motivation
e. information
e. inhibition
internal vs e. (I-E)
e. locus of control
e. meningitis
e. reality
e. reward
e. sense
e. source
e. speech
e. speech stimulus
e. spirit
e. stigma
e. stimulation
e. stressor
e. structure
e. support
e. support system
e. validity
e. world
e. world experience

externalization

externalize blame

externalized anger

externalizing behavior

externally
e. directed aggression
e. oriented thinking (EOT)

NOTES

E

externus
puer e.
exteroceptive
e. conditioning
e. exposure
exteroceptor
exteropsychic
extinction
differential e.
e. of ego
order of e.
perceptual e.
e. ratio
resistance to e.
sensory e.
tactile e.
visual e.
extinction-type pattern
extinguish
extirpate
extol
extra
fecundatio ab e.
extracellular contribution
extraception
extrachromosomal
extract
kava e.
natural herbal e.
extractive disorder
extrafamilial
e. sexual abuse
e. system
extraindividual behavior
extrajection
extramarital
e. affair
e. behavior
e. intercourse
e. relation
e. sex
e. sexuality
extraneous
e. movement
e. noise
extraocular motility
extrapolate
extrapsychic conflict
extrapunitive
extrapyramidal
e. disorder
e. dyskinesia
e. epilepsy
e. event
e. involvement (EPI)
e. medication side effect
e. motor system
e. rigidity
e. sign
e. symptom (EPS)
e. symptom potential
e. symptom sparing
e. syndrome (EPS)
e. syndrome symptom
e. system (EPS)
e. tract
extrasensory
e. perception (ESP)
e. projection (ESP)
e. thought transference
extraspective perspective
extratransference issue
extravagant
extraversion (*var. of* extroversion)
extravert (*var. of* extrovert)
extravisual
extreme
e. act of violence
e. agitation
e. anxiety
e. caloric fluctuation
e. level of violence
e. negativism
e. range
e. somatosensory evoked potential (ESEP)
e. stressor
e. trauma
extremis
in e.
extremist
extremity
phantom e.
swollen e.
extricate
extrinsic
e. constancy
e. cortex
e. epilepsy
e. harm
e. motivation
e. reward
extroceptor
extrospection
extroversion, extraversion
extrovert, extravert
extroverted
e. personality
e. type
exuberant
exultant
exultation
ex-wife
eye
e. accessing cue
black e.
e. blink
e. blink response

e. closure reflex
e. contact
e. contact avoidance
crossed e.'s
dancing e.
defected e.
deflected e.
e. dominance
evil e.
glassy e.'s
e. gouging
lusterless e.'s
e. memory
mind's e.
e. movement
e. movement abnormality
e. movement desensitization
e. movement desensitization and reprocessing (EMDR)
e. movement reprocessing
e. preference
e. psychogenic disorder
puffy e.
raccoon e.
e. roll sign
e. scan
e. scanning
swollen e.
e. tracking

eyeball-to-eyeball

eye-hand coordination

eyelash sign

eyelid

e. conditioning
drooping e.
insufficiency of e.

eye-opener

eye-to-eye

eye-voice span

Eysenck

E. and Gray biological theories of personality
E. model

eysenckian neuroticism

NOTES

E

F
form response
F+
good form response
F-
poor form response
f
frequency
fabricate
fabrication
fabulation
facade of competence
face
about f.
Albert's Famous F.'s
flushed f.
immobile f.
f. off
picking at f.
poker f.
f. recognition
save f.
f. saver
staring f.
unfamiliar f.
f. up
f. up to
f. validity
f. value
faced
face-saving behavior
facetious
face-to-face
f.-t.-f. advice
f.-t.-f. evaluation
f.-t.-f. meeting
facial
f. action coding system (FACS)
f. affect
f. agnosia
f. apraxia
f. asymmetry
f. deceit
f. diplegia
f. disfigurement
f. display
f. expression
f. expression automatism
f. expression interpretation
f. flushing
f. grimace
f. hemiatrophy
f. hemiplegia
f. identification
f. nerve
f. neuralgia
f. paralysis
f. paresis
f. perception
f. recognition
f. responsiveness
f. sensation
f. talk
f. tic
f. tremor
f. twitch
facialis phenomenon
facies, pl. **facies**
elfin f.
Hutchinson f.
mask f.
masked f.
masklike f.
myasthenic f.
myopathic f.
myotonic f.
facile
facilitated communication
facilitating environment
facilitation
associative f.
behavioral f.
f. of communication
intracortical inhibition and f.
reproductive f.
social f.
Wedensky f.
facilitory
facility
board-and-care f.
childcare f.
correctional f.
detention f.
emergency care f.
extended-care f.
health-related f.
inpatient psychiatric treatment f.
intermediate care f.
juvenile detention f.
long-term care f.
mental health treatment f.
psychiatric f.
rehabilitation f.
residential treatment f.
shelter f.
short-term care f.
substance abuse treatment f.
treatment f.
FACS
facial action coding system

fact
f. finding
f. giver
f. of life
matter of f.
f. seeker
faction
time f.
factitial dermatitis
factitious
f. disorder, combined type
f. disorder, physical type
f. disorder by proxy
f. disorder, psychological type
f. dissociative identity disorder
f. illness
f. illness by proxy
f. interface disorder
factitious-type neurotic hysteric disorder
facto
de f.
ex post f.
factor
activation f.
active risk f.
ADP ribosylation f.
adverse background f.
age-specific risk f.
aggression f.
alpha f.
f. analysis
antisocial psychopathic Q f.
arousability f.
assimilative f.
attitudinal risk f.
background f.
biologic risk f.
BPRS-E affect f.
BPRS-E anergia f.
BPRS-E disorganization f.
BPRS-E thought disturbance f.
C f.
causal f.
cellular immunity f.
ciliary neurotrophic f.
cleverness f.
cognitive-behavioral f.
cognitive risk f.
combined f.
f. comparison
f. comparison method
confounding f.
constitutional f.
corticotropin-releasing f.
Costa-McCrae f.
cultural f.
demographic risk f.
depression f.
disability risk f.
disorder due to combined f.'s
disorganized f.
DNA transcription f.
dysfunctional family f.
dysphoric Q f.
emotional f.
endogenous f.
endothelium-relaxing f.
endothelium-releasing f.
environmental f.
erectile disorder due to combined f.'s
erectile disorder due to psychological f.'s
ethnic f.
ethnocultural f.
etiological f.
exogenous f.
experiential f.
expressionism f.
familial risk f.
father f.
feedback inhibition f. (FIF)
foreseeable f.
Frankenstein f.
Frohman f.
G f.
general f.
genetic risk f.
geriatric f.
gestalt f.
growth hormone-releasing f.
hedonic tone f.
high-risk f.
histrionic Q f.
human growth f. (HGF)
impulsivity f.
interest f.
intrinsic strength f.
known organic f.
lethal f.
lifestyle f.
f. loading
f. matrix
mauve f.
method f.
motivation f.
motivational f.
negative f.
neurotic f.
noise f.
nonspecific neurotic f.
obsessional Q f.
organic f.
orthogonal depression f.
pathogenic f.
peer f.
perpetuating f.
personal f.

pharmacologic f.
phenotypic f.
physiologic risk f.
potential predisposing f.
potent risk f.
precipitating f.
predictive f.
predisposing f.
pregenital f.
preoedipal f.
pretraumatic risk f.
primary risk f.
protection f.
psychiatric risk f.
psychic f.
psychological stress f.
psychosexual f.
psychosis f.
psychosocial f.
psychotic f.
Q f.
f. reflection
religious orthodoxy f.
risk f.
rotated f.
f. rotation
S f.
f. of safety (FS)
schizoid Q f.
schizophrenic f.
f. score
seasonal f.
significant risk f.
social risk f.
spiritual f.
state f.
subjectivism f.
suicide risk f.
susceptibility f.
f. theory
f. theory of personality
thinking disturbance f. (TDF)
trait f.
uncertainty f.
uncertainty-arousal f.
unconscious f.
unspecified psychological f.
V f.
verbal comprehension f.
violence-promoting f.
will f.
within-family environmental f.

factor-1
steroidogenic f. (SF-1)

3-factor
3-f. dimensional model of schizophrenia
3-f. model of global rating

factorial
f. design
f. experiment
f. invariance
f. validity

2-factor theory of emotion

4-factor theory of etiology

factual
f. knowledge
f. memory

facultative

faculty
f. fusion
intellectual f.
language f.
mental f.
f. psychology

fad
f. activity
f. diet
illicit drug f.

faddish

faddism
food f.

fading
stimulus f.

FAE
fetal alcohol effect

failed
f. expectation
f. hope
f. relationship
f. suicide attempt

failing grade

failure
academic f.
f. to acquire
attentional f.
brain functional f.
f. to comply
f. to conform
f. to develop
f. to develop empathy
f. to develop relatedness
f. of drug trial
ejaculation f.
empathic f.

F

NOTES

failure *(continued)*
employment f.
erectile f.
f. to fulfill
functional f.
f. to gain weight
f. of lateralization
f. to marry
multiple-organ f.
f. of problem-solving
recall f.
reproductive f.
sense of f.
f. in social adaptation
f. to sustain consistent work behavior
f. to sustain a monogamous relationship
therapeutic f.
f. to thrive (FTT)
f. through success
f. to warm
f. to warn
failure-to-grow syndrome
failure-to-thrive syndrome
fain
faint
fight, flee, freeze, or f.
faint-hearted
fair sex
faire
savoir f.
fair-minded
Fairness in Treatment: Drug and Alcohol Addiction Recovery Act of 1999
fair-spoken
fair-weather friend
fait
f. accompli
déjà f.
faith
blind f.
f. conversion problem
f. cure
f. in God
good f.
f. healing
keeping f.
leap of f.
religious f.
f. in self
tenet of f.
faking
f. good
f. illness
fakir
fall
f. away
f. off
f. short
f. through
fallacious
fallacy
pathologic f.
fallible
falling
f. out
f. risk
f. sickness
false
f. accusation
f. arrest
f. association
f. attribution
f. belief
f. conditioning
f. euphoria
f. evaluation
f. fluency
f. friend
f. hearted
f. hermaphroditism
f. hope
f. identification
f. identity
f. image
f. imprisonment
f. masturbation
f. memory
f. memory syndrome
f. negative
f. paracusis
f. perception of movement
f. positive
f. pregnancy
f. pretense
f. promise
f. role disorder
f. sense of security
f. sensory experience
f. sensory perception
f. threshold
falsehood
false-negative
f.-n. case
f.-n. diagnosis
f.-n. response
false-positive
f.-p. answer
f.-p. diagnosis
f.-p. response
falsifiable hypothesis
falsification
memory f.
retrospective f.
falsify
falter

familial
f. aggregation
f. aggregation problem
f. bipolar mood disorder
f. clustering
f. correlation
f. deficiency
f. dementia
f. dysautonomia
f. encephalopathy
f. hemiplegic migraine
f. hormonal disorder
f. migraine headache
f. neuropathy
f. pattern
f. pediatric bipolar disorder
f. periodic paralysis
f. psychosis
f. pure depressive disease (FPDD)
f. risk factor
f. tendency
f. transmission
f. transmission of schizophrenia
f. tremor
f. unconscious
familiar
f. correlation coefficient
f. surroundings
familiarity
familism
famille
folie á f.
f. neuropathique
family
adoptive f.
alcoholic f.
f. ambiance
f. assessment
f. background
bilineal f.
birth f.
blended f.
f. burden
f. care
f. caregiver
close-knit f.
cohesive f.
f. conference (FC)
f. conflict
f. connectedness
f. constellation
f. counseling
f. counselor
f. court
f. disruption
drug f.
f. dynamics
dysfunctional f.
empowered f.
ethnically diverse f.
f. evaluation
extended f.
f. formation
f. fragmentation
f. group intake
f. group therapy
f. health insurance plan (FHIP)
high-conflict f.
f. history (FH)
f. history of mental illness (FHMI)
homeless f.
f. honor
f. identity
f. idiocy
f. incubus
f. interaction
f. intervention
f. involvement
Jukes f.
Kallikak f.
f. loyalty
matrilinear f.
matrilocal f.
f. medicine
f. member
f. member therapy
f. method
f. name
f. neglect
neolocal f.
f. neurosis
nuclear f.
f. obligation
occupational f.
patriarchal f.
patrilineal f.
patrilocal f.
f. pattern
f. perception
f. physician
f. planning
f. process
f. psychiatric history
f. psychotherapy
f. pursuit
reconstituted f.

NOTES

family *(continued)*
f. relation
f. relationship
rigid f.
f. risk study
f. romance
f. routine
runs in f.
f. sculpting
f. separation
single-parent f.
f. situation
f. sleeping arrangement
f. social integration
f. social work
f. stability
f. stress
f. strife
f. structural balance
f. support
f. support group
f. support network
f. support system
systemic f.
f. system interview
f. system research orientation
f. system theory
f. treatment
f. tree
f. turbulence
f. type
f. unit
f. unit therapy
f. violence
f. war trauma
zero f.
family-centered strategy
family-of-origin relationship
fanaticism
fanatic personality
fanciful
fancy free
fan sign
fantasize
fantasized sexual experience
fantasizing
active f.
fantastica, phantastica
paraphrenia f.
pseudologia f.
fantasy, phantasy
f. absence
affect f.
aggressive f.
anal rape f.
f. assessment
attachment f.
autistic f.
cannibalistic f.
f. cathexis
compensatory f.
directed violent f.
f. and dissociative disorder
erotic f.
eroticized f.
fellatio f.
f. figure
flight into f.
forced f.
grandiosity in f.
hero f.
hetaeric f.
homoerotic f.
id f.
incest f.
incestuous f.
intense sexual f.
internal world of f.
king-slave f.
f. life
magic f.
masochistic sexual f.
masturbation f.
night f.
nonpathological sexual f.
obsessive f.
online sexual f.
paraphiliac f.
paraphilic f.
pathognomonic f.
pathologic sexual f.
f. period
f. play
Pompadour f.
primal f.
f. process
rape f.
rebirth f.
rejuvenation f.
rescue f.
romance f.
romantic f.
schizoid f.
screen f.
secondary f.
sexual f.
sexually arousing f.
spider f.
unconscious f.
undirected violent f.
violent f.
voyeuristic sexually arousing f.
womb f.
world destruction f.
fantasy-based element of the doctor-patient relationship
fantod

FAP
fixed action pattern
far-field evoked potential
farflung
far-off
far-out
far-reaching
farseeing
farsightedness
FAS
fetal alcohol syndrome
fasciculation
fascinating
fascination
obsessional f.
fashion
cookbook f.
multiaxial f.
nonaxial f.
probabilistic f.
ritualistic f.
singsong f.
f. statement
fast
f. activity
anorexic f.
f. gradient-recalled spectroscopic imaging technique
f. speech
f. track
fast-acting agent
fastidious
fastidium
f. cibi
f. potus
fastigial pressor response (FPR)
fasting
religious f.
self-imposed f.
starvation f.
fast-talk
fast-track program
fat
body f.
f. body
f. depot
fatal
f. accident
f. attraction
f. complications of illicit drug use
f. consequence
f. hypothermia
f. mistake
f. overdose
fatale
femme f.
fatalism
fatalistic attitude
fatality
autoerotic f.
fata morgana
fate
f. analysis
law of common f.
f. neurosis
fated
father
abusive f.
adopted f.
adoptive f.
alleged f. (AF)
biologic f.
birth f.
f. complex
f. confessor
dysfunctional f.
f. factor
f. figure
f. fixation
foster f.
f. hypnosis
f. ideal
f. image
primal f.
f. substitute
surrogate f.
teenage f.
vaginal f.
father-child bond
father-daughter incest
fatherly
fatidic
fatigue
auditory f.
battle f.
chronic f.
cognitive f.
combat f.
f. condition
day f.
daytime f.
f. disease
disease-related f.
ease of f.
easy f.

NOTES

F

fatigue *(continued)*
emotional f.
excessive f.
idiopathic chronic f.
mental f.
nervous f.
f. neurosis
operational f.
overwhelming f.
persistent f.
pseudocombat f.
psychogenic f.
sense of f.
f. state
stimulation f.
f. strength
f. stress
sustained f.
f. symptom
f. syndrome
unusual f.
fatiguing vigil
fatness
feeling of f.
f. stimulus
fatuity
fatuous
fatuus
ignis f.
faucial paralysis
faugh
fault
find f.
to a f.
faulty judgment
fausse reconnaissance
faut
comme il f.
faute de mieux
faux pas
favor
sexual f.
favorable
favorite son
favoritism
faze
FC
family conference
formed response of colored area
foster care
frontal cortex
functional capacity
Fc
shading response to black areas
shading response to gray areas
FDA
Food and Drug Administration
FDA Modernization Act of 1997
fealty
FEAR
feeling frightened; expecting bad things to happen; attitudes and actions that help; results and reward
fear
f. of abandonment
f. appeal
f. association
bad-people f.
f. of bioterrorism
building f.
castration f.
childhood f.
cold f.
combat f.
f. conditioning
confinement f.
contamination f.
f. of contamination
f. of criticism
crowd f.
desire to instill f.
f. drive
f. of dying
eating f.
f. of embarrassment
emptiness f.
epidemic of f.
epilepsy f.
eternity f.
exaggerated f.
excrement f.
free-floating f.
f. hypnosis
hypochondriacal f.
image eliciting f.
impregnation f.
impulse f.
incapacitating f.
f. of infidelity
intense f.
interoceptive f.
irrational f.
lack of f.
life f.
lingering f.
marriage f.
masking f.
maturity f.
mirror f.
moisture f.
monster f.
morbid f.
motion f.
mouse f.
night f.
obligation f.
obsessional f.
obsessive f.

odor f.
overwork f.
paranoid f.
penis f.
performance f.
pleasure f.
point f.
pregnancy f.
f. reaction
realistic f.
reasonable f.
f. of rejection
rejection f.
f. response
f. of ridicule
f. of robbery
scratch f.
semen f.
sermon f.
sex f.
sexual f.
shock f.
sitting f.
skin disease f.
skin injury f.
skyscraper f.
sleep f.
snow f.
social f.
sound f.
sourness f.
star f.
story f.
strangeness f.
stranger f.
street f.
subjective f.
sudden f.
suffocation f.
sunlight f.
sunrise f.
talking f.
tapeworm f.
taste f.
f. of terrorism
f. of theft
f. thermometer
thinking f.
thought f.
time f.
tooth f.
train f.
f. of uncertainty
unreasonable f.
vehicle f.
virgin f.
void f.
vomiting f.
weakness f.
wind f.
writing f.

feared
f. disease
f. object
f. single performance situation
f. word

FearFighter computer program tailored for specific fear therapy

fearful C cluster

fearfulness
f. disorder of adolescence
f. disorder of childhood

fear-induced

fear-provoking object

fear-related
f.-r. belief
f.-r. thought

fearsome

feasible alternative treatment

feat

feature
age-related f.
age-specific f.
agitative f.
f. analysis
antisocial f.
associated descriptive f.
atypical f.
avoidant f.
behavioral f.
borderline personality disorder with histrionic f.
catatonic f.
characteristic f.
clinical f.
common shared f.
f. contrast process
culture-related f.
culture-specific f.
delusional f.
demographic f.
dependent f.
depression with psychotic f.
descriptive f.
diagnostic f.
dominant f.

F

NOTES

feature *(continued)*
dysautonomic f.
essential f.
gender f.
gender-specific f.
gross pathological f.
hysteroid f.
insomnia f.
inward expression of anger with ruminative f.
major depression with psychotic f.'s
manic f.
melancholic f.
mixed f.
mood-congruent psychotic f.
mood disorder with atypical f.'s
mood disorder with catatonic f.'s
mood disorder with melancholic f.'s
mood-incongruent psychotic f.
narcissistic f.
neurobehavioral f.
neuropsychiatric f.
neurotic f.
nondistinctive f.
obsessional f.
obsessive-compulsive f.
outward expression of anger with impulsive f.
paranoid f.
passive-aggressive f.
pathological f.
personality f.
phenomenological f.
predominant f.
prosodic f.
psychological f.
psychotic f.
schizoid f.
shared phenomenological f.
sociodemographic f.
specific culture, age, and gender f.'s
specific gender f.
suicidal f.
trait-like f.

febrifacient

febrile
f. delirium
f. psychosis
f. seizure

fecal
f. continence
f. incontinence

feces

feces-child-penis concept

feckless

fecundate

fecundatio ab extra

fecundation
artificial f.

fecundity

FED
first episode of depression

federal
F. Bureau of Prisons
f. statute

fed up

feeble-mindedness
affective f.-m.
primary f.-m.

feed
force f.

feedback
acoustic f.
afferent f.
alpha f.
altered auditory f. (AAF)
auditory f.
constructive f.
control f.
f. control
corrective f.
delayed auditory f.
efferent f.
haptic f.
information f.
f. inhibition factor (FIF)
inverse f.
kinesthetic f.
f. mechanism
negative f.
f. noise
physiologic f.
positive f.
proprioceptive f.
f. sensitivity
f. system
tactile f.
video f.

feeding
f. behavior
f. and eating disorder
fictitious f.
forced f.
f. habit
intravenous f.
parenteral f.
f. problem
f. psychogenic disorder
sham f.
f. system
f. technique
f. tube

feel-good molecule

feeling
f. of abandonment

absence of f.
affected by f.
ambivalent f.
f. analysis
f. of anger
antigovernment f.
f. of anxiety
f. apperception
ataxic f.
f. of attachment
avoidance of f.'s
f. of being detached from one's body
f. of being detached from one's mental processes
f. of being an outside observer of one's life
f. of boredom
choking f.
community f.
compassionate f.
conflicted f.
conflicting f.'s
f. of confusion
f. of control
covert f.
dammed-up f.
f. of depression
f. of despair
f. of desperation
f. of detachment
difficulty describing f.'s
difficulty identifying f.'s
f. of dirtiness
f. of disgust
f. of disloyalty
disturbing f.
f. of dominance
f. of doom
f. of dread
f. of electricity
f. of emptiness
f. of estrangement
exaggerated f.
expression of f.'s
expression with f.'s
f. of fatness
fellow f.
f. frightened; expecting bad things to happen; attitudes and actions that help; results and reward (FEAR)
f. of frustration
f. of grief
group f.
guilt f.
f. of hate
f. of helplessness
f. of hopelessness
inferiority f.
inner f.
f. of insecurity
intensified f.
f. of isolation
keyed-up f.
lack of f.
loving f.
maladaptive f.
negative f.
f. numb
f. of numbness
obsessive f.
oceanic f.
painful f.
f. panicky
positive f.
premonitory f.
premorbid inferiority f. (PIF)
f. of rage
rageful f.
range of f.'s
reflection of f.
f. of rejection
f. of remorse
repressed f.
f. of responsibility
f. of sadness
f. sensation
sexual f.
f. of shame
sinful f.
sinking f.
subjective emotional f.
subjectively unpleasant f.
substituting f.
superiority f.
suppression of f.'s
f. that self is not real
f. that things are not real
tone of f.
transference f.
tridimensional theory of f.'s
unacceptable f.
uncomfortable f.
f. of unreality
f. of unworthiness

NOTES

feeling *(continued)*
ventilation of f.'s
verbalization of f.'s
f. of worthlessness
wounded f.
feeling-talk
FEF
frontal eye field
Feighner criteria for alcoholism
feign
feigned
f. bereavement
f. symptom
feigning
conscious f.
death f.
deliberate f.
fraudulent f.
intentional f.
willful f.
Feingold diet
feint
feisty
felicific
felicitate
felicitous
felicity
fellatio fantasy
fellation
fellator
fellatorism
fellatrice, fellatrix
fellow
f. feeling
f. man
fellowship
felo-de-se, pl. **felones-de-se**
felon
felonious
felony
f. behavior
f. conviction
felt need
female
f. athlete triad
f. biological status
f. castration
f. circumcision
f. conditioning
f. dyspareunia
f. ejaculation
f. eunuchoidism
f. fantasy figure
f. gender identity
f. genitalia
f. genital mutilation
f. homosexuality
f. hypoactive sexual desire disorder
f. impersonator
f. imprinting
f. intersex
marasmic f.
f. menopause
f. orgasm
f. orgasmic disorder
f. patient
f. sexual arousal disorder
f. suffrage
f. system research orientation
f. therapist
f. victim
femaleness
female-to-male transgender identity
feminine
f. attitude
f. identification
f. identity
f. mannerism
f. masochism
f. social role
f. traits in males
femininity complex
feminism
feminist
feminization
feminize
feminizing testes syndrome
femme fatale
femora
coitus inter f.
fenestra
f. ovalis
f. rotunda
fenestration
feral children
Fere phenomenon
ferocious
ferocity
ferox
delirium f.
ferrugination
fertility
fertilization
fervent
fervid
fervor
FES
functional electrical stimulation
fester
festinant
festinating gait
festination
fetal
f. abuse
f. alcohol effect (FAE)
f. alcohol syndrome (FAS)
f. death
f. development

f. effect of alcohol
f. exposure
f. hydantoin syndrome
f. injury
f. movement
f. screening

fetalism

fetal-maternal exchange

fetation

fetched

feticide

fetish
f. object
rubber f.
sexual f.
shoe f.

fetishism
beast f.
latex f.
f. paraphilia
transvestic f. (TF)

fetishist

fetter

fetus
birth of malformed f.

feud

fever
cabin f.
high f.
low f.
stir f.

feverish

few friends

fey

FH
family history

FHIP
family health insurance plan

FHMI
family history of mental illness

FI
fixed interval

fiasco

fibrillary
f. chorea
f. myoclonia
f. tremor

fibrositic headache

fickle

fiction

fictitious
f. feeding
f. name

fiddle
second f.

fide
bona f.

fidelity

fidget

fidgetiness

fidgeting behavior

fiduciary duty

field
absolute f.
abuse f.
behavior f.
f. of consciousness
f. data
f. defect
f. dependence
f. dependence-independence
electric f.
excitatory f.
f. experiment
f. of fixation
f. force
frontal eye f. (FEF)
f. independence
minimal audible f. (MAF)
perceptual f.
phenomenal f.
play the f.
f. property
psychological f.
f. of regard
f. research
f. structure
terminal neuronal f.
f. theory
f. of vision
visual f.
f. work

field-cognition mode

field-tested criterion

FIF
feedback inhibition factor

fifth individuation in late adulthood

fight
domestic f.
f., flee, freeze, or faint
gang f.
physical f.
recurrent physical f.'s
f. for rights

fighting, injuries, sex, threats, self-defense (FISTS)

NOTES

F

fight-or-flight
f.-o.-f. reaction
f.-o.-f. response
f.-o.-f. stress
Figueira syndrome
figural
f. after-effect
f. cohesion
f. memory
figurative
f. blind spot
f. knowledge
f. meaning
figure
ambiguous f.
attachment f.
authority f.
childhood f.
empiric risk f.
fantasy f.
father f.
female fantasy f.
fortification f.
frightening attachment f.
f. and ground
identification f.
inability to trust authority f.
major attachment f.
mother f.
noise f.
simple f.
f. of speech
violent f.
figure-ground
f.-g. distortion
f.-g. perception
figurehead
file
computer f.
patient f.
protected f.
rank and f.
filial
f. generation
f. imprinting
f. piety
f. therapy
filiate
filicide
filioparental
Filipino, Filipina
filter
active f.
band-pass f.
perceptual f.
filthy
FIM
functional independence measure
finagle
final
f. analysis
f. diagnosis
f. tendency
finality
financial
f. abuse
f. crisis
f. incentive
f. obligation
f. strain
f. support
find fault
finding
associated laboratory f.
associated physical examination f.
case f.
clinical f.
comparable f.
empirical f.
equivocal f.
fact f.
neurophysiological f.
neuropsychologic f.
object f.
obtained f.
pathological f.
postmortem f.
spurious f.
tentative f.
fine
f. electric hair
f. motor
f. motor activity
f. motor coordination
f. motor dexterity
f. motor incoordination
f. motor movement
f. motor skill
f. postural tremor
f. resting tremor
f. tactile sensation
finesse
finger
f. agnosia
f. anomia
insane f.
jerk f.
lock f.
f. penetration
f. phenomenon
f. pointing
snap f.
f. snapping
f. spelling
spring f.
f. sucking
trigger f.
finger-biting behavior

fingerpaint
fingerprint
finger-tapping score
fingertip number-writing perception
finical
finicky eater
finite
finitude
fink
Finnish adoptive family study of schizophrenia
FIQ
full-scale intelligence quotient
fire
ball of f.
f. setter (FS)
f. setting
witnessed incoming f.
firearm
firebug
fired from work
fire-eater
fire-setting behavior
firing an anchor
firmly held belief
first
f. admission
f. aid
f. episode of depression (FED)
f. generation
f. impression
f. offense
f. psychotic episode
f. stage of anesthesia
firstborn
first-class
first-degree biological relative
first-episode
f.-e. patient
f.-e. psychosis
f.-e. schizophrenia
first-generation immigrant
firsthand
first-line
f.-l. agent
f.-l. medication
f.-l. therapy
first-order elimination kinetics
first-pass effect
first-rank
f.-r. psychotic symptom
f.-r. symptom (FRS)
f.-r. symptom of delusion
first-rate
first-signal system
fish scale
fissure
anal f.
central f.
cerebral f.
rolandic f.
f. of Rolando
fist
f. clenching
f. shaking
fistfight
FISTS
fighting, injuries, sex, threats, self-defense
fistula, pl. **fistulae, fistulas**
craniosinus f.
fit
f. of anger
f. of horrific temptation
parental f.
postdormital chalastic f.
psychomotor f.
pupil-teacher f.
running f.
uncinate f.
fitful sleep
fitness
inclusive f.
increased sense of physical f.
maternal f.
physical f.
fittest
survival of f.
fitting
fixate
fixation
affect f.
anxiety f.
authority figure f.
cannibalistic f.
child f.
child-parent f.
father f.
field of f.
freudian f.
gaze f.
f. hysteria
libido f.
line of f.
mother f.
f. neurosis

NOTES

fixation *(continued)*
oral f.
parent f.
f. pause
f. point
f. reaction
role f.
fixe
ideé f.
fixed
f. action pattern (FAP)
f. belief
f. delusion
f. delusional system
f. distribution
f. dosing
f. dosing arm
f. eye contact
f. hallucination
f. idea
f. income
f. interval (FI)
f. marker
f. model
f. pupil
f. ratio (FR)
f. reinforcement
fixed-dose stimulation
fixed-ended session
fixed-interval reinforcement schedule
fixed-ratio reinforcement schedule
fix and focus attention
flaccid
f. paralysis
f. speech
flaccidity
curarization-induced f.
flagellantism
flagellation
flagellomania
flagitious
flagrant
flair
flak
flamboyant behavior
flap
free bone f.
liver f.
sickle f.
flappable
flapping
f. movement
f. tremor
flare
flash
f. of color
hot f.
f. of light
flashback
acid f.
combat f.
f. hallucinosis
intrusive f.
marijuana f.
flashbulb memory
flasher
flashing pain syndrome
flashy
flat
f. affect
f. electroencephalogram
flatness
emotional f.
flattened sulcus
flattening
affective f.
emotional f.
flat-top wave
flaunt
flavor
emotional f.
flaw
character f.
fleer
fleeringly
fleeting
f. auditory hallucination
f. delusion
f. illusion
f. pain
f. visual hallucination
Flesch formula
Flesch-Kincaid method
fletcherism
flexibilitas
cerea f.
f. cerea
f. cerea schizophrenia
flexibility
behavioral f.
cognitive f.
waxy f.
flexible
f. neuroleptic dosing
f. treatment approach
flexor
f. spasticity
f. tetanus
flextime
flicker
chromatic f.
f. frequency
f. fusion
flicker-fusion point
flight
f. of color
f. from reality

f. of ideas (FOI)
f. into disease
f. into fantasy
f. into health
f. into illness

flighty

fling

flippancy

flippant

flirtation

flirtatious behavior

flirting and coquetting

flirty

flittering scotoma

floating-like sensation

floating transference

floccillation

flocculation

flog

flooding
emotional f.
imaginal f.
implosion f.

flopping tremor

florid
f. episode
f. psychosis
f. symptom

floridly
f. delusional
f. paranoid

flounder

Flourens
F. doctrine
F. theory

flout

flow
absolute f.
adventitious motor f.
anterior cingulate f.
brain blood f.
cerebral blood f. (CBF)
prefrontal f.
regional blood f.
regional cerebral blood f. (rCBF)
resting anterior cingulate f.
f. tracer
whole brain blood f.

fluanisone

flub

fluctuant

fluctuating
f. affect
f. cognitive symptoms
f. course
f. ego state
f. level of consciousness
f. mood disturbance

fluctuation
anxiety f.
attention f.
behavior f.
core temperature f.
extreme caloric f.
mood f.
subsyndromal bipolar mood f.
temperature f.

fluency
association f.
associative f.
basal f.
cross modal f.
f. disorder
f. disturbance
English language f.
false f.
intermodal f.
f. shaping therapy
speech f.
f. of thought
verbal f.
word f.

fluent
f. aphasia
f. aphasic seizure
f. aphasic speech
f. English
f. paraphasic speech

fluid
f. balance
body f.
cerebrospinal f. (CSF)
f. coordination
f. disturbance
f. imbalance
f. intake
f. output
f. overload
f. retention
f. retention syndrome (FRS)

fluidity
platelet membrane f.
f. value

fluke

flummox

flunky

NOTES

F

fluoxetine
f. intoxication
f. overdose
f. treatment
flupentixol
flush
flushed face
flushing
f. episode
facial f.
fluster
flutter
alar f.
ocular f.
flux
luminance f.
flyaway
Flynn-Aird syndrome
FMR1
fragile X syndrome
FMR1 gene mutation
FOC
frequency of contact
focal
f. ability
f. brain syndrome
f. conflict theory
f. contralateral routing of signals (FOCALCROS)
f. degeneration
f. dystonia
f. epilepsy
f. injury
f. lateralized dysfunction
f. neurological impairment
f. organic psychosyndrome
f. pathology
f. psychotherapy
f. sclerosis
f. seizure
f. suicide
f. twitch
FOCALCROS
focal contralateral routing of signals
focalize
focus, pl. **foci**
f. of anticipated danger
f. of anxiety
attention f.
characteristic paraphiliac f.
f. of clinical attention
f. of delusional system
epileptic f.
epileptogenic f.
f. group
inward f.
Loyola sensate f.
mirror f.
multiple foci
outward f.
paraphiliac f.
principal f.
restricted f.
sensate f.
somatic f.
f. of thought
unilateral f.
focused
f. analysis
f. delirium
f. expressive therapy
focus-execute component of attention
focusing mechanism
foe
fog
brain f.
mental f.
fogy, fogey
FOI
flight of ideas
foible
foist
folate deficiency
folie
f. á cinq
f. circulaire
f. communiquée
f. d'action
f. démonomaniaque
f. des persecutions
f. á deux
f. á double forme
f. á douze
f. du doute
f. du pourquoi
f. á famille
f. gémellaire
f. hypocondriaque
f. imitative
f. imposée
f. induite
f. morale
f. musculaire
f. paralytique
f. penitentiare
f. á plusieurs
f. á quatre
f. raisonnante
f. simulee
f. simultanée
f. à trois
f. vaniteuse
folk
f. diagnosis
f. diagnostic concept
f. healer
f. illness
f. medicine

f. psychiatry
f. psychology
f. soul
folklore
folksy
folkways
follicularis
follicular phase
follower role
following
f. behavior
gaze f.
f. movement
followup
f. counseling
f. data
f. examination
f. period
f. study
systematic f.
f. visit
folly
fomentation
fondle
fondling others
fondness
food
f. addict
f. addiction
f. additive
comfort f.
f. consumption pattern
f. craving
f. deprivation
F. and Drug Administration (FDA)
f. faddism
f. habit
hoard f.
f. insecurity
f. intake
f. intake abnormality
f. intake disorder
junk f.
f. poisoning
f. preference
restricted access to f.
f. satiation
f. therapy
tyramine-rich f.
food-related
f.-r. behavior
f.-r. obsessive-like symptom
foolery
foolhardy
foolish business investment
foolproof
foot
f. drop
f. reflex
footing
war f.
footloose
forage
foray
forbidden
f. fruit
f. impulse
force
antiinstinctual f.
catabolic f.
central f.
electromotive f. (EMF)
evil f.
external f.
f. feed
field f.
f. of habit
labor f.
f. majeure
nerve f.
outside f.
psychic f.
societal f.
unifying f.
US Air F.
work f.
forced
f. alimentation
f. attitude
f. cheerfulness
f. choice
f. cross-dressing
f. cross-gender
f. emigration
f. fantasy
f. feeding
f. hyperventilation
f. impulse
f. laughter
f. medication
f. movement
f. relationship
f. sex
f. sexual activity
f. sexual encounter
f. sleep

NOTES

forced *(continued)*
f. smile
f. treatment
f. vibration
f. whisper
forebrain
limbic f.
forecasting
drug use f. (DUF)
foreconscious
foredoom
foreign
f. body
f. custom
f. language
f. standard
f. value
foreign-born
forejudge
forensic
f. consultation
f. determination
f. medicine
f. mother
f. pathology
f. proof
f. psychiatrist
f. psychiatry
f. psychology
f. setting
foreperiod
foreplay
forepleasure
foreseeable factor
foreshortened future
foresight
foretell
forethought
forewarn
forfeit
forgery
prescription f.
forgetfulness
frequent f.
minor f.
forgetting
intentional f.
motivated f.
forgotten behavior
forked tongue
forlorn
form
Columbia suicide history f.
consent f.
depot f.
f. discrimination
equivalent f.
free f.
major f.
Medical Outcomes Study Short F.
minor f.
f. perception
f. of psychodrama
f. response (F)
f. of satisfactory relating
signed consent f.
thought f.
formal
f. contract
f. discipline
f. education
f. logic
f. method
f. operation
f. operational development
f. operations period
f. operation stage
f. testing
f. thought disorder
formalized contract
formant
format
nonaxial f.
self-report f.
f. treatment
formate
formation
amyloid plaque f.
brainstem reticular f.
compromise f.
concept f.
ego f.
family f.
friend f.
gender identity f.
habit f.
identity f.
f. of identity
inhibition f.
mesencephalic reticular f.
omen f.
pathologic character f.
personality f.
posttraumatic symptom f.
reaction f.
replacement f.
reversal f.
substitute f.
symptom f.
synapse f.
formative
formboard
forme
folie á double f.
f. fruste
f. tardive
formed
f. belief

f. image
f. opinion
f. response of colored area (FC)
f. visual hallucination

former
f. boyfriend
f. foster home
f. friend
f. identity
f. lover
f. marriage
f. partner
f. prisoner of war
f. relationship
f. treatment

formication
formicophilia
formidable
formula, pl. **formulae, formulas**
empirical f.
Flesch f.

formulary
formulate
formulation
case f.
clinical f.
cultural f.
dynamic f.
psychodynamic f.

fornicate
fornication
forte
forthcoming
forthright
fortification
f. figure
f. scotoma
f. spectrum

fortify
fortitude
fortuitous
fortuity
fortunate
fortune
f. hunter
soldier of f.

fortuneteller
forward
f. masking
f. planning

foster
f. care (FC)
f. care placement
f. care system
f. child
f. father
f. grandparent
f. home
f. mother
f. parent
f. parenting

fostering
fosterling
Fothergill neuralgia
foul-mouthed
foul play
foul-up
foundation
biologic f.
psychological f.
sociocultural f.
Washington Psychiatric F.

foundling
Fourier
F. analysis
F. law

foveal vision
FPDD
familial pure depressive disease

FPR
fastigial pressor response

FR
fixed ratio

fraction
ethanol volume f. (EVF)

fractional analysis
fractionation
fractious
fractured self-concept
frag
fragesucht
fragile
f. sense of self
f. X chromosome
f. X negative
f. X syndrome (FMR1)

fragment
fragmentary
f. delusion
f. dream image
f. hallucination
f. hallucination in schizophrenia
f. seizure

fragmentation
f. of ego
family f.

NOTES

fragmentation *(continued)*
sleep f.
f. of thinking
fragmented
f. communication
f. nighttime sleep
f. sense of self
f. social network
f. syndrome
frail elderly patient
frailty
human f.
frame
analytic f.
f. of reference
f. up
framework
ecologic f.
multidimensional f.
francomania
francophobe
frank
f. agitation
f. catatonic stupor
f. delirium
f. impotence
f. mental retardation
f. psychosis
f. psychotic symptom
Frankenstein factor
frantic
fraternal
f. twins
f. twins raised together
fraternize
fratricide
fraud
corporate f.
fraudulent feigning
fraught
FRC
functional residual capacity
freakish
freaky
free
f. access to processes
f. association
f. bone flap
f. and easy
fancy f.
f. field room
f. form
f. living
f. love
f. play
f. radical
f. radical scavenger
f. recall
f. recall bias
f. recall intrusion
f. rein
f. response
symptom f.
f. thought
f. will
free-access environment
freebase
cocaine f.
freebasing
freeborn
freedom
f. to choose
degree of f.
escape from f.
loss of f.
freed woman
free-floating
f.-f. anxiety
f.-f. attention
f.-f. fear
free-handed
free-hearted
freeload
free-running
freethinker
freezing
f. behavior
f. of movement
f. phenomenon
Fregoli
F. phenomenon
F. syndrome
French
F. classification for child and adolescent mental disorders
F. kiss
F. leave
frenetic
freneticism
Frenkel
F. movement
F. symptom
frenzied psychomotor activity
frenzy
en f.
presence of f.
frequency (f)
allele f.
alpha f.
f. of anxiety
band f.
f. combination
f. of contact (FOC)
critical flicker f.
f. curve
disease f.
f. distribution
f. disturbance

dominant waking f.
f. of drug use
expected f.
flicker f.
gambling f.
gene f.
intercourse f.
f. jitter
law of f.
f. masking
MOAS f.
f. of panic
relative f.
f. response
seizure f. (SF)
sexual f.
f. of treatment
f. of violent acts
waking f.

frequent
f. crying
f. decompensation
f. derailment
f. forgetfulness
f. nightly awakening
f. physical complaints
f. relocation
f. sadness

fretful

Freud
F. cathartic method
F. syndrome
F. theory
F. theory of depression
F. theory of dreams
F. view of depressive disorder

freudian
f. approach
f. censor
f. fixation
f. free association
f. psychoanalysis
f. psychotherapy
f. slip
f. theory
f. theory of personality

friability
skin f.

fribble

friction
interpersonal f.

Friedmann complex

Friedreich
F. ataxia
F. disease

friend
addict f.
death of close f.
fair-weather f.
false f.
few f.'s
f. formation
former f.
next f.
no f.'s

friendless

friendliness
active f.
attitude of active f.

friendship
f. in adulthood
f. model
platonic f.

fright
stage f.

frightened teen

frightening
f. attachment figure
f. circumstance
f. dream
f. stimulus

frigid

frigidity
sexual f.

fringe
f. of consciousness
radical f.
subliminal f.

frippery

frisk

fritter

frivolity

frivolous

Fröhlich syndrome

Frohman factor

frolicsome

frontal
f. aging hypothesis
f. brain region
f. cortex (FC)
f. eye field (FEF)
f. headache
f. lobe
f. lobe dementia
f. lobe dysfunction

NOTES

frontal *(continued)*
f. lobe function
f. lobe interstitial neuron
f. lobe neuronal density
f. lobe syndrome
f. lobe volume
f. metabolism
f. perceptual disorder
f. release sign
f. sulcus
frontal-based cognition
frontal-cerebellar-thalamic circuitry
frontalis
frontline combat experience
frontocortical
f. aphasia
f. area
f. dysfunction
f. function
frontolenticular aphasia
frontosubcortical
f. brain circuit
f. dementia
frontotemporal
f. brain atrophy
f. dementia
f. hypometabolism
Frostig-Horne training program
frottage
frotteur
frotteurism paraphilia
frozen watchfulness
FRS
first-rank symptom
fluid retention syndrome
frugal
fruit
forbidden f.
fruition
frumpy
fruste
forme f.
frustrate
frustration
control f.
f. dream
feeling of f.
level of f.
f. response
f. tolerance
frustration-aggression hypothesis
FS
factor of safety
fire setter
FSIQ
full-scale intelligence quotient
FTT
failure to thrive
fucosidosis
fuddle
Fuerstner disease
fugitive
fugue
dissociative f.
epileptic f.
hysterical f.
poriomanic f.
psychogenic f.
psychotic f.
f. state
Fukuda sign
fulfill
failure to f.
fulfilling
fulfillment
asymptotic wish f.
disguised wish f.
wish f.
fulgurating migraine
full
f. affect
f. blood
f. dependence
f. dose
f. psychotic decompensation
f. psychotic episode
f. recovery
f. relapse
f. remission
f. symptom criteria
f. syndrome
f. wakefulness
full-blown
f.-b. delirium
f.-b. depressive episode
f.-b. panic attack
f.-b. psychosis
f.-b. syndrome
full-dose-treated patient
full-fledged
full-mouthed
full-scale
f.-s. intelligence quotient (FIQ, FSIQ)
f.-s. IQ
full-time
fully organized belief
fulminant
fulminate
fulminating anoxia
fulsome
fumigation
function
affective f.
altered f.
arousal f.
autonomic f.
autonomous ego f.

axis f.
behavioral f.
below-average mental f.
biologic window on CNS f.
brain f.
brainstem f.
caloric stimulation test for vestibular f.
card-sorting f.
cerebral cortical f.
cognitive f.
communication f.
communicative f.
f. complex
complex cognitive f.
compromised f.
concept of brain f.
conflict-free f.
cortical f.
day-to-day f.
deteriorating f.
differential f.
diffuse f.
disordered personality f.
dream f.
ego f.
endocrine f.
f. engram
episodic memory f.
everyday f.
executive ego f.
existential ego f.
expressive f.
frontal lobe f.
frontocortical f.
global assessment of f. (GAF)
global intellectual f.
gnostic f.
higher cortical f.
higher intellectual f. (HIF)
higher level cognitive f.
higher neural f.
immune f.
impaired limbic-diencephalic f.
impaired sexual f.
impairment of cognitive f.
inability to f.
integrated f.
integrity of brain f.
intellectual f.
intrapsychical f.
inverted-U f.
isomeric f.
language f.
level of cognitive f.
localization of f.
localized f.
maintenance f.
mapping of cortical f.
marginal f.
mediated f.
memory f.
mental f.
motor f.
neurobehavioral f.
noradrenergic system f.
occupational f.
performance intensity f.
personal f.
phasic f.
f. pleasure
premorbid intellectual f.
preoccupation of bodily f.'s
primary autonomous f.
psychophysical f.
receptive f.
recovery of f.
reduced intellectual f.
referential f.
role f.
semantic memory f.
semiotic f.
sensory f.
seriatim f.
sexual f.
social f.
spiritual f.
splinter f.
symbolic f.
synthetic f.
thermoeffector f.
thermoregulatory f.
vicarious f.
f. word
working memory f.

functional

f. activation
f. activity
f. age
f. aid
f. ailment
f. analysis
f. anosmia
f. aphasia
f. aphonia
f. apoplexy

NOTES

functional *(continued)*
f. approach
f. assessment
f. assessment stage
f. assessment staging
f. asymmetry
f. autonomy
f. blindness
f. bradykinesia
f. brain imaging study
f. budgeting
f. capacity (FC)
f. cognitive impairment
f. component
f. conformance
f. contracture
f. deafness
f. death
f. decline
f. deficit zone
f. demand
f. deterioration
f. difference
f. disability
f. disease
f. distance
f. dyspareunia
f. dyspareunia psychosexual dysfunction
f. electrical stimulation (FES)
f. encopresis
f. failure
f. gain testing
f. headache
f. hearing impairment
f. illiteracy
f. illiterate
f. illness
f. imaging data
f. imaging technique
f. impotence
f. incapacity
f. independence measure (FIM)
f. invariant
f. irritation
f. leadership
f. limitation
f. loss
f. movement
f. neuropharmacology
f. neurosis
f. outcome
f. pain
f. pathology
f. plasticity
f. pragmatic procedure
f. psychiatric syndrome
f. psychogenic disorder
f. psychology
f. psychosis
f. relatedness
f. residual capacity (FRC)
f. shift
f. skill
socially f.
f. spasm
f. status
f. superego structure
f. symbolism
f. type
f. unity
f. vaginismus psychosexual dysfunction
f. voice disorder

functionalism

functionally impaired

functioning
adaptive f.
anxiety-induced impaired social f.
attentional f.
baseline cognitive f.
body f.
borderline intellectual f.
brain f.
cognitive f.
community f.
competent, optimal relational f.
decline in academic f.
disrupted, dysfunctional relational f.
disruptive family f.
f. disturbance
domain of f.
dysfunctional relational f.
educational f.
emotional f.
end state f.
executive f.
general verbal intellectual f.
global f.
good f.
grossly impaired f.
healthy f.
hierarchical f.
impaired attentional f.
impaired cognitive f.
impaired occupational f.
impaired social f.
independent f.
index of sexual f.
interpersonal f.
f. level
level of intellectual f.
major impairment of f.
marked decline in academic f.
f. measure
neurologic f.
neuropsychologic f.
normal neurological f.

occupational f.
optimal relational f.
overall cognitive f.
personality f.
premorbid level of f.
psychosocial f.
quality of sexual f.
receptor f.
school f.
self-rated f.
sensory f.
sexual f.
social f.
social-emotional f.
subaverage academic f.
subaverage intellectual f.
superego f.
superior f.
unequivocal change in f.
vasculogenic loss of erectile f.
verbal intellectual f.
visuospatial f.
in vivo brain f.
vocational f.
voluntary motor f.
voluntary sensory f.

fund
f. of information
f. of intelligence
f. of knowledge

fundamental
f. approach
f. attribution error
f. cognitive process
f. conceptual problem
f. defense mechanism
f. neural mechanism
f. predisposition
f. psychometric problem
f. response process
f. rule of psychoanalysis
f. social impulse
f. symptom
f. tone
f. wish

funiculitis
funk
funky
funnel plot
furious
furlough psychosis
furor
epileptic f.
f. epilepticus

furrowed brow
furtherance
furthest
furthest-neighbor analysis
furtive
fuse
short f.

fusion
faculty f.
flicker f.
instinctual f.
f. state
telencephalic f.
unity and f.

fusion-defusion cycle
fuss
fustigate
futile
futilitarian
futility
medical f.

future
f. danger
f. depression
f. episode
foreshortened f.
f. pace
sense of foreshortened f.
f. shock
f. suicidal act
f. suicidal behavior
f. suicide attempt

futuristic thinking
futurology
F-zero

NOTES

GA
Gamblers Anonymous
GABA
gamma amino benzoic acid
GABA receptor complex
GABAergic medication
GAD
generalized anxiety disorder
GAD-specific intervention
GAF
global assessment of function
gag reflex
GAI
guided affective imagery
gain
antipsychotic-induced weight g.
desire for personal g.
drug-associated weight g.
epinosic g.
expected weight g.
identifiable secondary g.
material g.
medication-related weight g.
paranosic g.
peak acoustic g.
primary g.
secondary g.
tertiary g.
weight g.
gainfully employed
gain-loss theory of attraction
Gairdner disease
gait
abnormal g.
g. abnormality
g. analysis
antalgic g.
g. apraxia
ataxic g.
cerebellar g.
clownish g.
g. disorder
g. disturbance
equine g.
festinating g.
halting g.
helicopod g.
hemiplegic g.
high steppage g.
hysterical g.
narrow-based g.
g. problem
retropulsion of g.
scissor g.
shuffling g.
slowed g.
spastic g.
staggering g.
steady g.
steppage g.
stuttering g.
swaying g.
uncoordinated g.
unsteady g.
waddling g.
wide-based g.
galectin-4
Gall craniology
gallery
rogue's g.
shooting g.
gallivant
gallomania
gallows humor
Galton law of regression
galvanic
g. skin reaction
g. skin reflex
g. skin resistance
g. skin response (GSR)
g. skin response biofeedback
g. vertigo
galvanometer
galvanotropism
GamAnon
Gamblers Anonymous
gamble
g. to escape from depression
lottery g.
urge to g.
gambler
adolescent g.
G.'s Anonymous (GA, GamAnon)
binge g.
compulsive g.
occasional g.
pathologic g.
problem g.
professional g.
recreational g.
regular g.
gambling
g. activity
g. addict
g. addiction
g. attitude
g. behavior
card game g.
casino g.
g. cessation

G

gambling *(continued)*
compulsive g.
convenience g.
g. cue
g. debt
g. disorder
dog track g.
excessive g.
g. experience
g. frequency
horserace g.
illegal g.
g. impact and behavior study
g. impulse
Indian casino g.
g. industry
Internet g.
g. involvement
legal g.
legalized g.
g. lifestyle
g. need
g. opportunity
pathological g. (PG)
personal skills g.
g. preoccupation
g. prevalence
professional g.
g. reduction
riverboat g.
g. screen
slot machine g.
social g.
sports betting g.
g. strategy
g. thought
underage g.
g. urge
video lottery terminal g.
youth g.

gambling-related
g.-r. difficulty
g.-r. infraction

game
choking g.
computer g.
dice g.
experimental g.
graphically violent video g.
hallucinatory g.
hate video g.
language g.
middle g.
mixed motive g.
model g.
g.'s people play
g. plan
play the g.
g. player
g. playing
point-and-shoot video g.
psychological g.
g. theory
video g.

gamine

gamma
g. alcoholism
g. amino benzoic acid (GABA)
g. band signal
g. movement
g. synchrony
g. wave

gammacism

gamomania

gamy

gang
g. attack
g. behavior
g. colors
g. encounter
g. fight
g. initiation
g. involvement
g. member
g. rape
street g.
g. up
g. war
g. warfare

ganja

Ganser syndrome

GAP
Group for Advancement of Psychiatry
growth-associated protein

gap
gender g.
generation g.
g. junction
memory g.
treatment g.

garbled articulation

gargoylism

garish

garnish

garnishment

garrote

garrulity

garrulous affect

GAS
general adaptation syndrome

gas
g. chamber
nerve g.
g. poisoning
tear g.
war g.

gasoline intoxication

gastric
g. bypass
g. lavage
g. neurasthenia
g. psychogenic disorder
g. varices
gastrin
gastrin-inhibiting peptide
gastritis
alcoholic g.
nervous g.
gastroesophageal reflux disorder (GERD)
gastrointestinal
g. disturbance
g. functional psychogenic disorder
g. symptom grouping
g. upset
gastroparalysis
gastroparesis
gastropathy
gastroplasty
GAT
group adjustment therapy
gate-control
g.-c. hypothesis
g.-c. theory
g.-c. theory of pain
gatekeeper emotion
gate theory
gateway drug
gathering
injustice g.
g. of intelligence
rave g.
gating
g. mechanism
sensorimotor g.
g. theory
gauche
Gaucher disease
gaudy
.410-gauge shotgun
Gault decision
gaunt
gauntlet anesthesia
gaussian
g. curve
g. distribution
gauze-wrapped glass capsule
gavage
gay
g. bashing
g. community
g. liberation
parents, family, and friends of lesbians and g.'s (PFLAG)
g. population
g. rights
gay/lesbian/bisexual/transgender (GLBT)
gayness
gaze
conjugate g.
consensual g.
g. deficit
downcast g.
g. fixation
g. following
g. impairment
g. paralysis
ping-pong g.
psychic paralysis of fixation of g.
spasticity of conjugate g.
tense g.
gazing
crystal ball g.
GBL
gamma butyrolactone
GC
gonococcus
geek
computer g.
geisha
gelasmus
gelastic epilepsy
Gelineau syndrome
gémellaire
folie g.
gemistocyte
gemistocytic reaction
gender
g. ambiguity psychosis
appropriate in g.
g. bias
boundaries and g.
g. comparison
g. difference
g. difference in anxiety
g. difference psychiatric syndrome
g. discrimination
g. dysphoria
g. dysphoria syndrome
g. exploitation
g. feature
g. gap
g. identification

NOTES

gender *(continued)*
g. identity
g. identity board
g. identity confusion
g. identity disorder (GID)
g. identity disorder in adolescence
g. identity disorder of adulthood
g. identity disorder in adults
g. identity disorder of childhood
g. identity disorder in children
g. identity formation
g. identity psychosexual development
g. issue in aging
multiple personalities and g.
g. neutrality
g. orientation
personality and g.
g. reassignment
g. role
g. role persistent discomfort
g. role reversal

gender-based
g.-b. attitude
g.-b. mental health differences

gender-linked attitude

gender-sensitive psychopharmacology

gender-specific
g.-s. feature
g.-s. intervention

gene
aberrant g.
g. arrangement
autosomal dominant g.
brain-derived neurotrophic factor g.
circadian clock g.
cytochrome P-450 2D6 g.
dominant g.
DRD4 g.
enzyme g.
g. expression
g. frequency
homeotic g.
g. marker
g. mutation
g. polymorphism
g. pool
recessive g.
structural g.
tryptophan hydroxylase g.

gene-environment interaction

general
g. adaptation reaction
g. adaptation syndrome (GAS)
g. adult psychopathology
g. anesthesia
g. anger disorder with aggression
g. anger disorder without aggression
g. clinical interview
g. cognitive status
g. component
g. factor
g. image
g. inquiry (GI)
g. knowledge
g. knowledge score
g. language disability
g. learning ability
g. medical condition (GMC)
g. medical etiology
g. medical impairment
g. medical physician
g. medical provider
g. medical treatment
g. medical use
g. memory index
g. mood state
g. paralysis
g. paresis
g. personality assessment
g. population
g. presentation
g. psychiatric practitioner
g. psychological distress
g. psychology
g. relaxation training
g. semantics
g. stress sensitivity
g. symptom
g. systems theory
g. transfer
g. value terms
g. verbal intellectual functioning
g. will

generalist

generality
glittering g.'s

generalization
g. gradient
g. response
stimulus g.
transfer by g.
verbal g.

generalized
g. amnesia
g. anxiety
g. anxiety disorder (GAD)
g. anxiety neurosis
g. auditory agnosia
g. flexion epilepsy
g. headache
g. hyperreflexia
g. intellectual impairment
g. neurotic anxiety state
g. pruritus
g. sexual dysfunction

g. tonic-clonic epilepsy
g. tonic-clonic seizure
generalized-type dyspareunia
generate
generation
g. of affect
baby-boom g.
baby-bust g.
beat g.
filial g.
first g.
g. gap
hypothesis g.
me g.
next g.
sandwich g.
second g.
silent g.
g. X
g. Y
g. Z
generational responsibility
generative
g. empathy
g. intervention
g. semantics
generativity versus stagnation
generic
g. negative symptom
g. question
g. skill
generosity
generous
genesial cycle
genesis
genetic
g.'s of alcoholics
g. alcoholism
g. association
g. basis
behavior g.'s
behavioral g.'s
g. block
g. code
g. component
g. counseling
g. counselor
g. defect
g. difference
g. directive
g. disease
g. disorder
g. drift
g. effect
g. endowment
g. engineering
g. equilibrium
g. error
g. heterogeneity
g. heterogenicity
g. history
g. influence
g. involvement
g. liability
g. linkage
g. linkage analysis
g. linkage study
g. loading
g. makeup
g. map
g. marker
g. material
g. memory
g. method
molecular g.'s
political g.'s
population g.'s
g. predisposition
psychiatric g.'s
g. psychology
g. redundancy
g. relationship
g. research
g. risk factor
g. schizophrenia vulnerability
g. screening
g. sequence
g. strategy
g. susceptibility
g. susceptibility to mental illness
g. technology
g. theory
g. tool
g. trait
g. transmission
g. typing
g. viewpoint
genetic-dynamic psychiatry
genetic-epidemiologic
geneticism
geneticist
genetotrophic disease
genetous idiocy
genial
geniculate

NOTES

genital
g. character
g. eroticism
g. herpes
g. intercourse
g. love
g. maturity
g. mutilation
g. organ
g. pain
g. phase
g. primacy
g. response
g. sensation
g. sexual contact
g. stage
g. stimulation
g. touching
g. trauma
g. zone
genitalia
ambiguous g.
external g.
female g.
male g.
genitalis
herpes g.
genitality
genitalization
genitourinary psychogenic disorder
genius
genocide
Armenian g.
genocopy
genogram
genome
g. scan
g. screen
genomic
g. DNA
g. event
g. imprinting
genotropism
genotype
COMT Val$^{108/158}$ Met g.
dominant g.
e4/e4 g.
schizophrenic g.
genotypical
genotypic programming
genotyping
ApoE g.
microsatellite g.
genteel
gentility
gentle assumption
genu, pl. **genua**
genuine epilepsy
geographic
g. displacement
g. mobility
geometric
g. design
g. hallucination
g. mean
geophagia, geophagy
geophasia
gephyromania
GERD
gastroesophageal reflux disorder
Gerhardt-Semon law
geriatric
g. abuse
g. delinquency
g. depression
g. depressive disorder
g. diagnosis
g. factor
g. healthcare setting
g. health outcome
g. medicine
g. need
g. neuropsychiatry
g. patient
g. population
g. psychiatrist
g. psychiatry
g. psychiatry inpatient service
g. psychologist
g. psychology
g. psychopharmacology
g. rehabilitation
geriatrics
geriopsychosis
germane
germanomania
germanophile
germ exposure
germinally affected
gerocomy, gerocomia
geromorphism
gerontological psychiatry
gerontologic psychiatry
gerontology
gerontophilia, gerophilia
geropsychiatry
geropsychology
Gesell developmental model
gesellschaft
gestalt
autochthonous g.
g. factor
g. phenomenon
g. psychiatry
g. psychology
g. psychotherapy
g. theory

g. therapy
g. therapy marathon
gestalten
gestaltism
gestaltist
gestate
gestational
g. diestrus
g. epilepsy
g. psychosis
gesticulate
gesticulation
gestural
g. automatism
g. communication
gestural-postural language
gesture
g. of affection
bizarre g.
body g.
clumsy g.
explicit g.
expressive g.
g. of good will
kinesic g.
g. language
obscene g.
overt g.
paucity of expressive g.'s
subtle g.
suicidal g.
suicide g.
gesturing communication pattern
G factor
GH
growth hormone
ghastly
GHB
gamma hydroxybutyrate
Gheel colony
ghetto
g. environment
psychiatric g.
ghettoize
ghostlike
GI
general inquiry
giantism
giant urticaria
gibberish aphasia
GID
gender identity disorder
giddy euphoria
gifted child
gigans
gigantea
gigantism
giggle
giggling
nervous g.
Gilles de la Tourette syndrome
ginger paralysis
Ginkgo biloba
ginseng
Chinese g.
Panax g.
girdle
g. anesthesia
g. pain
g. sensation
girl
call g.
phallus g.
girlfriend
girlish
given name
giver
fact g.
giving
transgenerational role of g.
Gjessing syndrome
glabellar tap
gladden
glance
expressive g.
gland
lacrimal g.
sublingual g.
glans
g. clitoridis
g. penis
glare of light
glass
rose-colored g.'s
glassy eyes
glazed look
GLBT
gay/lesbian/bisexual/transgender
glean
glib
glibness
Glick effect
glide
after g.
off g.
glissando technique

NOTES

G

glittering generalities
glitz
gloat
global
g. aggression score
g. amnesia
g. aphasia
g. assessment of function (GAF)
g. attractor state
g. bizarre delusion
g. brain lactate
g. change
g. clinical impression score
g. clinician rating
g. cognitive deficit
g. course
g. delay
g. dementia
g. deterioration
g. distress index
g. functioning
g. index of distress
g. intellectual function
g. loss of language
g. measure
g. measure of impairment
g. metabolism
g. outcome
g. paralysis
g. psychopathology
g. sociocultural trend
g. well-being
globi (*pl. of* globus)
globosa
dysphagia g.
globulin
sex-hormone binding g. (SHBG)
globus, pl. **globi**
g. hystericus
g. pallidus
gloomy
habitually g.
glorified self
glorify
glossodontotropism
glossodyniotropism
glossokinetic potential
glossolalia
glossolysis
glossopharyngeal
g. neuralgia
g. tic
glossoplegia
glossoptosis
glossospasm
glossosteresis
gloss over
glossy skin
glottal attack
glottidospasm
glove anesthesia
glucose
g. metabolism
g. test
glue
g. ear
g. sniffer's rash
g. sniffing
glue-sniffing habit
glutton
gluttonous
gluttony
GMA
gross motor activity
GMC
general medical condition
gnash
gnashing
gnosia
gnostic function
gnosticism
goal
g. attainment
common g.
g. gradient
gradient g.
latent g.
life g.
manifest g.
g. orientation
patient-generated g.
g. setting
g. setting in couples therapy
short-term g. (STG)
social g.
therapeutic g.
therapy g.
unattained g.
goal-directed
g.-d. activity
g.-d. behavior
goal-limited adjustment therapy
goal-oriented process
go-around
God
act of G.
belief in G.
G. complex
faith in G.
relationship with G.
G.'s will
godfather
godless
godlike
godly
godsend
go-getter
going

golden-ager
golden handshake
Goldenhar syndrome
Goliath syndrome
gonad
gonadal
g. agenesis
g. cycle
g. dysgenesis
g. hormone
gonadocentric
gonococcal
gonococcus (GC)
gonorrhea
good
bill of g.'s
g. faith
faking g.
g. form response (F+)
g. functioning
g. impression
g. kid violence
g. object
g. shape
g. sleep efficiency
good-enough
g.-e. mother
g.-e. mothering
good-for-nothing
good-looking
Goodman lock box
good-natured
good-tempered
goodwill
goody-goody
goon
goose bumps
Gordon
G. sign
G. symptom
gorger-vomiter
Gorlin sign
gormandize
gormless
gory
gospeler
gossip
gossipy
gouge
gouging
eye g.
gourmand
governess psychosis
Gowers
G. syndrome
vasovagal attack of G.
grabby
grace
impaired social g.
graceful
graceless
gracious
gradation method
grade
g. equivalent
failing g.
g. norm
g. rating
g. skipping
graded
g. activity
g. exposure
g. potential
gradient
approach g.
avoidance g.
axial g.
effect g.
excitation g.
generalization g.
goal g.
g. goal
g. slope
gradual topic shift
graduate
college g.
inmate g.
graffiti tagger
graft
cable g.
nerve g.
sleeve g.
grammar
g. development stage
g. formation stage
shared g.
grammatical equivalent
gramophone symptom
grand
g. mal epilepsy
g. mal seizure
g. mal status
grande attaque hystérique
grandeur
delusion of g.
grandfather complex

NOTES

grandiloquence
grandiose
g. concept
g. content
g. delirium
g. delusion
g. delusion of exceptional talent
g. expansiveness
g. idea
g. ideation
g. self
g. subtype
g. theme
g. type
g. word
grandiose-type
g.-t. delusional disorder
g.-t. paranoid disorder
g.-t. schizophrenia
grandiosity in fantasy
grandma rule
grandparent
foster g.
grandstand
granted
take for g.
granulated opium
granulatum
granulocytopenia
granulomatous
grape
grapevine
graphanesthesia
graphesthesia
graphic
g. aphasia
g. description
g. disorientation
g. impairment
g. violence
graphica
asemia g.
graphically violent video game
graphic-arts therapy
graphology
graphomania
graphomotor
g. aphasia
g. skill
g. technique
graphopathology
graphorrhea
graphospasm
grapple
Grashey aphasia
grasp
g. and reach
g. reflex
grasping and groping reflex
Grasset-Gaussel phenomenon
Grasset law
GRAT
Group ROI Analysis Trial
grate on nerves
gratification
delayed g.
g. of dependent wishes
immediate g.
inability to delay g.
material g.
oral g.
reduced g.
sexual g.
gratified
sexually g.
gratify
gratifying work
gratitude
priori expectation of g.
grave delirium
gravel voice
graven image
gravis
dementia paranoides g.
neurasthenia g.
oneirodynia g.
paranoia dementia g.
gravitate
gravity perception
gray
g. matter
g. matter area
g. matter lactate
g. matter lactate level
g. matter region
g. matter tissue
gray-out
g.-o. episode
g.-o. syndrome
gray-white matter difference
greed
greedy
gregarious
gregariousness
grenade shrapnel
gridiron abdomen
grief
animal loss g.
anticipatory g.
constellation of g.
g. counselor
delayed g.
denied g.
distorted g.
exposure to g.
expression of g.
feeling of g.
impacted g.

inhibited g.
g. management
mutual g.
prolonged g.
g. reaction
g. support group
g. therapy
traumatic g.
unresolved g.
g. work
grief-based attachment
grievance-seeker
grieve
grieving
inhibited g.
pathologic g.
grievous
g. assault
g. bodily harm
grimace
facial g.
tic-like facial g.
grimacing
prominent g.
grimly adhered-to routine
grimness
grin
sardonic g.
grinding
jaw g.
tooth g.
gripe
Griselda complex
grisette
grisi siknis
gristly
gritty
groaning
sleep-related g.
groomed
neatly g.
poorly g.
well g.
grooming
g. behavior
g. deterioration
excessive g.
unhygienic g.
groove
grope
groping others
gross
g. impairment
g. impairment of reality testing
g. insensitivity
g. medical error
g. motor activity (GMA)
g. motor deficit
g. motor skill
g. negligence
g. neurologic deficit
g. pathological feature
g. sensory deficit
g. stress reaction
grossly
g. disorganized behavior
g. impaired functioning
g. pathogenic care
grotesque
grouchy
ground
figure and g.
middle g.
g. rule
grounded
group
abstinence g.
g. acceptance
action g.
g. activity
g. adjustment therapy (GAT)
adolescent support g.
G. for Advancement of Psychiatry (GAP)
aftercare g.
age g.
all-women g.
amygdala nucleus g.
g. analysis
aspirational g.
attitudinal g.
g. behavior
bereavement support g.
blood g.
g. boundary
buzz g.
g. centered
charismatic g.
g. climate
closed g.
CNS disease g.
cognitive-behavioral coping skills training g.
g. cohesion
community action g.
g. composition

NOTES

G

group *(continued)*
g. consciousness
continuous g.
g. contract
control g.
g. counseling
g. counselor
couple skills g.
crisis g.
criterion g.
cultural reference g.
g. delinquency
g. delinquent reaction
diagnosis-related g.
diagnostic g.
g. difference
g. dimension
diverse g.
g. diversity
g. dynamics
encounter g.
equivalent g.
ethnic g.
ethnic reference g.
g. experience
experiential g.
experimental g.
family support g.
g. feeling
focus g.
grief support g.
g. harmony
hate g.
heterogeneous g.
high-risk g.
g. home
horizontal g.
human relations g.
g. identification
intake diagnostic g.
intake orientation g.
integrity g.
interact g.
interest g.
g. intervention
g. interview
laissez-faire g.
leaderless g.
g. living
mandated self-help g.
g. marriage
matched g.'s
g. medicine
militia g.
g. mind
minority g.
g. morale
multifamily skills g.
mutual aid g.
natural g.
g. norm
nurse support g.
online support g.
open g.
g. participation
peer g.
peer support g.
personal growth g.
g. phase
g. play
political g.
g. practice
g. pressure
primary support g.
g. problem-solving
g. process
psychoanalytic g.
psychoeducational g.
g. psychosis
g. psychotherapy
g. psychotherapy session
rank in peer g.
rap g.
reference g.
regressive inspirational g.
g. relations theory
G. ROI Analysis Trial (GRAT)
g. rule
self-help g.
sensitivity training g.
g. setting
social reference g.
socioeconomic g.
spiritual focus g.
splinter g.
g. stage
g. stress reaction
g. structure
structured interactional g.
study g.
substance g.
g. superego
support g.
symptom g.
T g.
task-oriented g.
thematically related g.'s
therapeutic play g. (TPG)
g. therapist
g. therapy
training g.
transient g.
g. treatment
work g.
g. work

grouping
clinical g.
DSM-IV-TR diagnostic g.

gastrointestinal symptom g.
heterogenous g.
homogeneous g.
homogenous g.
pain symptom g.
sexual symptom g.
symptom g.

groupthink
group-type conduct disorder
grovel
growing pain
growth
cognitive g.
continuous g.
existence, relatedness, and g. (ERG)
g. hormone (GH)
g. hormone-releasing factor
g. hormone-releasing hormone
mental g.
g. period
personal g.
surgent g.
tumultuous g.
zero population g. (ZPG)

growth-associated protein (GAP)
GROW The Marriage Enrichment Program
grudge bearing
grueling
gruesome
grumble
grumbling mania
grumpy
grunge look
grungy
grunt
grunting noise
GSR
galvanic skin response

GSW
gunshot wound

GSWH
gunshot wound to head

guaiac
g. negative
g. positive

Guam
guard
off g.
old g.
US Coast G.

guarded
g. manner
g. self-disclosure

guardedness
adolescent g.

guardian
g. ad litem
court-appointed g.
legal g.

guardianship
estate g.
individual g.
legal g.
required g.

Guatemalan refugee
guerrilla
g. tactics
g. warfare

guess
second g.

guidance
anticipatory g.
g. center
child g.
g. clinic
conscious g.
g. counselor
spiritual g.
vocational g.

guidance-cooperation model
guide
action g.
g. dog
medication g.
parental failure to g.
spiritual g.

guided
g. affective imagery (GAI)
g. meditation
g. mourning
g. smoking

guideline
practice g.

guidepost
guile
guileless
Guillain-Barré syndrome
guilt
g. by association
confession of g.
g. displacement
excessive g.
g. feeling

G

NOTES

guilt *(continued)*
inappropriate g.
initiative vs g.
lack of g.
mild g.
misattribution of g.
neurotic g.
g. obsession
pathologic g.
pervasive proneness to g.
preoccupation with g.
realistic g.
self-attribution of g.
self-reported g.
severe g.
survivor g.
g. theme
unconscious g.
guilt-induced hallucination
guiltless
guilty
g. rumination
g. verdict
Guinon
tic de G.
guise
Gulf War syndrome
gullwing pattern
gum
nicotine g.
g. opium
gumma
gumption
gun
access to g.
assault g.
carries a g.
g. control
hired g.
riot g.
stun g.
submachine g.
tommy g.
6-gun
gunfight
gunfire
gunman
gunned down
gunnery sergeant
gunrunner
gunshot
g. wound (GSW)
g. wound to head (GSWH)
gurney
guru
gushy
gustation
gustatism
gustatory
g. anesthesia
g. audition
g. aura
g. hallucination
g. hyperesthesia
g. nerve
g. seizure
gustatory-sudorific reflex
gusto
gutless
gutsy
Gwa Sha
Gwathmey anesthesia
gymnomania
gynander
gynandrism
gynandroid
gynandromorph
gynatresia
gynecic
gynecomania
gynomonoecism
gyrate
gyration
gyri (*pl. of* gyrus)
gyrosa
gyrospasm
gyrus, pl. **gyri**

h
human response
HA
harm avoidance
high anxiety
habeas corpus
habilitation
habit
acculturation problem with expression of h.
alcohol h.
benign h.
h. cessation
h. chorea
cocaine h.
compulsive h.
h. cough
h. deterioration
dietary h.
h. disorder
h. disturbance
drug h.
eating h.
h. exposure
feeding h.
food h.
force of h.
h. formation
glue-sniffing h.
h. hierarchy
inattention to proper dietary h.'s
inflexible h.
h. interference
kick the h.
laxative h.
motor h.
narcotic h.
nicotine h.
h. pattern
poor eating h.
responsible eating h.
h. reversal
h. reversal training (HRT)
h. spasm
h. strength
temporary h.
h. tic
h. training
h. treatment
unhygienic bathroom h.
habitability
habit-forming
habit-training
habitual
h. act
h. complaints
h. criminal
h. offender
h. pattern
h. runaway
h. sleep efficiency
habitually gloomy
habituate
habituation
caffeine h.
cocaine h.
electrical h.
habitude
habitué
habitus
abnormal h.
h. phthisicus
Hachinski ischemic score
hacker
computer h.
hackle
HACS
hyperactive child syndrome
Haeckel biogenic law
haggard appearance
hagiotherapy
hair
h. denuding
eating h.
fine electric h.
h. plucking
h. pulling
spiked h.
hair-pulling behavior
hair-raising
hairsplitting
half-brother
half-hearted attempt at suicide
half-life
drug h.-l.
elimination h.-l.
long h.-l.
short h.-l.
half-show
half-sister
half-truth
halfway
h. children
h. house
meet h.
halitosis
hallmark
Halloween effect
hallucinate
hallucinated voice

H

hallucinating patient
hallucination
accusatory h.
affective h.
alcoholic h.
alcohol-induced psychotic disorder with h.'s
amphetamine-induced psychotic disorder with h.'s
angel-of-death h.
anxiolytic-induced psychotic disorder with h.'s
auditory h.
autoscopic h.
blank h.
body image h.
cannabis-induced psychotic disorder with h.'s
cenesthetic h.
cocaine-induced psychotic disorder with h.'s
command h.
command auditory h.
complex h.
h. of conception
content of h.
daytime h.
depressive auditory h.
depressive olfactory h.
depressive visual h.
h. description
dreamlike h.
drug-induced h.
elementary h.
fixed h.
fleeting auditory h.
fleeting visual h.
formed visual h.
fragmentary h.
geometric h.
guilt-induced h.
gustatory h.
hallucinogen-induced psychotic disorder with h.'s
haptic h.
humiliating h.
hypnagogic h.
hypnopompic h.
hypnotic-induced psychotic disorder with h.'s
induced psychotic disorder with h.'s
inhalant-induced psychotic disorder with h.'s
intrusive h.
isolated auditory h.
kaleidoscope h.
kinesthesia h.
kinesthetic h.
Lilliputian h.
memory h.
methamphetamine-induced h.
microptic h.
mood-congruent h.
mood-incongruent h.
multimodal h.
nocturnal h.
nonaffective h.
nonpsychotic h.
olfactory h.
organic h.
overt h.
partial h.
h. of perception
phencyclidine-induced psychotic disorder with h.'s
posttraumatic h.
prominent h.
psychotic disorder with h.'s
reflex h.
running commentary h.
sedative-induced psychotic disorder with h.'s
self-destructive h.
simple h.
sleep-related h.
somatic h.
speech h.
structured h.
stump h.
tactile h.
tactual h.
teleologic h.
temporal h.
third-person auditory h.
threatening h.
transient auditory h.
transient tactile h.
transient visual h.
unformed auditory h.
unformed visual h.
unpleasant h.
vestibular h.
violent command h.
visceral h.
visual h.
vivid h.
hallucinatoria
paranoia h.
hallucinatory
h. behavior
h. dementia
h. drug
h. epilepsy
h. experience
h. game
h. image
h. mania

h. neuralgia
h. paranoia
h. state
h. transient organic psychosis
h. transient organic syndrome
h. verbigeration
hallucinatory-state drug psychosis
hallucinatory-type psychoorganic syndrome
hallucinogen
h. abuse
h. affective disorder
h. delusional disorder
h. dependence
designer h.
h. hallucinosis
h. intoxication delirium
h. persisting perception disorder
sedative h.
h. toxic effect
h. use disorder
hallucinogenesis
hallucinogenic
h. drug
h. drug dependence
h. hallucinosis
h. intoxication
h. overdose
h. potency
hallucinogen-induced
h.-i. delirium and anxiety disorder
h.-i. psychotic disorder with delusions
h.-i. psychotic disorder with hallucinations
hallucinogen-related
h.-r. disorder, NOS
h.-r. stroke
h.-r. subarachnoid hemorrhage
hallucinosis
acute h.
alcoholic h.
h. alcoholic psychosis
alcohol withdrawal h.
bromide h.
drug-induced h.
flashback h.
hallucinogen h.
hallucinogenic h.
organic h.
peduncular h.
psychoactive substance h.
withdrawal h.
halo
h. effect
h. of light
object h.
halogenated inhalation anesthesia
haloxazolam
HALT
Heroin Antagonist and Learning Therapy
halting
h. gait
h. manner
h. movement
h. speech
haltlose-type personality
hamartomania
hammered
hamper
hand
accoucheur's h.
alien h.
black h.
dead h.
dominant h.
laying on of h.'s
nondominant h.
h. preference
h. shaking
h. tremor
upper h.
h. waving
writing h.
handedness
handful
handgun
.22-caliber h.
.38-caliber h.
.44-caliber h.
concealed h.
h. control
licensed h.
9-mm h.
h. possession
unlicensed h.
hand-holding
handicap
emotional h. (EH)
severe emotional h. (SEH)
handicapped
educationally mentally h. (EMH)
emotionally h.
mentally h.
perceptually h.
trainable mentally h. (TMH)

NOTES

handshake
golden h.
hand-to-mouth reaction
hand-washing
h.-w. obsession
repeated h.-w.
h.-w. ritual
handwringing movement
handwriting analysis
hang
h. around
h. back
h. on
h. out
h. together
h. tough
hanged
hanging
accidental h.
h. arousal
h. attempt
erotized h.
suicide by h.
hangout
hangover
daytime sleep h.
h. effect
h. headache
hang-up
Hanoi
Tower of H.
hapax legomenon
haphalgesia
haphazard
hapless
haplology
happiness
excessive h.
h. measure
happy
h. childhood
h. puppet syndrome
happy-go-lucky
haptic
h. feedback
h. hallucination
h. perception
h. system
haptodysphoria
haptometer
haptophonia
harangue
harass
harassment
email h.
quid pro quo h.
same-sex h.
sexual h. (SH)
harbinger
hard
h. chancre
h. rock
hard-boiled
hard-drug use
harden
hardheaded
hardiness
hard-line
hardness
hard-of-hearing
hardy
Hardy-Weinberg equilibrium
harm
alcohol-related h.
h. avoidance (HA)
h. avoidance need
desire to inflict h.
extrinsic h.
grievous bodily h.
physical h.
harmaline
harm-avoidant trait
harmful
h. consequence
h. sexual relationship
h. side effect
socially h.
harmine
harming
h. baby
h. others
h. self
harmless wit
harmonic
h. analysis
h. mean
harmonious interaction
harmonizer
harmony
group h.
maintenance of h.
h. process
social h.
HARP
Harvard-Brown Anxiety Disorders Research Project
harria
harried
Harris migraine
Harrison Antinarcotic Act
harsh
h. discipline
h. reaction
Hartel technique
Hartnup disorder
Harvard-Brown Anxiety Disorders Research Project (HARP)
has-been

hashish
hassle
haste
hasten
hastened death
hatchet
h. job
h. man
hate
h. crime
ethnic h.
exposure to h.
feeling of h.
h. group
h. video game
hateful
Hatha yoga
hatred
haughty behavior
haunt
hauteur
haut mal epilepsy
haven
havoc
Hawaiian
hawk
Hawthorn effect
hazard
environmental h.
moral h.
occupational h.
hazardous treatment
haze
hazy
HBS
hyperkinetic behavior syndrome
HCA
heterocyclic antidepressant
HCD
higher cerebral dysfunction
HCl
hydrochloride
chlorphentermine HCl
diacetylmorphine HCl
HCR
hysterical conversion reaction
HDH
hostility and direction of hostility
HE
hepatic encephalopathy
head
h. banging
h. bobbing
h. consciousness
gunshot wound to h. (GSWH)
h. of household
h. injury
h. jerking
h. knocking
h. and neck tremor
perception of sound inside h.
perception of sound outside h.
h. rolling
h. shadow effect
sound inside h.
sound outside h.
H. Start program
swelled h.
swimming in h.
h. tetanus
h. tilt
h. trauma
h. turn technique
voice inside h.
voice outside h.
h. weaving
H. zone
headache
acute confusional migraine h.
bandlike h.
benign exertional h.
bifrontal h.
bilious h.
bioccipital h.
blind h.
cataclysmic h.
chronic h.
circumstantial migraine h.
classical migraine h.
cluster h.
coital h.
combination h.
common migraine h.
complicated migraine h.
confusional migraine h.
cyclic h.
disabling h.
essential h.
evening h.
exertional h.
familial migraine h.
fibrositic h.
frontal h.
functional h.
generalized h.
hangover h.

NOTES

H

headache *(continued)*
hemiparesthetic migraine h.
histaminic h.
Horton h.
ipsilateral h.
late-life migraine h.
migraine h.
Monday morning h.
muscle contraction h.
nitrite h.
nonpulsating h.
ocular migraine h.
organic h.
paroxysmal migraine h.
phobia-induced migraine h.
postcoital h.
postconcussion h.
posttraumatic h.
psychogenic h.
pulsating h.
rebound h.
recurrent migraine h.
reflex h.
seasonal migraine h.
sick h.
sleep-related cluster h.
suboccipital h.
sudden-onset h.
symptomatic h.
h. syndrome
temporal h.
tension migraine h.
tension vascular h.
traumatic h.
unilateral migraine h.
vacuum h.
vascular h.
vasomotor h.
weekend h.
head-banging behavior
head-bobbing doll syndrome
headlong
headquarters
headshrinker
HEADSS
home life, education level, activities, drug use, sexual activity, suicide ideation attempts
home life, education level, activities, drug use, sexual activity, suicide ideation or attempts
headstrong
head-to-head clinical trial
head-up tilt
heady
heal
healer
cultural h.
folk h.
religious h.
healing
Buddhist h.
concept of spiritual h.
faith h.
holistic h.
mental h.
h. prayer
h. process
h. ritual
spiritual h.
traditional h.
health
ASEAN Federation for Psychiatry and Mental H. (AFPMH)
h. behavior
behavioral h.
bill of h.
h. care
change in h.
community mental h.
delusion of ill h.
H., Education, and Welfare (HEW)
emotional h.
flight into h.
H. and Human Services (HHS)
h. insurance
h. issue
Joint Commission on Mental Illness and H. (JCMIH)
h. law
h. literacy skill
h. maintenance organization (HMO)
mental h.
National Institute of Mental H. (NIMH)
national longitudinal scale of adolescent h.
National Survey on Drug Use and H.
h. outcome
H. Plan Employer Data and Information Set
h. policy
President's New Freedom Commission on Mental H.
h. professional
psychological h.
h. psychology
public h.
h. risk
h. status
h. systems agency (HSA)
h. viewpoint
healthcare
h. bias
durable power of attorney for h.

h. informatics
h. proxy
healthful
health-related
h.-r. consequence
h.-r. facility
h.-r. psychology
h.-r. variable
healthy
h. adolescent behavior
h. aggression
h. approach
h. functioning
h. identification
h. individual
H. Lesbian, Gay, and Bisexual Students Project (HLGBSP)
h. lifestyle
h. patient
h. religious life
hearing
color h.
evidentiary h.
h. impairment
Riese h.
speech and h. (S&H)
h. theory
thought h.
visual h.
h. voices
hearsay
heart
broken h.
change of h.
h. disease
irritable h.
pounding h.
h. psychogenic disorder
purple h.
h. rate
soldier's h.
take h.
heartache
heartbreak
heartbroken
hearted
false h.
tender h.
heartless
heartrending
heartsick
heartstring
heat
h. defense
h. defense response
h. dissipation
h. effector
h. shock protein 90 (hsp90)
heated discussion
heat-induced asthenia
heat-loss
h.-l. apparatus
h.-l. mechanism
h.-l. pathway
heaviness
heavy
h. metal intoxication
h. metal music
h. metal screen
h. smoker
heavy-duty
hebbian
h. modification
h. property
Hebb rule
hebephilia
hebephrenia
manic h.
hebephrenic
h. dementia
h. schizophrenia
hebetic
hebetude
heboid
h. paranoia
h. praecox
heboidophrenia
heckle
hectic
hector
hedge
hedonic
h. capacity
h. drive
h. level
h. psychoactive effect
h. response
h. tone factor
h. volition
hedonism
hedonistic
h. activity
h. orientation
h. utilitarianism
hedonomania

NOTES

heed
heedless
heel
Achilles h.
heeltap
heeltap reaction
heightened
h. anxiety
h. attention
h. attention state
h. awareness
h. awareness state
h. emotional tone
h. sensory perception
h. sociability
height vertigo
Heinis constant
heinous
h. act
h. crime
h. event
heir of Oedipus complex
helicopod gait
helicopodia
heliencephalitis
heliomania
hell
raise h.
hellbent
hellcat
Heller
H. dementia
H. syndrome
hellion
hellish
helmet
neurasthenic h.
help
cry for h.
pastoral h.
plea for h.
professional h.
psychiatric h.
h. seeking
helper
magic h.
h. role
h. therapy
helping
h. behavior
h. model
h. relationship
helpless
helplessness
feeling of h.
learned h.
psychic h.
self-reported h.
helpmate
help-rejecting complainer
help-seeking behavior
hemiacrosomia
hemianalgesia
hemianesthesia
alternate h.
crossed h.
hemiapraxia
hemiasynergia
hemiataxia
hemiathetosis
hemiatrophy
facial h.
progressive lingual h.
hemiballismic movement
hemiballismus, hemiballism
hemifacial spasm
hemifield of vision
hemihyperesthesia
hemihypertonia
hemihypotonia
hemiopalgia
hemiparesthesia
hemiparesthetic migraine headache
hemiplegia
contralateral h.
crossed h.
double h.
facial h.
hysterical h.
infantile h.
h. migraine
nocturnal h.
spastic h.
hemiplegic gait
hemisensory loss
hemispasm
hemispatial arousal neglect
hemisphere
cerebral h.
dominant h.
language-dominant h.
left h.
right h.
hemispheric
h. dynamic
h. lateralization
h. reliance
hemispherical dysfunction
hemithermoanesthesia
hemitonia
hemitremor
hemizygous
hemlock
poison h.
H. Society
hemodynamic system
hemorrhage
hallucinogen-related subarachnoid h.

hemothymia
hemp
henbane
hepatic
h. coma
h. encephalopathy (HE)
h. encephalopathy tremor
h. injury
h. porphyria
h. steatosis
hepatitis
alcoholic h. (AH)
h. C
infectious h.
viral h.
hepatolenticular disease
hepatorenal syndrome
hepatosplenomegaly
hepatotoxicity
herbal
h. medicine
h. preparation
h. remedy
h. supplement
herbalism
herbalist
herbiceutical
herbivorous
herd instinct
hereafter
here-and-now approach
hereditaria
adynamia episodica h.
alopecia h.
hereditarian
hereditary
h. deficiency
h. disorder
heredity
environment and h. (E&H)
heredoataxia
heredofamilial
h. essential microsomia
h. psychosis
h. tremor
heredopathia atactica polyneuritiformis
heresiarch
heresy
heretic
heritability
broad h.
heritable
h. basis
h. component
h. influence
h. nature
h. symptom
heritage
mixed h.
hermaphrodite
hermaphroditism, hermaphrodism
bilateral h.
false h.
transverse h.
true h.
unilateral h.
hermeticism
hermetic medicine
hermit
hermitage
hero
h. daydream
h. fantasy
intellectual h.
negative h.
h. worship
h. worshiper
heroic act
Heroin Antagonist and Learning Therapy (HALT)
herpes
h. encephalitis
genital h.
h. genitalis
h. simplex virus
h. zoster
h. zoster meningitis
herpetic meningoencephalitis
Herrmann syndrome
hersage
hesitancy
patient h.
hesitant
h. communication
h. speech
hesitation phenomenon
Hess
trophotropic zone of H.
hetaeric fantasy
heteresthesia
heterocentric
heteroclite
heterocyclic
h. agent
h. antidepressant drug
heterodimer

NOTES

H

heteroeroticism, heteroerotism
heterogeneity
clinical h.
developmental h.
etiological h.
genetic h.
neurophysiological h.
heterogeneous
h. clinical presentation
h. condition
h. group
h. nuclear RNA
heterogenicity
genetic h.
locus h.
heterogenous
h. disorder
h. grouping
heterohypnosis
heterokinesis, heterokinesia
heterolalia
heteroliteral
heterologous stimulus
heteromorphic
heteronomous
h. psychotherapy
h. stage
h. superego
heteronomy
heteronymous
heteropathy
heterophasia
heterophemia, heterophemy
heterophonia
heterophoria
heteropsychologic
heteroreceptor
heterorexia
heterosexual
h. anxiety
h. behavior
h. incest
h. lover
h. marriage
h. orientation
h. pedophile
h. pedophilia
h. rape
h. relationship
h. sexual experience
heterosexuality
heterosexual sexual experience
heterosome
heterosuggestibility
heterosuggestion
heterotopia, heterotopy
heterotopic pain
heterotrimeric
h. G protein
h. postreceptor
heterozygote
heterozygous individual
heuristic
heutoscopy
HEW
Health, Education, and Welfare
hex, pl. **hexes**
h. doctor
hexacarbon
hexane
hexes (*pl. of* hex)
hexing
illness ascribed to h.
HFA
high-functioning autism
HGF
human growth factor
HHS
Health and Human Services
HI
hypoglycemic index
5-HIAA
hiccup, hiccough
psychogenic h.
hidden
h. agenda
h. meaning
h. message
h. observer
h. observer phenomenon
h. rage
h. self
hiding
h. behavior
h. symptoms
hidrosis
HIE
hypoxic-ischemic encephalopathy
hierarchical
h. functioning
h. organization
h. regression
h. regression analysis
h. structure
h. theory of instinct
hierarchy
anxiety h.
h. construction
corporate h.
dominance h.
exposure h.
habit h.
lifetime h.
Maslow h.
motivational h.
h. of motives

h. of needs
occupational h.
response h.
social h.

hieromania

hierotherapy

HIF
higher intellectual function

high
h. academic achiever
h. adaptive level
h. affectivity ratio
h. alcoholic elixir
h. alpha coefficient
h. anxiety (HA)
h. arousal
h. degree of competency
drug-induced h.
h. energy level
h. fever
h. impulsiveness high anxiety (HIHA)
h. impulsiveness low anxiety (HILA)
h. profile
h. roller
h. school adolescent
h. school diploma
h. school exit exam
h. sensitivity
h. steppage gait
h. suicide risk
h. tolerance potential
h. utilizer

high-altitude illness

high-anger individual

highbrow
ethical h.

high-calorie diet

high-conflict family

high-dose drug

high-emotion scene

high-energy
h.-e. bond
h.-e. cellular store

higher
h. being
h. brain center
h. cerebral dysfunction (HCD)
h. cortical dysfunction
h. cortical function
h. dementia
h. echelon
h. integrative language processing
h. intellectual function (HIF)
h. level cognitive function
h. level of consciousness
h. level skill
h. mental process
h. neural function
h. order conditioning
h. order emotion-related meaning
h. order interaction
h. power
h. state of consciousness
h. status

highest
h. grade achieved
h. ranking item

high-fat
h.-f. diet
h.-f. meal

high-fiber diet

high-frequency deafness

high-functioning
h.-f. autism (HFA)
h.-f. patient

high-grade
h.-g. defect
h.-g. heroin

high-intensity transition

high-level perceptual disturbance

high-pitched voice

high-potency
h.-p. antipsychotic
h.-p. D_2 antagonist
h.-p. medication
h.-p. neuroleptic treatment

high-profile
h.-p. case
h.-p. crime
h.-p. criminal
h.-p. patient

high-protein diet

high-quality
h.-q. education
h.-q. parenting

high-resolution MRI

high-risk
h.-r. approach
h.-r. drinking pattern
h.-r. drug behavior
h.-r. factor
h.-r. gambling situation
h.-r. group
h.-r. lifestyle

NOTES

H

high-risk *(continued)*
h.-r. patient
h.-r. population
h.-r. sexual activity
h.-r. sexual behavior
h.-r. study
high-spirited buoyancy
high-strung
high-volume hospital
HIHA
high impulsiveness high anxiety
hijacker
HILA
high impulsiveness low anxiety
Hilgard neodissociation theory
Hilton method
Hindu religion
Hinman syndrome
HIPAA
hip-hop
h.-h. culture
h.-h. music
hippie culture
hippocampal
h. activation
h. amnesia
h. complex
h. damage
h. epilepsy
h. formation subdivision
h. raw volume
h. sclerosis
h. sprouting
h. synaptic plasticity
h. volumetric loss
hippocratic oath
hippomania
hired gun
hirsutism
histaminic
h. cephalalgia
h. headache
historian
poor h.
historical
h. context
h. data
h. method
h. presentation
historicize
history
h. of abuse
h. of abusing animals
alcohol-positive h. (APH)
arrest h.
biopsychosocial h.
case h.
childhood mistreatment h.
clinical h.
criminal h.
h. of cult affiliation
cyclic h.
h. of delirium
depression h.
detailed h.
developmental h.
drinking h.
drug use h.
educational h.
family h. (FH)
family psychiatric h.
genetic h.
life h.
lifetime h.
marijuana use h.
marital h. (MH)
media h.
medical h.
military h.
h. of mistreatment
multigenerational h.
h. of neglect
no previous h. (NPH)
occupational h. (OH)
oral h.
pain h.
past h. (PH)
past personal h.
personal h. (PH)
personal psychiatric h.
personal and social h. (P&SH)
h. and physical (H&P)
poor job h.
postrelevant h. (PRH)
premorbid psychiatric h.
prenatal h.
h. of present illness (HPI)
previous h.
prison h.
psychiatric family h.
psychosexual h.
psychosocial h.
relationship h.
reliable h.
school h.
seizure h.
h. of self-mutilation
sexual abuse h.
smoking h.
social h. (SH)
h. of suicide attempt
suicide attempt h.
h. of tobacco use
value h.
h. of violence
violent h.
history-taking

histrionic
h. character
h. composite description
h. diagnostic category
h. neurotic personality disorder
h. paralysis
h. patient
h. personality
h. presentation
h. Q factor
h. quality
h. situation
h. spasm
hit
h. list
h. man
hit-and-run
hitting
h. own body
repetitive h.
HIV
human immunodeficiency virus
HIV dementia
HIV illness stage
HIV risk behavior
HIV-1-associated dementia
HIV-based dementia
HIV-induced dementia
HLGBSP
Healthy Lesbian, Gay, and Bisexual Students Project
HMO
health maintenance organization
Hmong refugee
hoard
h. food
weapon's h.
hoarding
h. character
h. and clutter
compulsive h.
h. orientation
h. personality
hoarseness
hoax
hockey stick strategy
hodomania
Hoffmann
H. phenomenon
H. sign
hold
choke h.
24-hour h.
sleeper h.
holding
h. environment
h. exercise
holiday
caffeine h.
h. depression
drug h.
Roman h.
h. syndrome
therapeutic drug h.
holier-than-thou attitude
holism
holistic
h. analysis
h. approach
h. healing
h. medicine
h. psychology
h. regimen
h. treatment
Holocaust survivor
holography
holophrase
homage
homatropine
home
adult foster h.
h. assessment
board-and-care h.
boarding h.
broken h.
h. care
h. caregiver
h. confinement
detention h.
domiciliary care h.
eloping from h.
h. environment
h. evaluation
former foster h.
foster h.
group h.
h. health aide
h. invasion victim
h. language
h. life, education level, activities, drug use, sexual activity, suicide ideation attempts (HEADSS)
h. management
personal care h.
h. placement

NOTES

H

home *(continued)*
- problem at h.
- rest h.
- returning to h.
- h. schooling
- h. service agency
- h. setting
- sheltered h.
- single-parent h.
- h. visit

home-based family management
homebody
homebound
homeland
homeless
- h. child
- h. family
- h. patient
- h. person
- h. shelter
- spiritually h.

homely
homemade
- h. drug paraphernalia
- h. pipe bomb

homemaking responsibility
homeopathic principle
homeopathy and depression
homeostasis
homeostatic
- h. balance
- h. equilibrium
- h. model
- h. principle

homeothermy
homeotic gene
homesick
homicidal
- h. behavior
- h. ideation
- h. intent
- h. plan
- h. preoccupation
- h. rumination
- h. state
- h. thought

homicide
- child h.
- justifiable h.

homicide-suicide
- h.-s. pact
- h.-s. protection contract
- h.-s. rate

homicidomania
hominem
- ad h.

homing
homochronous
homoerotic
- h. behavior
- h. fantasy

homoeroticism, homoerotism
homogamy
homogenate technique
homogeneity
- cross-cultural h.

homogeneous
- h. grouping
- h. reinforcement

homogenic love
homogenitality
homogenous
- h. grouping
- h. reinforcement
- h. scintillating scotoma

homogeny
homograph
homolateral
homologous stimulus
homonomy drive
homophile
homophobe
homophobia
- internalized h.
- pathological h.

homophobic cult
homorganic
homosexual
- h. behavior
- closet h.
- h. community
- h. complex
- h. conflict disorder
- effeminate h.
- h. incest
- h. lover
- h. marriage
- h. neurosis
- h. orientation
- h. panic
- h. pedophile
- h. pedophilia
- h. relationship
- h. sexual experience

homosexuality
- ego-dystonic h.
- female h.
- iatrogenic h.
- latent h.
- male h.
- masked h.
- overt h.
- situational h.
- unconscious h.

homotopic pain
homozygous individual
homunculus

honeymoon period
honor
court of h.
family h.
personal h.
point of h.
h. system
honorable discharge
hood
clitoral h.
hoodwink
hope
failed h.
false h.
misplaced h.
hopeful
hopelessness
degree of h.
h. delusion
h. and depression
feeling of h.
horizon
closed h.
open h.
horizontal
h. conflict
h. group
h. mobility
h. nystagmus
h. vertigo
hormism
hormonal
h. difference
h. level
h. maturation
h. sex reassignment
hormone
antidiuretic h. (ADH)
circadian h.
corticotropin-releasing h.
gonadal h.
growth h. (GH)
growth hormone-releasing h.
h. ingestion
luteinizing h. (LH)
luteinizing hormone-releasing h. (LHRH)
melanocyte-stimulating h.
h. replacement
resistance to thyroid h. (RTH)
sex h.
thyroid-stimulating h. (TSH)
thyrotropin-releasing h. (TRH)
thyrotropin-stimulating h. (TSH)
h. treatment
horrendous event
horrific
h. experience
h. impulse
h. mental imagery
h. temptation
horrify
horror story
hors de combat
horserace gambling
Horton headache
hospice care
hospital
h. addiction syndrome
h. admission
h. chaplain
h. and community psychiatry
day h.
high-volume h.
maximum-security forensic psychiatric h.
mental h.
h. mortality rate
night h.
open h.
open-door h.
private psychiatric h.
psychiatric h.
h. record
h. setting
state h. (SH)
state mental h. (SMH)
teaching h.
weekend h.
hospital-based psychiatry
hospitalism
hospitality
expression of h.
hospitalization
emergency h.
involuntary h.
long-term h.
multiple h.'s
partial h.
psychiatric h.
short-term h.
voluntary h.
weekend h.
hospitalize
hospital-treated mental disorder

NOTES

H

host
h. culture
h. mother
hostage
hostile
h. affect
h. aggression
h. attributional bias
h. behavior
h. challenge
h. identity
h. mania
h. motive
h. personality
h. response
h. tone
h. transference
h. work environment
hostility
aggressive h.
covert h.
h. and direction of hostility (HDH)
exposure to h.
expression of h.
open h.
paranoid h.
penalty, frustration, anxiety, guilt, h. (PFAGH)
hot
h. flash
h. line
h. temper
hot-blooded
hotheaded
hotline
abused child h.
abused spouse h.
abused wife h.
behavioral health h.
crisis h.
runaway h.
suicide h.
hot-seat technique
24-hour
24-h. hold
24-h. telephone help line
1-hour restraint rule
house
h. arrest
cooperative urban h.
halfway h.
h. physician
quarter-way h.
h. rule
transitional halfway h.
housebound
household
h. dysfunction
head of h.
h. product inhalant
h. responsibility
h. smoking
househusband
housemate
housewife
clingy h.
h. neurosis
h. psychosis
h. syndrome
housing
satellite h.
supportive h.
hovel
hover
howitzer
howler
H&P
history and physical
HPA
hypothalamic-pituitary-adrenal
HPI
history of present illness
HRT
habit reversal training
HSA
health systems agency
hsp90
heat shock protein 90
HT
hypertension
5-HT
5-hydroxytryptamine
5-hydroxytryptophan
5-HT agonist
5-HT antagonist
5-HT releasing agent
5-HT reuptake inhibitor
5-HT-1 receptor
5-HT-2 receptor
huang
hubris
hue
h. and cry
primary h.
human
h. cell death protein
h. communication
h. companionship
h. complexity
h. ecology
h. engineering
h. factor psychology
h. figure parts response
h. frailty
H. Genome Project
h. growth factor (HGF)
h. immunodeficiency virus (HIV)
h. motivation theory

h. movement response
h. nature
h. potential
h. potential model
h. potential movement
h. prion disease
h. problem
h. relations
h. relations group
h. relationship
h. relations training
h. resources
h. response (h)
h. rights
h. sexuality
h. strength
h. therapeutic experience

humane treatment
humanism
humanistic
h. concept
h. conscience
h. perspective
h. philosophy
h. psychology
h. school
h. theory
h. therapy

humanitarian
humanity
crime against h.

humanize
humankind
human-pet bonding
humble
humidity effect
humiliate
humiliating
h. event
h. hallucination

humiliation
humility
humor
anal h.
bitter h.
cynical h.
gallows h.
sense of h.

humoral
h. immunity
h. theory

humored
humorless
hunched posture
hunger
affect h.
air h.
h. drive
drug h.
h. edema
narcotic h.
h. pain
h. pang
paradoxic h.
psychogenic air h.
social h.
h. strike

hunter
fortune h.

hunting behavior
Huntington chorea organic psychosis
hurdle
hurtful
husband-to-wife aggression
hustler
bar h.

Hutchinson
H. facies
H. mask
H. pupil

HV
hyperventilation

HVA
homovanillic acid

HVS
hyperventilation syndrome

hwa-byung
wool h.-b.

hyalophagia
H-Y antigen
hydrargyromania
hydrate
hydration
intravenous h.

hydride
hydrocarbon
volatile h.

hydrocephalus ex vacuo
hydrochloride (HCl)
amitriptyline h.
azacyclonol h.
benactyzine h.
methadone h.
methamphetamine h.
methylamphetamine h.

hydrodipsomania

NOTES

H

hydrogenated alkaloid
hydromorphone
hydrophobica
agriothymia h.
hydrophorograph
hydrotherapy
hydroxylase
beta h.
tyrosine h.
5-hydroxytryptophan (5-HT)
hygieiolatry
hygiene
criminal h.
h. deterioration
inadequate sleep h.
inappropriate h.
industrial h.
mental h.
minimal personal h.
personal h.
poor h.
sleep h.
hygienic inducement
hymen
imperforate h.
hymenal membrane
Hyogo Institute for Aging Brain and Cognitive Disorders
hypacusic
hypacusis, hypoacusis
hypalgesia, hypoalgesia
hypalgia
hypapoplexia
hyperactive
h. affect
h. behavior
h. child syndrome (HACS)
h. impulse attention deficit disorder
h. impulsive behavior
h. sexual arousal
h. sexual desire
h. sympathetic response
hyperactivity
attention deficit disorder with h. (ADD-HA)
attention deficit disorder without h.
autonomic h.
developmental h.
h. disorder
dopaminergic h.
impulsive h.
h. index
motoric h.
norepinephrine h.
prefrontal h.
h. problem
sympathoadrenal h.
tactile h.
hyperactivity-impulsivity dimension
hyperacusis, hyperacusia
hyperadrenal constitution
hyperadrenalism
hyperadrenergic state
hyperadrenocorticism
hyperaesthetic (*var. of* hyperesthetic)
hyperaggressivity
hyperalert
hyperalgesia, hyperalgia
auditory h.
cutaneous h.
hyperamnesia
hyperaphia
hyperarousal
autonomic h.
physiologic h.
sensorial h.
h. symptom
hyperattentiveness to voice tone
hyperbaric medicine
hyperbulia
hypercarotenemia
hypercathexis
hypercompensatory
hypercortisolemia
hypercritical
hyperdynamia
hyperechema
hyperemotional
hyperemotionalism
hyperenergetic behavior
hyperergasia
hypereridic state
hyperesthesia
auditory h.
cerebral h.
gustatory h.
muscular h.
olfactory h.
tactile h.
hyperesthetic, hyperaesthetic
h. memory
h. personality
h. variant of schizoid temperament
h. zone
hyperevolutism
hyperexcitability
hyperfunction
hypergenitalism
hypergeusia
hypergnosis
hypergraphia
hyperhedonia
hyperhidrosis
Hypericum perforatum
hyperindependence
hyperintensity
h. change
deep white matter h.

MRI signal h.
periventricular h.
h. rating
h. severity
signal h.
subcortical gray matter h.
white matter h.

hyperirritability

hyperkinesis, hyperkinesia
antipsychotic-related h.
axial h.
developmental disorder associated with h.
h. index

hyperkinetic
h. behavior syndrome (HBS)
h. conduct disorder
h. conversion reaction
h. disturbance
h. dysphonia
h. encephalopathy
h. impulse disorder
h. reaction of childhood
h. speech
h. syndrome of childhood

hyperlexia

hyperlogia

hypermania

hypermanic

hypermetabolic effect

hypermetabolism
prefrontal h.

hypermetamorphosis

hypermetria

hypermimia

hypermnesia

hypermyesthesia

hypermyotonia

hypernatremia

hypernatremic encephalopathy

hypernoia

hypernomia

hypernomic

hypernyctohemeral syndrome

hyperontomorph

hyperoral behavior

hyperorexia

hyperosmia

hyperpathia

hyperpathic state

hyperphagia

hyperphagic obesity

hyperphoria

hyperphosphorylated tau protein

hyperphrasia

hyperphrenia

hyperphrenic

hyperpipecolatemia

hyperplasia
adrenal h.
cerebral h.
congenital adrenal h.

hyperplastic

hyperpolarization

hyperpolarize

hyperponesis

hyperpragia

hyperpragic

hyperpraxia

hyperprosexia

hyperprosody

hyperpsychosis

hyperpyrexia

hyperquantivalent idea

hyperreflexia
autonomic h.
generalized h.

hypersalivation

hypersensibility

hypersensitive

hypersensitivity
electromagnetic h.
sensorial h.
h. syndrome

hypersensitization

hyperserotonemia

hypersexual complex

hypersexuality

hypersomnia
h. associated with depression
depression-related h.
h. disorder
idiopathic h.
persistent h.
primary h.
transient h.

hypersomnia-type sleep disorder

hypersomnic depression

hypersomnolence disorder

hypertension (HT)
essential h.
idiopathic h.
masked h.
neurogenic h.
office h.
orthostatic h.

NOTES

H

hypertensive
h. crisis
h. encephalopathy
hyperthermalgesia
hyperthermia
ecstasy-associated malignant h.
psychostimulant-induced h.
rebound h.
hyperthermoesthesia
hyperthymia
hyperthymic
h. personality disorder
h. temperament
hyperthyroidism
hyperthyroxemia
hypertonia
sympathetic h.
treatment-emergent h.
hypertonic absence
hypertrophic
h. cervical pachymeningitis
h. interstitial neuropathy
hyperventilation (HV)
autonomic h.
central neurogenic h.
forced h.
hypocapnic h.
neurogenic h.
psychogenic h.
h. syndrome (HVS)
h. tetany
hypervigilance
hypervigilant narcissism
hypesthesia, hypoesthesia
olfactory h.
vaginal h.
hyphedonia
hypnagogic
h. hallucination
h. hallucination image
h. hallucination imagery
h. intoxication
h. jerk
h. perception
h. reverie
h. state
h. vision
hypnagogue
hypnapagogic
hypnic jerk
hypnoanalysis
hypnoanalytic
hypnoanesthesia
hypnocatharsis
hypnogenesis
hypnogenic, hypnogenous
h. spot
h. zone
hypnogram
hypnograph
hypnoidal
hypnoid state
hypnologist
hypnology
hypnonarcosis
hypnopompic
h. hallucination
h. image
h. perception
h. state
hypnosis
diagnostic use of h.
direct suggestion under h. (DSUH)
h. and dissociative disorder
father h.
fear h.
lethargic h.
major h.
minor h.
mother h.
questioning under h.
suggestion under h.
symptom relief through h.
waking h.
hypnosophy
hypnotherapy
hypnotic
h. abreaction
h. abuse
h. action
h. activity
h. agent
h. amnesia
h. analgesia
h. anesthesia
h. capacity
h. delirium
h. dependence
h. drug
h. induction
h. interview
h. intoxication
h. patient
h. psychotherapy
h. relationship
h. relaxation technique training
h. response
h. sleep
h. state
h. suggestion
h. trance
h. use disorder
h. withdrawal
h. withdrawal symptom
hypnotic-dependent
h.-d. patient
h.-d. sleep disorder

hypnotic-induced
h.-i. anxiety
h.-i. disorder
h.-i. persisting dementia
h.-i. psychotic disorder with delusions
h.-i. psychotic disorder with hallucinations
h.-i. sexual dysfunction
hypnotic-sedative drug
hypnoticus
status h.
hypnotism
hypnotist
hypnotizability
hypnotization
collective h.
hypnotize
hypoactive
h. affect
h. limbic structure
h. sexual arousal
h. sexual desire
h. sexual desire disorder
hypoactivity
hypoacusis (*var. of* hypacusis)
hypoalgesia (*var. of* hypalgesia)
hypocapnic hyperventilation
hypocathexis
hypochondria
hypochondriac
h. language
h. melancholia
h. neurosis
h. paranoia
h. psychoneurosis
h. psychoneurotic reaction
hypochondriaca
melancholia h.
hypochondriacal
h. complaint
h. fear
h. melancholia
h. neurosis
h. paranoia
h. preoccupation
h. psychogenic disorder
h. psychoneurosis
h. psychoneurotic reaction
h. psychosis
h. symptom
hypochondriasis
monosymptomatic h.
h. neurotic disorder
h. with poor insight type
hypocondriaque
folie h.
hypocrisy
hypocrite
hypodermic
h. injection
intracutaneous h.
intramuscular h.
intravenous h.
h. needle
hypodopaminergic state
hypoesthesia (*var. of* hypesthesia)
hypoesthetic
hypofrontality
h. hypothesis in schizophrenia
h. phenomenon
hypofunction
prefrontal h.
testicular h.
hypogeusia
idiopathic h.
hypoglycemia
hypoglycemic
h. delirium
h. encephalopathy
h. index (HI)
hypogonadism with anosmia
hypokinesia, hypokinesis
treatment-emergent h.
hypokinetic
h. anoxia
h. speech
h. syndrome
hypokrisia
hypologia
hypomania
treatment-emergent h.
hypomanic
h. behavior
h. disorder
h. episode
h. excitement
h. manic-depressive reaction
h. personality
h. phase
h. psychosis
h. quality
h. tendency
hypomanic-depressive reaction
hypomelancholia

NOTES

H

hypometabolism
frontotemporal h.
striatal h.
hypometria
hypomnesia
hypomotility
hyponatremia
hyponoia
hyponoic
hyponomic
hypoperfusion
bitemporal h.
cerebellar h.
parietooccipital h.
posterior frontal h.
hypophonia
hypophonic aphasia
hypophoria
hypophrasia
hypophrenic
hypophrenosis
hypophyseopriva
hypophysial, hypophyseal
hypophysiopriva
cachexia h.
hypophysis
catecholamine h.
hypoplasia
cerebral h.
hypoplasticus
status h.
hypopraxia
hypoprosody
hypopsychosis
hyporeflexia
hyposensitive
hyposexuality
hyposmia
hyposomnia
h. associated with anxiety
h. associated with depression
h. associated with psychosis
hyposomniac
hyposphresia
hyposthenia
hypostheniant
hyposthenic
hypotaxis
hypotension
intracranial h.
orthostatic h.
postural h.
hypothalamic
h. area
h. dysfunction
h. nucleus
h. obesity
h. regulatory input
hypothalamic-pituitary-adrenal (HPA)
hypothalamic-pituitary-adrenocortical system
hypothalamic-pituitary axis dysfunction
hypothalamus
anterior h.
lateral h.
medial h.
posterior h.
ventromedial h.
hypothermia
accidental h.
fatal h.
hypothermic disorder
hypothesis, pl. **hypotheses**
adaptive h.
alpha, beta, gamma hypotheses
anniversary h.
apertural h.
as-if h.
beta h.
biogenic amine h.
disconnection h.
dopamine h.
downward drift h.
drift h.
ethical risk h.
experimental h.
falsifiable h.
frontal aging h.
frustration-aggression h.
gate-control h.
h. generation
intergroup contact h.
matching h.
maturation h.
mediumistic h.
mnemic h.
monoamine h.
neurohumoral h.
null h.
quantal h.
segregation h.
self-medication h.
serotonergic deficiency h.
specificity h.
h. testing
topographic h.
up-regulation/down-regulation h.
hypothesize
hypothetical
h. continuum
h. deductive reasoning
h. deductive thinking
hypothymia
hypothymic personality disorder
hypothymism
hypothyroidism
hypoventilation
obesity h.

hypoxemia
hypoxia
cerebral h.
relative h.
short-term h.
tissue h.
toxic h.
hypoxic-ischemic encephalopathy (HIE)
hypoxyphilia
hypoxyphilia-caused death
hysteria
anxiety h.
Arctic h.
canine h.
Charcot grand h.
collective h.
combat h.
communicable h.
conversion h.
defense h.
dissociative h.
dissociative-type neurotic h.
epidemic h.
fixation h.
major h.
mass h.
minor h.
h. neurotic disorder
h. psychoneurosis
h. psychosis
St. Louis h.
h. study
hysterical, hysteric
h. abasia
h. amaurosis
h. amblyopia
h. amnesia
h. anesthesia
h. aphonia
h. ataxia
h. aura
h. behavior
h. blindness
h. character
h. character defense
h. chorea
h. coma-like state
h. conversion reaction (HCR)
h. convulsion
h. deafness
h. delirium
h. delirium depression
h. epilepsy
h. fugue
h. fugue state
h. gait
h. gait disorder
h. hearing impairment
h. hemiplegia
h. insanity
h. joint
h. laughter
h. lethargy
h. lithiasis
h. mania
h. movement disorder
h. mutism
h. myodynia
h. neurosis
h. paralysis
h. personality
h. personality disorder
h. polydipsia
h. pregnancy
h. pseudodementia
h. psychogenic disorder
h. psychomotor disorder
h. psychoneurotic reaction
h. psychosis
h. puerilism
h. seizure
h. stuttering
suffocation h.'s
h. syncope
h. torticollis
h. trance
h. tremor
h. vertigo
h. visual loss
h. voices
hystericum
delirium h.
hystericus
clavus h.
globus h.
hysteriform
hystérique
grande attaque h.
hysterocatalepsy
hysteroepilepsy
hysterogenic, hysterogenous
h. zone
hysteroid
h. defense
h. dysphoria
h. feature

NOTES

H

hysteroid *(continued)*
h. personality

I
I boundary
I complex
I marker
I tracing

IA
inactive alcoholic

IACPO
Inter-American Council of Psychiatric Organizations

IADL
instrumental activities of daily living

iamatology

iambic stress

iatric

iatrogenesis

iatrogenic
i. addiction
i. disorder
i. effect
i. homosexuality
i. illness
i. induction
i. instability
i. psychosis
i. schizophrenia
i. seizure

iatrogeny

iatrology

iatrophysics

IB
index of body build

ibotenic acid

IBS
irritable bowel syndrome

IBW
ideal body weight

ICD
impulse control disorder

ICD-9
International Classification of Diseases, Ed. 9
ICD-9 code
ICD-9 diagnostic codes for Medicare reimbursement

ICD-10
International Classification of Diseases, Ed. 10
ICD-10 psychiatric diagnosis

ICD-9CM
International Classification of Diseases, Clinical Modification, Ed. 9

iceberg
tip of i.

ice block theory

Iceland disease

ichnogram

ichthyohemotoxism

ichthyomania

ichthyophagia

ichthyosarcotoxin

ichthyotoxin

icon
corporate i.

iconic
i. memory
i. sign
i. storage

iconicity

iconoclasm

iconoclast

iconology

iconomania

ICP
intracranial pressure

ICPS
interpersonal cognitive problem-solving

ICS
intracranial stimulation

ICSD
International Classification of Sleep Disorders: Diagnostic and Coding Manual

ICSW
International Committee on Social Welfare

ictal
i. amnesia
i. automatism
i. confusional seizure
i. depression
i. depression phase of seizure
i. emotion
i. period
i. symptomatic zone

icteric

icterogenic

icterohepatitis

icteroid

icterus

ictus
i. epilepticus
i. paralyticus

ICU
intensive care unit
ICU psychosis

ID
identification

id
id anxiety

id *(continued)*
id fantasy
id interpretation
id psychology
id resistance
id sadism
id wish
idea
abstract i.
associated i.
i. association
autochthonous i.
bizarre i.
i. chase
complex of i.'s
compulsive i.
delusion-like i.
disconnected i.
dominant i.
expansion i.
expansive i.
fixed i.
flight of i.'s (FOI)
grandiose i.
hyperquantivalent i.
imperative i.
inappropriate i.
i. of influence
intruding i.
intrusive distressing i.
morbid i.
obliquely related i.
obsessional i.
obtrusive i.
overcharged i.
overvalued i.
permanent dominant i.
persecutory i.
persistent inappropriate i.
persistent intrusive i.
poverty of i.'s
pressure of i.'s
psychotic-like i.
recurring i.
i. of reference
referential i.
repetitive i.
ruminative i.
strongly held i.
i. of unreality
unreasonable i.
unwarranted i.
ideal
i. beau
body i.
i. body weight (IBW)
ego i.
father i.
i. masochism
narcissistic ego i.
i. personality
transient ego i.
idealism
idealist
idealistic notion
idealization
i. defense mechanism
primitive i.
idealize
idealized
i. image
i. parental imago
i. self
i. value
idealizing transference
ideation
adolescent sexual i.
delusional i.
elopement i.
grandiose i.
homicidal i.
incoherent i.
lethality of suicidal i.
overvalued i. (OVI)
paranoid i.
persecution i.
recurrent suicidal i.
stress-related paranoid i.
suicidal i.
suspicious i.
transient stress-related paranoid i.
violent i.
ideational
i. agnosia
i. apraxia
i. shield
i. style of coping
ideatory apraxia
ideé fixe
idem
identical
i. element
i. twins
identifiable
i. antecedent
i. psychiatric illness
i. secondary gain
i. stress
i. stressor
identification (ID)
anthropometric i.
cause of i.
cosmic i.
cross-gender i.
deep trance i.
i. defense mechanism
empathic i.
facial i.

- false i.
- feminine i.
- i. figure
- gender i.
- group i.
- healthy i.
- letter-word i.
- multiple i.'s
- object i.
- i. phenomenon
- phenomenon i.
- primary i.
- i. process
- projective i.
- secondary i.
- social i.
- i. transference
- trial i.
- i. with aggressor
- i. with dead

identified trait

identifier

identify

identifying

- i. data
- i. with aggression

identity

- adolescent personal i.
- adolescent sexual i.
- alteration in i.
- i. alteration
- alternate i.
- assumption of new i.
- belief about i.
- body i.
- controlling i.
- i. crisis
- cultural i.
- i. by descent
- i. disorder
- i. disorder of adolescence
- i. disorder of childhood
- i. disturbance
- ego i.
- ethnic i.
- i. experience
- i. experience integer
- false i.
- family i.
- female gender i.
- female-to-male transgender i.
- feminine i.
- i. formation
- formation of i.
- former i.
- gender i.
- hostile i.
- inflated i.
- intrapsychic i.
- loss of i.
- male gender i.
- male-to-female transgender i.
- masculine i.
- multiple distinct i.'s
- i. need
- new i.
- personal i.
- place i.
- primary i.
- i. problem
- protector i.
- psychosexual i.
- sense of i.
- sexual i.
- social i.
- i. state
- i. theme
- vocational i.
- i. vs role confusion
- i. vs role diffusion

identity-disordered children

ideodynamism

ideogram

ideographic

ideokinetic

- i. apraxia
- i. praxis

ideological

- i. commitment
- i. orientation

ideology

ideometabolic

ideometabolism

ideomotion

ideomotor

- i. aphasia
- i. apraxia
- i. signal

ideophrenia

idiocrasy

idiocy

- amaurotic axonal i.
- amaurotic familial i. (AFI)
- axonal i.
- Aztec i.
- Bielschowsky i.

NOTES

idiocy *(continued)*
cretinoid i.
developmental i.
diplegic i.
epileptic i.
erethismic i.
family i.
genetous i.
infantile i.
intrasocial i.
Kalmuk i.
microcephalic i.
moral i.
paralytic i.
plagiocephalic i.
profound i.
scaphocephalic i.
sensorial i.
spastic amaurotic axonal i.
torpid i.
traumatic i.
Vogt-Spielmeyer i.
idiodynamic control
idiogenesis
idiogenetic
idiogenous
idioglossia
idiogram
idiographic approach
idiohypnotism
idiolalia
idiologism
idiom
personal i.
idiomatic usage
idioneurosis
idiopathic
i. chronic fatigue
i. dystonia
i. encephalopathy
i. epilepsy
i. hypersomnia
i. hypertension
i. hypogeusia
i. insomnia
i. language retardation
i. neuralgia
i. psychosis
idiopathy
idiophrenic
i. insanity
i. psychosis
idiopsychologic
idioreflex
idiospasm
idiosyncrasy
idiosyncratic
i. alcohol intoxication
i. behavior
i. material
i. meaning
i. process
i. reaction
i. reasoning
i. side effect
i. thinking
i. topic shifting
idiot
erethismic i.
oxycephalic i.
pithecoid i.
i. prodigy
i. savant
superficial i.
torpid i.
idiotrophic
idiotropic type
idiovariation
idle
idol
idolatrous
idolatry
idolism
idolize
idolomania
IDT
interdisciplinary team
IDU
injecting drug user
I-E
internal vs external
IER
Institute of Educational Research
IFROS
ipsilateral frontal routing of signals
ignipedites
ignis fatuus
ignoble
ignominious
ignominy
ignorance
social i.
ignorant
ignore
IHS
Indian Health Service
I-it relationship
ikota
I-labeled cocaine analog
ill
i. at ease
chronically mentally i.
mentally i.
terminally i.
i. will
ill-advised
ill-bred

illegal
i. behavior
i. drug
i. drug sale
i. drug synthesis
i. drug use
i. gambling
illegible
illegitimate
ill-fated
ill-humored
illicit
i. drug abuse
i. drug distribution
i. drug fad
i. drug synthesis
i. drug use
i. drug use in family member
i. lover
i. opiate use
i. opioid
i. psychoactive drug
i. psychoactive substance
illimitable
illiteracy
functional i.
i. screening
technological i.
illiterate
functional i.
ill-mannered
ill-natured
illness
advantage by i.
affective i.
i. ascribed to hexing
i. as self-punishment
autoimmune i.
i. behavior
bipolar i. (BPI)
brain i.
catastrophic i.
chronic factitious i.
chronic mental i.
chronic psychotic i.
comorbid psychiatric i.
course of i.
cyclic i.
debilitating i.
dementing i.
disabling mental i.
dysautonomic i.
early-onset mental i.
emotional i.
escape into i.
factitious i.
faking i.
family history of mental i. (FHMI)
flight into i.
folk i.
functional i.
genetic susceptibility to mental i.
high-altitude i.
history of present i. (HPI)
iatrogenic i.
identifiable psychiatric i.
Kraepelin classification of mental i.
legitimate i.
length of i.
life-threatening i.
major mental i.
manic-depressive i.
mass psychogenic i.
mass sociogenic i.
medical i.
mental i.
model of i.
multifactorial i.
neurologic i.
neurotic i.
new-onset mental i.
no mental i. (NMI)
nonschizophrenic i.
objective severity of i.
outcome of i.
petition of mental i. (PMI)
i. phase
preexisting i.
present i. (PI)
progressive dementing i.
psychiatric i.
psychogenic i.
psychosomatic i.
psychotic i.
refractory mental i.
schizophrenic i.
significant medical i.
social class and mental i.
stress-related i.
underlying medical i.
untreated psychiatric i.
usual childhood i.
illogical
i. attitude
i. communication

NOTES

illogical *(continued)*
i. reasoning
i. thinking
illogicality
ill-tempered
ill-treat
illumination condition
illuminism
ill-use
illusion
bodily i.
i. des sosies
i. of doubles
dream i.
fleeting i.
memory i.
movement i.
narcissistic i.
i. of omnipotence
optic i.
optical i.
i. of orientation
Poggendorf i.
i. of power
i. of power over others
recurrent i.
tactile i.
temporal lobe i.
transient auditory i.
transient tactile i.
transient visual i.
visual i.
windmill i.
Zollner i.
illusional
illusionary misconception
illusory conjunction
illustrate
illustration
pornographic i.
IM
intramuscular
image
accidental i.
i. agglutination
body i.
body i. perception
changed body i.
cohesive i.
concrete i.
i. control
dangerous i.
depersonalized i.
direct i.
distorted body i.
eidetic i.
i. eliciting disgust
i. eliciting fear
i. eliciting neutral emotion
erotic i.
false i.
father i.
formed i.
fragmentary dream i.
general i.
ghost i.
graven i.
hallucinatory i.
hypnagogic hallucination i.
hypnopompic i.
idealized i.
imperfect i.
inappropriate i.
incidental i.
i. intensifier
intrusive obsessional i.
inverted i.
i. issue
memory i.
mental i.
mirror i.
mother i.
motor i.
negative body i.
neutral i.
nurturant i.
obsessional mental i.
parent i.
percept i.
perception of body i.
peripheral field i.
persistent inappropriate i.
persistent intrusive i.
personal i.
poor body i.
positive i.
primary mental i.
proteome i.
i. pseudohallucination
public i.
real i.
recurrent i.
i. registration
sensory i.
tactile i.
trailing i.
transient i.
unformed i.
visual i.
vivid dream i.
image-distorting level
imageless thought
imagery
affective i.
auditory i.
i. code
eidetic i.
emotive i.

i. exercise
guided affective i. (GAI)
horrific mental i.
hypnagogic hallucination i.
intrusive i.
mental i.
paraphiliac i.
pictorial i.
smell i.
tactile i.
taste i.
i. therapy
visual i. (VI)

imaginable process

imaginal
i. desensitization
i. exposure
i. flooding
i. process

imaginary
i. companion
i. companionship
i. language
i. relationship

imagination
creative i.

imaginative play

imagined
i. abandonment
i. body defect
i. loss
i. physical appearance defect
i. transgression
i. ugliness

imagines (*pl. of* imago)

imaging
brain i.
cerebral dynamic i.
Diffusion Tensor I. (DTI)
2-dimensional proton echo-planar spectroscopic i.
in vivo i.
magnetic resonance i. (MRI)
i. method
i. modularity
morphometric magnetic resonance i.
neuroreceptor i.
structural brain i.
structural magnetic resonance i.
i. study

imagining
active i.
involuntary active i.
voluntary active i.

imago, pl. **imagines**
idealized parental i.

imbalance
autonomic i.
biochemical i.
central language i.
developmental i.
effort-reward i.
electrolyte i.
fluid i.
intellectual i.
language i.
sympathetic i.
vasomotor i.

imbecile
moral i.

imbecility
old-age i.
senile i.

imbibe

imbibition

imbroglio

IMC
information memory concentration

imitation
elicited i.
morbid i.
repetition by i.
spontaneous i.

imitative
i. behavior
i. dissociative identity disorder
folie i.
i. speech
i. tetanus

immaculate

immanence theory

immature
i. coping mechanism
i. defense
i. personality
i. personality disorder

immaturity
emotional i.
emotionally unstable i.
perceptual i.
i. reaction
social i.

immediacy behavior

immediate
i. allergy

NOTES

immediate *(continued)*
i. anxiety
i. control
i. danger
i. echolalia
i. ejaculation
i. environment
i. experience
i. gratification
i. memory
i. memory deficit
i. posttraumatic automatism
i. posttraumatic convulsion
i. recall
immediately
immedicable
immerge
immersion
immigrant
first-generation i.
Kosovo i.
i. status
imminent
i. justice
i. risk
immissio penis
immobile
i. face
i. state
immobility
motor i.
motoric i.
immobilization paralysis
immobilize
immodest
immoral imperative
immoralist
immortalize
immovable
immune
i. body
i. deficiency
i. deficiency syndrome
i. function
i. response
i. system
i. system regulation
immunity
active i.
humoral i.
passive i.
stress i.
immunoassay
enzyme-multiplied i.
immunoblot analysis
immunocompromised
immunodeficiency
sexually acquired i. (SAID)
immunofluorescence assay
immunogen
behavioral i.
immunologic
i. abnormality
i. aspect
i. dysfunction
immunological paralysis
immunology
clinical i.
immunomodulatory
immunosorbent assay
immunosuppression
immunosuppressive effect
immure
immutable
impact
i. analysis
developmental i.
disruptive i.
pharmacologic i.
potential i.
psychological i.
systemic i.
impacted grief
impaired
i. abstraction ability
i. abstract thinking
i. affect
i. affect modulation
i. arousal
i. attention
i. attentional functioning
i. balance
i. cognitive functioning
communicatively i.
i. concentration
i. concentration ability
i. connectedness
i. consciousness
i. development
i. driving ability
i. effective communication
emotionally i.
functionally i.
i. impulse control
i. insight
i. language
learning i.
i. limbic-diencephalic function
i. memory
mentally i.
i. migration of brain neurons
i. occupational functioning
i. orgasm satisfaction
i. orientation
i. performance
i. recognition
i. recovery effect
i. relationship

i. repetition
i. self-care
i. self-image
i. self-soothing
severely mentally i. (SMI)
i. sexual desire
i. sexual function
i. sexual performance
i. sleep
i. social functioning
i. social grace
i. social interaction
i. social judgment
i. social manners
speech and language i. (SLI)
i. thinking ability
i. vision

impairment
acute i.
age-associated memory i. (AAMI)
aphasic phonological i.
i. of attention
attention i.
attentional i.
basic i.
cerebral i.
clinically significant i.
cognitive i.
i. of cognitive function
communication i.
i. of consciousness
i. criterion
degree of i.
i. of dementia
depression-induced cognitive i.
disproportionate i.
early speech i.
emotional i.
employment i.
focal neurological i.
functional cognitive i.
functional hearing i.
gaze i.
generalized intellectual i.
general medical i.
global measure of i.
graphic i.
gross i.
hearing i.
hysterical hearing i.
i. index
initial spoken language i.
intellectual i.
interpersonal i.
language i.
level of i.
life i.
major i.
marked i.
measurable i.
medical i.
memory i.
mental i.
motivation i.
motor i.
musical appreciation i.
narrative speech perception i.
neurocognitive i.
neurologic i.
neuropsychologic i.
nonlanguage cognitive i.
occupational i.
organic i.
perceptual-motor i.
permanent residual i.
phonological assembly i.
physical i.
psychogenic hearing i.
reading comprehension i.
residual i.
reversible memory i.
school functioning i.
sensory i.
serious i.
severe i.
sexual i.
significant i.
sleep-induced respiratory i.
social functioning i.
speech processing i.
spiritual i.
spoken language i.
stress-induced cognitive i.
i. symptom
verbal memory i.
visual memory i.
visuomotor i.
volitional control i.

impartial

impasse
therapeutic i.

impassible

impassion

impassive

impassivity

impatience

NOTES

impatient
impedance
i. matching
i. method
impel
impend
impending
i. death
i. decompensation
i. doom
i. relapse
i. suicide attempt
i. violence
impenetrable
imperative
categorical i.
i. conception
ethical i.
i. idea
immoral i.
i. mood
imperceptible
imperception
imperfect
i. image
i. image registration
imperfection
imperforate hymen
imperious act
impersistence
impersonal
i. factual knowledge
i. projection
i. relationship
i. unconscious
impersonation
impersonator
female i.
impertinent
imperturbable
impervious
impetuous
impetus
impinge
implant
breast i.
silicone i.
implausible phenomenon
implementation
standards i.
implication
clinical i.
legal i.
policy i.
social i.
societal i.
theoretical i.
implicit
i. behavior
i. language
i. learning
i. memory
i. personality theory
i. process
i. response
i. role
implied criticism
implore
implosion
i. flooding
i. therapy
implosive therapy
impolite
import
personal i.
importance
clinical i.
diagnostic i.
exaggerated sense of i.
importune
impose
imposée
folie i.
impostor
juvenile i.
i. psychotic manifestation
i. syndrome
impotence, impotency
anal i.
anatomic i.
atonic i.
ejaculatory i.
erectile i.
frank i.
functional i.
organic i.
orgastic i.
paretic i.
penile i.
primary i.
psychic i.
psychogenic i.
relative i.
secondary i.
sexual i.
symptomatic i.
impotent
impotentia
i. coeundi
i. erigendi
impoverished
i. community
i. early environment
i. fantasy life
i. speech
i. thought
impoverishment
intellectual i.

personality i.
i. in thinking
impractical
imprecate
imprecise
impregnation fear
impressible
impression
absolute i.
clinical i.
diagnostic i.
erroneous i.
first i.
good i.
i. management
mental i.
i. method
sensory i.
impressionable
impression-bipolar
clinical global i.-b. (CGI-BP)
impressive aphasia
imprinting
female i.
filial i.
genomic i.
male i.
imprison
imprisonment
false i.
improbable
improper
i. diet
i. dose
impropriety
improved communication skills
improvement
clinical i.
cognitive i.
life-changing i.
OCD i.
plateau in i.
practice-based learning and i.
pronounced i.
self-rated i.
spontaneous i.
statistically significant i.
i. training
transference i.
improvisation
imprudent
impudent
impudicity
impugn
impuissant
impulse
aggressive i.
base i.
i. control
i. control conduct disorder
i. control disorder (ICD)
i. control disorder NOS
i. control issue
i. control problem
cruel i.
disinhibited sexual i.
excitatory i.
i. fear
forbidden i.
forced i.
fundamental social i.
gambling i.
horrific i.
inappropriate i.
inhibitory i.
intrusive i.
irresistible i.
libidinal i.
i. life
maladaptive i.
morbid i.
nervous i.
i. neurosis
nociceptive i.
obsessional i.
obsessive i.
oral i.
persistent inappropriate i.
persistent intrusive i.
i. regulation
repressed i.
self-destructive i.
sexual i.
stealing i.
strong i.
unacceptable i.
unconscious instinctual i.
voluntary i.
wandering i.
impulsion
impulsive
i. act
i. activity
i. aggression
i. behavior
i. character

NOTES

impulsive *(continued)*
i. dyscontrol
i. hyperactivity
i. insanity
i. lifestyle decision
i. madness
i. neurosis
i. obsession
i. outburst
i. overactivity
i. petit mal epilepsy
i. raptus
i. spectrum
i. suicide
i. tendency
i. trait of personality
impulsive-aggressive trait
impulsive-compulsive psychopathology
impulsiveness
low i.
impulsivity
counteracting i.
i. factor
lifetime i.
self-damaging i.
impunity
impurity
imputability
impute
in
in absentia
acting in
in ano
in articulo mortis
being locked in
in character
in charge
in control
in crisis
in extremis
in loco parentis
in prison
in propria persona
run in
shut in
sit in
turn in
in vivo
in vivo brain functioning
in vivo imaging
in vivo observation
inability
i. to concentrate
i. to cry
i. to delay gratification
i. to ejaculate
i. to enjoy interests
i. to experience emotion
i. to finish work
i. to function
i. to function independently
i. to trust authority figure
inaccessibility
inaccessible
inaction
inactive alcoholic (IA)
inactivity
alert i.
behavioral i.
physical i.
inadequacy
intellectual i.
personal i.
social i.
inadequate
i. discipline
i. impulse control
i. information
i. literacy
i. parenting
i. personality
i. personality disorder
i. rapport
i. response
i. school environment
i. sleep hygiene
i. stimulus
i. therapy
i. treatment
inadmissible
inadvertent
inadvisable
inalterable (*var. of* unalterable)
inamorata
inane
inanimate learning device
inanition
inappetence
inappropriate
i. activity
i. affect
i. appearance
i. attitude
i. circumstance
i. clothing
i. crying
i. defense mechanism
i. dependent care
i. disrobing
i. dressing
i. guilt
i. handling of objects
i. hygiene
i. idea
i. image
i. impulse
i. language
i. laughing

i. laughter
i. posture
i. quality of obsession
i. relationship
i. religious training
i. response
i. sexual expression
i. sexuality
i. social behavior
i. social relatedness
i. thought
i. touching
i. urge
i. verbalizing
i. voiding

inappropriateness
sexual i.
social i.

inarticulate

inassimilable

inattention
i. dimension
i. to proper dietary habits
selective i.
sensory i.
visual i.

inattentive behavior

inattentiveness
social i.

inattentive-type attention deficit hyperactivity disorder

inaudible

inborn
i. error of metabolism
i. reflex

inbred

inbreeding
coefficient of i.

incapacitating
i. drowsiness
i. fear

incapacity
functional i.
i. to sustain social bonds

incaprettamento

incarcerate

incarcerated
i. patient
i. youth

incarceration
drug-related i.

incarnata
Passiflora i.

incendiare
monomanie i.

incendiarism

incendiary arsonist

incense

incentive
aversive i.
external i.
financial i.
i. learning
i. motivation
positive i.
i. system
i. theory

inception

incertitude

incessantly
i. reiterated obscenities
i. reiterated thoughts
i. reiterated words

incessant speech

incest
i. barrier
i. fantasy
father-daughter i.
heterosexual i.
homosexual i.
mother-daughter i.
mother-son i.
i. taboo

incestuous
i. behavior
i. desire
i. fantasy
i. relationship
i. ties

incidence
i. rate
suicide i.

incident
i. case
original i.
parasuicidal i.
sexual i.

incidental
i. image
i. learning
i. learning language
i. learning language retardation
i. memory
i. stimulus

NOTES

incipient
i. schizophrenia
i. schizophrenic psychosis
incisive
incite
incitement premium
incivility
inclement
inclination
philosophical i.
religious i.
spiritual i.
inclusion
class i.
inclusive fitness
incoercible
incogitant
incognito
incognizant
incoherence
incoherent
i. behavior
i. ideation
i. patient
i. speech
income
fixed i.
low i.
incommunicado
incomparable
incompatibility
incompatible
i. behavior
i. response
incompetence
ejaculatory i.
level of i. (LOI)
subjective i.
incompetency
certificate of i.
i. proceeding
incompetent
mentally i.
incomplete alexia
incompleteness
incomprehensible
i. speech
i. thinking
i. thought
incomputable
inconceivable
inconclusive
incongruity
insensitivity to i.
incongruous affect
inconsequential
inconsiderate behavior
inconsistent
i. historical information
i. manner
i. parental discipline
i. recall
i. response
inconsolable
inconsonance
inconspicuous
inconstancy
inconstant
incontestable
incontinence, incontinentia
active i.
affective i.
bowel i.
emotional i.
fecal i.
overflow i.
paradoxical i.
passive i.
reflex i.
urge i.
urinary i.
incontinent
incontrovertible
i. evidence
i. proof
inconvenient
inconvincible
incoordinate
incoordination
fine motor i.
incorporation defense mechanism
incorrect
i. diagnosis
i. inference
politically i.
incorrigible
incorruptible
increase
differential i.
metabolic i.
increased
i. anxiety
i. appetite
i. arousal
i. dependence
i. energy
i. interpersonal conflict
i. irritability
i. mortality
i. responsibility
i. sense of physical fitness
i. sexual desire
i. sexual interest
i. signal
i. speech
i. speed of thought
incredible
incredulous

I

increment
sensation i.
increscent
incriminate
incrimination
incrustation
incubation of avoidance
incubus
family i.
inculcate
inculpable
incult
incurable problem drinker (IPD)
incurious
incursion
IND
investigational new drug
indagation
indebted
indecency
indecent
i. assault
i. exposure
indecision
indecisive
indecisiveness
parental i.
indecorous
indefatigable
indefensible
indefinable
indefinite
indelible
indelicate
indemnify
independence
field i.
loss of i.
moral i.
physical i.
independent
i. action
i. event
i. functioning
i. group experimental study design
i. interviewer
i. living
i. physical reality
i. play
i. predictor
i. relationship
i. variable
independently
inability to function i.
i. motivated
indescribable
indestructible
indeterminate
i. sex
i. sleep
index, pl. **indices, indexes**
active hostility i. (AHI)
adolescent alienation i. (AAI)
air pollution i.
allergy i. (AI)
alpha i.
ambulation i.
anterior horn i. (AHI)
anxiety i. (AI)
articulation i.
association i.
beta i.
i. of body build (IB)
body mass i. (BMI)
BPRS-E immediate memory i.
case i.
i. case
cephalic i.
cerebrospinal i.
child posttraumatic stress reaction i.
Colorado symptom i.
composite i.
Crown crisp experiential i.
delayed recall i.
delta i.
deterioration i. (DI)
i. of discrimination
Elixhauser comorbidity i.
empathic i.
i. episode
i. episode of sexual abuse
i. of forecasting efficiency
general memory i.
global distress i.
hyperactivity i.
hyperkinesis i.
hypoglycemic i. (HI)
impairment i.
maturation i.
memory i.
multiitem i.
narrow therapeutic i.
national death i.
neighborhood stress i.

NOTES

index *(continued)*
neurocognitive i.
overall risk i.
perceptual organizational i.
physiologic sleepiness i.
positive symptom distress i.
posttraumatic stress disorder reaction i.
pressure-volume i.
putative i.
referential i.
response i.
schizophrenia i.
i. of sexual functioning
shift referential i.
i. of spouse abuse
spouse abuse i.
status i.
stimulation i. (SI)
switch referential i.
tabular i.
therapeutic i.
theta i.
thought disorder i.
total response i. (TRI)
i. variable
verbal comprehension i.
Whiteley i.

indexical
i. communication
i. sign

Indian
American I.
I. casino gambling
I. folk medicine
I. Health Service (IHS)

indicant

indicatio
i. causalis
i. curativa
i. symptomatica

indication
causal i.
off-label i.
symptomatic i.

indicative mood

indicator
direct tension i.
risk i.
single-item i.
skill i. (SKI)
status i.
type i.

indices (*pl. of* index)

indicis

indict

indictment
bill of i.

indifference
maternal i.
i. to pain syndrome
parental i.
paternal i.
i. point
i. reaction
sexual i.

indifferénce
la belle i.

indifferent
i. euphoria
i. to surroundings

indigenous
i. family culture
i. worker

indigent

indigestion
nervous i.

indignant

indignation
sense of righteous i.

indignity

indirect
i. aggression
i. association
i. evidence
i. genetic transmission
i. life-threatening behavior
i. mechanism
i. method of therapy
i. motor system
i. object
i. probe
i. self-destructive behavior (ISDB)
i. striatopallidal pathway
i. wit

indiscernible

indisciplinable

indiscreet

indiscretion
sexual i.

indiscriminate sexual encounter

indisposed

indisposition

indisputable

indistinct

indistinguishable

individual
affected i.
age-matched i.
alcohol-dependent i.
i. analysis
androgynous i.
caffeine-intolerant i.
caffeine-sensitive i.
i. care
cocaine-dependent i.
i. comprehensive assessment

i. counseling
i. counselor
i. depressive symptom
i. differences
drug-dependent i.
i. guardianship
healthy i.
heterozygous i.
high-anger i.
homozygous i.
low-anger i.
i. marital therapy
normal i.
predisposed i.
i. program
i. psychology
i. psychotherapy
i. psychotherapy session
i. response
i. response specificity
i. responsibility
schizophrenia-prone i.
i. subsystem
susceptible i.
i. therapist
i. therapy (IT)
i. treatment
i. war trauma
i. with schizophrenia

individualist

individualistic
i. motive
i. reward structure

individuality

individualized
i. contract
i. education program
i. instruction

individual-specific environment

individuation stage

Indochinese refugee

indoctrination while captive

indolalkylamine

indole derivative

indolence

indolent

indomitable

indubitable

induced
i. abortion
i. anxiety disorder
i. association
i. delusional disorder
i. factitious symptom
i. insanity
i. lethargy
i. mood disorder
i. paranoid disorder
i. persisting amnestic disorder
i. persisting dementia
i. psychosis
i. psychotic disorder
i. psychotic disorder with delusions
i. psychotic disorder with hallucinations
i. sadness
i. schizophrenia
i. sexual dysfunction
i. sleep disorder
i. trance

inducement
hygienic i.

inductance

induction
i. coil
dream i.
emotion i.
enzyme i.
hypnotic i.
iatrogenic i.
i. loop
mood i.
negative mood i.
perceptual i.
positive i.

inductive
i. problem-solving
i. reactance
i. reasoning

inductor

induite
folie i.

indulgence
plenary i.

indulgent

indurate

industrial
i. hygiene
i. organizational psychologist
i. psychiatry
i. psychology
i. psychopath
i. rehabilitation counselor
i. sociology
i. therapy

industrialized culture

NOTES

industrious
industriousness
industry
gambling i.
i. vs inferiority
inebriant
inebriate
American Association for the Cure of I.'s (AACI)
inebriation
inebriety
ineducable
ineffable
ineffective
i. anger
i. communication pattern
i. decision-making
i. stimulus
i. treatment
ineffectively treated
ineffectiveness
sense of i.
ineffectual parent
inefficient
inelasticity of thought
ineligible
inenarrable
ineptness
social i.
inept parenting
inequality
inequity
inertia
motor i.
principle of i.
psychic i.
i. time
inescapable pain
inevitability
sensation of ejaculatory i.
inevitable
inexorable
inexperience
inexplicable
inexpressible
inexpressive
inexpugnable
inexpungible
infallible
infamous
infamy
infancy
adjustment reaction of i.
anal phase of i.
attachment in i.
attachment disorder of i.
bonding in i.
i. developmental stage
i. and early childhood disturbance
i. research
rumination disorder of i.
infant
i. at risk
i. behavior record
i. mortality
i. narcotic withdrawal
i. psychiatry
psychological birth of human i.
i. stimulation program
infanticide
infantile
i. affect
i. amnesia
i. aphasia
i. articulation
i. autism
i. behavior
i. convulsion
i. dementia
i. diplegia
i. dynamics
i. Gaucher disease
i. hemiplegia
i. idiocy
i. masturbation
i. paresis
i. perseveration
i. psychosis
i. sadism
i. seduction
i. seizure
i. sexuality
i. spasm
i. spastic paraplegia
i. speech
i. tetany
infantilis
dementia i.
mania phantastica i.
infantilism
Brissaud i.
cachectic i.
regressive i.
sex i.
sexual i.
static i.
infantilistic
infantilize
infantum
autismus i.
infarct
cerebral i.
lacunar i.
infarction
migrainous i.
nonhemorrhagic cerebral i.
silent cerebral i.
watershed i.

Infatabs
infatuation
infection
cerebral i.
pediatric autoimmune neuropsychiatric disorder associated with streptococcal i. (PANDAS)
recurrent urinary tract i.
infection-exhaustion psychosis
infection-organic psychosis
infection-triggered OCD
infectious
i. disease-associated dementia
i. hepatitis
i. insanity
infectious-exhaustive
i.-e. psychosis
i.-e. syndrome
infective psychosis
infecundity
infelicitous
infelicity
inference
clinical i.
incorrect i.
logical i.
statistical i.
i. strategy
inferential
i. behavioral monitoring
i. behavioral monitoring distortion
i. perception
i. perception distortion
i. statistic
i. thinking
inferior
i. frontal sulcus
i. orbitofrontal complex
i. parietal region
i. prefrontal cortex
i. sibling lifestyle
i. temporal cortex (ITC)
i. temporal sulcus
inferiority
i. complex
constitutional psychopathic i.
i. feeling
industry vs i.
organ i.
psychopathic i.
infernal
inferred
i. conflict
i. delusional conviction
infertile
infertility
infestation delusion
infibulation
infidel
infidelity
delusion of i.
fear of i.
marital i.
infighting
infiltration
i. anesthesia
perineural i.
infinity neurosis
infirmity
inflammatory disease-associated dementia
inflated
i. appraisal
i. appraisal of talent
i. identity
i. knowledge
i. power
i. relationship to deity
i. relationship to famous person
i. self-esteem
i. self-worth
i. wealth
i. worth
i. worth theme
inflection
speech i.
inflexibility
enduring pattern of i.
inflexible
i. attitude
i. habit
i. perception pattern
i. personality trait
inflict
influence
additive environmental i.
additive genetic i.
contextual i.
cultural i.
delusion of i.
developmental i.
direct genetic i.
driving under i. (DUI)
environmental i.
evil i.

NOTES

influence *(continued)*
genetic i.
heritable i.
idea of i.
media i.
mystical i.
outside i.
passive i.
putative i.
i. of religion
religious i.
sleep i.
influenced
easily i.
i. psychosis
influential
informal
i. admission
i. contract
i. method
i. retention
informant report
informatics
biomedical i. (BMI)
healthcare i.
Psychiatric Society for I.
information
afferent thermosensory i.
assimilating i.
i. assimilation
autobiographical i.
biochemical i.
circumstantial i.
collateral i.
i. collection
contradictory i.
drug i. (DI)
educational i.
emotional i.
emotionally arousing i.
external i.
i. feedback
fund of i.
inadequate i.
inconsistent historical i.
i. input process
job i.
kinetic i.
learning i.
i. memory concentration (IMC)
neurocognitive i.
nonverbal i.
i. optimization position
i. overload
personal i.
phonetic i.
privileged i.
i. processing
i. processing bias
i. processing deficit
rapidity of analyzing i.
rapidity of assimilating i.
release of i.
reliability of patient i.
i. retrieval
sensory i.
structured verbal i.
tangential i.
i. technology
i. theory
thermosensory i.
thirdhand i.
unbiased i.
i. underload
unstructured verbal i.
valid i.
verbal i.
informational support
informed
i. consent
i. decision
informer
infraclass
infraction
disciplinary i.
gambling-related i.
prison disciplinary i.
infradian rhythm
infrapsychic
infrequent interpersonal conflict
infringe
infuriate
infusion
continuous i.
lactate i.
ingenious
ingenuity
ingestion
acute i.
caffeine i.
caustic i.
drug i.
hormone i.
pill i.
ingrain
ingrate
ingratiate
ingratiating
i. attitude
i. behavior
ingratiation
ingratitude
ingredient
psychoactive i.
toxic i.
in-group
inhabit

inhalant-induced
i.-i. delirium
i.-i. dementia
i.-i. disorder
i.-i. psychotic disorder with delusions
i.-i. psychotic disorder with hallucinations
inhalant-related
i.-r. death
i.-r. disorder
inhalation
CO_2 i.
cocaine i.
i. convulsive treatment
i. of drug
intentional i.
xenon i.
inhaled anesthesia
inhaler
amphetamine i.
nasal i.
nicotine i.
inharmonious
inherent
inheritability
disorder i.
inheritable
inheritance
archaic i.
autosomal dominant i.
mendelian rules of i.
mode of i.
multifactorial i.
nonmendelian pattern of i.
polygenic i.
inherited
i. abnormality
dominantly i.
i. releasing mechanism (IRM)
inhibit
inhibited
i. communication
emotionally i.
i. female orgasm
i. female orgasm psychosexual dysfunction
i. grief
i. grieving
i. male orgasm
i. male orgasm psychosexual dysfunction
i. mania
i. person
i. sexual arousal
i. sexual desire
i. sexual desire psychosexual dysfunction
i. sexual excitement (ISE)
i. sexual excitement psychosexual dysfunction
i. sexual response
inhibited-type reactive attachment disorder of infancy or early childhood
inhibition
academic i.
aim i.
antidepressant i.
associative i.
behavioral i.
central i.
chronic antidepressant i.
conditioned i.
i. of delay
dopaminergic i.
emotional i.
i. epilepsy
external i.
i. formation
internal i.
i. mechanism
motor i.
occupational i.
pervasive i.
prepulse i.
proactive i. (PI)
i. profile
reactive i.
reciprocal i.
retroactive i. (RI)
sexual i.
social i.
specific academic or work i.
work i.
inhibition-action balance
inhibitor
carbonic anhydrase i.
dual reuptake i.
excitatory amino acid receptor i.
5-HT reuptake i.
MAO i.
nonselective phosphodiesterase i.
physiologic hyaluronidase i. (PHI)
reuptake i.
reversible cholinesterase i.

NOTES

inhibitor *(continued)*
secretase i.
selective norepinephrine reuptake i.
selective serotonin reuptake i. (SSRI)
serotonin-norepinephrine reuptake i.
serotonin reuptake i. (SRI)
inhibitory
i. control
i. effect
i. epilepsy
i. impulse
i. obsession
i. postsynaptic potential (IPSP)
i. regulatory input
i. tone
in-home crisis stabilization
inhospitable
in-house evaluation
inhuman
inhumane
inhumanity
inimical
iniquity
initial
i. disinhibition
i. interview
i. lag
i. masking
i. onset
i. phase of insomnia
i. spoken language impairment
i. spurt
i. stage
i. stress reaction
i. teaching alphabet
initiate relationship
initiating
i. insomnia
i. structure
initiation
i. of action
gang i.
i. of goal-directed behavior
sleep i.
treatment i.
initiative
lack of i.
research i.
i. vs guilt
initiator
initio
ab i.
injectable
i. drug
i. medication
injected sclera
injecting drug user (IDU)
injection
cerebral i.
conjunctival i.
death by lethal i.
depot medication i.
hypodermic i.
intracutaneous i.
intradermal i.
intramuscular i.
intrathecal i.
intravascular i.
intravenous i.
lethal i.
long-acting i.
subcutaneous i.
injector
injunction
paradoxical i.
injury
accidental i.
alcohol-related i.
birth i.
blood injection i.
brain i.
closed head i. (CHI)
current of i.
deceleration i.
dementia due to brain i.
diffuse axonal i.
fetal i.
focal i.
head i.
hepatic i.
narcissistic i.
open head i.
past head i.
physical i.
i. potential
self-induced i.
self-inflicted bodily i.
self-inflicted chemical i.
self-inflicted physical i.
self-inflicted thermal i.
structural i.
toxic i.
traumatic i.
traumatic brain i. (TBI)
i. of war
whiplash i.
injustice
i. collecting
i. gathering
inmate
i. graduate
i. personality
prison i.
innate
i. behavior
i. drive

i. reflex
i. releasing mechanism
i. response system
innateness theory
inner
i. barrenness
i. belief
i. child issue
i. city adolescent
i. city community
i. conflict
i. control
i. directed
i. estrangement
i. experience
i. feeling
i. language
i. life
i. need
i. self-helper
i. slight
i. space
i. tension
i. thought
i. vision
i. world
inner-directed person
innermost
innervate
innervation
i. apraxia
motor i.
innocence
childlike i.
innocent act
innocuous
i. environmental cue
i. object
innominata
substantia i.
innovative
innoxious
innuendo
innutrition
inoculation
emotional i.
stress i.
inoperable
inopportune
inordinate
inorganic mercury salt
inotropic component
inpatient
acute psychotic i.
aggressive psychotic i.
i. care
i. drug treatment
psychiatric i.
i. psychiatric institution
i. psychiatric setting
i. psychiatric treatment facility
psychotic i.
schizophrenic i.
i. service
i. stay
i. unit
i. violence
input
acoustic i.
afferent i.
behavioral i.
cortical i.
emotional i.
hypothalamic regulatory i.
inhibitory regulatory i.
phonetic i.
regulatory i.
input-output mechanism
inquest
inquiry
character education i. (CEI)
general i. (GI)
systematic i. (SI)
inquisition
inquisitive
inquisitor
inroad
insalubrious
insane
criminally i.
i. delusion
i. finger
paralysis of i.
insania lupina
insanity
acute confusional i.
adolescent i.
affective i.
alcoholic i.
alternating i.
American Law Institute formulation of i.
basedowian i.
choreic i.
circular i.

NOTES

insanity *(continued)*
climacteric i.
communicated i.
compulsive i.
confusional i.
consecutive i.
constitutional i.
criminal i.
cyclic i.
i. defense
degenerative i.
delusional i.
double i.
doubting i.
dread of i.
drug i.
emotional i.
hysterical i.
idiophrenic i.
impulsive i.
induced i.
infectious i.
intermittent i.
interpretation i.
interpretational i.
legal i.
manic-depressive i.
moral i.
i. of negation
not guilty by reason of i. (NGI, NGRI)
partial i.
periodic i.
plea of i.
religious i.
senile i.
simultaneous i.
subacute confusional i.
toxic i.
triple i.
insatiable appetite
insect
insecticide
organophosphate i.
insecure attachment
insecurity
feeling of i.
food i.
social i.
insemination
artificial i.
insenescence
insensate
insensible thirst
insensitive
insensitivity
gross i.
i. to incongruity
insentient
inseparability
linear i.
inseparable
insertion
delusion of thought i.
thought i.
insertion-deletion polymorphism
inside density
insidious onset
insight
absence of i.
analytic i.
emotional i.
exploratory i.
impaired i.
intellectual i.
judgment and i.
lack of i.
i. learning
limited i.
myopic i.
poor i.
sudden i.
therapeutic i.
i. therapy
true i.
insightful
psychologically i.
insight-oriented
i.-o. approach
i.-o. psychotherapy
i.-o. treatment
insignificant
insinuate
insipid
insistent
insolation
insolent
insomnia
alcohol-related i.
i. associated with anxiety
i. associated with depression
i. associated with psychosis
bout of i.
childhood-onset i.
chronic i.
i. diagnostic interview
drug-dependent i.
drug-related i.
i. due to nonorganic origin
i. feature
idiopathic i.
initial phase of i.
initiating i.
intermittent i.
long-term i.
maintenance i.
middle i.
midwinter i.

nonorganic origin i.
persistent i.
i. phase
primary i.
psychophysiological i.
rebound i.
i. related to another mental disorder
short-term i.
situational i.
sleep disorder i.
sleep-onset i.
stimulant-induced i.
i. symptom
terminal i.
transient i.
withdrawal i.

insomniac

insomnia-type

i.-t. sleep disorder due to general medical condition
i.-t. substance-induced sleep disorder

insouciance

inspersion

inspirate

inspiration

inspirational

i. appeal
i. group therapy

instability

affect i.
affective i.
autonomic i.
emotional i.
iatrogenic i.
i. in interpersonal relationships
job i.
living i.
marital i.
postural i.
vasomotor i.
vertebral cervical i.

instantaneous power

instigate

instigation therapy

instigator

instillation

instillator

instinct

acquisitive i.
aggressive i.
complementary i.
death i.
destructive i.
ego i.
erotic i.
herd i.
hierarchical theory of i.
life i.
mother i.
i. need
part i.
partial i.
i. representative
i. ridden
sexual i.
social i.

instinctive

i. behavior
i. reaction

instinct-training interlocking

instinctual

i. aim
i. anxiety
i. drive
i. dyscontrol
i. fusion
i. renunciation
i. tension
i. vicissitude

Institute

I. of Educational Research (IER)
I. of Medicine (IOM)
New York State Psychiatric I.
I. of Personality and Research (IPAR)

institution

inpatient psychiatric i.
mental i.
religious i.
state psychiatric i.

institutional

i. abuse
i. care
i. commitment
i. environment
i. peonage
i. review board
i. setting
i. transference

institutionalize

instruction

competency-based i.
individualized i.
unable to follow i.'s

NOTES

instructional objective
instrument
(Hymovich) Chronicity Impact and Coping I. (CICI)
instrumental
i. activities of daily living (IADL)
i. ADL measurement
i. affair
i. aggression
i. avoidance act
i. conditioning
i. dependence
i. need
i. relativist orientation
i. response
i. support
i. task
instrumentalism
insubordinate
insuccation
insufferable
insufficiency
adrenocortical i.
corticoadrenal i.
i. of eyelid
mental i.
muscular i.
role i.
vertebrobasilar i.
insufficient
i. nocturnal sleep
i. stimulation
insufflation anesthesia
insular
i. cortex tissue
i. sclerosis
insularity
insulation
i. anesthesia
emotional i.
insulator
insulin-dependent diabetic
insult
nutritional i.
putative i.
verbal i.
insuperable
insupportable
insurable
insurance
i. carrier
disability i.
extended-care i.
health i.
liability i.
malpractice i.
short-term i.
traditional indemnity i.
unemployment i.
insured patient
insurgent
insurmountable
insusceptibility
intact
cognitively i.
judgment, orientation, memory, abstraction and calculation i. (JOMACI)
naming i.
intake
abnormal energy i.
abnormal food i.
caffeine i.
caloric i.
cocaine i.
i. diagnostic group
excessive alcohol i.
excessive food i.
family group i.
fluid i.
food i.
intranasal drug i.
i. orientation group
i. worker
intangible
integer
identity experience i.
integral role
integrate
integrated
i. community
i. ECT system
i. function
i. psychological therapy
integration
biosocial i.
cerebral i.
community i.
ego i.
family social i.
message i.
personality i.
primary i.
secondary i.
sensory i.
social i.
structural i.
integrative
i. agnosia
i. approach
i. aspect
i. learning
integrity
i. of brain function
ego i.
i. group
physical i.
i. vs despair

I

intellect
ambivalence of i.
structure of i. (SI)
intellection
intellectual
i. ability
i. activity
i. agony
i. aphasia
i. aura
i. capacity
i. deterioration
i. development
i. exercise
i. faculty
i. function
i. function deficit
i. functioning level
i. hero
i. imbalance
i. impairment
i. impoverishment
i. inadequacy
i. insight
i. maturity
i. monomania
i. resource
i. rigidity
i. skill
i. superiority
intellectualism
intellectualization communication pattern
intellectualize
intellectualized terms
intellectually sharp
intelligence
above-average i.
abstract i.
aura i.
biologic i.
coefficient of i. (CI)
concrete i.
crystallized i.
i. disorder
fund of i.
gathering of i.
low i.
marginal i.
measured i.
mechanical i.
psychomotor i.
i. quotient (IQ)
representative i.
i. score
social i.
subnormal i.
superior i.
verbal i.
intelligibility threshold
intelligible
intemperance
intended victim
intense
i. affect
i. affiliation
i. anger
i. anxiety
i. apprehension
i. autonomic arousal
i. depression
i. desire
i. energy
i. episodic dysphoria
i. fear
i. interpersonal relationship
i. intoxication
i. longing
i. preoccupation
i. psychological distress
i. sexual behavior
i. sexual fantasy
i. sexual urge
i. startle response
i. wish
intensification
intensified
i. action
i. feeling
intensifier
image i.
intensity
affective i.
delusional i.
i. of mood
pain i.
i. of reaction
i., severity, and discharge (ISD)
i. of trauma
treatment i.
intensive
i. care community residence
i. care syndrome
i. care unit (ICU)
i. case management
i. day treatment program
i. habit pattern

NOTES

intensive *(continued)*
i. psychotherapy
i. treatment unit (ITU)
intent
criminal i.
homicidal i.
malicious i.
i. rating
severity of i.
sex, age, depression, previous attempt, ethanol, rational thinking loss, separated, divorced, widowed, organized plan, no social support, stated future i. (SAD PERSONS)
suicidal i.
suicide i.
violent i.
intention
i. to deceive
paradoxical i. (PI)
i. spasm
suicidal i.
i. tremor
intentional
i. death
i. feigning
i. fire setting
i. forgetting
i. inhalation
i. overdose
i. process
i. stereotyped movement
i. tremor
intentionality
intentionally produced symptom
intent-to-treat analysis
interact group
interacting
i. cognitive subsystem
i. medications
interaction
accelerated i.
affective i.
afferent stimulus i.
alcohol-methadone i.
amygdala-prefrontal cortex-locus ceruleus i.
communicative i.
complementarity of i.
complex social i.
demanding i.
differential i.
drug i. (DI)
drug-drug i.
i. effect
family i.
gene-environment i.
harmonious i.
higher order i.
impaired social i.
interpersonal i.
marital i.
mother-infant i.
negative peer i.
neurochemical i.
occupational i.
peer i.
person-environment i.
i. process analysis
reciprocal social i.
sexual i.
social i.
state-trait i.
i. term
i. territory
treatment intensity by time i.
interactional
i. childhood psychosis
i. contract
i. group psychotherapy
i. theory of personality
interaction-oriented group therapy
interactive
i. effect
i. measurement
i. phenomenon
i. voice response system
Inter-American Council of Psychiatric Organizations (IACPO)
interbody
interbreed
intercalation
intercede
intercept
intercession
interchange
intercommunicate
interconnect
interconnected cerebral region
interconnection
intercostal neuralgia
intercourse
age at first i.
anal i.
i. anxiety
attempted i.
buccal i.
extramarital i.
i. frequency
genital i.
painful i.
psychosexual i.
puritanical aversion to i.
sexual i.
simulated i.
unprotected i.
intercurrent anxiety

I

interdependence
interdependent
interdigitate
interdisciplinary
i. approach
i. environment
i. environmental design
i. team (IDT)
interest
i. blank
conflict of i.
cross-gender i.
decreased i.
diminished sexual i.
diminished social i.
i. factor
i. group
inability to enjoy i.'s
increased sexual i.
interpersonal i.
lack of i.
loss of i.
low sexual i.
markedly diminished i.
precocious sexual i.
range of i.'s
religious i.
restricted i.
i. schedule
sex i.
sexual i.
social i.
stereotyped i.
interface
acoustic i.
emotion-cognition i.
motor i.
sensory i.
interfamily
interfere
interference
anterograde memory i.
background i.
habit i.
i. modification
i. pattern of discharge
retrograde memory i.
sleep i.
theme i.
i. theory
treatment i.
intergang
intergenerational
i. activity
i. relation
i. transmission
i. trauma
intergradation
intergrade
intergroup
i. contact hypothesis
i. exercise
interhemispheric
i. asymmetry
i. transfer
interictal
i. behavior
i. behavior syndrome
i. depression
i. period
i. psychosis
intérieur
milieu i.
interindividual variation
interject
interjudge reliability
interleaved learning
interlocking
instinct-training i.
interlocutor
interlude
intermarriage
intermediary
intermediate
i. brain syndrome
i. brain syndrome due to alcohol
i. care facility
i. hemispheric dynamic
i. sex
i. structure
intermenstrual
intermenstruum
intermetamorphosis
intermingle
intermittent
i. aphonia
i. emotional conflicts or reactions
i. explosive behavior
i. explosive disorder
i. explosive disturbance
i. insanity
i. insomnia
i. melancholia
i. pain
i. psychosis

NOTES

intermittent *(continued)*
i. reinforcement
i. reinforcement schedule
i. wakefulness
intermodal fluency
intermorbid
internal
i. architecture neuronal size
i. conflict
i. consistency
i. cue
i. decompression
i. demand
i. drive
i. inhibition
i. locus of control
i. model
i. representation
i. respiration
i. second messenger system
i. selection
i. sensation of anxiety
i. state
i. stimulus
i. stressor
i. validity
i. value
i. vs external (I-E)
i. world of belief
i. world of expectation
i. world of fantasy
i. world of perception
internal-external control
internalization
internalize
internalized
i. anger
i. homophobia
i. sense
i. speech
i. validity
internalized-state rating
internalizing
international
i. adoption
I. Association of Group Psychotherapy
i. child pornography ring
I. Classification of Diseases, Clinical Modification, Ed. 9 (ICD-9CM)
I. Classification of Diseases, Ed. 9 (ICD-9)
I. Classification of Diseases, Ed. 10 (ICD-10)
I. Classification of Sleep Disorders: Diagnostic and Coding Manual (ICSD)
I. College of Psychosomatic Medicine
I. Committee on Social Welfare (ICSW)
I. Price Foundation Genetic Study of Bulimia Ner vosa
I. Psychoanalytical Association (IPA)
I. Society for Adolescent Psychiatry
I. Society for Mental Health Online (ISMHO)
I. Society for the Psychological Treatment of Schizophrenics
I. Society for Sexually Transmitted Disease Research
I. Society for Traumatic Stress Studies
I. Statistical Classification of Diseases and Related Health Problems
I. Transactional Analysis Association (ITAA)
internecine
Internet
I. addiction
I. addiction disorder
adolescent use of I.
I. child pornography
I. counseling
I. gambling
I. psychotherapy
I. relationship
I. sex
I. suicide chat room
Internet-addicted adolescent
interneuronal connection
internuncial
interobserver reliability
interoception
interoceptive
i. awareness
i. conditioning
i. cue
i. exposure
i. fear
interoceptor
interpersonal
i. accommodation
i. behavior
i. cognitive problem
i. cognitive problem-solving (ICPS)
i. concern
i. conflict
i. consequence
i. control
i. crisis
i. dependence
i. difficulty

i. distrust
i. dysfunction
i. effectiveness skill
i. environmental determinant
i. exploitation
i. friction
i. functioning
i. impairment
i. interaction
i. interest
i. issue
i. loss
i. morality
i. network
i. pathology
i. personality trait
i. process
i. psychiatry
i. psychotherapy (IPT)
i. radar
i. rapport
i. realm
i. rejection
i. relations
i. relationship
i. relationship deficit
i. relationship problem
i. research orientation
i. responsibility
i. role
i. self-consciousness
i. sensitivity
i. sensitivity measure
i. spacing communication pattern
i. strain
i. style
i. theory
i. therapy (IPT)
i. trust
i. withdrawal

interpersonally exploitive

interplay

interpose

interpretation
abstract i.
action i.
anagogic i.
analytic i.
aura i.
cognitive i.
defense i.
i. delusion
distortion of i.
dream i.
facial expression i.
id i.
i. insanity
loose proverb i.
mutative i.
personalized i.
proverb i.
psychoanalytic i.
psychodynamic i.
test i.

interpretational insanity

interpreter role

interpretive
i. leap
i. therapy

interracial marriage

interrater reliability

interrelate

interrelationship

interrogate

interrupted tracing

interrupter device

interruption
evidence of i.
repeated REM sleep i.'s
sleep i.
i. of thought

interruptus
coitus i.

intersensory
i. disorder
i. transfer

intersex
i. condition
female i.
male i.
true i.

intersexual disorder

intersexuality

intersociety

interstimulation

interstitial
i. neuritis
i. neurosyphilis

intersubjective

intertwine

interval
class i.
confidence i. (CI)
fixed i. (FI)
lucid i.
i. psychosis

NOTES

interval *(continued)*
i. reinforcement
time i.
variable i. (VI)
intervene
intervening
i. act
i. validity
i. variable
intervention
active i.
adjunctive i.
alternative i.
associated i.
barrier to i.
behavioral i.
biologic i.
clinical facilitated i.
cognitive-behavioral i.
community i.
community-based i.
crisis i.
culture-specific i.
drug i.
drug-specific i.
early pharmacological i.
early psychotherapeutic i.
educational i.
educative i.
emergency i.
employment i.
evolutionary i.
experimental i.
exposure-based i.
family i.
GAD-specific i.
gender-specific i.
generative i.
group i.
lifestyle i.
medical i.
optimal therapeutic i.
outpatient i.
paradoxical i.
pharmacologic i.
pharmacotherapeutic i.
postdisaster psychosocial i.
preventive i.
psychiatric i.
psychological i.
psychopharmaceutical i.
psychopharmacologic i.
psychosocial i.
psychotherapeutic i.
religious i.
remedial i.
i. research
school-based i.
selective preventive i.
spiritual i.
stop, look and listen i.
strategic i.
targeted i.
therapeutic i.
verbal i.
interventionist
early i.
interview
adolescent-parent i.
amobarbital i.
Amytal i.
axis I, II i.
barbiturate-facilitated i.
burden i.
clinical i.
composite international diagnostic i. (CIDI)
confidential i.
conjoint i.
counseling i.
delirium symptom i.
diagnostic i.
direct i.
drug-facilitated i.
employment i.
evaluation i.
exit i.
family system i.
general clinical i.
group i.
i. group psychotherapy
hypnotic i.
initial i.
insomnia diagnostic i.
job i.
i. method
nonconfrontational i.
open-ended i.
patient i.
patterned i.
pilot i.
i. protocol
psychiatric i.
psychodynamic i.
psychological i.
research i.
semistructured diagnostic i.
stress i.
structural clinical i.
structured clinical i.
i. technique
i. therapy
unstructured i.
interviewer
i. effect
independent i.
i. training
interviewing technique

interview-related parental environment item
interview-revised
inter vivos
intestinal psychogenic disorder
intimacy
i. in aging
delusional belief in i.
i. maintenance
physical i.
i. principle
rejection of i.
relationship i.
sense of i.
sexual i.
i. vs isolation
i. vs self-absorption
intimate
i. attachment to caregiver
i. attachment to mother
i. experience
i. human relations
i. partner violence
i. relationship
sexually i.
i. zone
intimidate
intimidating
i. behavior
i. others
intolerable
i. behavior
i. inner conflict
i. side effect
intolerance
alcohol i.
caffeine i.
cold i.
drug i.
i. of stress
intonation
voice i.
intoxicant
intoxicated
driving while i. (DWI)
legally i.
intoxication
acute alcohol i.
alcohol i.
amphetamine i.
anticonvulsant i.
anxiolytic i.
arylcyclohexylamine i.
barbiturate i.
bromide i.
Burundanga i.
caffeine i.
cannabis i.
carbon dioxide i.
carbon disulfide i.
carbon monoxide i.
chronic i.
cocaine i.
i. delirium
drug i.
i. episode
ethanol i.
fluoxetine i.
gasoline i.
glutethimide i.
hallucinogenic i.
heavy metal i.
hypnagogic i.
hypnotic i.
idiosyncratic alcohol i.
inhalant i.
intense i.
level of i.
i. level
marijuana i.
metal i.
narcotic chemical i.
nicotine i.
opioid i.
i. organic psychosis
organic psychosis drug i.
pathological i.
pathologic alcohol i.
pathologic drug i.
phencyclidine i.
i. phenomenon
physiologic i.
psychoactive substance i.
reversible i.
sedative i.
severe i.
sign of alcohol i.
substance i.
substance-induced i.
sympathomimetic i.
i. syndrome
water i.
intoxication-related phenomenology
intoxication-type organic psychosis
intracellular
i. contribution

NOTES

intracellular *(continued)*
i. energy metabolism
i. metabolic process
i. second messenger
i. second messenger system
intraception
intracisternal
intraclass correlation
intraconscious personality
intracortical inhibition and facilitation
intracranial
i. brain volume
i. disorder
i. hypotension
i. infection organic psychosis
i. pressure (ICP)
i. raw volume
i. self-stimulation
i. stimulation (ICS)
intracrine
intractable
i. grand mal epilepsy
i. mania
i. pain
intracutaneous
i. hypodermic
i. injection
intracytoplasmic protein deposit
intradermal injection
intrafamilial
i. conflict
i. relationship
i. sexual abuse
intramedullary canal
intramuscular (IM)
i. absorption
i. administration
i. hypodermic
i. injection
intranasal
i. cocaine use
i. drug intake
i. heroin
intraneuronal argentophilic Pick inclusion body
intransigent
intrapersonal conflict
intrapopulation
intrapsychic
i. ataxia
i. change
i. conflict
i. distortion
i. distress
i. identity
i. origin
i. personality trait
i. style
i. world
intrapsychical function
intrapsychology
intrasocial idiocy
intrathecal injection
intravaginal
intravascular injection
intravenous (IV, I.V.)
i. cocaine
i. drug
i. drug abuse (IVDA)
i. drug use
i. drug user
i. feeding
i. hydration
i. hypodermic
i. injection
i. medication
i. treatment
intra vitam
intrepid
intricate
intrigue
romantic i.
sexual i.
intriguing
intrinsic
i. asthma
i. behavior
i. capacity
i. constancy
i. damage
i. motivation
i. reflex
i. relationship
i. religiosity
i. reward
i. strength factor
introject
introjection defense mechanism
introjective-projective cycle
intropunitive response
introspect
introspection
phenomenalistic i.
introspectionism
introspective method
introtensive
i. personality style
i. problem-solving style
introversion
passive i.
social i. (SI)
introversion-extroversion continuum
introversive
i. problem-solving style
i. tendency
i. trait
introvert

introverted
i. disorder of adolescence
i. disorder of childhood
i. personality disorder
i. schizoid personality
i. schizothymia
i. type
intrude
intruding idea
intrusion
ego-dystonic i.
free recall i.
i. score
intrusive
i. behavior
i. distressing idea
i. flashback
i. hallucination
i. imagery
i. impulse
i. memory
i. obsessional image
i. recollection
i. sexual disorder
i. sexual proposition
i. symptom
i. thought
i. treatment
i. urge
i. wandering
intubation
intuition
intuitive
i. encounter
i. judgment
i. stage
i. type
inure
invade
invalid
invalidating environment
invalidism
invaluable behavior
invariable behavior
invariance
factorial i.
invariant
functional i.
invasion
aggressive i.
personal space i.
i. of privacy
invasive treatment
invective
inveigh
inveigle
inventory
i. adjustment
i. of loss
inverse
i. agonist
i. feedback
i. relationship
inversion
absolute i.
affect i.
amphigenic i.
occasional i.
i. relationship
sex role i.
sexual i.
sleep i.
inverted
i. image
i. Oedipus complex
i. radial reflex
inverted-U function
invested
emotionally i.
investigate
investigation
drug under i.
eating disorder i. (EDI)
empirical i.
postmortem i.
principal i.
psychoanalytic i.
investigational new drug (IND)
investigatory reflex
investing
investment
emotional i.
foolish business i.
inveterate drinking
invidious
invincible
inviolable
inviolacy motive
invisible
i. college
i. wound
inviting
invocational psychosis
invoke
involuntary
i. active imagining

NOTES

involuntary *(continued)*
i. admission
i. behavior
i. civil commitment
i. discharge
i. ECT
i. emotional expression
i. hospitalization
i. manslaughter
i. medication
i. motion
i. motor movement
i. outpatient commitment
i. pause in speech
i. premonitory urge
i. response
i. restraint
i. retention
i. seclusion
i. state of trance
i. time-out
i. treatment
i. twitch
i. vocalization
i. whispering
involution
senile i.
involutional
i. depression
i. melancholia
i. paranoia
i. paranoid psychosis
i. paranoid reaction
i. paranoid state
i. paraphrenia
i. period
i. psychotic reaction
involved
sexually i.
involvement
brain i.
ego i.
emotional i.
extrapyramidal i. (EPI)
family i.
gambling i.
gang i.
genetic i.
lack of i.
personal i.
subcortical brain i.
invulnerable
inward
i. aggression
i. expression of anger with ruminative feature
i. focus
i. picture
inwardly directed anger
IOM
Institute of Medicine
ionic transduction alteration
iotacism
Iowa Case Management Project
IPA
International Psychoanalytical Association
IPAR
Institute of Personality and Research
IPD
incurable problem drinker
I-persona
ipsation
ipsilateral
i. cerebellar ataxia
i. deficit
i. frontal routing of signals (IFROS)
i. headache
i. loss
i. reflex
IPSP
inhibitory postsynaptic potential
IPT
interpersonal psychotherapy
interpersonal therapy
IQ
intelligence quotient
full-scale IQ
IR
insulin receptor
IR specificity
Iraq veteran
irascible
irate
ire
irk
irksome
IRM
inherited releasing mechanism
ironclad
ironic aspect
irony
irradiation-induced mental deterioration
irrational
i. action
i. anger
i. argument
i. behavior
i. desire
i. doubt
i. fear
i. type
irrationality
irreality level
irreconcilable
irrecoverable
irrecusable

irredeemable
irreformable
irrefragable
irrefutable
irregular
i. movement
i. sleep pattern
i. sleep-wake pattern
i. sleep-wake rhythm
irregularity
irrelevant
i. answer
i. external stimulus
i. language
i. pair
irreparable
irrepressible
irreproachable
irresistibility
irresistible
i. apprehension
i. impulse
i. sleep
irresoluble
irresolute
irresponsibility
consistent i.
criminal i.
irresponsible
i. acting out
i. parenting
i. work behavior
irresponsive
irretrievable
irreverence
irreverent communication
irreversibility
irreversible
i. coma
i. dementia
i. shock
irritability
acoustic i.
electric i.
increased i.
marked i.
irritable
i. bowel
i. bowel syndrome (IBS)
i. heart
i. mania
i. mood
i. morosity
i. temperament
i. testis
irritant
irritate
irritation
cerebral i.
functional i.
i. therapy
irritative zone
irrumation
irruption
IRT
item response theory
IS
IS total score
IS900 VET tracking system
Isakower phenomenon
ischemia
total cerebral i.
ischemia organic psychosis
ischemic pathology
ISD
intensity, severity, and discharge
ISDB
indirect self-destructive behavior
ISE
inhibited sexual excitement
island
i. of control
i. of memory
social i.
Islander
Asian American Pacific I.
Pacific I.
islet of precocity
Isle of Wight study
ISMHO
International Society for Mental Health Online
isocaloric diet
isochronal
isochronism
law of i.
isodynamic
isoeffect
isolate
social i.
isolated
i. auditory hallucination
i. delusion
emotionally i.
i. explosive disorder
i. explosive disturbance

NOTES

isolation
- i. of affect
- alcoholism in i.
- i. amentia
- i. aphasia
- autistic i.
- i. effect
- feeling of i.
- intimacy vs i.
- social i.
- i. syndrome

isolative behavior
isomeric
- i. ballast
- i. function

isomorphism
isopathic principle
isophilic
isoproterenol
isosexual
isotypical
Israeli-Palestinian issue
issue
- aging i.
- biologic i.
- boundary i.
- confidentiality i.
- cosmetic i.
- cross-culture i.
- custody i.
- end-of-life i.
- extratransference i.
- health i.
- image i.
- impulse control i.
- inner child i.
- interpersonal i.
- Israeli-Palestinian i.
- late-life substance abuse i.
- legal i.
- lifestyle i.
- medicolegal i.
- moral i.
- nature-nurture i.
- Northern Ireland i.
- personal i.
- preexisting underlying emotional i.
- process i.
- psychological i.
- psychosocial i.
- public health i.
- reality i.
- recovery i.
- rehabilitative i.
- reimbursement i.
- skirt the i.
- spiritual i.
- take i.
- termination i.
- theologic i.
- treatment i.
- treatment-relevant i.
- underlying emotional i.
- weight i.
- workforce i.

IT
individual therapy

ITAA
International Transactional Analysis Association

ITC
inferior temporal cortex

itching
item
- i. analysis
- axis I, II i.
- cultural i.
- i. difficulty
- i. discrimination parameter
- highest ranking i.
- interview-related parental environment i.
- jargon-free i.
- parental environment i.
- personality-descriptive i.
- i. response theory (IRT)
- scale i.
- i. scaling
- i. selection
- SWAP-200 i.
- i. validity
- i. weighting

item-total correlation
iterate
iterative
- i. behavior
- i. tendency

I-thou relationship
itinerate
ITU
intensive treatment unit

IV, I.V.
intravenous
- IV drug abuse
- IV drug use

IVDA
intravenous drug abuse

ivory tower

jabber
jacket
jackknife seizure
jack-of-all-trades
Jackson
J. epilepsy
J. law
J. rule
J. sign
jacksonian
j. convulsion
j. epilepsy
j. seizure
Jacobson view of depressive disorder
jactatio
j. capitis nocturna
j. capitis nocturnus
jactitation, jactation
periodic j.
jaded
jag
arousal j.
crying j.
j. drinker
j. drinking
jail
j. cell
j. days per year
j. diversion program
j. sentence
j. term
jail-based treatment program
JaK
Janus kinase
Jakob-Creutzfeldt disease organic psychosis
Jamaica ginger paralysis
jamais
j. phenomenon
j. vu
j. vu aura
James-Lange-Sutherland theory
James-Lange theory of emotion
Janet disease
Janus-faced
janusian thinking
Janus kinase (JaK)
Japanese erection ring (JER)
jape
jargon
j. agraphia
j. aphasia
organ j.
organic j.
j. paraphasia
semantic j.
jargon-free item
jargonistic
jaundice
nuclear j.
jaunty
jaw
j. grinding
j. jerk
j. reflex
jaw-jerk reflex
jaw-working reflex
JCAHO
Joint Commission on Accreditation of Healthcare Organizations
JCMIH
Joint Commission on Mental Illness and Health
jealous
j. delusion
j. rage
j. subtype
j. type
jealousness
jealous-type
j.-t. delusion
j.-t. delusional disorder
j.-t. paranoid disorder
j.-t. schizophrenia
jealousy
alcoholic j.
j. delusion
delusional j.
morbid j.
projected j.
retrospective ruminative j.
sexual j.
sibling j.
jeer
Jekyll and Hyde personality
Jenny Craig diet
jeopardize
JER
Japanese erection ring
jerk
Achilles j.
ankle j.
chin j.
crossed adductor j.
crossed knee j.
j. finger
hypnagogic j.
hypnic j.
jaw j.

jerk *(continued)*
knee j.
supinator j.
jerking
head j.
j. movement
jest
jester
jet
j. lag
j. lag phenomenon
j. lag sleep disorder
j. lag-type dyssomnia
j. set
jet-setter
jewelry
excessive j.
Jewish
jilt
jinx
jitter
frequency j.
jittery
JLO
judgment of line orientation
JND
just noticeable difference
job
j. analysis
j. change
j. component method
j. demand
j. design
j. dimension
j. enrichment
j. evaluation
hatchet j.
j. information
j. instability
j. interview
j. loss
j. performance
j. placement
j. pressure
j. reinstatement
j. retirement
j. satisfaction
snow j.
j. specification
j. stability
j. strain
j. stress
j. tenure
job-hopping
jobless
job-related stress
job-sample experience
Jocasta complex
jock
jocose
jocosity
jocular
jocularity
excessive j.
Joffroy sign
joiner
joint
J. Commission on Accreditation of Healthcare Organizations (JCAHO)
J. Commission on Mental Illness and Health (JCMIH)
j. custody
hysterical j.
neuropathic j.
j. play
j. psychogenic disorder
j. sense
joker
joking mania
Jolly reaction
jolt
JOMACI
judgment, orientation, memory, abstraction and calculation intact
Jonah word
jong
shook j.
Joubert syndrome
journaling exercise
journalize
journey
jovial
joyless
joyous
Juan
Don J.
Juanism
Don J.
jubilation
judaism
judge
judgmatic
judgment
automatic j.
clinical j.
comparative j.
critical j.
diagnostic j.
faulty j.
impaired social j.
j. and insight
intuitive j.
j. of line orientation (JLO)
moral j.
negative j.
j., orientation, memory, abstraction and calculation intact (JOMACI)
personal j.

poor j.
qualitative j.
quantitative j.
social j.
j. standard
value j.

judgmental attitude
judicature
judicial process
judicious
juggle
jugular bulb
Jukes family
jumble
jumbo
mumbo j.

jumper
jumper disease of Maine
jumping Frenchmen of Maine syndrome
jumpy
junction
gap j.

juncture
closed j.
open j.

Jung
J. method
J. theory

jungian
j. psychoanalysis
j. psychology
j. theory

junk food
juramentado
jurisdiction
jurisprudence
dental j.
medical j.

jury
special j.
traverse j.
trial j.

jus primae noctis
justice
imminent j.
juvenile j.
J. in Mental Health Organization
social j.
j. system

justifiable
j. homicide
j. reaction

justified
therapeutically j.

justify
just noticeable difference (JND)
juvantibus
diagnosis ex j.

juvenescence
juvenile
j. aggression
antisocial j.
j. chorea
j. competence
j. court
j. court consultant
j. criminal
j. delinquency
j. delinquent
j. detention facility
j. drug user
j. era
j. impostor
j. justice
j. justice case
j. justice system
j. myoclonic epilepsy
j. nonneuropathic Niemann-Pick disease
j. offender
j. officer
j. paralytic dementia
j. paresis
j. psychosis
j. residential facilities census
j. tabes
j. violence

juvenilis
dementia paralytica j. (DPJ)

juvenilism
juvenility

J

NOTES

KAB
knowledge, attitude, behavior
kahuna
kainomania
kakergasia
kakosmia
kakotrophy
kaleidoscope hallucination
Kallikak family
Kallmann syndrome
Kalmuk idiocy
Kanner
K. autism
K. syndrome
kappa
k. coefficient
k. opiate receptor
k. opioid
k. opioid receptor
Kapseals
Dilantin K.
karma
bad k.
katasexuality
kathisomania
katzenjammer
kava
k. extract
kava k.
kavain
kavalactone
kavapyrone
Kayser-Fleischer ring
K complex
Keeler polygraph
keenly aware
keep
recognize, empathize, think, hear, integrate, notice, k. (RETHINK)
keeping faith
keirospasm
Kemadrin
Kempf disease
kempt
Kendell classification
kernel complex
Kernig sign
ketanserin
ketazolam
ketoacidosis
alcoholic k. (AKA)
diabetic k. (DKA)
ketoaciduria
ketogenic diet
ketorolac
ketosteroid
key
k. concept
k. question
k. symptom
keyed-up feeling
keying
empirical criterion k.
kg
kilogram
khat
Khmer Rouge
kick
k. around
k. the habit
k. out
kicking
k. objects
k. people
kiddie porn
kidnapper
killed
witnessed someone being k.
killer
k. cult
detection of adolescent k.
serial k.
teen k.
time k.
killing
mercy k.
kilogram (kg)
kilounit (ku)
kilovolt (kV)
kilovoltage peak (kVp)
kin
next of k.
kinanesthesia, cinanesthesia
kinase
Janus k. (JaK)
mitogen-activated protein k.
protein k. C (PKC)
kindergarten
kindhearted
kindling
k. effect
K. pattern
kindly
kindness
kinephantom
kinesalgia
kinesia paradoxica
kinesiatrics

K

kinesic
k. behavior
k. gesture
kinesics
kinesigenic ataxia
kinesiology
kinesioneurosis
kinesiotherapy
kinesipathy
kinesis
kinesomania
kinesthesia, kinesthesis
k. hallucination
kinesthesiometer
kinesthetic
k. analysis
k. apraxia
k. aura
k. cue
k. feedback
k. hallucination
k. method
k. perception
k. sensation
k. sense
k. technique
kinetic
k. analysis
k. ataxia
chemical k.'s
k. drive
k. energy
first-order elimination k.'s
k. information
k. model
k. modeling
k. tremor
zero-order elimination k.'s
kinetism
kinetogenic
kinetosis
kinetotherapy
king-slave fantasy
kinky-hair disease
kinship
k. network
k. system
KIPS
knowledge information processing system
kiss
French k.
tongue k.
kissing behavior
kit
QIAamp blood k.
kitchen
soup k.
kitten
sex k.
klazomania
Klein
K. death wish
K. suffocation alarm theory
K. theory of depression
K. view of depressive disorder
Kleine-Levin syndrome
kleptolagnia
kleptomaniac
kleptomania in children
kleptomanic behavior
Klinefelter syndrome
Klippel-Feil syndrome
klismaphilia
Klüver-Bucy syndrome
knavery
knee
k. jerk
k. phenomenon
kneippism
knight move
knismogenic
knismolagnia
knocked up
knocking
head k.
knockout drops
knot
love k.
lover's k.
slip k.
know-how
know-it-all
knowledge
acquired k.
k., attitude, behavior (KAB)
carnal k.
competence k.
factual k.
figurative k.
fund of k.
general k.
impersonal factual k.
inflated k.
k. information processing system (KIPS)
lack of k.
source of sexual k.
k. structure
k. theme
knowledgeable
known
k. group validity
k. organic factor
know-nothing
knuckle under
Kohlberg developmental model
kohlbergian theory of moral reasoning development

Kohnstamm phenomenon
Kohut theory of depression
kolyphrenia
kolytic
Korean War veteran
koro
k. psychosis
k. syndrome
Korsakoff
K. alcoholic psychosis
K. amnesia
K. disease
K. nonalcoholic psychosis
K. syndrome
Kosovo immigrant
Krabbe syndrome
Kraepelin
K. classification of mental illness
K. diagnostic system
K. disease
K. schema
K. theory of depression
kraepelinian
k. subtype
k. view of psychosis
Kraepelin-Morel disease
krauomania
Kretschmer type
ku
kilounit
kuru
Kussmaul
K. aphasia
K. coma
Kussmaul-Landry paralysis
kV
kilovolt
kVp
kilovoltage peak
kymatism
kymogram
kymograph

K

NOTES

LA
low anxiety
la
la belle indifferénce
la belle indifferénce phenomenon
la dolce vita
LAAM
LAAM maintenance therapy
label
designer l.
social l.
labeling theory
labialism
labial paralysis
labile
l. emotionality
l. mood
l. personality disorder
l. range of affect
lability
affective l.
emotional l.
mood l.
labiochoreic stuttering
labiorum
morsicatio l.
labor
l. camp
l. force
laboratory
l. abnormality
basement l.
clinical l.
l. data
l. diagnosis
diagnostic l.
l. method model
NIDA-certified forensic toxicology l.
personal growth l.
l. study
l. test
l. training
laborer
manual l.
labyrinthine
l. disorder
l. righting reflex
l. sense
l. speech
lachrymose
lacing agent
lack
l. of academic success
l. of confidence
l. of control
l. of courage
l. of efficacy
l. of empathy
l. of energy
l. of expressiveness
l. of family support
l. of fear
l. of feeling
l. of future planning
l. of guilt
l. of initiative
l. of insight
l. of interest
l. of interoceptive awareness
l. of involvement
l. of knowledge
l. of mature defense
l. of memory
l. of motivation
l. of patience
l. of penetrance
l. of performing to potential
l. of perseverance
l. of premeditation
l. of reactivity
l. of remorse
l. of restraint
l. of self-confidence
l. of self-discipline
l. of speech
l. of structure
l. of vocational success
l. of will
lacking social resources
laconic speech
laconism
lacrimal gland
lacrimation
lactate
brain l.
global brain l.
gray matter l.
l. infusion
regional brain l.
sodium l.
white matter l.
lactation
lactational diestrus
lactic acidosis
lactoovovegetarian diet
lactotrophic
lactovegetarian diet
lacuna, pl. **lacunae**

lacuna *(continued)*
l. cerebri
superego l.
lacunaire
lacunar
l. amnesia
l. dementia
l. infarct
l. state
l. stroke
l. syndrome
lacunaris
status l.
LAD
language acquisition device
ladder
abstraction l.
counseling l.
Laennec cirrhosis
Lafayette pegboard
lag
cultural l.
initial l.
jet l.
maturational l.
terminal l.
laid back
laissez-faire
l.-f. group
l.-f. leader
l.-f. leadership pattern
laliatry
lallation
lalling
lalochezia
lalognosis
lalomania
laloneurosis
lalopathology
lalopathy
laloplegia
lalorrhea
lamarckian theory
lambaste
lambdacism
lame
lament
lancinating
Landau-Kleffner syndrome
landmark
l. agnosia
developmental l.
land mine victim
Landry-Guillain-Barré syndrome
Landry paralysis
language
l. ability
abusive l.
l. acquisition
l. acquisition device (LAD)
l. area
artificial l.
l. arts
l. assessment
automatic l.
l. barrier
l. behavior
behavior l.
bizarre l.
body l.
l. boundary
l. center
l. change
l. and communication
l. and communication distortion
communication in sign l.
l. comprehension
l. comprehension and production
l. content
daughter l.
l. deficit
l. delay
delayed l.
l. development
l. developmental delay disorder
deviant l.
l. difficulty
l. disability
l. disorder in dementia
l. disturbance
dominant l.
l. dysfunction
egocentric l.
emotive l.
English as second l. (ESL)
l. enrichment therapy (LET)
erotic l.
exaggerated body l.
executive l.
l. experience approach (LEA)
explicit l.
expressive l.
l. faculty
foreign l.
l. function
l. function deterioration
l. game
gestural-postural l.
gesture l.
global loss of l.
home l.
hypochondriac l.
imaginary l.
l. imbalance
impaired l.
l. impairment
implicit l.
inappropriate l.

incidental learning l.
inner l.
irrelevant l.
l. lateralization
legal l.
lewd l.
l. localization
loss of l.
l. manipulation
metaphoric l.
mixed receptive-expressive l.
negotiating l.
nonspecific l.
nonverbal l.
obscene l.
oral l.
organic l.
l. origin
l. pathology
primary l.
primitive psychosomatic l.
l. problem
l. processing
l. processing model
l. purist
l. quotient
l. recovery
religious l.
scatological l.
school l.
l. screening
shared l.
sign l.
l. skills learning retardation
l. and speech disorder
spoken l.
subcultural l.
syntaxic l.
target l.
l. theory
l. therapist
l. therapy
twin l.
unknown l.
unusual l.
vulgar l.
written l.
l. zone

language-associated cortex
language-dominant hemisphere
languid
languish
languor
languorous
lanugo
Laotian refugee
laparotomaphilia
lapse
attention l.
l. of awareness
memory l.

lapsus
l. calami
l. lingua
l. memoriae

larcenist
larcenous
larceny
large
at l.

larval
l. epilepsy
l. sadism
l. schizophrenia

larvated epilepsy
laryngeal
l. anesthesia
l. chorea
l. crisis
l. epilepsy
l. paresthesia
l. psychophysiologic reaction
l. syncope
l. vertigo

laryngoparalysis
LAS
laxative abuse syndrome

lascivia
lascivious
l. forced laughter
l. hysterical laughter

Lasègue syndrome
lashing
lassitude
last
l. chance
l. word

latah, lata
l. syndrome

latchkey
l. child
l. children
l. status

late
l. adulthood
l. life

NOTES

late *(continued)*
l. luteal phase dysphoric disorder
l. paraphrenia
l. reaction
l. speech development
l. stage in adolescence
l. traumatic epilepsy
late-age trauma
late-emerging medical side effect
late-life
l.-l. depression
l.-l. developmental stage
l.-l. migraine
l.-l. migraine headache
l.-l. schizophrenia
l.-l. substance abuse issue
latency
Erickson theory of l.
mean sleep l.
l. period (LP)
l. period psychosexual development
l. phase
prolonged sleep l.
rapid eye movement l.
reduced rapid eye movement l.
reflex l.
l. of reply
l. of response
short REM l.
short sleep l.
sleep l.
l. stage
latency-age children
late-night activity
latent
l. class analysis
l. content
l. epilepsy
l. goal
l. homosexuality
l. learning
l. meaning
l. period
l. psychosis
l. reflex
l. response
l. schizophrenia
l. schizophrenic reaction
l. tetany
l. thought
l. zone
late-onset
l.-o. category
l.-o. schizophrenia
later
l. life
l. reading disorder
lateral
l. dominance
l. geniculate nucleus (LGN)
l. hemispheric dynamic
l. hypothalamus
l. orbitofrontal cortex
l. rostral supplementary motor area
l. ventricle
l. vertigo
laterality
crossed l.
dominant l.
mixed l.
lateralization
cortical l.
failure of l.
hemispheric l.
language l.
lateralized dysfunction
lateralizing abnormality
lateriflora
Scutellaria l.
lateropulsion
latex fetishism
lathyrism
Latin
L. American
L. American guide for psychiatric diagnosis
Latino, Latina
laudable
laudanum
laugh
nervous l.
l. off
sardonic l.
laughing
l. disease
excessive l.
inappropriate l.
l. sickness
laughter
compulsive l.
drawn l.
forced l.
hysterical l.
inappropriate l.
lascivious forced l.
lascivious hysterical l.
obsessive l.
pathologic l.
l. reflex
spasmodic l.
spontaneous l.
uncontrollable l.
uncontrolled l.
Laurence-Biedl syndrome
Laurence-Moon-Bardet-Biedl syndrome
Laurence-Moon-Biedl syndrome
Laurence-Moon syndrome

lavage
gastric l.
law
l. abiding
l. of advantage
American Academy of Psychiatry and L. (AAPL)
l. of assimilation
l. of association
autonomic affective l.
l. of avalanche
l. of average localization
biogenetic mental l.
Briggs l.
Charpentier l.
l. of closure
l. of coercion to biosocial mean
l. of cohesion
l. of combination
command l.
l.'s of commitment
l. of common fate
l. of constancy
l. of contiguity
l. of contrast
court of l.
cyberstalking l.
Dale l.
l. of denervation
l. of diminishing return
l. of effect
effect l.
empirical l.
enclosure l.
l. enforcement agency
equality l.
equipotentiality l.
eugenic sterilization l.
l. of exercise
Fourier l.
l. of frequency
Gerhardt-Semon l.
Grasset l.
Haeckel biogenic l.
health l.
l. of isochronism
Jackson l.
Leyden l.
martial l.
Megan L.
mendelian l.
mental health l.
Merkel l.
Müller l.
Murphy's l.
natural l.
Ohm l.
parallel l.
Pitres l.
poor l.
l. of precision
l. of referred pain
l. of relativity
restraint l.
l. of retrogenesis
Ritter l.
Rosenbach l.
seclusion l.
Semon l.
Semon-Rosenbach l.
stalking l.
3-strikes l.
talion l.
three strikes l.
van der Kolk l.
Weber-Fechner l.
Yerkes-Dodson l.
law-abiding citizen
law-and-order orientation
lawbreaker
lawful behavior
lawless
lawsuit
lawyer
trial l.
laxative
l. abuse
l. abuse syndrome (LAS)
l. addiction
l. of choice (LOC)
l. dependence
l. habit
l. misuse
lay analysis
layer
arachnoid l.
tangential l.
laying on of hands
layman
lazy listening
LCU
life change unit
LD
learning disability
lethal dose

NOTES

LEA
language experience approach
LEAD
longitudinal expert evaluation using all available data
lead
l. encephalopathy
l. exposure
l. neuropathy
l. palsy
l. paralysis
l. pipe contraction
l. poisoning
leaden paralysis
leader
authoritarian l.
laissez-faire l.
l. match
l. role
team l. (TL)
leaderless
l. group
l. group discussion (LGD)
l. group therapy
leadership
l. behavior
dual l.
functional l.
l. potential
l. power struggle
l. role
spiritual l.
l. theory
l. training
lead-pipe rigidity
leaf
cassina l.
coca l.
leakage
verbal l.
leap
l. of faith
interpretive l.
Lear complex
learned
l. autonomic control
l. drive
l. dysfunctional behavior
l. helplessness
material previously l.
learner
auditory l.
slow l.
learning
l. ability
l. aptitude
associate l.
association l.
associative l.
attachment l.
avoidance and escape l.
cognitive theory of l.
concept l.
conceptual l.
contingency l.
l. cue
l. curve
l. defect
l. development
l. development disorder
l. difficulty
l. disabilities specialist
l. disability (LD)
l. disabled
discrimination l.
dissociated l.
dissociation of l.
l. by doing
emotional l.
escape l.
l. experience
l. impaired
implicit l.
incentive l.
incidental l.
l. information
insight l.
integrative l.
interleaved l.
latent l.
l. material
l. mechanism
l. model
l. new information disturbance
observational l.
operant l.
paired-associates l.
l. paradigm
passive l.
passive-avoidance l.
perceptual l.
perceptual-motor l.
probability l.
l. problem
problem-based l.
propositional l.
l. psychogenic disorder
l. retardation
reversal l.
rote verbal l.
self-directed l. (SDL)
sensate focus l.
serial list l.
l. session
l. set
sexual l.
state-dependent l.
l. strategy

stress effect on l.
subliminal l.
systems-based l.
l. task
test of memory and l. (TOMAL)
l. theory
Thorndike trial-and-error l.
transfer of l.
trial-and-error l.
verbal l.
vicarious l.
visceral l.

least
l. noticeable
l. preferred
l. resistance
l. restrictive alternative

least-effort principle

leather restraint

leave, pl. **leaves**
l. of absence (LOA)
absent without l. (AWOL)
authorized l.
extended sick l.
French l.
medical l.
l. on pass (LOP)
sick l.
unauthorized l. (UL)

leaving

Leboyer method

lecanomancy

lecher

lecherous

lechery

left
l. hemisphere
l. hemisphere dominance
l. parietal association metabolism

left-hand dominant

left-handedness

left-out sibling profile

leftward asymmetry

leg
cold mottled insensate l.
l. phenomenon
restless l.

legal
l. age
l. approach
l. blindness
l. capacity
l. commitment
l. consequence
l. contract
l. counselor
l. criteria for competency
l. decision
l. deliberation
l. determination
l. dilemma
l. divorce
l. drug
l. gambling
l. guardian
l. guardianship
l. implication
l. insanity
l. issue
l. language
l. marriage
l. medicine
l. opioid
l. problem
l. psychiatry
l. psychology
l. punishment
l. responsibility
l. sanction
l. separation
l. standard

legality

legalized gambling

legally
l. committed
l. drunk
l. intoxicated
l. separated (LS)

Legatrin PM

legendary

Legendre sign

legislation
mental health l.

legitimacy

legitimate illness

legitimize

legomenon
hapax l.

Leichtenstern
L. phenomenon
L. sign

leisure
l. activity
l. awareness
l. skill
l. time

NOTES

length
cycle l.
l. of episode
l. of illness
l. of patient stay (LOPS)
l. of stay (LOS)
telomere l.
lengthened off-time (LOT)
lengthening reaction
leniency
lenient
lenticular aphasia
leprosy
dry l.
leprotica
alopecia l.
leptin
l. level
l. secretion
l. signal
leptophonia
leptophonic
Leri sign
lesbianism
lesbian population
Lesch-Nyhan syndrome
lesion
erythroplastic l.
self-inflicted l.
unexplained skin l.
less
l. pervasive disorder
l. than maximal effect
lesson
object l.
trial l.
LET
language enrichment therapy
let down
lethal
l. blow
l. catatonia
l. dose (LD)
l. factor
l. injection
l. means
l. overdose
lethality
l. rating
severity of l.
l. of suicidal ideation
suicide l.
lethargic
l. hypnosis
l. patient
l. stupor
lethargica
encephalitis l.
lethargy
hysterical l.
induced l.
lucid l.
profound l.
letheomania
lethica aphasia
lethologica
letter
l. blindness
Dear John l.
scarlet l.
suicide l.
letter-number sequencing
letter-word identification
leukocytosis
emotional l.
levallorphan
level
l. of abstraction
action l.
activity l.
aggression l.
agitation l.
alcohol l.
l. of alertness
alertness l.
alpha l.
androgen l.
annoyance l. (AL)
l. of anxiety
anxiety l.
l. of arousal
aspiration l.
l. of aspiration
automatic phrase l.
basal resistance l.
below detectable l. (BDL)
beta l.
blood alcohol l. (BAL)
l. of care
circulating leptin l.
cognitive awareness l.
l. of cognitive function
cognitive impairment l.
cohesiveness l.
l. of cohesiveness
comfort l.
l. of confidence
confidence l.
l. of conflict
conflict l.
conscious l.
l. of consciousness (LOC)
l. of cooperativity
criterion l.
current defense l.
defense l.
l. of defensive dysregulation

delta l.
denervation l.
l. of depression
depressive symptom l.
desire l.
l. of development
developmental l.
difficulty l.
disability l.
disavowal l.
discomfort l.
l. of disruption
dissociation l.
distress l.
l. of disturbance
drug l.
dyadic l.
l. of education
education l.
educational l.
effective l.
effort l.
endurance l.
energy l.
engagement l.
l. of exhaustion
l. of expressed emotion
l. of frustration
functioning l.
gray matter lactate l.
hedonic l.
high adaptive l.
high energy l.
hormonal l.
image-distorting l.
l. of impairment
l. of incompetence (LOI)
l. of intellectual functioning
intellectual functioning l.
intoxication l.
l. of intoxication
irreality l.
leptin l.
l. of liability
lithium l.
low educational l.
low energy l.
maintenance l.
major image-distorting l.
medication l.
mental inhibition l.
minor image-distorting l.
morning cortisol l.
native language l.
occupation l.
occupational l.
operant l.
l. of pain tolerance
pathological l.
peak plasma l.
peak and trough l.'s
perceptual l.
performance l.
phallic l.
plasma C-peptide l.
plasma leptin l.
posttest l.
pragmatic l.
preconscious l.
predominant current defense l.
l. of premeditation
preoedipal l.
primitive emotional l.
l. of psychological pain
psychopathology l.
l. of psychosocial stress
reduced aggression l.
reference zero l.
resistance l.
l. of response
risk l.
sensory l.
sentential language l.
serotonin l.
serum l.
significance l.
social functioning l.
society l.
stress l.
symptom l.
therapeutic blood l.
theta l.
tolerance l. (TL)
toxic l.
uncertainty l.
vegetative l.
white matter lactate l.

leveling
leveling-sharpening
level-of-care criterion
levirate
levitation
levity
lewd language
lewdness

NOTES

Lewy body variant of Alzheimer disease
lexica concept
lexical
l. agraphia
l. ambiguity
l. processing
lexicon
unique l.
lexicosemantic processing
lex talionis
Leyden
L. ataxia
L. law
L. neuritis
LFT
liver function test
LGD
leaderless group discussion
LGN
lateral geniculate nucleus
LH
luteinizing hormone
LHRH
luteinizing hormone-releasing hormone
liability
abuse l.
l. abuse
genetic l.
l. insurance
level of l.
vicarious l.
weight l.
liaison
l. nursing
l. psychiatrist
l. psychiatry
sexual l.
liar
pathologic l.
libation
liberal cutoff score
liberate
liberation
gay l.
women's l.
liberomotor
libidinal
l. cathexis
l. development
l. drive
l. energy
l. impulse
l. object constancy
l. phase
l. transference
l. type
libidinization
libidinous
libido
l. analog
l. binding
bisexual l.
change in l.
dammed-up l.
decreased l.
diminished l.
displaceability of l.
ego l.
l. fixation
loss of l.
mobility of l.
normal l. (NL)
object l.
organ l.
l. organization
plasticity of l.
primal l.
l. quantum
sexual l.
l. stasis
l. theory
traumatization of l.
viscosity of l.
l. wish
Libritabs
lice (*pl. of* louse)
license
revocation of driver's l.
licensed
l. handgun
l. marriage and family therapist
l. professional counselor (LPC)
l. psychologist
licentious
Lichtheim
L. aphasia
L. sign
licking
Liddle psychomotor poverty
LIDO
longitudinal investigation of depression outcomes
lid tic
lie
bald-faced l.
l. detection
l. detector
life l.
white l.
liebestod
Liepmann apraxia
lieutenant
life, pl. **lives**
adaptation to l.
adjustment reaction of later l.
adult l.
appetite for l.

l. change
change of l.
l. change unit (LCU)
l. circumstance problem
l. course
l. crisis
l. cycle
dating l.
deprived early l.
l. difficulty
direct threat to l.
dysfunctional home l.
l. energy
l. event
everyday activities in l.
l. expectancy
expectation of l.
l. experience
fact of l.
fantasy l.
l. fear
feeling of being an outside observer of one's l.
l. goal
healthy religious l.
l. history
l. history calendar
l. impairment
impoverished fantasy l.
impulse l.
inner l.
l. instinct
late l.
later l.
l. lie
love l.
mental l.
noon of l.
l. organization
overstimulated home l.
l. of party
phase of l.
philosophy of l.
l. plan
prayerful l.
prime of l.
purpose in l. (PIL)
quality of l.
reading activities in l.
real l.
religious l.
right to l.
l. satisfaction
l. script
l. sentence
sexual l.
sheltered l.
l. space
l. span
l. stage
l. stress
l. stressor
l. support system
sustenance of l.
l. table
threat to l.
tumultuous l.
vegetative l.
vicissitudes of l.
l. years

Life-BREF
World Health Organization Quality of L.-B. (WHOQOL-BREF)

life-changing
l.-c. improvement
l.-c. spiritual experience

life-cycle
l.-c. adjustment
l.-c. change
l.-c. theory
l.-c. transition

life-event stress theory

lifeless

lifeline

lifelong
l. affiliation
l. behavior pattern
l. obesity
l. personality disorder
l. sexual dysfunction

lifelong-type
l.-t. dyspareunia
l.-t. vaginismus

lifespan development

lifestyle
alternative l.
antisocial l.
balanced l.
l. change
disciplined l.
l. factor
gambling l.
healthy l.
high-risk l.
inferior sibling l.
l. intervention

NOTES

lifestyle *(continued)*
l. issue
l. modification
nomadic l.
nontraditional l.
l. prejudice
sedentary l.
traditional l.
unstable l.
life-threatening
l.-t. behavior (LTB)
l.-t. condition
l.-t. danger
l.-t. disease
l.-t. event
l.-t. experience
l.-t. illness
lifetime
l. aggression
l. anxiety disorder
l. behavior
l. depression criterion
l. episode
l. expectancy
l. hierarchy
l. history
l. impulsivity
l. personality
l. prevalence
l. risk
l. risk for alcohol
l. sex partner
l. social phobia
lifter
mood l.
weight l.
ligand selection
ligature
strangulation l.
light
l. diet
l. drinking
flash of l.
glare of l.
halo of l.
l. sleep (LS)
l. therapy
l. therapy-induced mood disorder
l. touch sensation
l. trance
l. treatment
l. treatment for winter depression
lighter fluid dependence
lightheaded
likability
peer l.
likable
likelihood
l. of recurrence
l. of violence
Lilliputian hallucination
limb
abnormal position of distal l.
l. kinetic apraxia
phantom l.
l. psychogenic disorder
limbi (*pl. of* limbus)
limbic
l. activation
l. brain region
l. circuit
l. circuitry
l. dopamine receptor
l. dysregulation
l. effect
l. epilepsy
l. forebrain
l. leucotomy for treatment of OCD
l. lobe
l. structure
l. system
l. system disorder
l. zone
limbic-related region
limbus, pl. **limbi**
limen, pl. **limina**
difference l.
liminal stimulus
liminometer
limit
class l.
medication l.
method of l.'s
normal l.'s
off l.'s
physiologic l.
set l.'s
l. setting
within normal l.'s (WNL)
limitation
adolescent l.
conceptual l.
empirical l.
functional l.
l. of movement (LOM)
sex l.
technical l.
technological l.
limited
l. activity
l. attention span
l. diet
l. effect
l. insight
l. responsibility
l. social support

l. symptom attack
l. war
limited-capacity retrieval
limiting decision
limit-setting
l.-s. for adolescent
l.-s. parenting
limit-testing behavior
limophoitas
limophthisis
limosis
limotherapy
lineage
linear
l. causality
l. inseparability
l. perspective
l. thought process
l. type
line of expression
linen
liner
lingering fear
lingua, pl. **linguae**
lapsus l.
lingual delirium
linguistic
l. approach
l. determinism
l. disorganization
l. disturbance
l. savant
l. style
linguistic-kinesic method
linguistics
anthropological l.
lining
silver l.
link
causal l.
pathophysiologic l.
linkage
associative l.
l. disequilibrium
genetic l.
l. object
sex l.
l. worker
liothyronine (L-T_3)
lip
l. biting
l. eroticism
l. puckering
l. pursing
l. reading
l. reflex
l. smacking
lipolytic enzyme
lipophilic
liquefied heroin
liquidation of attachment
liquid diet
liquor
malt l.
lisping
Lissauer dementia paralytica
Lissauer-type paresis
lissencephaly, lissencephalia
list
hit l.
l. preoccupation
sleep-awake experience l. (SWEL)
listen
unable to l.
listening
l. attitude
diotic l.
l. language quotient
lazy l.
passive l.
l. with third ear
listless
litem
guardian ad l.
literacy
l. deficiency
inadequate l.
low l.
patient l.
visual l.
literal
l. agraphia
l. alexia
l. meaning
l. paraphasia
l. paraphrasia
literalis
paralalia l.
lithiasis
hysterical l.
lithium
l. action on first messenger
l. action on membranes
l. action on second messenger
l. dose
l. level

NOTES

Lithizine
litigious
l. delusional state
l. environment
l. paranoia
litigiousness
littering
live
l. birth
l. on welfare
l. in the project
l. together
will to l.
live-in relationship
liver
l. cirrhosis
cirrhotic l.
l. damage
l. disease
l. disease organic psychosis
l. enzymes
l. flap
l. function test (LFT)
palpable l.
l. span
lives (*pl. of* life)
livid
living
activities of daily l. (ADL)
ambivalence about l.
l. arrangement
basic activities of daily l. (BADLs)
capacity for independent l.
daily l.
existential l.
free l.
group l.
independent l.
l. instability
instrumental activities of daily l. (IADL)
reason for l.
simulated activities of daily l. (SADL, SADLs)
l. situation
standard of l.
task of independent l.
vicarious l.
l. wage
l. will
LOA
leave of absence
loosening of associations
load
sensory l.
loading
factor l.
genetic l.
salient l.
l. strategy
loafer
loath, loth
loathe
loathsome
lobar
l. dysfunction
l. sclerosis
lobata
Pueraria l.
lobe
contralateral parietal l.'s
l. dysfunction
frontal l.
limbic l.
occipital l.
parietal l.
posterodorsal temporal l.
prefrontal l.
temporal l.
lobectomy
temporal l.
transorbital l.
lobotomy
prefrontal l.
l. syndrome
transorbital l.
LOC
laxative of choice
level of consciousness
locus of control
loss of consciousness
local
l. convulsion
l. epilepsy
l. excitatory state
l. potential
l. response
l. sign
l. syncope
l. tic
l. vasoconstrictive action
localis paracusis
locality attachment
locality-specific pattern of aberrant behavior
localization
l. agnosia
auditory l.
l. of behavior
cerebral l.
l. of function
language l.
law of average l.
point l.
spatial l.
l. of symptoms
localization-related epilepsy

localized
l. amnesia
l. epilepsy
l. function
l. weakness
location
action l.
brain l.
cerebral l.
l. constancy
LOC-C
locus of control-chance
LOC-E
locus of control-external
LOC-I
locus of control-internal
loci (*pl. of* locus)
lock
l. finger
scalp l.
locked
l. cell
l. door seclusion
l. hospital unit
l. room
l. in state
l. ward
locking
phase l.
locoism
locomotion
locomotive
locomotor
l. activity
l. arrest
l. ataxia
locomotor-genital stage
locomotorium
loco plant
LOC-PO
locus of control-powerful others
locum tenens
locus, pl. **loci**
l. ceruleus
l. ceruleus neuron
chromosomal l.
l. of control (LOC)
l. of control-chance (LOC-C)
l. of control-external (LOC-E)
l. of control-internal (LOC-I)
l. of control-powerful others (LOC-PO)
l. heterogenicity
l. minoris resistentiae
quantitative trait loci (QTL)
single major l. (SML)
susceptibility l.
locution
Lofexidine
logagnosia
logagraphia
logamnesia
logaphasia
logarithm of odds score
logasthenia
logic
formal l.
perverted l.
trance l.
logical
l. analysis of automatic thought
l. inference
l. memory
l. memory subtest score
l. operation
l. positivism
logistic
l. curve
l. regression
l. regression analysis
l. regression equation
logoclonia
logographic
logokyphosis
logomachy
logomania
logoneurosis
logopathy
logoplegia
logorrhea
logospasm
logotherapy
LOI
level of incompetence
loiterer
lolling
LOM
limitation of movement
loss of movement
London
Drexel Tour of L.
loneliness
lonely
loner
psychological l.
lonesome

NOTES

L

long
l. half-life
l. hot summer effect
l. latency response
long-acting
l.-a. barbiturate
l.-a. injectable medication
l.-a. injection
long-circuiting
longevity
marital l.
long-half-life anxiolytic substance
longing
intense l.
passive-receptive l.
longitudinal
l. assessment
l. course
l. course specifier
l. experimental study design
l. expert evaluation using all available data (LEAD)
l. exploration of psychosocial factors in sickle cell disease
l. investigation of depression outcomes (LIDO)
l. mental status examination
l. method
l. observation
l. scan
l. study
long-lasting drug effect
long-lived
long-stay ward
long-suffering
long-term
l.-t. abstinence
l.-t. associative memory
l.-t. care
l.-t. care facility
l.-t. care placement
l.-t. commitment
l.-t. consequence
l.-t. course
l.-t. course of abuse
l.-t. danger
l.-t. data
l.-t. declarative memory
l.-t. dependence
l.-t. detoxification program
l.-t. disability (LTD)
l.-t. disease
l.-t. effect
l.-t. effectiveness
l.-t. effects of trauma
l.-t. heavy use
l.-t. hospitalization
l.-t. insomnia
l.-t. maintenance treatment
l.-t. management
l.-t. memory (LTM)
l.-t. mental health program
l.-t. mortality rate
l.-t. naturalistic study
l.-t. outcome
l.-t. pattern
l.-t. potentiation (LTP)
l.-t. psychotherapy
l.-t. recovery
l.-t. recurrent depression
l.-t. risk
l.-t. storage
l.-t. storage of memory
l.-t. therapy
look
glazed l.
grunge l.
paranoid l.
look-alike
amphetamine l.-a.
looking-glass self
loop
basal ganglia-cingulate gyrus-frontal lobe l.
calibrated l.
induction l.
loose
l. association
l. proverb interpretation
looseness of association
loosening of associations (LOA)
LOP
leave on pass
LOPS
length of patient stay
loquacious
loquaciousness
loquacity
LOS
length of stay
loser
losing
l. control
l. time
loss
age-related hearing l.
amygdala volumetric l.
l. of appetite
appetite l.
approval l.
l. of autonomy
autonomy l.
l. of belief
l. of biographical memory
l. of boundaries of ego
l. of breadwinner
central sensory l.
cognitive l.

l. of consciousness (LOC)
l. of control
cortical sensory l.
dense sensory l.
l. discrimination
dissociated sensory l.
l. of effect
l. of ego boundary
ego boundary l.
l. of energy
evidence of weight l.
l. experience
l. of freedom
functional l.
hemisensory l.
hippocampal volumetric l.
hysterical visual l.
l. of identity
imagined l.
l. of independence
l. of interest
l. of interest in usual activities
interpersonal l.
inventory of l.
ipsilateral l.
job l.
l. of language
l. of libido
l. of loved one
major l.
mechanical functional l.
memory l.
minor weight l.
monocular visual l.
l. of motivation
motor l.
l. of movement (LOM)
multiple l.'s
nerve l.
neuronal l.
nonnormative hair l.
object l.
l. of orientation
parental l.
past l.
perceived l.
peripheral sensory l.
personal l.
l. of pleasure
postsurgical l.
pregnancy l.
psychogenic hearing l.
real l.
recent l.
l. of relationship
l. of response
self-induced hair l.
semen l.
l. of semen
l. of sensation
l. of sensitivity
significant l.
significant weight l.
sleep l.
social l.
soul l.
spousal l.
stocking-and-glove sensory l.
symbolic l.
threat of job l.
l. of touch with reality
unresolved l.
volumetric l.
weight l.
l. of zest

lost
l. privileges (LP)
l. in thought

LOT
lengthened off-time

loth (*var. of* loath)

lottery gamble

loud
l. music
l. speech

Louis-Bar syndrome

Louisiana Psychiatric Medical Association

loup-garou

louse, pl. **lice**

love-hate relationship

loveless

lovely

lovemaking

lover
distraught former l.
former l.
heterosexual l.
homosexual l.
illicit l.
l.'s knot

lovesick

loving
l. behavior
delusional l.

NOTES

loving *(continued)*
l. feeling
l. parenting
low
l. alpha coefficient
l. anger threshold
l. anxiety (LA)
l. back pain psychogenic disorder
l. delirium
l. dose
l. education
l. educational level
l. energy
l. energy level
l. fever
l. frustration tolerance
l. impulsiveness
l. income
l. intelligence
l. literacy
l. profile
l. self-confidence
l. sensory environment
l. sexual desire
l. sexual interest
l. social desirability
l. stimulation environment
l. threshold of competency
l. tolerance potential
low-activity situation
low-anger individual
low-calorie diet
low-carbohydrate diet
low-complexity movement
low-dose
l.-d. antipsychotic
l.-d. strategy
l.-d. treatment
lowered mood
lower-intensity treatment
low-fat diet
low-grade
l.-g. heroin
l.-g. thought disorder
low-key response
lowlife
low-minded
low-potency D_2 antagonist
low-salt diet
low-spirited
low-stimulation situation
low-tyramine diet
Loxapac
loxia
loyalty
doubt of l.
family l.
unjustified doubt of l.
Loyola sensate focus
LP
latency period
lost privileges
LPC
licensed professional counselor
LS
legally separated
light sleep
LSD
lysergic acid diethylamide
LSD dependence
LSD reaction
LSD-type perception
LTB
life-threatening behavior
LTD
long-term disability
LTM
long-term memory
LTP
long-term potentiation
lubricant
lubricious
lucid
l. interval
l. lethargy
lucidification
lucidity
lucrative
lucubrate
ludic
ludicrous
lues
luetic curve
lugubrious
lumbarization
luminance flux
luminescence of object
lump in throat
lunacy
lunatic
Lunesta
lung
trench l.
lupina
insania l.
lure
Luria
L. hand sequence
L. technique
lurid
lush
lust
l. dynamism
l. murder
lusterless eyes
lustful

luteal
l. phase
l. phase assessment
luteinizing
l. hormone (LH)
l. hormone-releasing hormone (LHRH)
Luvox
luxuriate
lycanthropy
lycomania
lycorexia
lygophilia
lying
pathologic l.
repetitive l.
Lyme disease
lymphatic psychogenic disorder
lymphoblastoid cell
lymphocyte
peripheral l.
lynch
lysatotherapy
lysergic
l. acid amide
l. acid diethylamide (LSD)
l. acid monoethylamide
lyssa
lytic cocktail
lz R
total response

NOTES

L

MA
mental age
migraine with aura
M/A
mood and/or affect
MAB
management of assaultive behavior
MAC
maximum allowable cost
macabre
MacArthur violence risk assessment study
mace
macerate
maceration
Macewen
M. sign
M. symptom
machiavellian
machiavellianism
machinate
machination
machinator
machinery
machismo
macho manner
macrobiotic diet
macrocranium
macroencephalon
macroesthesia
macrographia, macrography
macrogyria
macromania
macromaniacal delirium
macropsia
macrostereognosis
maculocerebral
Madame Butterfly syndrome
madcap
MADD
mixed anxiety depression disorder
madden
maddening
made-to-order dream
Mad Hatter syndrome
madhouse
madly
madman
madness
impulsive m.
raving m.
Madonna complex
Madonna-prostitute complex
madwoman
MAF
minimal audible field
magazine
sexually charged m.
Magenblase syndrome
magersucht
magic
black m.
m. bone
communication m.
compulsive m.
cursing m.
m. fantasy
m. helper
m. mushroom
m. omnipotence
m. phase
m. thinking
magical
m. meaning
m. thinking
magisterial
magna
cisterna m.
Magnan
M. sign
M. trombone movement
magnanimity
magnet
m. reaction
m. reflex
magnetic
m. apraxia
m. attraction
m. crisis
m. personality
m. resonance imaging (MRI)
m. resonance spectroscopy (MRS)
m. seizure therapy
magnetism
animal m.
magnetometer
magnific
magnification
magnificent
magnify
magniloquence
magniloquent
magnitude
perturbation m.
maid
old m.
maidenhair tree
maiden name

M

maidica
psychoneurosis m.
maim
main
m. d'accoucheur
m. effect
m. en crochet
M. syndrome
m. treatment modality
mainline
mainlining heroin
mainstream
mainstreaming
maintenance
m. dose
m. drug
m. drug therapy
m. function
m. of harmony
m. insomnia
intimacy m.
m. level
m. medication
methadone m.
minimum m.
perceptual m.
physiologic m.
short-term m.
m. striving
m. treatment
m. treatment program
weight m.
weight loss m.
maitre de plaisir
majeure
force m.
major
m. affective disorder
m. attachment figure
m. break
chorea m.
m. depression
m. depression with psychotic features
m. depressive affective psychosis
m. depressive disorder (MDD)
m. depressive disorder, recurrent
m. depressive episode (MDE)
m. epilepsy
m. form
m. hypnosis
m. hysteria
m. image-distorting level
m. impairment
m. impairment of functioning
m. life activity
m. life change
m. life stress
m. loss
m. mental illness
m. mood disorder
m. mood swinging
m. motor aphasia
m. motor seizure
m. psychiatric disorder
m. psychiatric syndrome
m. risk period
m. role obligation
m. role therapy (MRT)
m. solution
m. tranquilizer
majority society
make
m. believe
m. love
m. out
m. sense
make-believe
m.-b. play
m.-b. world
maker
surrogate decision m.
makeup
excessive m.
genetic m.
mental m.
making
attachment in m.
tyrannical decision m.
mal
comitial m.
m. de la rosa
m. de ojo
m. de pelea
m. d'orient
petit m.
m. puesto
m. rosso
malabsorption
maladaptation, maladaption
social m.
maladaptive
m. behavioral change
m. coping
m. coping mechanism
m. coping strategy
m. defense mechanism
m. feeling
m. illness behavior
m. impulse
m. pattern of behavior
m. pattern of emotion
m. pattern of motivation
m. pattern of substance abuse
m. pattern of thought
m. personality
m. personality pattern
m. personality trait

m. problem-solving strategy
m. psychological change
m. reaction
m. reaction to stressor
m. response
m. thought
m. way
maladaptively aggressive youth
maladie
m. des tics
m. du doute
m. du pays
maladjusted
sexually m.
maladjustment
sexual m.
social m.
vocational m.
malady
royal m.
malaise
postexertional m.
malapert
malaria
cerebral m.
therapeutic m.
malcontent
maldevelopment
male
m. alcoholism subtype
m. biological status
m. bond
m. castration
m. circumcision
m. climacteric syndrome
m. dyspareunia
m. erectile disorder
m. erectile dysfunction
feminine traits in m.'s
m. gender identity
m. genitalia
m. homosexuality
m. hypoactive sexual desire disorder
m. imprinting
m. intersex
m. menopause
m. orgasm
m. orgasmic disorder
m. patient
m. pattern alopecia
m. rape
m. therapist
m. victim
malediction
malefaction
malefactor
maleficence
maleficent
maleness
male-to-female
m.-t.-f. ratio
m.-t.-f. transgender identity
malevolence
malevolent
m. behavior
m. concern
m. distrust
m. thought system
malfeasance
malfunction
malice
malicious
m. intent
m. mischief
malign
malignancy
malignant
m. brain neoplasm
m. narcissism
m. neurosis
m. psychosis
m. stupor
m. trend
malinger
malingered dissociative identity disorder
malingerer
malingering
m. behavior
m. disorder
test of memory m. (TOMM)
malleability
malleable
malleation
mallet
anger m.
mall treatment concept
malnourished child
malnutrition
malodorous
malpractice
m. insurance
m. stress syndrome
malternative drink
malt liquor

NOTES

maltreat
maltreatment
child m.
childhood m.
elder m.
malvaria
malversation
mammalian
m. teratology
m. tissue
mammalingus
mammonist
mammotroph
man, pl. **men**
drug-using m.
eight stages of m.
enlisted m.
Erikson 8 stages of m.
fellow m.
hatchet m.
hit m.
medicine m.
men who have sex with men (MSM)
non-drug-using m.
personal m.
wise old m.
manacle
manage
difficult to m.
manageable
managed
m. care
M. Care Appropriateness Protocol
m. care environment
management
adolescent anger m.
anger m.
anxiety m.
m. of assaultive behavior (MAB)
behavioral m.
clinical m.
conflict m.
conservative m.
contingency m.
craving m.
crisis m.
cue m.
diet m.
drug m.
exhaustion m.
grief m.
home m.
home-based family m.
impression m.
intensive case m.
long-term m.
medication m.
multidimensional pain m.
nonmedical m.
obesity m.
pain m.
participative m.
pharmacological m.
psychological m.
psychosocial m.
reflux m.
seizure m.
stress m.
style of leadership and m.
symptomatic m.
task m.
weight m.
manager-style appraisal
managing behavior
Manchester
M. and Salford self-harm project
mandate
mandated self-help group
mandatory treatment
mandibular dystonia
maneuver
body concept-exploration m.
body contact-exploration m.
passive-aggressive m.
tactical m.
manganese
m. exposure
m. mask
manhandle
manhood
manhunt
mania
absorbed m.
acute alcoholic m.
acute bipolar m.
acute hallucinatory m.
adolescent m.
akinetic m.
alcoholic m.
anxious m.
atypical m.
biting m.
chronic alcoholic m.
classic euphoric m.
collecting m.
compulsive m.
copying m.
dancing m.
delirious m.
depressed m.
doubting m.
drug-induced m.
dysphoric m.
ephemeral m.
epileptic m.
grumbling m.
hallucinatory m.

hostile m.
hysterical m.
inhibited m.
intractable m.
irritable m.
joking m.
peracute m.
periodic m.
periodical m.
m. phantastica infantilis
political m.
pornographic m.
postpartum m.
poststroke m.
m. á potu
prepubertal m.
process m.
puerperal m.
pure m.
m. rating score
reactive m.
reasoning m.
recommencement m.
recurrent episode chronic m.
religious m.
seaman m.
m. secandi
secondary m.
self-absorbed m.
senile m.
single-episode chronic m.
squander m.
stage 3 m.
steroid-induced m.
stupor m.
transitory m.
traumatic brain injury-associated m.
unipolar m.
unproductive m.
m. with rapid cycling

maniacal grief reaction

maniac catatonia

manic

acutely m.
m. agitation
m. bipolar disorder
m. child
m. delirium
m. depression
m. excitement
m. feature
m. hebephrenia
m. mood
m. mood episode
m. mood theme
m. patient
m. phase
m. psychosis
m. reaction
schizoaffective disorder, m.
m. speech
m. stare
m. state
m. stupor
m. symptom
m. syndrome
m. temperament

manic-depressive

m.-d. affective psychosis
m.-d. disorder
m.-d. illness
m.-d. insanity
perplexed-type m.-d.
m.-d. reaction
m.-d. syndrome

manic-like episode

manie

m. de perfection
m. de rumination

manifest

m. anxiety
m. content
m. destiny
m. dream
m. goal
m. symptom
m. tetany

manifestation

behavioral m.
characteristic m.
clinical m.
m. of depression
m. of emotion
impostor psychotic m.
neuroimaging m.
neuropsychiatric m.
neuropsychologic m.
neurotic m.
objective m.
overt physical m.
physiologic m.
psychiatric m.
psychogenic physiological m.
psychophysiologic m.
psychotic m.
m. of resistance

NOTES

manifestation *(continued)*
subjective m.
underlying psychological m.
m. of violence
manifested disability
manifestly observable symptom
manifold
manipulability
manipulable
manipulate
manipulation
m. communication pattern
emotional m.
environmental m.
language m.
m. stage
m. tendency
manipulative
m. behavior
m. device
m. drive
m. pseudohallucination
m. technique
manipulatory task
manliness
manly
man-machine system
man-made disaster
manner
allosteric m.
authoritative m.
bellicose m.
condescending m.
detached m.
m.'s deterioration
devious m.
elementary m.
evil m.
guarded m.
halting m.
impaired social m.'s
inconsistent m.
macho m.
part-object m.
patronizing m.
secretive m.
superior m.
sustained m.
unkempt m.
unusual m.
mannered
mannerism
bizarre repetitive m.
childlike m.
feminine m.
speech m.
mannish
Mannkopf sign
mannosidosis
manslaughter
involuntary m.
manslayer
mansuetude
mantic
mantle sclerosis
mantra
manual
m. communication
m. dexterity
diagnostic m.
m. dominance
International Classification of Sleep Disorders: Diagnostic and Coding M. (ICSD)
m. laborer
m. sadism
self-help m.
m. stimulation
manual-based interpersonal psychotherapy
manumit
many-sided
many-valued
MAO
monoamine oxidase
MAO inhibitor
MAOI
monoamine oxidase inhibitor
MAOI-serotonergic agent
MAOI-tricyclic agent
map
cognitive m.
genetic m.
personal skills m.
Z-score m.
maple sugar syrup urine disease
maplike skull
mapping
behavior m.
brain m.
brain electrical activity m. (BEAM)
cognitive m.
cortical m.
m. of cortical function
speech and motor m.
topographic m.
maprotiline
mar
marasmic
m. female
m. state
marasmus
nutritional m.
Marateaux-Lamy disease
marathon
drug-fueled music m.
gestalt therapy m.

m. group psychotherapy
m. session
marauder
Marcé study
Marchant zone
Marchiafava-Bignami disease
mareos
marginal
m. consciousness
m. function
m. intelligence
m. thinking
m. transvestite
marginalis
alopecia m.
marginalization
marginalized
marginally therapeutic dose
Marie ataxia
Marie-Robinson syndrome
Marines
US M.
mariposia
marital
m. adjustment
m. conflict
m. counseling
m. counselor
m. discord
m. disharmony
m. disruption
m. dissatisfaction
m. group therapy
m. history (MH)
m. infidelity
m. instability
m. interaction
m. longevity
m. problem
m. satisfaction
m. schism
m. skew
m. stability
m. status
m. stress
m. turbulence
m. violence
mark
belt m.
easy m.
marked
m. anger
m. anxiety
m. decline in academic functioning
m. depression
m. impairment
m. irritability
m. motor agitation
m. tension
markedly
m. diminished interest
m. diminished participation
marker
biochemical phenotypic m.
biologic m.
circadian m.
emotional m.
fixed m.
gene m.
genetic m.
I m.
phenotypic m.
psychological m.
somatic m.
X-chromosome m.
m. X syndrome
market
sex m.
marketing personality
marketplace
sexual m.
marking
analog m.
marriage
arranged m.
civil m.
cluster m.
common law m.
companionate m.
compassionate m.
consanguineous m.
m. contract
m. of convenience
m. counseling
m. counselor
m. encounter
experimental m.
m. fear
former m.
group m.
heterosexual m.
homosexual m.
interracial m.
legal m.
mixed m.
multiple m.'s

M

NOTES

marriage *(continued)*
nonconsanguineous m.
open m.
open-end m. (OEM)
m. response
m. ritual
same-sex m.
sandbox m.
shotgun m.
stability of m.
starter m.
symbiotic m.
synergic m.
m. therapy
traditional m.
trial m.
troubled m.
unconsummated m.
m. vows
married
never m.
marry
failure to m.
marshal
sky m.
martial
m. arts
m. law
Martin-Bell syndrome
martyr complex
martyrdom
marvelous
marxism
marxist
masculation
masculine
m. attitude
m. attitude in female neurotic
m. identity
m. protest
m. social role
masculinity
masculinization
masculinize
masher
Masini sign
mask
death m.
m. discipline
Hutchinson m.
manganese m.
masked
m. affection
m. anxiety
m. depression
m. deprivation
m. epilepsy
m. facies
m. homosexuality
m. hypertension
m. obsession
masking
background m.
backward visual m.
behavioral m.
central m.
effective m.
m. efficiency
m. fear
forward m.
frequency m.
initial m.
maximum m.
m. pain
perceptual m.
peripheral m.
m. stimulus
upward m.
masklike facies
Maslow hierarchy
masochism
erotogenic m.
feminine m.
ideal m.
mental m.
moral m.
sexual m.
social m.
verbal m.
masochist
masochistic
m. behavior
m. character
m. character defense
m. component
m. personality
m. personality disorder
m. ritual
m. sabotage
m. sexual activity
m. sexual fantasy
m. sexual urge
m. solution
m. stance
m. wish
m. wish dream
masquerade
mass
m. action theory
apperceptive m.
m. behavior
black m.
m. hysteria
m. media
m. method
m. movement
m. murderer
m. polarization

m. psychogenic illness
m. psychology
m. reflex
m. sociogenic illness
m. terrorism
m. therapy
thermogenic tissue m.
m. violence

massacre

massacrer

massage
autoerotic m.
electrovibratory m.
nerve-point m.
m. parlor
tremolo m.
vibratory m.

massager

masse
en m.

massed negative practice

masseur

masseuse

massive seizure

massotherapy

master
m. of avoidance
M.'s and Johnson study
M. of Science in Nursing (MSN)
M. of Social Work (MSW)

masterful

mastermind

mastery
motive m.
m. motive
sense of m.
symbolic m.

masticatoria
monoplegia m.

masticatory
m. diplegia
m. spasm

Mast syndrome

masturbate

masturbation
anal m.
m. behavior
compulsive m.
m. equivalent
false m.
m. fantasy
infantile m.
mutual m.
psychic m.
public m.
symbolic m.

masturbator

masturbatory
m. activity
m. pain

matatabi

match
leader m.
perceptual-motor m.

matchbox sign

matched groups

matching
m. hypothesis
impedance m.
prototype m.
sexual m.

matchmaker

mate
soul m.
stressful m.

materfamilias

material
clinical m.
emotional m.
evidence of intrusion of idiosyncratic m.
evidence of intrusion of private m.
m. gain
genetic m.
m. gratification
m. home condition
idiosyncratic m.
learning m.
neutral m.
occupational exposure to toxic m.
m. previously learned
m. symbolism
unstructured verbal m.
verbal m.

materialism

materialistic

materialization

materialize

maternal
m. abuse
m. age
m. attachment
m. attitude
m. behavior
m. childrearing
m. competency

NOTES

maternal *(continued)*
m. depression
m. deprivation
m. deprivation syndrome
m. desertion
m. drive
m. dysfunction
m. fitness
m. indifference
m. neglect
m. overprotection
m. problem-solving strategy
m. rejection
m. relationship
m. role
m. stress
maternity blues
mathematical
m. ability
m. skill
m. symbol
mathematics, math
m. achievement
assessment in m.
m. disorder
mating
assortative m.
assortive m.
m. behavior
nonrandom m.
random m.
matriarch
matriarchy
Matricaria recutita
matrices (*pl. of* matrix)
matrices-R
Raven progressive m.-R (RPM-R)
matricide
matrilinear family
matrilocal family
matrimony vine
matrix, pl. **matrices**
factor m.
therapeutic m.
matroclinous
matrocliny
matron
matter
central gray m. (CGM)
cortical gray m.
deep white m.
dorsal gray m.
m. of fact
gray m.
midbrain m.
parahippocampal white m.
periaqueductal gray m.
periventricular white m.
sclerosis of white m.
subcortical gray m.
subcortical white m.
theologic m.
white m.
mattoid
maturate
maturation
cognitive m.
emotional m.
hormonal m.
m. hypothesis
m. index
mitosis, migration, and m.
neurologic m.
principle of anticipatory m.
psychological m.
m. rate
retarded m.
social m.
maturational
m. change
m. crisis
m. lag
mature
m. defense
m. defense mechanism
m. minor rule
maturity
biologic m.
cognitive m.
emotional m.
m. fear
genital m.
intellectual m.
mental m.
motor m.
psychological m.
m. rating
matutinal epilepsy
maudlin drunkenness
Maudsley theory of depression
maul
maunder
mauve factor
maven, mavin
maverick
mawkish
maximal
m. contrast
m. effect
m. electroshock
m. electroshock seizure (MES)
m. stimulus
maximization
ego m.
maximum
m. acoustic output
m. allowable cost (MAC)
m. intent rating

m. lethality rating
m. masking
m. permissible dose
m. recommended human dose (MRHD)
m. security
m. tolerable amount
maximum-intensity projection
maximum-security
m.-s. forensic psychiatric hospital
m.-s. prison
m.-s. prisoner
m.-s. unit
Mayberg limbic-cortical dysregulation model
mayhem
maze
m. behavior
m. coordination
proteus m.
MBD
minimal brain dysfunction
McCarthyism
McCullough-Pitts
M.-P. model
M.-P. neuron
MCE
medical care evaluation
McLean study of adult development
MCR
mother-child relationship
MD
mentally deficient
MDA
methylenedioxyamphetamine
MDD
major depressive disorder
MDE
major depressive episode
MDMA
methylenedioxymethamphetamine
MDSO
mentally disordered sex offender
me
bad me
meager
meal
high-fat m.
skip m.'s
mealy-mouthed
mean
m. age
m.'s for anxiety
arithmetic m.
assumed m.
m. deviation
geometric m.
harmonic m.
m. intracranial raw volume
law of coercion to biosocial m.
lethal m.'s
m. normalized whole brain volume
regression of m.
m. sleep latency
standard error of m. (SEM)
statistical m.
suicide m.'s
m. total weighted sum score
m. years of education
meaning
affect-related m.
conflict of m.
double m.
effort after m.
emotion-related m.
figurative m.
hidden m.
higher order emotion-related m.
idiosyncratic m.
latent m.
literal m.
magical m.
psychological m.
m. reframing
sliding of m.
subtle m.
symbolic m.
transferred m.
unknown m.
will to m.
meaningful
m. conversation
m. encounter
m. interpersonal relationship
meaningfulness
theoretical m.
meaningless
m. syllable sequence
m. word association
meanness
measurable impairment
measure
abuse m.
achievement identification m.
adjustment m.
affect intensity m.

NOTES

M

measure *(continued)*
assessment m.
attentional m.
avoidance m.
m. of balance
baseline m.
behavioral assessment m.
biologic m.
m. of central tendency
central tendency m.
cognitive m.
m. of competence
course of illness m.
diagnostic m.
dissociation m.
functional independence m. (FIM)
functioning m.
global m.
happiness m.
interpersonal sensitivity m.
neglect m.
neurocognitive m.
neuropsychologic m.
number-recency m.
objective m.
outcome m.
overall cognitive m.
phenomenological m.
physiologic m.
pretreatment m.
psychometric m.
psychometrically established m.
psychopathology m.
psychotherapeutic m.
quality of life m.
quantitative m.
reactive m.
Schutz m.
self-report m.
sensitive m.
social adjustment m.
sociodemographic m.
state-dependent m.
symptom m.
therapeutic m.
unambiguous m.
unobtrusive m.

measured
m. capacity
m. dose
m. intelligence

measurement
absolute m.
educational m.
EEG activity m.
m. effect
m. error
error of m.
instrumental ADL m.
interactive m.
mental m.
psychomotor m.

Mebaral

MEC
minimum effective concentration

mecca

mechanical
m. anosmia
m. aptitude
m. asphyxia
m. functional loss
m. intelligence
m. vertigo

mechanics
body m.

mechanism
abnormalities in sleep-wake timing m.
acting-out defense m.
adaptation m.
adaptive defense m.
adaptive ego m.
adaptive involuntary coping m.
adjustment m.
alerting m.
analogous brain m.
arousal boost m.
arousal reduction m.
association m.
attentional m.
balance m.
basic brain m.
biobehavioral m.
brain metabolic m.
causal m.
causative m.
circadian pacemaker m.
cognitive m.
compensation defense m.
compensatory m.
conversion defense m.
coping m.
cross-correlation m.
defense m.
denial defense m.
de novo m.
direct causative pathophysiological m.
displacement defense m.
dissociation defense m.
ego defense m.
emotional m.
endogenous brain m.
escape m.
feedback m.
focusing m.
fundamental defense m.
fundamental neural m.

gating m.
heat-loss m.
idealization defense m.
identification defense m.
immature coping m.
inappropriate defense m.
incorporation defense m.
indirect m.
inherited releasing m. (IRM)
inhibition m.
innate releasing m.
input-output m.
introjection defense m.
learning m.
maladaptive coping m.
maladaptive defense m.
mature defense m.
mediating m.
mental m.
metabolic m.
neural m.
neurobiological m.
neutralizing m.
outgoing m.
pain m.
pathologic defense m.
pathophysiologic m.
perceptual cognitive m.
pharmacological m.
physiologic m.
plastic compensatory m.
Pollyanna m.
postsynaptic compensatory m.
primary m.
projection defense m.
rationalization defense m.
reaction formation defense m.
regression defense m.
relapse m.
rescue m.
sex arousal m. (SAM)
shared m.
sleep m.
sour grapes m.
specific pathophysiological m.
sublimation defense m.
substitution defense m.
sweet-lemon m.
symbolization defense m.
thermogenic m.
triggering m.
undoing defense m.

mechanistic approach
mechanize
mechanoreflex
mechanotherapy
mechanothermy
meconism
meddle
meddlesome behavior
meddling
Medea complex
media (*pl. of* medium)
medial
m. frontal cortex
m. frontal lobe syndrome
m. hemispheric dynamic
m. hypothalamus
m. orbitofrontal cortex
m. prefrontal cortex
m. rostral supplementary motor area
m. temporal memory system
m. temporal structure

median
center m.
m. sagittal plane
statistical m.

mediate
mediated
m. function
m. response

mediating
m. effect
m. mechanism

mediation
cognitive m.
conflict m.
peer m.
verbal m.

mediators of social support (MOSS)
Medica
Excerpta M.

medicable
Medicaid
medical
m. advice
m. anesthetic
m. anthropology
m. assistance
m. attention
m. audit
m. care
m. care evaluation (MCE)
m. center
m. comorbidity

NOTES

medical *(continued)*
m. complication of obesity
m. condition
m. consultant
m. contraindication
m. deliberation
m. discharge
m. doctor
m. effect
m. emergency
m. ethics
m. etiology
m. examiner
m. futility
m. history
m. identification tag
m. illness
m. impairment
m. intervention
m. jurisprudence
m. leave
m. model
m. morbidity
m. necessity
M. Outcomes Study (MOS)
M. Outcomes Study Short Form
m. power of attorney
m. problem
m. profession
m. professional
m. provider
m. psychoanalyst
m. psychology
m. psychotherapy
m. reason
m. record
m. record correction
m. review
m. sociology
m. staff
m. staff member
m. stress
m. symptom
m. syndrome
m. treatment
m. use
m. utilization
m. value system
medically compromised
medicament
medicamentosa
alopecia m.
Medicare supplement
medicaster
medicate
medicated patient
medication
m. abuse
active antidepressant m.
adjunctive m.
adolescent m.
agonist m.
antagonist m.
antianxiety m.
anticholinergic m.
antidepressant m.
antiepileptic m.
antihypertensive m.
antipsychotic m.
antiretroviral m.
antiseizure m.
anxiolytic m.
attitude to m. (AM)
beta adrenergic m.
black-market m.
m. change
cheeking m.
conservative m.
continuous antipsychotic m.
continuous maintenance m.
m. contraindication
conventional antipsychotic m.
cyclic m.
depot m.
m. dosage
m. error
experimental m.
first-line m.
forced m.
GABAergic m.
m. guide
high-potency m.
injectable m.
interacting m.'s
intravenous m.
involuntary m.
m. level
m. limit
long-acting injectable m.
maintenance m.
m. management
mood-stabilizing m.
multiple daily m.'s
neuroleptic m.
m. nonadherence
m. noncompliance
over-the-counter m.
parenteral m.
patient guide to m.
peripherally acting anticholinergic m.
poor response to m.
prescription m.
psychiatric m.
psychoactive m.
psychotropic m.
m. reduction
m. refractoriness

m. refusal
m. regimen
second-line m.
m. side effect
m. stigma
sublingual m.
substitutive m.
supportive m.
m. tapering
m. taper schedule
targeted m.
m. treatment
m. trial
unnecessary m.
up-to-date m.
weight-neutral psychotic m.

medication-induced
m.-i. delirium
m.-i. dementia
m.-i. disorder
m.-i. movement
m.-i. tardive dyskinesia
m.-i. tremor

medication-related weight gain
medication-resistant schizophrenia
medication-taking behavior
medicinal
patent m.'s

medicine
Academy of Psychosomatic M. (APM)
alternative m.
American Academy of Pain M. (AAPM)
American Academy of Psychosomatic M.
American Academy of Sleep M. (AASM)
American Board of Sleep M.
American Society of Addiction M. (ASAM)
artificial intelligence in m. (AIM)
aviation m.
Band-Aid m.
behavioral m.
Chinese m.
clinical m.
comparative m.
complementary and alternative m. (CAM)
compound m.
m. concept
constitutional m.
diploma in psychological m. (DPM)
domestic m.
dosimetric m.
emergency m.
environmental m.
evidence-based m. (EBM)
experimental m.
family m.
folk m.
forensic m.
geriatric m.
group m.
herbal m.
hermetic m.
holistic m.
hyperbaric m.
Indian folk m.
Institute of M. (IOM)
International College of Psychosomatic M.
legal m.
m. man
mental m.
modern Western m.
National Center for Complementary and Alternative M.
neo-hippocratic m.
nutritional m.
Office of Alternative M. (OAM)
patent m.
physical m.
preclinical m.
prescription-only m. (POM)
preventive m.
psychologic m.
psychosomatic m. (PSMed)
rational m.
sleep m.
social m.
socialized m.
suggestive m.
Western m.
m. woman

medicolegal issue
medicomechanical
medicopsychological
medicopsychology
medicosocial
medievalism
mediocrity
meditate
meditatio mortis

NOTES

M

meditation
guided m.
mindfulness m.
principle of Buddhist m.
qi gong movement-based m.
transcendental m. (TM)
meditation-based stress reduction
meditative tradition
medium, pl. **media**
electronic media
media history
media influence
mass media
spiritual m.
m. trance
media violence
violent media
mediumistic hypothesis
medium-security prisoner
medley
chance m.
medulla, pl. **medullae**
m. oblongata
medullary
m. canal
m. narcosis
m. syndrome
medullovasculosa
zona m.
meek
meet halfway
meeting
face-to-face m.
12-step m.
megacephalic, megacephalous
megacolon
psychogenic m.
megalgia
megaloencephalic
megaloencephalon
megaloencephaly
megalographia, megalography
megalomania
megalomaniac
megalomanic
Megan Law
megavitamin therapy
me generation
megrim
meiosis
melancholic, melancholiac
m. constitutional type
m. depression
m. feature
m. involutional reaction
m. mood
m. personality
m. sign
melancholicus
raptus m.
melancholium
omego m.
melancholy, melancholia
acute m.
affective m.
m. affective psychosis
agitated m.
m. attonita
chronic m.
climacteric m.
convulsive m.
hypochondriac m.
melancholia hypochondriaca
hypochondriacal m.
intermittent m.
involutional m.
menopausal m.
panphobic m.
paranoid m.
paretic m.
puberty m.
puerperal m.
reactive m.
recurrent m.
melancholia religiosa
senile m.
sexual m.
melancholia simplex
melancholia stuporosa
stuporous m.
suicidal m.
melancholia vera
m. with delirium
m. zoanthropy
melanocyte-stimulating hormone
melatonin
melee
meliorism
melioristic
Melissa officinalis
melitracen
Mellanby effect
mellitus
diabetes m.
mellow
mellowness
melodramatic
melodramatize
melomania
meltdown
member
adolescent gang m.
couple m.
m. of coven
cult m.
family m.
gang m.

illicit drug use in family m.
medical staff m.
neo-Nazi gang m.
skinhead gang m.
staff m.
surviving family m.
team m. (TM)

membrane
hymenal m.
lithium action on m.'s
neuronal m.
m. phenotype

memento mori

memoir

memorabilia

memorable

memoration
amnesic m.

memoriae
lapsus m.

memorial

memorialist

memorialize

memorize

memory
m. ability
accuracy of m.
affect m.
m. afterimage
m. amplification
angry m.
anterograde loss of m.
associative m.
auditory m.
autobiographic m.
automatic m.
behavioral m.
m. bias
biographical m.
blocked m.
body m.
Bower model of mood-congruent m.
m. buffer
childhood m.
coast m.
conscious m.
m. consolidation
constructive m.
m. decay
declarative m.
decreased m.
m. defect
delayed m.
m. for design (MFD)
m. deterioration
m. difficulty
digit-symbol and incidental m.
m. disability
m. disorder
m. distortion
distributed m.
m. disturbance
disturbance of m.
echoic m.
m. by emotion
emotional m.
emotionally loaded event m.
m. encoding
enhance m.
episodic m.
euthymic m.
event m.
explicit m.
eye m.
factual m.
false m.
m. falsification
figural m.
flashbulb m.
m. function
m. function deficit
m. gap
genetic m.
m. hallucination
hyperesthetic m.
iconic m.
m. illusion
m. image
immediate m.
impaired m.
m. impairment
implicit m.
incidental m.
m. index
m. intrusion error
intrusive m.
island of m.
lack of m.
m. lapse
logical m.
long-term m. (LTM)
long-term associative m.
long-term declarative m.
long-term storage of m.
m. loss

M

NOTES

memory *(continued)*
loss of biographical m.
minute m.
mirthful m.
nondeclarative m.
m. organization
overconsolidation of m.'s
painful m.
panoramic m.
m. paradigm
m. passage
m. performance
permanent m.
personal m.
photographic m.
physiologic m.
pleasant m.
primary m.
priming m.
procedural m.
m. process
m. processing
prospective m.
m. quotient (MQ)
racial m.
m. recall
recent m.
recognition m.
m. reconstruction
recovered m.
recurrent m.
recurring trauma m.
recursive autoassociative m.
m. reference
remote episodic m.
replacement m.
m. retention
m. retrieval strategy
retrograde loss of m.
retrospective gaps in m.
m. romance
rote m.
m. score
m. screen
secondary verbal m.
selective m.
semantic m.
senile m.
sequence m.
sequential m.
short-term m. (STM)
short-term declarative m.
m. skill
somatic m.
m. span
state-dependent m.
m. storage
story m.
stress effect on m.
subconscious m.
m. symbol
m. for symbolic unit (MSU)
m. system
m. task
m. theory
TOMAL facial m.
top-down organization of m.
m. trace
m. training
m. transfer
traumatic m.
unconscious m.
unhappy m.
m. variable
verbal working m.
visuospatial m.
working m.

memory-continuous performance
Memphis Educational Model Providing Handicapped Infant Services (MEMPHIS)
men (*pl. of* man)
menace
menacing
menage à trois
menarche
mendacious
mendacity
mendelian
m. law
m. rules of inheritance

Mendel instep reflex
mendelism
mendicancy
pathologic m.

mendicant
menial
meningeal neurosyphilis
meninges (*pl. of* meninx)
meningism
meningismus psychosis
meningitis, pl. **meningitides**
external m.
herpes zoster m.
occlusive m.
syphilitic m.

meningoencephalitis
herpetic m.
syphilitic m.

meningomyelitis
meningovascular syphilis
meninx, pl. **meninges**
Menninger Clinic Treatment Intervention Project
menopausal
m. depression
m. distress
m. melancholia

m. paranoid psychosis
m. paranoid reaction
m. paranoid state
m. paraphrenia
m. status

menopause

adjustment reaction of m.
m. and aging
female m.
male m.
m. neurosis

Mensa

menses

altered m.

mens rea

menstrual

m. cramp
m. cycle
m. disturbance
m. psychogenic disorder

menstrual-associated syndrome

menstruation

psychogenic painful m.

mensuration

mental

m. aberration
m. ability
m. abnormality
m. abuse
m. act
m. activity
m. age (MA)
m. agitation
m. agraphia
m. alertness
m. anesthesia
m. apparatus
m. arousal
m. asthenia
m. asymmetry
m. ataxia
m. audition
m. blind spot
m. block
m. capacity
m. capacity evaluation
m. chemistry
m. chronometry
m. clouding
m. competence
m. competency
m. concept
m. confusion
m. control
m. data
m. defect
m. deficiency
m. deficit
m. depression
m. derangement
m. deterioration
m. development
m. disability
m. discipline
m. disease
m. disorder due to alcoholism
m. disorder due to general medical condition
m. disorganization
m. distress
m. disturbance
m. dynamism
m. eclipse
m. ego
m. energy
m. evolution
m. excitement
m. exercise
m. exhaustion
m. faculty
m. fatigue
m. fog
m. function
m. growth
m. healing
m. health
m. health advocate
M. Health Association (MHA)
m. health care
m. healthcare professional
m. health clinic (MHC)
m. health community
m. health counseling
m. health counselor
m. health court
m. health diagnostic interview schedule
M. Health Early Intervention, Treatment, and Prevention Act of 2000
M. Health Equitable Treatment Act of 2001
m. health expert
m. health information system
m. health law
m. health legislation

M

NOTES

mental *(continued)*
M. Health Parity Act of 1998
m. health practitioner
m. health professional
m. health provider
m. health reform
m. health resource
m. health service
m. health specialist
m. health treatment
m. health treatment facility
m. health worker
m. hospital
m. hygiene
m. hygiene clinic
m. illness
m. image
m. imagery
m. impairment
m. impression
m. inhibition level
m. institution
m. insufficiency
m. life
m. makeup
m. masochism
m. maturity
m. measurement
m. mechanism
m. medicine
m. metabolism
m. model
m. obtundation
m. pain
m. patient organization
m. patient sterilization
m. patient warehousing
m. phenomenon
m. pressure
m. process
m. psychoneurotic disorder
m. retardation (MR)
m. retardation, severity unspecified
m. scotoma
m. sensation
m. set
m. shock
m. skill
m. speed
m. stability
m. state
m. status
m. status assessment
m. status change
m. status examination (MSE)
m. status examination record
m. status examination report (MSER)
m. status schedule (MSS)
m. stress
m. structure
m. subnormality
m. subnormality disorder
m. suffering
m. symptom
m. tension
m. testing
m. topography
m. upset
m. urge
m. workload

mentalis

mentalism

mentalist

mentalistic

mentality
dominant m.

mentally
m. competent
m. defective
m. deficient (MD)
m. deranged
m. disabled
disordered m.
m. disordered offender
m. disordered sex offender (MDSO)
m. handicapped
m. ill
m. ill from war
m. impaired
m. incompetent
m. obtunded
m. retarded
m. retarded child
m. retarded persons' rights

mentation
altered m.
change in m.
normal m.
m. rate
subjective m.

menticide

mentis
abalienatio m.
alienatio m.
compos m.
non compos m.

mentoring program

mentulomania

MEP
motor evoked potential
multimodality evoked potential

meperidine

mephenesin

mephobarbital

mercenary

merciful

merciless
mercurial
m. behavior
m. tremor
mercurialis
erethism m.
mercuric chloride
mercury
elemental m.
m. encephalopathy
m. exposure
mercy killing
mere-exposure effect
merergasia
meretricious
merger state
merit
m. ranking
m. rating
meritocracy
meritorious
Merkel law
merosmia
merycism
MES
maximal electroshock seizure
mescal button
mescalism
mesencephalic reticular formation
mesencephalitis
mesencephalon
mesial
m. prefrontal cortex
m. prefrontal cortical area
mesmeric crisis
mesmerism
mesmerize
mesmeromania
mesoblastic sensibility
mesocortical dopamine pathway
mesolimbic
m. dopamine
m. dopamine pathway
m. selectivity
mesolimbic-mesocortical tract
mesomorph
mesomorphic constitutional type
mesoneuritis
mesontomorph
mesopsychic
message
conflicting m.
covert m.
cryptic m.
dichotic m.
diotic m.
hidden m.
m. integration
mixed m.
overt m.
2-sided m.
subliminal m.
threatening m.
messenger
chemical m.
external chemical m. (ECM)
intracellular second m.
lithium action on first m.
lithium action on second m.
m. RNA
second m.
messiah complex
messianic
messianism
mesylate
meta-analysis
metabolic
m. abnormality
m. acidosis
m. activation
m. activity
m. alkalosis
m. anomaly
m. anoxia
m. asymmetry
m. capability
m. change
m. coma
m. conversion
m. defect
m. derangement
m. difference
m. disease organic psychosis
m. disorder
m. disturbance
m. dysperception
m. effect
m. encephalopathy
m. energy
m. increase
m. mechanism
m. nutritional model
m. process
m. rate
m. response
m. syndrome

M

NOTES

metabolic *(continued)*
m. syndrome X
m. tolerance
m. tremor
m. variability
m. volume depletion
metabolism
abnormal m.
alcohol m.
m. at rest
basal m.
brain glucose m.
caffeine m.
carbohydrate m.
cerebellar m.
cerebral glucose m.
cortical m.
cytochrome P-450 m.
dopamine m.
energy m.
frontal m.
global m.
glucose m.
inborn error of m.
intracellular energy m.
left parietal association m.
mental m.
methadone m.
mineral m.
myelin m.
neuronal m.
parallel pathways of m.
prefrontal m.
psychotropic m.
purine m.
pyrimidine m.
regional brain glucose m.
striatal m.
striatus-orbitofrontal m.
metabolite
active m.
dopamine m.
neurotransmitter m.
metabolizer
ultrarapid m.
metacognitive
m. capacity
m. training
metacommunication
metaethics
metaevaluation
metagenesis
metakinesis
metal
m. intoxication
m. neurotoxin
m. object
metalanguage
metalinguistic
metallic tremor
metamemory
metamorphic paralogia
metamorphopsia
metamorphose
metamorphosis
behavioral m.
m. sexualis paranoica
metamotivation
metaneed
metapathology
metapelet
metaphase
metaphor
religious m.
metaphoric
m. language
m. paralogia
m. symbolism
metaphrenia
metaphysics
metapsyche
metapsychiatry
metapsychic
metapsychological profile
metapsychology
metasyncrisis
metatarsalgia
metatropism
metempirical
metempsychosis
metenkephalin
meter
biofeedback m.
methadone hydrochloride
methamphetamine hydrochloride
methamphetamine-induced hallucination
method
adjustment m.
m. of administration
adoptee family m.
alternative m.
m. analysis
analytic m.
anecdotal m.
approximation m.
aristotelian m.
m. of ascertainment
assessment m.
behavior m.
biofeedback m.
biographical m.
bisensory m.
brain imaging m.
Brasdor m.
case m.
cathartic m.
chewing m.
classification m.

clinical m.
cognitive m.
complete learning m.
concentration m.
confluence m.
m. of constant stimuli
Cooper m.
correlation m.
correlational m.
cross-sectional m.
m. of defining criteria
m. of delivery
diagnostic m.
dose reduction m.
Dubois m.
equal-and-unequal-cases m.
equal-appearing intervals m.
equivalent m.
exosomatic m.
experimental m.
expression m.
m. factor
factor comparison m.
family m.
Flesch-Kincaid m.
formal m.
Freud cathartic m.
genetic m.
gradation m.
Hilton m.
historical m.
imaging m.
impedance m.
impression m.
informal m.
interview m.
introspective m.
job component m.
Jung m.
kinesthetic m.
Leboyer m.
m. of limits
linguistic-kinesic m.
longitudinal m.
mass m.
metric m.
Milligan annihilation m.
minimal change m.
minimum separable m.
Montessori m.
Moore m.
need-press m.
nonpurging m.
numerical cipher m.
observational m.
obstruction m.
operant m.
optimal m.
part-learning m.
Pavlov m.
pedigree m.
plateau m.
preferred m.
proband m.
purging m.
Purmann m.
Q m.
Q-Sort m.
rating m.
recall m.
reconstruction m.
relearning m.
review m.
rhythm m.
Rochester m.
Scarpa m.
scientific m.
m. of self-injury
sibship m.
steady-state m.
suicide m.
swallow-belch m.
synthetic m.
systematic m.
Tadoma m.
Taylor series linearization m.
torture m.
Trager m.
Wardrop m.
Xe clearance m.

methodical chorea
methodologic
methodology
Q m.
methomania
3-methoxy-4-hydroxyphenylglycol (MHPG)
methoxymethylenedioxyamphetamine (MMDA)
methylamphetamine hydrochloride
methylated spirit addiction
methyldopa
methylenedioxyamphetamine (MDA)
methylenedioxymethamphetamine (MDMA)
3,4-methylenedioxymethamphetamine

M

NOTES

Methylin
M. chewable tablet
M. oral solution
methylphenidate-induced change
***N*-methyl-4-phenyl-1,2,3,6,-tetrahydropyridine (MTPT)**
methyprylon
meticulous
metonymic distortion
metonymy
metopoplasty
Metrazol
metric method
metromania
metronoscope
mettle
mettlesome
Mexiletine
Meyer
M. theory
M. theory of depression
MF
multifactorial model
MFD
memory for design
MH
marital history
MHA
Mental Health Association
MHC
mental health clinic
MHPG
3-methoxy-4-hydroxyphenylglycol
MIA
missing in action
miasma theory
micrencephalous
micrencephaly, micrencephalia, microencephaly
microarray
microcephalic idiocy
microcephalus
microcephaly
schizencephalic m.
microcheilia
microcosm of words
microdysgenesia
microelectrode technique
microencephaly (*var. of* micrencephaly)
microgeny
microglia
microgliomatosis
microgliosis
micrography
microgyria
microinjection
micromania
micromaniacal delirium
micromelia
microorganism
microphonia
micropsia, micropsy
micropsychophysiology
micropsychosis
micropsychotic
m. dimension
m. episode
microptic
m. delirium
m. hallucination
microsatellite genotyping
microsleep
microsomia
heredofamilial essential m.
microsurgery
microsuture
microtia
micturate
micturition
m. psychogenic disorder
m. syncope
Midas punishment
midazolam
midbrain
m. deafness
m. dysfunction
m. matter
midchildhood
middle
m. adulthood
m. age
m. age pedophilia
m. class
m. frontal sulcus
m. game
m. ground
m. insomnia
play both ends against m.
m. school
m. school adolescent
m. stage in adolescence
middle-aged
middle-class
m.-c. community
m.-c. youth
middleman
midfrontal
midlife
m. crisis
m. transition
midline nucleus
midpontine wakefulness
mid-potency D_2 antagonist
Midtown Manhattan study
midwinter insomnia
mien
mieux
faute de m.

Mifeprex
mifepristone-RU486
Mignon delusion
migraine
abdominal m.
aphasic m.
Bickerstaff m.
classic m.
cluster m.
common m.
familial hemiplegic m.
fulgurating m.
Harris m.
m. headache
hemiplegia m.
late-life m.
ocular m.
ophthalmic m.
ophthalmoplegic m.
paroxysmal m.
m. personality
seasonal m.
tension m.
unilateral m.
vestibular m.
m. with aura (MA)
m. without aura
migraineur
migrainoid
migrainous
m. infarction
m. neuralgia
migrant
migrate
migration
m. adaptation
adjustment following m.
cultural adjustment following m.
m. psychosis
migratory
mild
anxiety reaction, m. (ARM)
m. ataxia
m. delusion
m. depression
m. disability
m. eccentricity in demeanor
m. guilt
m. neurocognitive disorder
m. sleep disturbance
Miles Nervine Nighttime Pain Relief
milestone
developmental m.
m. event
milieu
m. environment
m. extérieur
m. intérieur
religious m.
sociocultural m.
structured m.
therapeutic m.
m. therapy
militant
militaristic
militarize
military
m. chaplain
m. combat
m. forensic psychiatry
m. history
m. neurosis
m. psychology
m. rank
m. sexual assault
militate
militia group
militiaman
milk
m. ejection reflex
heroin mixed with powdered m.
Millard-Gubler syndrome
Milles syndrome
Milligan annihilation method
milling crowd
milnacipran
Milton model
mime
mimesis
mimetic
m. chorea
m. paralysis
m. seizure
mimic
m. convulsion
m. seizure
m. spasm
m. speech
m. tic
mimica
asemia m.
mimicked
mimicry
mimmation

NOTES

M

minatory
mind
m. blindness
m. control
disharmonious state of m.
m.'s eye
group m.
miniature m.
mortal m.
open m.
m. pain
m. power
prelogical m.
m. reader
m. reading
m. set
state of m.
subconscious m.
theory of m.
m. theory
1-track m.
wandering m.
mind-altering
m.-a. drug
m.-a. substance
mind-bending
mind-blowing
mind-body
m.-b. dualism
m.-b. problem
mind-boggling
minded
absent m.
mindedness
psychological m.
mind-expanding
mindful
mindfulness
m. meditation
m. skill
mindfulness-based stress reduction
mindless
mindset
mineral metabolism
miner's cramp
mingy
miniature
m. mind
m. system
minimal
m. audible field (MAF)
m. audible pressure
m. brain damage
m. brain dysfunction (MBD)
m. change method
m. cue
m. personal hygiene
m. provocation
m. residual symptom
m. risk
m. spontaneous speech
minimalist
minimization of emotional detail
minimize responsibility
minimizing stimulation
minimum
m. dose
m. duration
m. effective concentration (MEC)
m. maintenance
m. separable method
minimum-change therapy
minimum-intensity projection
minimum-security prisoner
minion
mini-psychotic episode
minister
ministry
minor
m. analysis
m. asylum seeker
chorea m.
m. depressive disorder
emancipated m.
m. epilepsy
m. forgetfulness
m. form
m. hypnosis
m. hysteria
m. image-distorting level
m. penalty
m. stimulus
m. tranquilizer
m. weight loss
minority
m. community
m. discrimination
ethnic m.
m. group
m. group psychiatry
racial m.
underrepresented m.
minute
m. memory
m. object
7-minute screen
miosis
paralytic m.
spastic m.
miracle
miraculous
mirage
mirror
m. checking
m. drawing
m. exercise
m. fear
m. focus

m. image
m. movement
m. reading
m. sign
m. speech
m. technique
m. transference
1-way m.
m. writing

mirroring
crossover m.
m. transference

mirror-writing

mirth

mirthful memory

miryachit, myriachit

misaction

misalignment

misalliance

misandry

misanthropy, misanthropia

misapplication

misattribution of guilt

misbehave

misbehaving child

misbehavior
sexual m.

misbelief

miscalculate

miscarriage

miscast

miscegenation

mischance

mischief
malicious m.

mischievous behavior

misclassify

miscode

miscommunication

misconception
illusionary m.

misconduct
sexual m.

misconstrue

miscreant

misdemeanor
m. assault
m. conviction

misdiagnose

misdiagnosis

misdirection phenomenon

miser

miserable

miserliness

miserly

miserotia

misery
emotional m.

misfit

misfortune

misgiving

mishandle

mishap

misidentification
delusion of m.

misinformation effect

misinterpret

misjudge

mislead

mismatch

misnomer

misocainia

misogamy

misogynist

misogynistic

misogyny

misology, misologia

misoneism

misopedia, misopedy

misophonia

misperception
sleep state m.

misplace

misplaced hope

misprision

mispronounce

misquote

misrepresent

missed
m. abortion
m. diagnosis
m. dose
m. school

missexual

missile

missing in action (MIA)

mistake
basic m.
category m.
fatal m.

mistreat

mistreatment
history of m.

mistress

NOTES

M

mistrust
basic m.
trust vs m.
mistrustful attitude
misty-eyed
misuse
alcohol m.
diuretic m.
laxative m.
Mitchell treatment
mitgehen
mitigate
mitigated echolalia
mitis
catatonia m.
dementia paranoides m.
epilepsia m.
mitissima
mitochondrial
mitochondrion, pl. **mitochondria**
Mitofsky-Waksberg random digit dialing procedure
mitogen-activated protein kinase
mitosis, migration, and maturation
Mitran
mitten pattern
mix
case m.
mixed
m. anxiety depression disorder (MADD)
m. aphasia
m. bag
m. bipolar affective psychosis
bipolar I disorder, most recent episode m.
m. bipolar state
bipolar type, m.
m. cerebral dominance
m. chancre
m. compulsive states psychasthenia
m. dementia
m. design
m. developmental delay disorder
m. disturbance stress reaction
m. drink
m. feature
m. heritage
m. laterality
m. mania episode
m. manic-depressive psychosis
m. marriage
m. message
m. model
m. mood disorder
m. mood episode
m. mood state
m. motive game
m. neurosis
m. paralysis
m. paralytic conversion reaction
m. personality disorder
m. presentation
m. psychoneurosis
m. psychoneurotic disorder
m. psychopathic personality
m. race
m. receptive-expressive language
m. receptive-expressive language disorder
m. reinforcement
m. schizophrenia
m. schizophrenic-affective psychosis
m. specific developmental disorder
m. substance abuse
m. type
m. up
mixed-foot dominant
mixed-sex group composition
mixed-type
m.-t. delusion
m.-t. delusional disorder
m.-t. epilepsy
m.-t. psychopathic personality
m.-t. schizophrenia
mixoscopia bestialis
mixoscopy
mixture
m. approach
color m.
m. theory
MMDA
methoxymethylenedioxyamphetamine
MMECT
multimonitored electroconvulsive treatment
9-mm handgun
MMT
methadone maintenance treatment
MMUS
multiple medically unexplained symptoms
M'Naghten rule
mneme
phylogenetic m.
mnemic, mnemenic
m. hypothesis
m. theory
mnemism theory
mnemonic
m. strategy
m. system
m. trace
MO
modus operandi
MOAS
modified overt aggression scale

MOAS frequency
MOAS severity

mob
m. behavior
m. psychology

mobile
m. crisis outreach team
m. spasm
upwardly m.

mobility
m. disability
geographic m.
horizontal m.
m. of libido
tongue m.
upward m.
vertical m.

mobilization reaction

mobilize

mobocracy

mock

mockery

modafinil

modal dose

modality
main treatment m.
sensory m.
suboptimal treatment m.
tactile sensory m.
therapeutic m.
treatment m.
visual sensory m.

modality-specific

mode
Actigraph zero-crossing m.
enactive m.
field-cognition m.
m. of inheritance
parataxic m.
prototaxic m.
quiet wakefulness m.
syntaxic m.

model
active-passive m.
adversary m.
affective schematic mental m.
affect-related schematic mental m.
affect trauma m.
awareness training m.
behavioral m.
biomedical m.
biopsychosocial m.
Blos developmental m.
Bowen m.
Bowlby developmental m.
brain m.
categorical m.
cognitive m.
contingency m.
cost-reward m.
developmental-vulnerability m.
dimensional m.
dual-arousal m.
ecological system m.
educational-socialization m.
ego m.
Erickson developmental m.
executive function m.
Eysenck m.
fixed m.
friendship m.
m. game
Gesell developmental m.
guidance-cooperation m.
helping m.
homeostatic m.
human potential m.
m. of illness
internal m.
kinetic m.
Kohlberg developmental m.
laboratory method m.
language processing m.
learning m.
Mayberg limbic-cortical dysregulation m.
McCullough-Pitts m.
medical m.
mental m.
metabolic nutritional m.
Milton m.
mixed m.
multifactorial m. (MF)
multimodal treatment m.
multiple-regression m.
Munich cooperative m.
mutual participation m.
nicotine dependency m.
nonaffective schematic mental m.
parent-child m.
m. penal code
m. of personality
PLISSIT m.
psychodynamic-experiential m.
psychological m.
m. psychosis

NOTES

model *(continued)*
public health m.
random m.
role m.
schematic mental m.
single major locus m.
SML m.
social integration-disintegration m.
socially intimate m.
standard kinetic m.
stress-diathesis m.
subcortical dysfunction m.
teacher-student m.
treatment m.
vulnerable populations conceptual m. (VPCM)
modeled behavior
modeling
abstract m.
behavioral m.
covert m.
m. exercise
kinetic m.
multilevel m.
participant m.
moderate
m. ataxia
m. difficulty
m. mental retardation
m. mental subnormality
m. to severe depression
moderator variable
modern
m. psychiatry
m. Western medicine
modernize
modest
modesty
modification
active m.
behavior m.
body m.
carbonyl m.
dietary m.
environment m.
environmental m.
hebbian m.
interference m.
lifestyle m.
mood m.
posttranslational m.
modified
m. Bonferroni adjustment
m. ECT therapy
m. overt aggression scale (MOAS)
m. Stroop effect
modularity
imaging m.
modulated affect
modulating
modulation
affect m.
amplitude m. (AM)
dopaminergic m.
emotional m.
impaired affect m.
modulator
module
modus operandi (MO)
mogiarthria
mogigraphia
mogilalia
mogiphonia
mogul
moiety
moil
moisture fear
MOJAC
mood, orientation, judgment, affect, content
molar
m. approach
m. behavior
mold
molecular
m. behavior
m. genetic analysis
m. genetics
m. neuropathology
m. psychiatry
molecule
feel-good m.
molest
molestation
child m.
molester
child m.
serial child m.
molilalia
molimen, pl. **molimina**
m. climactericum virile
moll
mollify
molluscum, pl. **mollusca**
Molotov cocktail
mom
deadbeat m.
moment
m. of aggression
m. of epiphany
m. of truth
momentarily
momentary tearfulness
momentous
moment-to-moment mood change
momentum
momism
monandry

monarchical
monastic
monathetosis
Monday morning headache
monde
beau m.
monesthetic
monestrous
money
ability to manage m.
old m.
monism
monistic
monition
monitor
body m.
monitoring
arrestee drug abuse m. (ADAM)
baseline m.
behavioral m.
clinical m.
close clinical m.
distortion of inferential behavioral m.
electronic m.
exaggeration of inferential behavioral m.
inferential behavioral m.
seizure m.
m. technique
therapeutic drug m.
treatment compliance m.
monk
monkey
m. love
m. therapist
monoamine
m. hypothesis
m. neurotransmitter
m. oxidase (MAO)
monochorea
monocular visual loss
monocyclic antidepressant
monoecious
monoecism
monoethylamide
lysergic acid m.
monogamist
monogamous relationship
monogamy
monogynous
monogyny
monoideic somnambulism
monoideism
monolithic adult block
monologue
collective m.
monomania
affective m.
emotional m.
intellectual m.
monomaniac
monomanie
m. du vol
m. érotique
m. incendiare
monomoria
monomyoplegia
mononeuralgia
mononeuritis multiplex
mononoea
mononuclear
monoparesis
monoparesthesia
monophagia, monophagism
monophagic
monophasia
monophasic
monophosphate
adenosine m.
monoplegia masticatoria
monoplegic psychogenic disorder
monopolar depression
monopolization communication pattern
monopolize
monopsychosis
monorecidive chancre
monoscenism
monosexual
monospasm
monosyllabic speech
monosymptom
monosymptomatic
m. circumscription
m. hypochondriacal psychosis
m. hypochondriasis
m. neurosis
monotheism
Moses and m.
monotherapy
antidepressant m.
monotone
m. speech
m. voice
monotonic

NOTES

monotonous
m. emotion
m. speech
m. voice
monotony
monotropic
monoxide
carbon m.
monozygotic twins (MZ)
monster fear
monstrosity
monstrous
Montessori method
month
abstinent days per m.
monumental
mood
abnormal m.
absence of depressed m.
absence of elevated m.
adjustment disorder with angry m.
adjustment disorder with anxious m.
adjustment disorder with mixed anxiety and depressed m.
m. and/or affect (M/A)
anxious m.
m. balance
blunted m.
m. brightening
m. change
m. chart
m. cluster score
m. congruent
consistent m.
m. control system
dark m.
dejected m.
depressed m.
depth of m.
m. deterioration
m. disorder due to general medical condition
m. disorder patient
m. disorder with atypical features
m. disorder with catatonic features
m. disorder with melancholic features
m. disorder with postpartum onset
m. disorder with rapid cycling
m. disorder with seasonal pattern
m. disturbance
duration of m.
dysphoric m.
elated m.
elevated m.
m. elevation
m. elevator
endoreactive m.
m. episode
erratic m.
euphoric m.
euthymic m.
excited m.
expansion m.
expansive m.
m. fluctuation
imperative m.
indicative m.
m. induction
intensity of m.
irritable m.
labile m.
m. lability
m. lifter
lowered m.
manic m.
melancholic m.
m. modification
morbid m.
nondepressed m.
normal range of m.
m., orientation, judgment, affect, content (MOJAC)
persistently expansive m.
m. profile
prominent irritable m.
public health m.
pure m.
quality of m.
m. reactivity
m. regulation
m. regulator
m. responsivity
rhythmic m.
sad m.
self-reported m.
m. shift
shift in m.
somber m.
m. spectrum disorder
m. stabilization
m. stabilizer
m. stabilizing agent
m. state
subjunctive m.
m. swing
m. swing affective psychosis
m. swing syndrome
m. symptom
m. symptomatology
unpleasant m.
unstable m.
usual m.
vascular dementia with depressed m.
mood-altering
m.-a. chemical

m.-a. drug
m.-a. substance
mood-congruent
m.-c. delusion
m.-c. hallucination
m.-c. psychosis
m.-c. psychotic feature
m.-c. theme
mood-cyclic disorder
mood-elevating drug
mood-incongruent
m.-i. delusion
m.-i. hallucination
m.-i. psychosis
m.-i. psychotic feature
moodiness
developmental m.
mood-stabilizing
m.-s. drug
m.-s. medication
moody
Moonies
mooning
moon phase
moon-phase study
moonshine
moonstruck
Moore
M. method
M. syndrome
moot point
mope
mora
moral
m. action
m. anxiety
m. assessment
m. ataxia
m. attitude
m. behavior
m. code
m. component
m. conduct
m. conflict
m. consistency
m. decision
m. deficiency
m. deficiency personality disorder
m. development
m. dilemma
m. emotion
m. hazard
m. idiocy
m. imbecile
m. independence
m. insanity
m. issue
m. judgment
m. masochism
m. objection
m. oligophrenia
m. outrage
m. philosophy
m. precept
m. pride
m. principle
m. realism
m. relativism
m. right
m. theory
m. thought
m. treatment
m. turpitude
m. value
m. worry
m. wrongdoing
morale
acquired folie m.
folie m.
group m.
moralism
moralist
morality
m. of constraint
m. of conventional role conformity
m. of cooperation
interpersonal m.
m. of self-accepted moral principle
sphincter m.
moralize
morally
morass
moratorium
psychosexual m.
psychosocial m.
morbid
m. anxiety
m. dependence
m. desire
m. doubt
m. fear
m. idea
m. imitation
m. impulse
m. jealousy
m. mood

NOTES

morbid *(continued)*
m. obesity
m. perplexity
m. response
m. risk
m. rumination
m. thirst
morbidity
medical m.
persistent m.
psychiatric m.
psychosocial m.
secondary m.
morbidostatic
mordancy
mordant
MORE
multiple outcomes of raloxifene evaluation
mores
sexual m.
social m.
Morgagni syndrome
morgana
fata m.
mori
memento m.
moria
moribund state
Morita
M. psychotherapy
M. therapy
Mormon religion
morning
m. after
m. bright light therapy
m. cortisol level
m. drinking
m. glory seed dependence
morning-after pill
moron
moronity
morose
morosity
irritable m.
morpheme
circumfix m.
morphine-like action
morphinism
morphinist
morphinistic
morphinization
morphinomania, morphiomania
morphinomaniac
morphogenetic
morphological
m. deformation
m. difference
m. rule
morphologic teratogenicity
morphology
planum temporale m.
morphometric
m. abnormality
m. analysis
m. magnetic resonance imaging
m. technique
morphometry
deformation-based m.
morphosynthesis
morsicatio
m. buccarum
m. labiorum
mortal
m. mind
m. sin
mortality
actual m.
drug-associated m.
increased m.
infant m.
prediction of m.
m. rate
reproductive m.
m. risk
risk factor for m.
m. trend
mortally
mort douce
mortification
mortify
mortis
in articulo m.
meditatio m.
mortisemblant
MOS
Medical Outcomes Study
mosaicism
Moses and monotheism
mosque
MOSS
mediators of social support
mother-child
m.-c. attachment
m.-c. bond
m.-c. dyad
m.-c. experience
m.-c. relationship (MCR)
mother-daughter incest
mother-infant
m.-i. attachment
m.-i. bonding
m.-i. interaction
m.-i. proximity
m.-i. relationship
mothering
good-enough m.
multiple m.

motherly
mother-son incest
Mother Superior complex
motile
motility
m. disorder
extraocular m.
m. psychosis
motion
m. agnosia
brownian m.
m. fear
involuntary m.
m. perception
phenomenal m.
m. picture violence
set in m.
m. sickness
voluntary m.
motivate
motivated
m. error
m. forgetting
independently m.
sexually m.
motivating operation
motivation
achievement m.
adult m.
m. analysis
m. analysis testing
characteristic pattern of m.
childhood m.
competence m.
competing theories of m.
m. for cross-dressing
decreased m.
deficiency m.
m. deterioration
expressed m.
external incentive m.
extrinsic m.
m. factor
m. impairment
incentive m.
intrinsic m.
lack of m.
loss of m.
maladaptive pattern of m.
personal m.
positive m.
primary m.
prosocial m.
psychological m.
reduced m.
m. research
secondary m.
m. for self-injury
sexual m.
suicide m.
true m.
unconscious m.
work m.
motivational
m. enhancement approach
m. enhancement therapy
m. factor
m. hierarchy
m. process
m. selectivity
motive
abundant m.'s
m. achievement
achievement m.
aroused m.
autonomy of m.'s
competitive m.'s
conflicting m.'s
cooperative m.'s
deficiency m.
hierarchy of m.'s
hostile m.
individualistic m.
inviolacy m.
m. mastery
mastery m.
personal social m.
physiologic m.
safety m.
ulterior m.
m. for violent act
motley
motor
m. ability
m. abreaction
m. activity
m. agraphia
m. alexia
m. amusia
m. aphasia
m. apraxia
m. area
m. ataxia
m. aura
m. behavior
m. clumsiness

M

NOTES

motor *(continued)*
m. compliance
m. control of ego
m. conversion symptom
m. coordination
m. cortex
m. cortical center
m. dapsone neuropathy
m. deficit
m. depressant
m. development
m. disability
m. disinhibition
m. evoked potential (MEP)
fine m.
m. function
m. habit
m. image
m. immobility
m. impairment
m. inertia
m. inhibition
m. innervation
m. interface
m. loss
m. maturity
m. movement
m. nerve
m. nerve conduction
m. neurosis
m. passivity
m. performance
m. perseveration
m. persistence
m. phenomenon
m. planning
m. point
m. psychogenic disorder
m. psychosis
m. region
m. response
m. restlessness
m. retardation
m. routine
m. sign
m. skill
m. skill disturbance
m. skills disorder
m. slowing
m. speed
m. system
m. tension
m. theory of thought
m. threshold
m. tic
m. tic disorder
m. vocalization
m. zone

motoric
m. abnormality
m. hyperactivity
m. immobility
m. reproduction process
m. restlessness

motorium

motor-verbal
m.-v. tic
m.-v. tic disorder

motor-vocal tic disorder

moulage

mount

mourn

mourning
guided m.
m. work

mouse fear

mouth
m. blemish
downturned corners of the m.
dry m.
poor m.
twisted m.

mouthing
object m.

mouthy

movable, moveable

move
knight m.
opening m.

movement
abnormal eye m.
abnormal involuntary m.
m. abnormality
active m.
adventitious m.
alpha m.
anomalous m.
arcuate m.
associated m.
automatic m.
ballistic m.
beta m.
bodily m.
body m.
brownian m.
cardinal ocular m.
choreic m.
choreiform m.
clonic m.
compensatory m.
complex whole body m.
constraint of m.
decomposition of m.
discordance of m.
m. disorder
m. disorder effect
dyskinetic m.

dysmetric hand m.
dyspraxic m.
dysrhythmic m.
dystonic m.
encounter m.
episodic body m.
epsilon m.
exaggerated m.
expressive m.
extraneous m.
eye m.
false perception of m.
fetal m.
fine motor m.
flapping m.
following m.
forced m.
freezing of m.
Frenkel m.
functional m.
gamma m.
halting m.
handwringing m.
hemiballismic m.
human potential m.
m. illusion
intentional stereotyped m.
involuntary motor m.
irregular m.
jerking m.
limitation of m. (LOM)
loss of m. (LOM)
low-complexity m.
Magnan trombone m.
mass m.
medication-induced m.
mirror m.
motor m.
myoclonic m.
neurobiotactic m.
nonproductive m.
nonrapid eye m. (non-REM, NREM)
nonrhythmic stereotyped motor m.
passive m.
paucity of m.
perseverative m.
picking m.
poverty of m.
purposeful m.
purposeless m.
purposive m.
quasi-purposive m.
random m.
rapid alternating m.'s (RAM)
rapid eye m. (REM)
rapid fine m.
rapid motor m.
rapid repetitive m.
recurrent motor m.
reflex m.
reflexive m.
repetitive imitative m.
rhythmic slow eye m.
rotatory jaw m.
roving eye m.
roving ocular m.
saccadic eye m.
sleep m.
smooth pursuit eye m. (SPEM)
spontaneous m.
stereotyped body m.
stereotyped motor m.
stereotypic motor m.
sudden motor m.
m. symptom
synkinetic motor m.
m. therapist
m. therapy
tonic-clonic m.
tremulous m.
unusual hand m.
vermicular m.
vestibular m.
visual pursuit m.
volitional m.
voluntary muscle m.
withdrawal m.
women's liberation m.
writhing m.

movie
sexually charged m.

moving object

moxa

moxibustion

Moynahan syndrome

Mozart effect

MPD
multiple-personality disorder

MPS
mucopolysaccharidosis

MQ
memory quotient

MR
mental retardation

NOTES

MRHD
maximum recommended human dose
MRI
magnetic resonance imaging
blood oxygenation level dependent MRI
BOLD MRI
high-resolution MRI
MRI signal hyperintensity
structural MRI
MRI volumetry
MRS
magnetic resonance spectroscopy
MRT
major role therapy
MSE
mental status examination
MSER
mental status examination report
MSIS
multistate information system
MSM
men who have sex with men
MSN
Master of Science in Nursing
MSS
mental status schedule
MST
multisystemic therapy
MSU
memory for symbolic unit
MSW
Master of Social Work
multiple stab wounds
MT
music therapy
MTP
multidisciplinary treatment plan
MTPT
N-methyl-4-phenyl-1,2,3,6,-tetrahydropyridine
MTR
Music Therapist, Registered
mucinosa
alopecia m.
muck
muckrake
mucopolysaccharidosis, pl. **mucopolysaccharidoses (MPS)**
muddle through
muddling
mudslinger
Muenzer-Rosenthal syndrome
muffle
mugged
mugger
mulato
muliebrity
mulish
mull
Müller law
multiaxial
m. classification
m. classification system
m. evaluation
m. fashion
multicomponent
m. behavioral treatment
m. program
multicultural environment
multidetermination
multidimensional
m. assessment
m. assessment of outcome
m. construct
m. family therapy
m. framework
m. health locus and control
m. pain management
m. scale for rating psychiatric patients
multidirectional
multidisciplinary
m. assessment
m. group psychiatry
m. treatment plan (MTP)
multidrug
multifacet circumplex
multifaceted nature
multifactorial
m. etiology
m. event
m. illness
m. inheritance
m. model (MF)
multifamilial
multifamily skills group
multifarious
multifocal thought
multiforme
multiforme-like
multifunctional
multigenerational history
multiimpulsivity syndrome
multiinfarct dementia
multiinfarct psychosis
multiitem index
multilayered
multilevel modeling
multilingual aphasia examination visual naming
multimodal
m. behavior therapy
m. hallucination
m. therapeutic approach
m. treatment model
multimodality evoked potential (MEP)

multimonitored electroconvulsive treatment (MMECT)
multiorgasmic
multiphase
multiple
m. affairs
m. agentry
m. analyses
m. anxiety comorbidities
m. arrests
m. associations
m. baseline designs
m. births
m. cognitive deficits
m. correlations
m. daily medications
m. delusions
m. distinct identities
m. domains of self
m. ego states
m. foci
m. hospitalizations
m. identifications
m. life difficulties
m. losses
m. marriages
m. medically unexplained symptoms (MMUS)
m. mothering
m. neuritides
m. outcomes of raloxifene evaluation (MORE)
m. personalities and gender
m. personality
m. personality crime
m. psychotherapies
m. regressions
m. regression technique
m. reinforcements
m. relationships
m. sclerosis-type organic psychosis
m. sexual partners
m. spontaneous orgasms
m. stab wounds (MSW)
m. surgeries
m. surgical scars
m. target behaviors
m. tics with coprolalia
m. victimizations
multiple-choice
m.-c. assessment
m.-c. testing
multiple-dose regimen
multiple-episode patient
multiple-family therapy
multiple-organ failure
multiple-personality disorder (MPD)
multiple-regression model
multiple-system atrophy
multiple-tracer approach
multiplex
dysostosis m.
mononeuritis m.
myoclonus m.
multiplication of personality
multiplicity
target m.
multipolarity
multisensory
multispeaker phonetic noise
multistate
m. drug distribution ring
m. information system (MSIS)
multisynaptic
multisystemic
m. therapy (MST)
m. therapy approach
multitalented
multitude
multitudinous
multivalence
multivariable
multivariate
m. analysis
m. study
m. technique
multiversity
mum
mumble
mumbling automatism
mumbo jumbo
mummery
mummy attitude
Munchausen
M. disease by proxy
M. by proxy syndrome
M. syndrome by proxy
mundane realism
Munich cooperative model
munificent
mu opiate receptor
murder
lust m.
m. rampage
revenge m.
m. suspect

M

NOTES

murder *(continued)*
m. trial
witness to m.
murderer
mass m.
serial m.
murderess
murky
murmur
brain m.
Murphy's law
muscaria
Amanita m.
muscarine
m. agonist-induced
m. blockade
muscarinic
m. cholinergic receptor
m. receptor blockade
muscle
buccinator m.
m. contraction headache
m. dysmorphia
m. dysmorphism
m. eroticism
m. pleasure
m. psychogenic disorder
m. reflex
m. rigidity
m. spasm
m. strength
m. tension
m. tone
m. twitch
m. twitching
vascular m.
muscle-relaxing effect
musculaire
folie m.
muscular
m. anesthesia
m. body
m. hyperesthesia
m. insufficiency
m. quiver
m. reflex
m. sense
m. tension
muscular-anal stage
muscularis
musculoskeletal psychogenic disorder
musculospiral paralysis
muse
mushroom
magic m.
music
background m.
m. blindness
m. deafness
heavy metal m.
hip-hop m.
loud m.
punk m.
rap m.
spatial m.
M. Therapist, Registered (MTR)
m. therapy (MT)
musical
m. agraphia
m. alexia
m. appreciation impairment
m. stimulus
m. therapy
musician's cramp
musicogenic epilepsy
musicomania, musomania
musicotherapy
Muslim religion
musomania (*var. of* musicomania)
mussitans
delirium m.
mussitation
mustard
nitrogen m.
mutable
mutacism
mutagenicity
mutal consent
mutation
deleterious m.
FMR1 gene m.
gene m.
m. rate
testicular feminization m. (TFM)
mutative interpretation
mute
m. patient
m. state
muted voice
muteness
mutilate
mutilation
female genital m.
genital m.
sadistic m.
mutism
akinetic m.
catatonic m.
elective m.
hysterical m.
relative elective m.
selective m.
traumatic m.
voluntary m.
mutter
muttering delirium
Mutt and Jeff approach

mutual
m. accommodation
m. affective responsiveness
m. aid group
m. grief
m. help services
m. masturbation
m. participation model
m. pretense awareness
m. regard
m. respect
m. trust
mutualism
mutuality
mutually exclusive
myalgia
myasthenia
myasthenic
m. facies
m. reaction
m. syndrome
mycophagy
mycosis
spastic m.
mydriasis
alternating m.
paralytic m.
spasmodic m.
spastic m.
springing m.
mydriatic rigidity
myelapoplexy
myelatelia
myelauxe
myelin metabolism
myeloplegia
myelosyphilis
myobradia
myocardiopathy
alcoholic m.
myocarditis
toxic m.
myocelialgia
myoclonia
fibrillary m.
myoclonic
m. absence
m. astatic epilepsy
m. convulsion
m. movement
m. seizure
myoclonica
dementia m.
dyssynergia cerebellaris m.
myoclonus
m. epilepsy
m. multiplex
nocturnal m.
stimulus-sensitive m.
myodynia
hysterical m.
myodystony
myofascial pain
myogenic paralysis
myoglobin
myoinositol
myokymia
myoneuralgia
postural m.
myoneurasthenia
myoneuroma
myopalmus
myoparalysis
myoparesis
myopathic
m. facies
m. paralysis
myopathy
acute alcoholic m.
alcoholic m.
myopic insight
myorhythmia
myosalgia
myoseism
myotone (*var. of* myotony)
myotonia neonatorum
myotonic facies
myotony, myotone
myriachit (*var. of* miryachit)
mysophilia
mysophobic
mystic
m. paranoia
m. union
mystica
unio m.
mystical
m. experience
m. influence
m. remedy
m. state of consciousness
mysticism
purveyor of m.
mystification

NOTES

M

mystify
mystifying behavior
mystique
mytacism
myth
personal m.
sexual m.
mythical
mythological theme
mythomania
myxedema depression
myxedematous
MZ
monozygotic twins

N
numerical aptitude
N protein
NA, NarcAnon
Narcotics Anonymous
N/A
not applicable
n-Ach
achievement need
nadir
nag
nagger
nail
n. biter
n. biting
n. polish remover
NAIP
National Association of Inpatient Physicians
naiveté
naive wit
nakedness
name
birth n.
family n.
fictitious n.
given n.
maiden n.
name-calling
name-dropping
naming
n. intact
multilingual aphasia examination visual n.
nance
napalm burn
NAPHS
National Association of Psychiatric Health Systems
naphtha
napping phenomenon
narcissism
acquired situational n.
body n.
covert n.
deflated n.
ego n.
hypervigilant n.
malignant n.
primary n.
primitive n.
secondary n.
vulnerable n.
narcissistic
n. character
n. character structure
n. composite
n. diagnosis
n. dynamic
n. ego ideal
n. equilibrium
n. feature
n. illusion
n. injury
n. neurotic personality disorder
n. object choice
n. personality
n. personality disorder (NPD)
n. Q score
n. quality
n. rage
n. self-concept
n. self-peeping
n. tendency
n. transference
n. vulnerability
n. wounding
narcoanalysis
narcoanesthesia
narcocatharsis
narcohypnia
narcohypnosis
narcolepsy
n. experience
non-REM n.
narcolepsy-associated sleep apnea
narcolepsy-cataplexy syndrome
narcoleptic tetrad
narcomania
narcomatous
narcose
narcosis
basal n.
continuous n.
medullary n.
nitrogen n.
narcosomania
narcostimulant
narcosuggestion
narcosynthesis
narcotherapy
narcotic
n. abuse
n. addict
n. addiction
n. agonist drug
n. analgesic
N.'s Anonymous (NA, NarcAnon)
n. antagonist
n. antagonist drug

narcotic *(continued)*
n. blockade
n. chemical intoxication
n. drug dependence
n. habit
n. hunger
n. poisoning
n. withdrawal
narcotic-blocking drug
narcotism
narcotize
narrative
n. account
n. data
n. description
patient illness n.
n. speech
n. speech perception
n. speech perception impairment
n. therapy
narrow
straight and n.
n. therapeutic index
narrow-based gait
narrowed attention span
narrow-minded
nasal inhaler
nasality
assimilated n.
nascentium
national
N. Association of Inpatient Physicians (NAIP)
N. Association of Psychiatric Health Systems (NAPHS)
N. Association of Social Workers
N. Association of Veterans Affairs Chiefs of Psychiatry (NAVACP)
N. Center for Complementary and Alternative Medicine
N. Center for Health Statistic
N. Center for Injury Prevention and Control
n. character
N. Comorbidity Study (NCS)
N. Council on Sexual Addiction and Compulsivity (NCSAC)
n. death index
N. Depressive and Manic-Depressive Association (NDMDA)
n. epithet
N. Guild of Catholic Psychiatrists (NGCP)
N. Institute of Mental Health (NIMH)
N. Institute of Mental Health-Diagnostic Interval Schedule (NIMH-DIS)
N. Institute of Mental Health-Epidemiologic Catchment Area (NIMH-ECA)
N. Institute of Neurological and Communicative Disorders and Stroke
N. Institute of Neurological Disorders and Stroke-Association Internationale pour la Recherche et l'Enseignement en Neurosciences (NINDS-AIREN)
N. Institute on Drug Abuse (NIDA)
n. longitudinal scale of adolescent health
N. Mental Health Association (NMHA)
N. Mental Illness Screening Project
N. Nuclear Energy Commission
N. Population Register
n. psyche
N. Psychological Association for Psychoanalysis
N. Rehabilitation Association (NRA)
N. Resource Center on Domestic Violence
N. Survey on Drug Use and Health
N. Vietnam Veterans Readjustment Study (NVVRS)
native
N. American
n. language level
nativism
nativist theory
natural
n. disaster
n. emotion
n. environment
n. group
n. herbal extract
n. law
n. selection
n. theology
naturalism
naturalistic
n. design
n. followup study
n. stressor
naturalized citizen
naturalness
nature
adaptive n.
demanding in n.
dilatory n.
heritable n.
human n.
multifaceted n.

negative n.
pathologic n.
pejorative n.
sexual n.
sexually violent n.
n. vs nurture

nature-nurture issue
naturopath
naturopathy
nauseam
ad n.
nauseant
nauseate
nausea and vomiting (N&V)
nauseous
nautomania
NAVACP
National Association of Veterans Affairs Chiefs of Psychiatry
Navy
US N.
naysayer
nazism, naziism
NCP
NeuroCybernetics Prosthesis
NCP programming wand
NCS
National Comorbidity Study
NCSAC
National Council on Sexual Addiction and Compulsivity
ND
nondirective
NDCHealth health information service company
N-desmethylclozapine
NDMDA
National Depressive and Manic-Depressive Association
near-death experience
neatly groomed
nebbish
nebulous
necessary
as n.
n. condition
n. task
necessitate
necessitous
necessity
medical n.
neck
buffalo n.
n. reflex
stiff n.
wry n.
necking
necromancy
necromania
necromimesis
necrophagous
necrophile
necrophilia, necrophilism, necrophily
necrophilous
necrosadism
necrosis
n. negation
neuronal n.
occlusal n.
necrotic cell death
need
achievement n. (n-Ach)
n. for admiration
adolescent educational n.
affective n.
affiliation n.
blithely ignored n.
n. for care
certificate of n.
changing n.'s
clinical n.
cognitive n.
community n.
n. for constant attention
n. to control
diverse n.
emotional n.
esteem n.
excessive n.
exhibitionist n.
existence n.
felt n.
gambling n.
geriatric n.
harm avoidance n.
hierarchy of n.'s
identity n.
inner n.
instinct n.
instrumental n.
love n.
oral n.
personal n.
physiologic n.
primary n.
psychological n.

NOTES

need *(continued)*
n. for punishment
repressed n.
seclusion n.
n. for sleep
special education n.
submerged individual n.
succorance n.
togetherness n.
transcendence n.
unmet dependency n.
n. to vomit
needed
as n. (p.r.n., PRN)
need-fear dilemma
needle
contaminated n.
dirty n.
hypodermic n.
n. sharing
n. stick
n. track
n. user
needle-related HIV risk behavior
needless repetition
need-press method
nefarious
Neftel disease
negate
negation
délire de n.
delirium of n.
delusion of n.
n. delusion
n. of ego
insanity of n.
necrosis n.
negative
n. affect
n. attitude
n. behavior
n. body image
n. change
chromatin n.
n. command
n. conditioning
n. correlation
n. delusion
n. diagnosis
n. emotion
n. emotionality
n. eugenics
n. evaluation
n. expectation
n. factor
false n.
n. feedback
n. feeling
fragile X n.
guaiac n.
n. hero
n. immunosuppressive effect
n. judgment
n. life consequence
n. life event
n. mood induction
n. mood state
n. nature
n. Oedipus complex
n. outcome
n. peer interaction
n. picture-caption pair
n. practice
n. predictive power
n. quality
n. race-related experience
n. reinforcement
n. reinforcer
n. relation
n. relationship
n. response
n. ruler of soul
n. score
n. scotoma
n. self-comparison
n. self-concept
n. self-image
n. symptom
n. symptomatology
n. symptom dimension
n. therapeutic reaction
n. transference
true n.
n. utilitarianism
n. variation
n. voice
n. word
negative-affect alcoholism
negatively
n. bathmotropic
n. correlated region
n. tuned rearing environment
negative-symptom schizophrenia
negativism
active n.
adolescent n.
catatonic n.
command n.
extreme n.
sexual n.
toddler n.
negativistic
n. behavior
n. bias
n. personality disorder
n. response
negativity
endogenous n.

neglect
adult survivor of n.
child n.
n. of child
n. of duty
elder adult n.
emotional n.
family n.
hemispatial arousal n.
history of n.
maternal n.
n. measure
organic n.
parent n.
paternal n.
perceived n.
personal n.
problems related to n.
psychosocial n.
sensory n.
spatial n.
subcortical n.
survivor of n.
n. syndrome
unilateral organic n.
unilateral spatial n.
unilateral visual n.
visual n.
neglecta
self-inflicted dermatitis n.
neglected child
neglectful
negligence
contributory n.
gross n.
professional n.
negligent
negligible routine
negotiable
negotiate
negotiating
n. language
n. routine skill
n. rules skill
negotiation
contract n.
problem-solving n.
negrophile
neighborhood stress index
nemesis
NEO
neuroticism, extroversion, openness
neoassociationism
neoatavism
neoconnectionism
neocortex
neocortical
n. association area
n. region
neofreudian
neographism
neography
neo-hippocratic medicine
neo-kraepelian classification
neolalia
neolallism
neolocal family
neologism
neomimism
neomnesis
neomyerian era
neonatal abstinence syndrome
neonaticide
neonatorum
myotonia n.
tetanus n.
neo-Nazi gang member
neophasia
polyglot n.
neophilia, neophilism
neophrenia
neophyte
neoplasia
neoplasm
malignant brain n.
neopsychic
neosleep
neoteny
Neotrofin
nepenthe
nepenthic
nepotism
nerve
accommodation of n.
acoustic n.
auditory n.
autonomic n.
n. cell death
n. cell survival
n. conduction
n. conduction study
n. conduction velocity
cranial n.
n. deafness
efferent n.
facial n.

NOTES

nerve *(continued)*
n. force
n. gas
n. graft
grate on n.'s
gustatory n.
n. loss
motor n.
n. pain
n. root
sensory n.
trigeminal n.
vagus n.
vestibular n.
war of n.'s
nerveless
nerve-point massage
nerve-racking
nervimotility, neurimotility
nervimotion
nervimotor, neurimotor
nervine
nervios
ataque de n.
nervosa
anorexia n. (AN)
bulimia n.
chronic anorexia n.
dysphagia n.
dysphoria n.
International Price Foundation Genetic Study of Bulimia N.
reverse anorexia n.
nervosus
status n.
nervous
n. asthma
n. bladder
n. breakdown
n. chill
n. clucking
n. consumption
n. debility
n. depression
n. disease
n. exhaustion
n. fatigue
n. gastritis
n. giggling
n. impulse
n. indigestion
n. laugh
n. stomach
n. system
n. tension
n. vomiting
nervousness
nervy
nest
empty n.
n. syndrome
network
altered memory n.
artificial neural n.
attention n.
body awareness resource n. (BARN)
communication n.
cortical n.
delusional n.
Drug Abuse Warning N. (DAWN)
family support n.
fragmented social n.
interpersonal n.
kinship n.
neural n.
Practice Research N.
social n.
Stanley Foundation bipolar n.
n. therapy
Neumann syndrome
neural
n. activation
n. darwinism
n. deficit
n. efficiency
n. mechanism
n. network
n. plasticity
n. structure
n. substrate
n. system
neuralgia
atypical n.
epileptiform n.
facial n.
n. facialis vera
Fothergill n.
glossopharyngeal n.
hallucinatory n.
idiopathic n.
intercostal n.
migrainous n.
periodic migrainous n.
reminiscent n.
stump n.
suboccipital n.
supraorbital n.
symptomatic n.
trigeminal n.
neuralgic pain
neuralgiform
neuramebimeter
neuranagenesis
neurapraxia
neurasthenia, neurosthenia
acoustic n.

angiopathic n.
aviator's n.
experimental n.
gastric n.
n. gravis
n. neurotic disorder
n. praecox
primary n.
professional n.
pulsating n.
sexual n.
traumatic n.

neurasthenic
n. helmet
n. neurosis
n. personality
n. psychoneurosis
n. psychoneurosis reaction
n. psychoneurotic reaction

neuremia

neurergic

neurexeresis

neuriatria, neuriatry

neurility

neurimotility (*var. of* nervimotility)

neurimotor (*var. of* nervimotor)

neuritic
n. atrophy
n. plaque

neuriticum
atrophoderma n.

neuritis, pl. **neuritides**
axial n.
central n.
descending n.
Eichhorst n.
endemic n.
interstitial n.
Leyden n.
multiple neuritides
optic n.
parenchymatous n.
peripheral n.
segmental n.
suboccipital n.
toxic n.
traumatic n.

neuroadaptation

neuroallergy

neuroanalysis

neuroanatomic
n. circuit
n. connection

neuroanatomy
behavioral n.

neuroaugmentation

neuroaugmentive

neurobehavioral
n. assessment
n. cognitive status examination
n. consequence
n. feature
n. function
n. readaptation
n. symptom
n. syndrome

neurobiochemistry

neurobiological
n. cause
n. mechanism
n. perspective

neurobiology
behavioral n.
n. of early childhood development

neurobiotactic movement

neuroborreliosis

neurocardiac

neurochemical
n. change
n. disequilibrium
n. interaction
n. pathway
n. research

neurochemistry
behavioral n.

neurocirculatory
n. asthenia
n. psychogenic disorder

neurocladism

neurocognition

neurocognitive
n. alteration
n. deficit
n. disorder
n. impairment
n. index
n. information
n. measure
n. process

neurocristopathy

neurocutaneous syndrome

NeuroCybernetics Prosthesis (NCP)

neurodegeneration

neurodegenerative
n. disease
n. process

NOTES

neurodevelopmental
n. disorder
n. dysfunction
n. pattern
n. telencephalic ontogenic process
neurodynia
neuroendocrine abnormality
neuroethological symptom
neuroethology
neurofeedback training (NT)
neurofibrillary tangle
neurogenic
n. atrophy
n. bladder
n. hypertension
n. hyperventilation
n. reaction
n. shock
n. shock syndrome
neurogenous
neurogram
neurography
neurohormone
neurohumor
neurohumoral
n. hypothesis
n. transmission
neurohypophysis
neuroimaging
n. approach
n. assessment
n. manifestation
structural n.
neuroinduction
neurointerventional
neurokym
neuroleptic
n. adjunct
n. agent
n. anesthesia
conventional n.
n. dosage
n. dose
n. dose-dependent akathisia
n. dosing
n. drug
n. exposure
n. malignant syndrome (NMS)
n. medication
n. responsivity
traditional n.
n. treatment
n. treatment of childhood conduct disorder
typical n.
n. use
neuroleptic-free patient
neuroleptic-induced
n.-i. acute dystonia
n.-i. acute movement disorder
n.-i. akathisia
n.-i. akinesia
n.-i. dysmentia
n.-i. dysphoria
n.-i. postural tremor
n.-i. tardive dyskinesia
neuroleptic-naive patient
neuroleptic-related event
neuroleptic-resistant schizophrenic
neuroleptization
rapid n.
neurolinguistic
n. assessment
n. deficit
n. programming
neurologic, neurological
n. amnesia
n. cognition
n. condition
n. control
n. defect
n. disorder
n. dysfunction
n. evaluation
n. examination
n. functioning
n. illness
n. impairment
n. maturation
n. restitution
neurology
American Board of Forensic Psychiatry and N. (ABFPN)
American Board of Psychiatry and N. (ABPN)
behavioral n.
neurolysis
neuromessenger
neurometric analysis
neuromimesis
neuromodulator
neuromotor
neuromuscular rehabilitation
neuromyasthenia
neuron
A9 n.
ballooned n.
bipolar n.
cholinergic n.
cold-sensitive n.
n. doctrine
excitability of n.
frontal lobe interstitial n.
n. II
impaired migration of brain n.'s
locus ceruleus n.
McCullough-Pitts n.
nonsynaptic n.

noradrenergic n.
pain transmission n.
presynaptic n.
primary afferent n.
projection n.
sensory n.
serotonergic n.
swollen n.
upper motor n.
warm-sensitive n.

neuronal
n. activation
n. activity
n. circuit
n. damage
n. enkephalin
n. loss
n. membrane
n. metabolism
n. necrosis
n. plasticity
n. process
n. size
n. somata

neuronopathy
sensory n.

neuronophage

neuronyxis

neuro-optimized IGE LX System scanner

neuropathic
n. diathesis
n. joint
n. pain

neuropathique
famille n.

neuropathogenesis

neuropathological alteration

neuropathologic examination

neuropathology
Alzheimer disease n.
molecular n.

neuropathy
alcoholic peripheral n.
alcohol-induced peripheral n.
asymmetric motor n.
autonomic n.
buffer n.
familial n.
hypertrophic interstitial n.
lead n.
motor dapsone n.
onion bulb n.
peripheral autonomic n.
segmental n.
symmetric distal n.
vitamin B12 n.

neuropharmacology
functional n.

neurophilic

neurophonia

neurophthalmology

neurophysin

neurophysiological
n. assessment
n. finding
n. heterogeneity
n. study
n. testing

neurophysiology

neuroplegic

neuroprotective

neuropsychiatric
n. condition
n. feature
n. manifestation
n. movement disorder
n. psychiatry

neuropsychiatrist (NP)
American College of N.'s

neuropsychiatry (NP)
geriatric n.
schedule for clinical assessment in n.

neuropsychic

neuropsychologic, neuropsychological
n. area
n. assessment
n. characteristic
n. disorder
n. domain
n. evaluation
n. finding
n. functioning
n. impairment
n. manifestation
n. measure
n. performance
n. resource
n. testing

neuropsychologically relevant task

neuropsychology
clinical n.
cognitive n.

neuropsychopathic

neuropsychopathy

NOTES

neuropsychopharmacology
neuropsychophysiological
neuropsychosis
neuroreceptor imaging
neurorecidive
neurorecurrence
neuroregulator
neurorelapse
neuroscience
behavioral n.
cognitive n.
National Institute of Neurological Disorders and Stroke-Association Internationale pour la Recherche et l'Enseignement en N.'s (NINDS-AIREN)
psychotherapeutic n.
neuroscientist
clinical n.
neurosis, pl. **neuroses**
accident n.
actual n.
acute conditioned n. (ACN)
acute posttraumatic n.
analytic n.
anancastic n.
anxiety n.
artificial n.
association n.
asthenic n.
battle n.
cardiac n.
cardiovascular n.
character n.
chronic posttraumatic n.
climacteric n.
collective n.
combat n.
compensation n.
compulsion n.
compulsive n.
conversion hysteria n.
conversion-type hysterical n.
countertransference n.
craft n.
death n.
decompensative n.
depersonalization n.
depressive n.
dissociative-type hysterical n.
ego n.
environmental n.
esophageal n.
existential n.
expectation n.
experimental n.
family n.
fate n.
fatigue n.
fixation n.
functional n.
generalized anxiety n.
homosexual n.
housewife n.
hypochondriac n.
hypochondriacal n.
hysterical n.
impulse n.
impulsive n.
infinity n.
malignant n.
menopause n.
military n.
mixed n.
monosymptomatic n.
motor n.
neurasthenic n.
noogenic n.
obsessional n.
obsessive-compulsive n.
occlusal n.
occupational n.
oedipal n.
organ n.
organic n.
pain-type anxiety n.
panic-type anxiety n.
pension n.
performance n.
phobic-anxiety-depersonalization n.
phobic obsessional n.
postconcussion n.
posttraumatic n.
prison n.
professional n.
progredient n.
promotion n.
psychasthenic n.
psychoanalytic n.
railroad n.
regression n.
regressive transference n.
retirement n.
senile n.
sexual n.
situation n.
situational posttraumatic n.
success n.
Sunday n.
suppression n.
symptom n.
transference n.
traumatic n.
uprooting n.
vagabond n.
vegetative n.
visceral n.

war n.
weekend n.
neurospasm
neurosteroid
neurosthenia (*var. of* neurasthenia)
neurostimulator
neurosyphilis
asymptomatic n.
cerebral n.
congenital n.
ectodermogenic n.
interstitial n.
meningeal n.
parenchymatous n.
vascular n.
neurosyphilis-associated dementia
neurotension
neurothekeoma
neurotherapeutic, neurotherapy
neurotic
n. acting out
n. anxiety state
n. delinquency
n. depression
n. depressive state
n. direction profile
n. excoriation
n. factor
n. feature
n. guilt
n. hysteric disorder
n. illness
n. manifestation
masculine attitude in female n.
n. mental disorder
passive-aggressive n.
n. personality
n. personality disorder
n. process
n. reaction
n. reaction brain syndrome
n. resignation
n. rumination
n. state with depersonalization
n. style
neurotica
alopecia n.
neurotic-depressive reaction
neuroticism
n., extroversion, openness (NEO)
eysenckian n.
neuroticum
neurotization
neurotize
neurotmesis
neurotogenic
neurotonic
neurotony
neurotoxic
neurotoxicant exposure
neurotoxicant-related
n.-r. ataxia
n.-r. cholinergic crisis
n.-r. encephalopathy
neurotoxin
metal n.
therapeutic botulinum n.
neurotransmission
chemical n.
dopamine n.
dysregulated n.
serotonergic n.
neurotransmitter
n. abnormality
acetylcholine as n.
biogenic amine n.
catecholamine n.
coexistence of n.
excitatory n.
n. metabolite
monoamine n.
peptide n.
putative n.
n. receptor
specific n.
n. synthesizing enzyme
n. system
neurotrauma
neurotripsy
neurotrophasthenia
neurotrophic atrophy
neurotrophy
neurotropic effect
neurotrosis
neurovegetative
n. sign
n. symptom
neutral
n. attitude
n. image
n. material
n. party
socially n.
n. spirit
n. stimulus
n. word

NOTES

neutrality
gender n.
therapeutic gender n.
neutralization rule
neutralized anxiety
neutralizer
neutralizing mechanism
never
n. married
n. smoked
never-medicated patient
nevoid amentia
new
n. age
n. age suicide prevention
n. evidence
N. Hampshire rule
N. Haven study
n. identity
n. normal
n. responsibility
n. treatment
n. wave
N. York longitudinal study (NYLS)
N. York State Psychiatric Institute
newborn
n. abuse
n. drug withdrawal
Newcastle classification
new-generation
n.-g. antipsychotic
n.-g. antipsychotic drug
newly
n. abstinent alcoholic
n. diagnosed
n. emergent categorical change
new-onset
n.-o. mental illness
n.-o. seizure
next
n. friend
n. generation
n. of kin
nexus, pl. **nexus**
NGCP
National Guild of Catholic Psychiatrists
NGI, NGRI
not guilty by reason of insanity
niacin deficiency
Nicaragua
niche
quiet n.
social n.
nickel exposure
nickname
nicotine
n. abstinence
n. abuse
n. addiction
n. administration
n. craving
n. dependence
n. dependency model
n. habit
n. inhalation system
n. inhaler
n. intoxication
n. nasal spray
n. organic brain disorder
n. pharmacology
n. poisoning
n. reinforcement process
n. replacement product
n. replacement therapy
n. transdermal system
n. use
n. use disorder
n. user
n. withdrawal
n. withdrawal symptom
nicotine-induced disorder
nicotine-related disorder, NOS
nicotinic
n. acid deficiency
n. cholinergic receptor
n. receptor blockade
nictation
nictitans
spasmus n.
nictitate
nictitating spasm
nictitation
NIDA
National Institute on Drug Abuse
NIDA-certified forensic toxicology laboratory
Nielsen syndrome
niente
niggling
night
n. eating syndrome
n. fantasy
n. fear
n. hospital
n. pain
n. palsy
n. residue
n. rider
slept all n. (SAN)
n. terror
wedding n.
nightmare
n. disorder
recurrent n.
vivid n.
nightshade
deadly n.
n. poisoning

nighttime
n. activity
n. agitation
n. awakening
nigra
substantia n.
nihilism
n. theme
therapeutic n.
nihilistic delusion
NIMH
National Institute of Mental Health
NIMH-DIS
National Institute of Mental Health-Diagnostic Interval Schedule
NIMH-ECA
National Institute of Mental Health-Epidemiologic Catchment Area
NINDS-AIREN
National Institute of Neurological Disorders and Stroke-Association Internationale pour la Recherche et l'Enseignement en Neurosciences
Ninjitsu
nipping
Niravam
nirvana principle
nisus
nitpick
nitpicking
nitrite
cyclohexyl n.
n. headache
n. inhalant
nitrocellulose
nitrogen
blood urea n. (BUN)
n. mustard
n. narcosis
nitrous oxide dependence
NL
normal libido
NLC&C
normal libido, coitus, and climax
NMHA
National Mental Health Association
NMI
no mental illness
NMS
neuroleptic malignant syndrome
N,N-dimethyltryptamine
NNS
nonspecific neurotic syndrome
NO
nitric oxide
no
no friends
no mental illness (NMI)
no previous history (NPH)
no response
no sense
no trauma personality disorder
noc
nocere
primum non n.
nociassociation
nociceptive
n. impulse
n. nerve pain
nociceptor
nociinfluence
nociperception
noctambulism, noctambulation
noctimania
noctis
jus primae n.
nocturna
enuresis n.
jactatio capitis n.
nocturnal
n. agitation
n. confusion
n. diarrhea
n. drinking syndrome
n. eating syndrome
n. emission
n. epilepsy
n. fragmentation disorder
n. hallucination
n. hemiplegia
n. myoclonus
n. panic
n. panic attack
n. paralysis
n. paroxysmal dystonia
n. penile tumescence (NPT)
n. penile tumescence study
n. restlessness
n. seizure
n. sleep episode
n. sleep-related eating disorder
n. vertigo
nocturnus
jactatio capitis n.
pavor n.
nocuous

NOTES

nodal behavior
nodding
n. off
n. spasm
noematachograph
noematachometer
noematic
noesis
noetic anxiety
no-fault
no-good
noire
bęte n.
noiseless
noisiness
noisome
noisy
noli me tangere
nolo contendere
nomad
nomadic lifestyle
nomadism
nomenclature
psychiatric n.
standard psychiatric n.
nominal aphasia
nominalism
nominalist
nominalization
nomogram
d'Ocagne n.
nomograph
nomological
nomothetic approach
non
n. compos mentis
n. possumus
n. sequitur
sine qua n.
nonability
cognitive n.
nonabrasive
nonacceptable
nonadaptive
nonaddicting
nonadherence
medication n.
nonaffective
n. hallucination
n. psychosis
n. schematic mental model
nonage
nonaggressive objectionable behavior
nonaggressive-type undersocialized conduct disorder
nonalcoholic
nonattentive
nonautistic
nonaxial
n. fashion
n. format
nonbarbiturate
nonbelief
religious n.
nonbeliever
nonbipolar major depression
nonbizarre
n. delusion
n. symptom
noncaloric
noncausal possibility
nonchalance
nonchalant
noncharismatic
noncoherent
noncoital stimulation
noncombatant
noncommissioned officer
noncommittal
noncomparable
noncomplementary role
noncompliance
medication n.
n. with medical treatment
noncompliant behavior
noncomprehension
nonconclusive
nonconcur
nonconflicting
nonconformist
nonconformity, nonconformance
nonconfrontational
n. communication skill
n. interview
nonconfrontive therapy
nonconsanguineous marriage
nonconsenting
n. adult
n. partner
n. patient
noncontrastive distribution
noncontributory
noncontroversial
nonconvulsive status epilepticus
noncooperative
noncued memory pattern
noncustodial parent
nondeclarative memory
nondefense
nondeficit schizophrenia
nondegenerative nonvascular dementia
nondemented
nondependent adult abuse
nondepressed mood
nondescript
nondirective (ND)
n. approach

n. psychotherapy
n. therapy
nondisclosure
nondiscretionary
nondiscriminatory
nondisease
psychogenic cardiac n.
nondistinctive feature
nondominant hand
nondopaminergic
nondrinker
non-drug-using
n.-d.-u. man
n.-d.-u. woman
nonegalitarian
nonentity
nonesuch
nonevent
nonexistence
nonexistent
nonextrapyramidal neurologic sign
nonfatal
nonfattening
nonfearful panic disorder
nonfeasance
nonfluency
nonfluent
n. aphasia
n. aphasic seizure
n. aphasic speech
nonfocal elevation
nonfunctional
nongambling partner
nongeneral
nongeriatric
nonhazardous
nonhemorrhagic cerebral infarction
nonhereditary
nonhero
non-24-hour
n.-24-h. sleep-wake cycle
n.-24-h. sleep-wake syndrome
nonictal
nonidentical
noninvasive
n. brain imaging study
n. operation
noninvolvement
nonjudgmental attitude
nonketotic
nonkraepelinian chronic schizophrenia
nonlanguage cognitive impairment
nonlinear
n. developmental curve
n. distortion
nonlinguistic
nonmajor depression
nonmaleficence
nonmedical
n. management
n. personnel
nonmendelian pattern of inheritance
nonmoral
nonnarcotic analgesic
nonnegative
nonnegotiable
non-neuroleptic-induced tremor
nonneuronal
nonnormative hair loss
nonobjective
no-nonsense
nonopioid
nonorganic
n. origin
n. origin insomnia
psychogenic paranoid psychosis, n.
n. psychosis
n. steep disorder
nonorgasmic
nonorthodox
no-no tremor
nonparametric test of significance
nonparaphilic compulsive sexual behavior
nonparkinsonian tremor
nonparticipant observer
nonparticipatory
nonpartisan
nonpathological
n. amnesia
n. anxiety
n. dissociation
n. reaction
n. sexual fantasy
n. substance use
nonpersistent
nonperson
nonpharmacologically induced tremor
nonphobic anxiety behavior therapy
nonplus
nonplussed
nonpredictive
nonprescription
n. drug

N

NOTES

nonprescription *(continued)*
n. drug abuse
n. drug addiction
nonproband
nonproblematic drinking
nonproductive
n. activity
n. behavior
n. movement
nonpsychotic
n. Alzheimer patient
n. anxiety
n. hallucination
n. mental disorder
n. onset of symptoms
n. posttraumatic brain syndrome
n. psychiatric disorder
n. psychoorganic syndrome
n. signs and symptoms
n. unipolar depression
unspecified mental disorder, n.
nonpsychotropic drug
nonpublic residential treatment center
nonpulsating headache
nonpurging method
nonrandom
n. mating
n. rating
nonrapid eye movement (non-REM, NREM)
nonreactive depression
nonreader
nonrecall
nonrecognition
spatial n.
nonrecurrent
nonreduplicated babbling
nonregressive schizophrenia
non-REM
nonrapid eye movement
non-REM narcolepsy
nonreporting
nonresidency
nonresistant
nonrespondent
nonresponder
nonresponsive state
nonrestorative sleep
nonrestraint
nonrestrictive
nonrhythmic
n. stereotyped motor movement
n. vocalization
nonrigid
nonschizophrenic illness
nonscientific
nonselective phosphodiesterase inhibitor
nonself source
nonsense
n. syndrome
n. in wit
nonsensical
n. speech
n. statement
nonsensuous
nonserotonergic
nonsexist
nonsexual boundary violation
nonshivering thermogenesis
nonsignificant
n. difference
n. protective effect
n. trend
nonsmoker (NS)
nonsocial
nonspeaking
nonspecific
n. abnormality
n. abnormality on EEG
n. arousal
n. benefit
n. binding
n. effect
n. language
n. neurotic factor
n. neurotic syndrome (NNS)
n. research
n. response rate
n. stress
n. syndrome
n. system
nonstandard
nonstarter
nonstress-induced personality disorder
nonsubstance-induced mental disorder
nonsuffocation panicker
nonsuicidal depressed patient
nonsupport
nonsymbolic
nonsynaptic neuron
nonsystematic schizophrenia
nonsystematized delusion
nontherapeutic
non-tic-related obsessive-compulsive disorder
nontoxic substance
nontraditional lifestyle
nontranssexual cross-gender disorder
nontrivial value
nonturning against self (NTS)
nonunique
nonuser
ethanol n.
nonverbal
n. abstractive ability
n. behavior
n. communication

n. cue
n. expression
n. information
n. intellectual capacity
n. language
n. reasoning
n. synthesizing ability
n. task
nonviable
nonviolence
nonviolent
n. behavior
n. crime
n. delinquent
n. stalker
nonvocal communication
noogenic neurosis
nookleptia
noology
noon of life
noopsyche
noose
noothymopsychic ataxia
nootropic
noradrenaline dementia of Alzheimer type
noradrenergic
n. drug
n. effect
n. neuron
n. receptor
n. synapse
n. system
n. system function
norepinephrine
n. hyperactivity
n. neurotransmitter systems
peripheral n.
n. transporter
norepinephrine-selective
norm
age n.
age-appropriate societal n.
cultural n.
culture n.
deviation from physiological n.
grade n.
group n.
occupational n.
percentile n.
physiologic n.
social n.
societal n.
subculture n.
n. violator
normal
n. affect
n. affective processing
n. aging
n. anxiety
n. autistic phase
n. child
n. childhood development
n. circuitry
n. curve
n. distribution
n. grief reaction
n. heat defense
n. individual
n. libido (NL)
n. libido, coitus, and climax (NLC&C)
n. limits
n. mentation
n. neurological functioning
new n.
n. personality
n. range
n. range of mood
n. sadness
n. subject
n. thermogenesis
n. thinking
n. transition
n. valence
n. voluntary napping phenomenon
normalcy
normality
normalization principle
normalize
normalized whole brain volume
normalizing boundary
norm-assertive stance
normative
n. aging process
n. aspect
n. behavior
n. crisis
n. data
n. ethics
n. standard
normative-referenced
normatologically
normatological research
normatology
normethadone

NOTES

normothymatic
normotonic
normotype
norpseudoephedrine
Northern
N. California Psychiatric Society
N. Ireland issue
North Pacific Society of Neurology, Neurosurgery and Psychiatry
NOS
not otherwise specified
NOS category
impulse control disorder NOS
PDD NOS
personality disorder NOS
phencyclidine-related disorder NOS
nose
runny n.
noser
nosey (*var. of* nosy)
nosh
nosocomial
nosogenesis
nosogeny
nosological
nosology
psychiatric n.
nosomania
nosophilia
nosotropic
n. drug
n. drug dementia of Alzheimer type
nostalgia
nostalgic
nostalgist
nostomania
nostrum
nosy, nosey
not
n. applicable (N/A)
n. guilty by reason of insanity (NGI, NGRI)
n. otherwise specified (NOS)
n. prisoner of war (NPOW)
n. significant (NS)
n. supportive
n. turning against self
notable
notably
notanencephalia
notation
note
n. blindness
suicide n.
noteworthy
nothingness
Nothnagel syndrome
noticeable
least n.
notifiable
notion
idealistic n.
notoriety
notorious
noumenal
noumenon
nourish
nourishment
nous
nouveau riche
nouvelle vague
novation
novel
n. antipsychotic
n. antipsychotic drug
n. environment
n. stimulus
n. task performance
novelistic
novelty seeking
novelty-seeking trait
novice
no-win relationship
noxa
noxious
n. agent
n. stimulus
NP
neuropsychiatrist
neuropsychiatry
NPD
narcissistic personality disorder
NPH
no previous history
NPOW
not prisoner of war
NPT
nocturnal penile tumescence
NRA
National Rehabilitation Association
NREM
nonrapid eye movement
NREM sleep
NS
nonsmoker
not significant
Nicotrol NS
NT
neurofeedback training
NTS
nonturning against self
nuance
nubile
nubility
nuchal rigidity

nuclear
n. depression
n. family
n. jaundice
n. problem
n. schizophrenia
n. transsexual
n. transvestite
n. war
nuclei (*pl. of* nucleus)
nucleopetal
nucleotide
nucleus, pl. **nuclei**
anterior n.
n. basalis
cell n.
central tegmental n.
cerebellar n.
dorsal raphe n.
Edinger-Westphal n.
ego n.
hypothalamic n.
lateral geniculate n. (LGN)
midline n.
pontine n. (PN)
pulvinar n.
reticular thalamic n.
n. reuniens
serotonergic raphe n.
spinal trigeminal n.
subthalamic n.
superior salivary n. (SSN)
suprachiasmatic n.
supraoptic n.
nude
nudism
nudist
nudity
public n.
nudomania
nugatory
nuisance
n. behavior
n. complaint
null hypothesis
nullify
numb
emotionally n.
feeling n.
number-recency measure
900-number sex
numbing
emotional n.
psychic n.
n. sensation
sense of n.
n. symptom
numbness
emotional n.
feeling of n.
psychic n.
sleep n.
waking n.
numen
numerical
n. aptitude (N)
n. cipher method
n. reasoning skills
n. score
n. thinking
numerologist
numerology
numinous
nunnation
nuptial
nurse
n. practitioner
psychiatric n.
school n.
n. support group
visiting n.
nurses' aide
nursing
n. home placement
liaison n.
Master of Science in N. (MSN)
nurturant image
nurture
nature vs n.
nurturer
nurturing
n. environment
n. relationship
nut
betel n.
nutans
chorea n.
epilepsia n.
spasmus n.
nutation
nutriceutical
n. data
n. product
nutrient
nutriment
emotional n.

N

NOTES

Nutri/System diet
nutrition
American Institute of N. (AIN)
autotrophic n.
total parenteral n. (TPN)
n. treatment
nutritional
n. adequacy
n. amblyopia
n. amenorrhea
n. change
n. deficiency
n. deficiency disorder
n. edema
n. insult
n. marasmus
n. medicine
n. polyneuropathy
n. status
n. therapy
nutritional-type cerebellar atrophy
nutritionist
nutritious
nutritive
n. enema
n. equilibrium
nutriture
N&V
nausea and vomiting
NVVRS
National Vietnam Veterans Readjustment Study
nyctalgia
nyctalopia
nyctophilia
NYLS
New York longitudinal study
nymph
nymphet
nympholepsy
nymphomania
active n.
platonic n.
nymphomaniac
nymphomaniacal
nystagmus
downbeat n.
horizontal n.
retraction n.
rotary n.
toxic n.
vertical n.
Nytol Quick Caps

OA
object assembly
Overeaters Anonymous
O-A
objective-analytic
OAM
Office of Alternative Medicine
OAP
occupational ability pattern
oath
hippocratic o.
OBD
organic brain disease
organic brain disorder
obdormition
obduracy
obdurate
OBE
out-of-body experience
obedience
automatic o.
deferred o.
destructive o.
obedient behavior
obese
o. adolescent
o. body
o. child
o. patient
obesity
adult-onset o.
alimentary o.
o. care
endocrine o.
endogenous o.
exogenous o.
hyperphagic o.
hypothalamic o.
o. hypoventilation
lifelong o.
o. management
medical complication of o.
morbid o.
psychogenic o.
simple o.
o. treatment
obesogenous
obfuscate
obfuscation
terminological o.
obfuscatory
object
o. addict
o. addiction
agent, action, and o.
aggression toward o.'s
o. agnosia
analytic o.
anxiety o.
o. of arousal
o. assembly (OA)
o. attachment
o. attitude
bad o.
o. blindness
o. cathexis
o. choice
o. concept
o. constancy
o. of delusion
feared o.
fear-provoking o.
fetish o.
o. finding
good o.
o. halo
o. identification
inappropriate handling of o.'s
indirect o.
innocuous o.
kicking o.'s
o. lesson
o. libido
linkage o.
o. loss
love o.
luminescence of o.
metal o.
minute o.
o. mouthing
moving o.
paraphiliac o.
part o.
o. perception
o. permanence
physical aggression against o.'s
pointed o.
primary transitional o.
o. relation
o. relationship
o. relations theory
religious o.
secondary transitional o.
sex o.
o. shadow
sharp o.
substitute o.
test o.
transitional o.
twirling of o.

O

objectifying attitude
objection
moral o.
objectionable behavior
objectivation
objective
o. anxiety
o. assessment
o. behavior
behavioral o.
o. correlative
o. criticism
o. examination
instructional o.
o. manifestation
o. measure
operational o.
o. orientation
o. pain
performance o.
principal o.
o. psychobiology
o. psychology
o. psychotherapy
o. reality
o. scoring
o. self-awareness
o. sensation
o. severity
o. severity of illness
o. sign
o. sleep parameter
social o.
o. sociogram
o. symptom
o. trauma characteristic
o. type
o. vertigo
objective-analytic (O-A)
objectivism
objectivity
object-love
primary o.-l.
objurgate
obligate
obligation
ethical o.
family o.
o. fear
financial o.
major role o.
patient o.
role o.
therapist o.
obligatory
o. occurrence
o. perception
o. relay station
oblige
obliquely related idea
obliquity
obliterate
obliterative
oblivion
obliviousness to social cues
oblivious to surroundings
oblongata
medulla o.
obloquy
obmutescence
obnoxious
obnubilation
OBS
organic brain syndrome
obscene
o. expression
o. gesture
o. language
o. phone call
o. sexual comment
o. telephone caller
o. wit
obscenity
incessantly reiterated o.'s
obscenity-purity complex
obscurantism
obscure
obscuring fundamental truth
observable disability
observant
scrupulously o.
observation
around-the-clock o.
behavioral o.
careful o.
clinical o.
clinician o.
close o.
o. commitment
continuous o.
covert o.
cross-sectional o.
o. delusion
direct o.
evaluation and o. (E&O)
longitudinal o.
participant o.
o. period
preclinical o.
quantified clinical o.
random o.
receptive-expressive o. (REO)
research o.
serial o.
systematic quantitative o.
o. technique
unselective o.
in vivo o.

observational
- o. learning
- o. learning theory
- o. method

observer
- o. drift
- hidden o.
- nonparticipant o.
- participant o.
- o. position

obsession
- aggressive o.
- alien o.
- contamination o.
- counting o.
- ego-dystonic o.
- erotic o.
- guilt o.
- hand-washing o.
- impulsive o.
- inappropriate quality of o.
- inhibitory o.
- masked o.
- o. psychasthenia
- pure o.
- quality of o.
- religious o.
- revenge o.
- rooted o.
- rotted o.
- sexual o.
- somatic o.
- suicidal o.
- symmetry o.
- o. syndrome

obsessional
- o. anxiety
- o. brooding
- o. character
- o. fascination
- o. fear
- o. feature
- o. idea
- o. impulse
- o. mental image
- o. neurosis
- o. personality
- o. personality disorder
- o. psychoneurosis
- o. psychoneurotic reaction
- o. Q factor
- o. rehearsal
- o. rumination
- o. slowness
- o. state
- o. syndrome
- o. thinking
- o. thought
- o. type

obsessionalism

obsessionality

obsessive
- o. attack
- o. behavior
- o. doubt
- o. fantasy
- o. fear
- o. feeling
- o. feelings of responsibility
- o. impulse
- o. laughter
- o. neurotic style
- o. personality
- o. personality disorder
- o. preoccupation
- o. psychogenic disorder
- o. psychoneurotic reaction
- o. rumination
- o. thought

obsessive-compulsive
- o.-c. behavior
- o.-c. disorder (OCD)
- o.-c. disorder with poor insight type
- o.-c. feature
- o.-c. inventory (OCI)
- o.-c. neurosis
- o.-c. neurotic disorder
- o.-c. personality
- o.-c. personality disorder (OCPD)
- o.-c. psychoneurosis
- o.-c. reaction
- o.-c. symptom

obsessively bitter

obsessiveness

obsessive-ruminative tension state

obsolescence
- role o.

obstacle sense

obstinate progression

obstipation

obstipatio paradoxa

obstreperous

obstruction
- o. box
- o. drive

NOTES

obstruction *(continued)*
o. method
thought o.
visual o.
obstructionism
obstructive
o. sleep apnea
o. sleep apnea-hypopnea syndrome (OSAHS)
o. sleep apnea syndrome (OSAS)
obstruent
obtained finding
obtrude
obtrusive idea
obtundation
mental o.
obtunded
mentally o.
obtundent
obturator
obtuse
obtusion
obvious
o. distress
o. proof
ocaperidone
occasional
o. gambler
o. inversion
o. sexual aversion
occipital
o. association
o. association cortical area
o. cortex
o. cortex tissue
o. lobe
o. metabolic disturbance
o. sulcus
occipitotemporal cortex
occiput
occlusal
o. necrosis
o. neurosis
occlusion
artery o.
occlusive meningitis
occult
o. blood
o. head trauma
occultism
occupancy
D_2 o.
preferential o.
receptor o.
occupation
British Manual of the Classification of O.'s
o. level
sedative o.
stimulating o.
occupational
o. ability
o. ability pattern (OAP)
o. activity
o. adjustment
o. analysis
o. choice
o. cramp
o. crisis
o. deafness
o. delirium
o. disease
o. drinking
o. dysfunction
o. exposure
o. exposure to toxic material
o. family
o. function
o. functioning
o. hazard
o. hierarchy
o. history (OH)
o. impairment
o. inhibition
o. interaction
o. level
o. neurosis
o. neurotic disorder
o. norm
o. problem
o. psychiatry
o. psychogenic disorder
o. psychoneurosis
o. rehabilitation
o. safety regulation
o. skills training
o. spasm
o. stability
o. stress
o. therapist (OT)
o. therapy (OT)
o. tic
o. violence
occupationally effective
occurrence
obligatory o.
OCD
obsessive-compulsive disorder
anterior capsulotomy for treatment of OCD
anterior cingulotomy for treatment of OCD
augmentation agent overactivity in OCD
behavioral avoidance test for OCD
bilateral anterior capsule deep brain stimulation for OCD

caudate nucleus overactivity in OCD
cingulate gyrus overactivity in OCD
OCD improvement
infection-triggered OCD
limbic leucotomy for treatment of OCD
OCD patient
OCD responsiveness
ritual injury in OCD
OCD spectrum disorder
thalamus overactivity in OCD

oceanic feeling
ochlomania
OCI
obsessive-compulsive inventory
ocnophile
O'Connor vs Donaldson
OCPD
obsessive-compulsive personality disorder
ocular
o. apraxia
o. bobbing
o. dominance column
o. flutter
o. migraine
o. migraine headache
o. paralysis
ocularis
angor o.
oculogyric crisis
oculomotor
o. apraxia
o. disturbance
o. response
odaxesmus
odaxetic
ODD
oppositional defiant disorder
odd
o. behavior
o. belief
o. eccentric cluster
o. man out
o. posturing
o.'s ratio (OR)
o. speech
o. word choice
odd-even method reliability coefficient
oddity
odious
odium
odogenesis
odonterism
odontoneuralgia
odontoprisis
odor
body o. (BO)
o. fear
o. of solvent on breath
o. of solvent on clothing
odorant
odoriferous, odorous
odorivection
ODS
Operation Desert Storm
odynometer
odynophagia
odynophonia
Odysseus pact
odyssey
oedipal
o. behavior
o. complex
o. conflict
o. neurosis
o. period
o. phase
o. situation
o. stage
oedipism
Oedipus
O. complex
O. period
OEM
open-end marriage
oenomania
Oenothera biennis
off
o. balance
better o.
carry o.
cooling o.
o. effect
face o.
fall o.
o. glide
o. guard
laugh o.
o. limits
nodding o.
shrug o.
slough o.
snapping o.

O

NOTES

off *(continued)*
throw o.
touch o.
offbeat
offender
adolescent sex o.
convicted sex o.
criminal o.
habitual o.
juvenile o.
mentally disordered o.
mentally disordered sex o. (MDSO)
registered sex o.
repeat sex o.
sex o. (SO)
special sex o.
status o.
Task Force on Sexually Dangerous O.'s
violent o.
offending agent
offense
alcohol o.
alcohol-related o.
capital o.
first o.
sex o.
sexual o.
sexually violent o.
statutory o.
violent o.
offensive chat-room dialogue
office
O. of Alternative Medicine (OAM)
o. hypertension
O. of Juvenile Justice and Delinquency Prevention
O. of National Drug Control Policy
o. seclusion
office-based opioid treatment
officer
juvenile o.
noncommissioned o.
probation o.
officinalis
Melissa o.
officious
offish
off-label indication
off-putting
offscouring
offset
offsetting
off-the-cuff
off-the-record
off-the-wall
off-time
lengthened o.-t. (LOT)
off-track betting
ogle
ogler
ogre
OH
occupational history
OHIO
only handle it once
OHIO rule
Ohm law
OI
orientation inventory
oikiomania
oikiotropic
oikofugic
oikomania
oinomania
ojo
mal de o.
Okinawan
olanzapine-associated DKA
old
o. age
o. guard
o. maid
o. money
old-age
o.-a. dementia
o.-a. imbecility
o.-a. psychiatry
o.-a. therapy
old-fashioned
old-sergeant syndrome
olfactie (*var. of* olfacty)
olfaction
olfactism
olfactory
o. amnesia
o. anesthesia
o. aura
o. eroticism
o. hallucination
o. hyperesthesia
o. hypesthesia
o. pathway
o. perception
o. psychomotor seizure
o. reference syndrome
o. stimulation
olfacty, olfactie
oligergasia
oligodendrite
oligodendroblastoma
oligodendrocyte
oligodendroglioma
oligodipsia
oligodontia
oligomania
oligomenorrhea

oligophrenia
moral o.
phenylpyruvic o.
polydystrophic o.
oligophrenic
oligopsychia
oligoria
oligosthenic
oligothymia
oligothymic
oligotrophia
oligotropy
olivopontocerebellar
ombudsman
OMD
organic mental disorder
omega sign
omego melancholium
omen formation
ominous
omission
o. of duty
o. in wit
omissive
omnipotence
illusion of o.
magic o.
o. of thought
omnipotency
omnipotent infantile sadism
omnipotently
omnipresent dysphoria
omniscience
omniscient
omnisexual
omnisexuality
omophagia
OMS
organic mental syndrome
organic mood syndrome
on
carry on
cast on
on edge
on effect
hang on
set eyes on
set foot on
on the skin
on top of the world
onanism
buccal o.
onanist
once
only handle it o. (OHIO)
oncocytoma
oncogene
Ondine curse
one
day o.
o. day at a time
loss of loved o.
number o.
Oneida community
oneiric, oniric
o. delirium
oneirique
délire o.
oneirism
oneiroanalysis
oneirocritical
oneirodelirium
oneirodynia
o. activa
o. gravis
oneirogenic
oneirogmus
oneirogonorrhea
oneirogonos
oneiroid
o. schizophrenia
o. state
oneirology
oneiromancy
oneironanalysis
oneironosus
oneirophrenia
oneiroscopy
one-on-one supervision
onerous
oneself
burning o.
cutting o.
dangerous to o.
play with o.
will to be o.
one-sided
one-to-one situation
one-upmanship
ongoing
o. cognitive process
o. neuroleptic treatment
oniomania
onion bulb neuropathy
oniric (*var. of* oneiric)

O

NOTES

online
o. counseling
o. education
o. encounter
International Society for Mental Health O. (ISMHO)
o. mental health care
o. pharmacy
o. pornography
o. relationship
o. sexual activity
o. sexual addiction
o. sexual experience
o. sexual fantasy
o. support community
o. support group
o. therapy
only handle it once (OHIO)
only-handle-it-once rule
onology
onomatomania
onomatopoeia
onomatopoiesis
onotoanalysis
onotogenesis
onset
abrupt o.
acute o.
adolescent o.
age at o.
o. of agitation
childhood o.
dementia of Alzheimer type, with early o.
dementia of Alzheimer type, with late o.
initial o.
insidious o.
mood disorder with postpartum o.
schizophrenia with childhood o.
o. of sleep
sleep o.
sudden o.
o. of symptoms
on-task behavior
on-the-job bias
on-the-wagon
ontoanalysis
ontogenesis
ontogenic process
ontogeny
psychic o.
ontological
ontology
onus
onychophagia
onychotillomania
OOB
out of bed
OOC
out of control
oophagia
OP
outpatient
opacity
open
o. awareness
o. discussion
o. group
o. head injury
o. horizon
o. hospital
o. hostility
o. juncture
o. marriage
o. mind
o. place
o. posture
o. quotient
o. seclusion restriction
o. space
o. up
o. ward
open-cue situation
open-door
o.-d. hospital
o.-d. policy
open-ended
o.-e. interview
o.-e. question
o.-e. session
open-end marriage (OEM)
opener
opening
o. move
o. sound
o. statement
open-label trial
openness
o. to experience
neuroticism, extroversion, o. (NEO)
open-ward status
operandi
modus o. (MO)
operant
autoclitic o.
o. behavior
o. behaviorism
o. conditioning
o. learning
o. level
o. method
o. reserve
o. therapy
operation
O. Anaconda
concrete o.
decompression o.

O. Desert Storm (ODS)
dissectible cognitive o.
effector o.
formal o.
logical o.
motivating o.
noninvasive o.
rescue o.
o.'s research (OR)
security o.
sensor o.

operational
o. checklist for psychotic disorders
o. definition
o. evaluation
o. fatigue
o. objective
o. planning
o. research
o. sign
o. thought

operative behavior

opératoire
pensée o.

ophidiomania

ophidiophilia

ophryosis

ophthalmia

ophthalmic migraine

ophthalmoplegic migraine

opiate
o. abstinence
o. abstinence syndrome
o. addict
o. addiction
o. antagonist
o. overdose
o. poisoning
o. poppy
o. receptor
o. withdrawal

opiate-free urine screen

opiate-induced emergency

opinion
formed o.
personal o.
o. poll
second o.

opinionated

opinionnaire

opioid
o. abuse
o. antagonist
o. dependence
endogenous o.
illicit o.
o. intoxication
o. intoxication delirium
kappa o.
legal o.
o. overdose
o. peptide
o. poisoning
o. receptor
o. replacement therapy
o. substitute
o. tolerance
o. use
o. use disorder
o. withdrawal

opioid-dependent
o.-d. mother
o.-d. patient

opioid-induced
o.-i. delirium
o.-i. psychotic disorder
o.-i. sexual dysfunction

opioid-positive urine

opiomania

opiophagism

opiophagorum

opisthoporeia

opisthotonic

opisthotonoid

opium
belladonna and o. (B&O)
Boston o.
cannabis and o.
crude o.
deodorized o.
granulated o.
gum o.
powdered o.
pudding o.

opiumism

opotherapy

Oppenheim syndrome

opportunist

opportunity
educational o.
equal employment o.
gambling o.
sexual o.
social o.
o. for theft

O

NOTES

opposed
diametrically o.
opposite
o. affect state
o. biological sex
o. phase
polar o.
relational o.
o. sex peer
o. sex sexual experience
opposition
o. breathing
passive o.
o. respiration
oppositional
o. attitude
o. behavior
o. defiance
o. defiant disorder (ODD)
o. disorder
o. disorder of adolescence
o. disorder of childhood
o. thinking
oppress
oppression artifact disorder
oppressive
opprobrium
public o.
opsomania
optative
optesthesia
optic
o. agnosia
o. agraphia
o. aphasia
o. apraxia
o. ataxia
o. illusion
o. neuritis
optical
o. alexia
o. illusion
o. projection
Optifast diet
optimal
o. care
o. development
o. diet
o. group size
o. interpersonal distance
o. method
o. relational functioning
o. relationship
o. stimulation principle
o. therapeutic intervention
o. treatment
o. treatment strategy
optimism
excessive o.
oral o.
period of o.
therapeutic o.
optimistic
o. atmosphere
o. expectation
o. relapser
optimize
optimum dose
option
activity, interest, o.'s (AIO)
therapeutic o.
treatment o.
opulent
OR
odds ratio
operations research
oral
o. administration
o. aggression
o. anxiety
o. apraxia
o. behavior
o. biting period
o. character
o. coitus
o. communication
o. contraceptive
o. crisis
o. dependence
o. dose
o. ego
o. eroticism
o. eroticism phase
o. fixation
o. gratification
o. history
o. impulse
o. incorporative phase
o. language
o. language skill
o. need
o. optimism
o. orientation
o. penetration
o. personality
o. pessimism
o. primacy
o. route
o. sadism
o. sensory ability
o. sex
o. stage
o. stage psychosexual development
o. state
o. stereotypy
o. stimulation
o. supplementation
o. triad

oral-aggressive character
oralism
orality
oral-nasal acoustic ratio
oral-passive character
oral-receptive character
oral-sadistic cathexis
oral-sensory stage
orange
Agent O.
O. County Psychiatric Society
Orap
Orbeli effect
orbicularis
sign of o.
tic o.
orbital
o. decompression
o. prefrontal cortex
orbitofrontal
o. activity
o. area
o. cortex
o. pathway
o. region
orbitomedial syndrome
orchidomania
order
birth o.
chronological o.
court o.
o. of extinction
outpatient commitment o.
pecking o.
putting affairs in o.
rank o.
restraining o.
ordering and arranging
orderliness
compulsive o.
organic o.
o. preoccupation
orderly behavior
ordinal position
ordinate
ordure
orectic
Oregon Adolescent Depression Project
orexia
orexigenic
oreximania
Orexin (ORX)
Orexis
organ
auxiliary o.
o. donation
end o.
o. eroticism
executive o.
o. failure-associated dementia
genital o.
o. inferiority
o. inferiority complex
o. jargon
o. libido
o. neurosis
o. pleasure
o. speech
target o.
o. transplantation
organic
o. affective syndrome
o. amnesia
o. amnestic syndrome
o. anxiety
o. anxiety disorder
o. approach
o. brain disease (OBD)
o. brain disorder (OBD)
o. brain dysfunction
o. brain syndrome (OBS)
o. contracture
o. deafness
o. defect
o. delirium
o. delusion
o. delusional disorder
o. dementia
o. dyscontrol
o. epilepsy
o. etiology
o. factor
o. hallucination
o. hallucinosis
o. hallucinosis syndrome
o. headache
o. impairment
o. impotence
o. jargon
o. language
o. mental disorder (OMD)
o. mental syndrome (OMS)
o. mood disorder
o. mood syndrome (OMS)
o. neglect
o. neurosis

O

NOTES

organic *(continued)*
o. orderliness
o. pain
o. persona
o. personality disorder
o. personality syndrome
o. pleasure
o. psychiatric disorder
o. psychiatry
o. psychosis
o. psychosis drug intoxication
o. psychosyndrome
o. psychotic condition
o. psychotic state
o. reaction
o. repression
o. speech
o. therapy
o. variable
o. vertigo
organica
alalia o.
organic-functional dilemma
organicism
organicist
organicity screening
organism
empty o.
organismic
o. causation
o. psychology
o. variable
organization
action o.
borderline personality o.
care o.
cytoarchitectural o.
defense o.
disrupted sleep o.
health maintenance o. (HMO)
hierarchical o.
Inter-American Council of Psychiatric O.'s (IACPO)
Joint Commission on Accreditation of Healthcare O.'s (JCAHO)
Justice in Mental Health O.
libido o.
life o.
memory o.
mental patient o.
peer review o. (PRO)
perceptual o.
personality o.
preferred provider o.
pregenital o.
o. preoccupation
Professional Standards Review O. (PSRO)
psychic o.
religious o.
sleep o.
social welfare o.
spatial o.
temporal o.
topographical o.
trait o.
welfare o.
World Health O. (WHO)
organizational
o. chaos
o. entry
o. plan
o. psychology
o. skills
o. structure
organized
o. activity
o. care psychiatry
o. play
o. religion
organizer
decision-making o.
organizing
o. principle
o. task
organogenesis
organogenic, organogenetic
organoleptic
organophosphate
o. insecticide
o. pesticide
organotherapy
organ-specific symptom
orgasm
coital o.
o. delay
delayed o.
dry o.
o. dysfunction
female o.
inhibited female o.
inhibited male o.
male o.
multiple spontaneous o.'s
paradoxical o.
pharmacogenic o.
premature female o.
premature male o.
o. satisfaction
vaginal o.
orgasmic
o. anhedonia
o. capacity
o. cephalalgia
o. deficiency
o. disorder
o. dysfunction
o. phase

o. phase of sexual response cycle
o. platform
o. problem
o. reconditioning
orgasmus deficiens
orgastic
o. impotence
o. potency
o. release
orgiastic
orgone therapy
orgy
oriental nightmare death syndrome
orientation
academic o. (AO)
autopsychic o.
behavioral research o.
biologic research o.
bisexual o.
cognitive research o.
coronal o.
o. cue
delusion of o.
o. disorder
disturbed o.
double o.
eclectic theoretical o.
ego-dystonic o.
exploitative o.
family system research o.
female system research o.
gender o.
goal o.
hedonistic o.
heterosexual o.
hoarding o.
homosexual o.
ideological o.
illusion of o.
impaired o.
instrumental relativist o.
interpersonal research o.
o. inventory (OI)
judgment of line o. (JLO)
law-and-order o.
loss of o.
objective o.
oral o.
psychodynamic research o.
reality o. (RO)
receptive o.
religious o.
reverse o.
reversed o.
sagittal o.
same-sex o.
o. session
sexual o.
spatial o.
spiritual o.
subjective o.
temporal o.
theoretical o.
transverse o.
whole focus o.
oriented
achievement o.
alert and o.
alert, cooperative, and o. (ACO)
o. in all spheres
awake, alert, and o. (AAO)
past o.
o. to person, place, and time
present o.
reality o. (RO)
o. to time and place
well o.
orienting
o. reflex
o. response
orifice
body o.
o. picking
origin
bleeding of undetermined o. (BUO)
bruising of undetermined o. (BUO)
culture of o.
insomnia due to nonorganic o.
intrapsychic o.
language o.
nonorganic o.
psychodynamic o.
psychogenic o.
tic disorder of organic o.
undetermined o. (UO)
o. of violence
original
o. citizenship
o. incident
o. response
o. trauma
originaria
paranoia o.
ornery
ornithinemia
ornithomania

O

NOTES

orofacial dyskinesia
orofaciodigital syndrome
orogenital
o. activity
o. contact
o. sex
orolingual apraxia
oromotor apraxia syndrome
orphan
diagnostic o.
o. drug
o. train
O. Train Heritage Society
orthergasia
orthobiosis
orthodox
orthogenesis
orthogenetic
orthogenic
orthogonal
o. combination
o. depression factor
orthograde degeneration
orthographic
orthography
orthomolecular psychiatry
orthonasia
orthophrenia
orthopsychiatry
orthostasis
orthostatic
o. hypertension
o. hypotension
orthosympathetic
orthothaniasia
ORX
Orexin
OSAHS
obstructive sleep apnea-hypopnea syndrome
OSAS
obstructive sleep apnea syndrome
oscillating tremor
oscillation
o. of attachment
behavioral o.
rhythmic o.
osmoceptor (*var. of* osmoreceptor)
osmodysphoria
osmolagnia
osmolality
osmoreceptor, osmoceptor
osmotherapy
osphresia
osphresiolagnia
osphresiophilia
osphresis
ossification
ossify
ostentatious
osteoplastic
osteoporosis
posttraumatic o.
senile o.
ostracism
peer o.
ostracize
OT
occupational therapist
occupational therapy
OTC
over the counter
Othello
O. delusion
O. syndrome
other
avoidance of o.'s (AO)
contempt for o.'s
danger to o.'s
dangerous to o.'s
o. directed
fondling o.'s
groping o.'s
harming o.'s
illusion of power over o.'s
o. interpersonal problems
intimidating o.'s
locus of control-powerful o.'s (LOC-PO)
physical aggression against o.'s
relating to o.'s
significant o.
o. specified family circumstance
o. type personality disorder
o. woman
other-directed person
otiose
otohemineurasthenia
otoneurasthenia
Ouija board
oust
out
acting o.
asocial acting o.
o. of bed (OOB)
blacking o.
o. of the blue
o. of bounds
o. of character
chill o.
o. of closet
o. of control (OOC)
dry o.
exacerbation of acting o.
excessive acting o.
falling o.
hang o.
irresponsible acting o.

kick o.
make o.
neurotic acting o.
odd man o.
passive-aggressive acting o.
rub o.
rule o. (R/O)
sexual acting o.
shut o.
sign o.
sit o.
skip o.
social acting o.
o. of sorts
speak o.
spell o.
stand o.
take o.
talk o.
talking it o.
thought o.
throw o.
time o.
o. of touch
o. of touch with reality
tripped o.
violent acting o.
washed o.
o. of wedlock
wipe o.
working o.

outburst
aggressive o.
o. of anger
anger o.
angry o.
behavioral o.
explosive o.
impulsive o.
tearful o.
temper o.
uncharacteristic o.
verbal o.
violent o.

outcast
social o.

outcome
o. assessment
clinical o.
o. domain
o. expectancy
functional o.
geriatric health o.
global o.
health o.
o. of illness
longitudinal investigation of depression o.'s (LIDO)
long-term o.
o. measure
multidimensional assessment of o.
negative o.
Permanency Planning: Service Use and Child O.'s
poor work o.
primary efficacy o.
psychosocial symptom o.
o. study
therapeutic o.
treatment o.
untoward o.
o. variable
vocational o.
well-formed o.

outcome-based therapy

outdoing wit

outer-provider

outframing

outgoing mechanism

outlandish

outlet
creative o.
o. for success

outlier

outlook
pessimistic o.

out-of-body
o.-o.-b. experience (OBE)
o.-o.-b. sensation

out-of-control
o.-o.-c. adolescent
o.-o.-c. behavior

out-of-mind sensation

outpatient (OP)
o. basis
o. care
o. clinic
o. commitment order
o. intervention
o. mental health clinic setting
o. patient population
o. program
o. psychiatric help seeking
o. psychotherapy
o. treatment

outpatient-based psychiatry

NOTES

output
o. disability
energy o.
fluid o.
maximum acoustic o.
reduced verbal o.
sympathetic o.
outrage
moral o.
outrageous
outre
outreach
assertive o.
o. program
o. services
outside
o. activity
o. activity avoidance
o. control
o. density
o. force
o. influence
o. range of normal human experience
o. stimulus
outward
o. expression of anger with impulsive feature
o. focus
ovalis
fenestra o.
over
bind o.
blow o.
o. the counter (OTC)
gloss o.
slough o.
talk o.
throw o.
working o.
overachiever
overact
overactivity
impulsive o.
psychomotor o.
overadequate-inadequate reciprocity
overage
overall
o. cognitive functioning
o. cognitive measure
o. defensive functioning score
o. depressive symptom
o. disability
o. psychopathology
o. risk index
overanxious
o. disorder
o. disorder of adolescence
o. disorder of childhood
o. reaction
overbearance
phallic o.
overbearing
overbreathing
voluntary hysterical o.
overburden
overcharged idea
overcome
overcommit
overcommitment to work
overconcern
overconcrete speech
overconfident
overconscientious personality disorder
overconsciousness
overconsolidation of memories
overcontrolled eating plan
overcorrection
overcrowding
overdependence
social o.
overdependency
overdependent attitude
overdetermination
overdominance
overdominant
overdose
accidental o.
amphetamine o.
barbiturate o.
benzodiazepine o.
down from o.
drug o.
fatal o.
fluoxetine o.
hallucinogenic o.
heroin o.
intentional o.
lethal o.
opiate o.
opioid o.
paregoric o.
sedative o.
stimulant o.
talk down from o.
Overeaters Anonymous (OA)
overeating
over-elaborate speech
overestimation
overexertion
overextension
overflow
o. encopresis
o. incontinence
overgrooming
overidentification
overinclusion

overinclusiveness
overinclusive thinking
overindependence
overindulge
overinvolvement
overlap
DSM disorder o.
symptom o.
overlapping agitation
overlay
emotional o.
psychogenic o.
supratentorial o.
overlearning
overload
attention o.
fluid o.
information o.
sensory o.
stimulus o.
overly stimulating treatment
overmanning
overmedicated
overmedication
overmobilization
overoptimistic
overplay
overpopulation
overpower
overprescribed
overproduction
overprotection
maternal o.
parental o.
o. score
overprotective parent
overreaction
emotional o.
overreactive disorder
overrepresented
o. characteristic
o. experience
overresponse
oversee
oversensitive
oversexed
overshadow
overshadowing
diagnostic o.
oversimplify
oversleeping
oversoul
overspending
overstatement
overstep
overstimulated home life
overstimulation
overstrain
overstress
overt
o. aggressive act
o. agitation
o. behavior
o. behavior consequence of divorce
o. compliance
o. compliance masking covert resistance
o. criticism
o. gesture
o. hallucination
o. homosexuality
o. message
o. physical manifestation
o. rage
o. response
o. self-esteem
o. sensitization
o. sign of anger
o. sign of depression
o. sign of powerlessness
o. sign of shame
o. sign of sorrow
o. weeping
overtalkative
over-the-counter
o.-t.-c. drug abuse
o.-t.-c. drug addiction
o.-t.-c. drug-related disorder
o.-t.-c. medication
overthrow
overtly sexual
overtone
psychic o.
overture
overvaluation of shape
overvalued
o. idea
o. ideation (OVI)
overventilation
overweight
overwhelm
overwhelmed subjectivity
overwhelming
o. anxiety
o. childhood experience
o. depression

O

NOTES

overwhelming *(continued)*
o. fatigue
o. intimate experience
o. stress
overwork fear
overwrought
OVI
overvalued ideation
ovovegetarian diet
ovulation
paracyclic o.
ownership
sense of o.
oxidant
oxidase
monoamine o. (MAO)
platelet monoamine o.
oxidative
oxide
nitric o. (NO)
oxotremorine
oxyaphia
oxyblepsia
oxycephalia
oxycephalic idiot
oxyesthesia
oxygen
o. deficiency
o. deprivation
o. therapy
oxygen-carrying capacity
oxygen-deprived sexual arousal
oxygen-depriving activity
oxygeusia
oxylalia
oxylate
oxyopia
oxyosmia
oxyosphresia
oxypathia
oxypertine
oxyphonia
oxyphresia
ozoline

PA
paranoia
passive-aggressive
physician's assistant
psychoanalysis
psychoanalyst
psychogenic aspermia
psychosocial assessment
PAB
positive attention behavior
pace
change of p.
future p.
pacemaker
cerebral p.
endogenous circadian p.
pachygyria
pachyleptomeningitis
pachymeningitis
hypertrophic cervical p.
pyogenic p.
pacification
Pacific Islander
pacifism
pacifist
pacify
pacing
p. behavior
ceaseless p.
restless p.
6-pack
package testing
pack-per-day smoker
packs per day (PPD)
PACT
program of assertive community treatment
pact
devil's p.
homicide-suicide p.
Odysseus p.
suicide p.
PAD
primary affective disorder
psychoaffective disorder
pad
visuospatial scratch p.
padded
p. cell
p. room
paddled
pagan
paganism
paganize
pagophagia
pain
abdominal p.
anatomic site of p.
atypical p.
p. avoidance
p. behavior
burning p.
central p.
chest p.
chronic p.
p. clinic
p. complaint
p. control
core p.
degree of p.
deliberate infliction of p.
diminished response to p.
p. disorder
p. disorder, chronic
p. and distress score
dream p.
p. dysfunction syndrome (PDS)
ecstatic p.
ejaculatory p.
endogenous p.
p. exacerbation
fleeting p.
functional p.
gate-control theory of p.
genital p.
girdle p.
growing p.
heterotopic p.
p. history
homotopic p.
hunger p.
inescapable p.
p. intensity
p. intensity threshold
intermittent p.
intractable p.
law of referred p.
level of psychological p.
p. management
p. management team
masking p.
masturbatory p.
p. mechanism
mental p.
mind p.
myofascial p.
nerve p.
neuralgic p.
neuropathic p.
night p.

P

pain *(continued)*
nociceptive nerve p.
objective p.
organic p.
pathologic p.
pelvic p.
p. perception
phantom limb p.
physical manifestation of p.
posttraumatic p.
pounding p.
prepsychotic p.
p. presentation
p. principle
psychic p.
psychogenic chest p.
psychogenic pelvic p.
psychogenic penis p.
psychogenic precordial p.
psychogenic testicular p.
psychogenic testis p.
psychogenic uterus p.
psychological p.
psychosocial p.
pulsating p.
p. reaction
recalcitrant p.
p. receptor
referred p.
p. relief
residual p.
response to p.
rest p.
scrotal p.
searing p.
secondary p.
sexual p.
shooting p.
somatoform p.
soul p.
spiritual p.
stabbing p.
p. state
stinging p.
p. stricken
subjective p.
superficial p.
p. symptom
p. symptom grouping
p. tolerance
p., touch and stroke psychiatric syndrome
p. transmission neuron
unendurable psychological p.
unexplained p.
unrelenting p.
vice-like p.
wandering p.

painful
p. affect
p. anesthesia
p. consequence
p. feeling
p. intercourse
p. memory
p. paraplegia
p. point
p. ritual
p. stimulus
p. symptom
p. thought

paining
painkiller
pain-pleasure principle
painstaking
paint
spray p.
p. thinner

painter's encephalopathy
painting
action p.

pain-type
p.-t. anxiety
p.-t. anxiety neurosis

pair
p. bond
p. bonding
coherent negative picture-caption p.
coherent positive picture-caption p.
control picture-caption p.
irrelevant p.
negative picture-caption p.
picture-caption p.
positive picture-caption p.
reference picture-caption p.

paired
p. associates
p. dreams

paired-associates learning
palatoplegia
palaver
paleopsychology
paleosensation
paligraphia
palikinesia, palicinesia
palilalia
palimony
palindrome
palindromia
palindromic encephalopathy
palinesthesia
palingnosticum
palingraphia
palinmnesis
palinopsia
palinphrasia palipraxia
paliopsy

paliphrasia
palipraxia
palinphrasia p.
pallanesthesia
pallesthesia
pallesthetic
palliate
palliative care
pallid
pallidal
p. cell
p. syndrome
pallidectomy
pallidoamygdalotomy
pallidoansotomy
pallidotomy
pallidum
pallidus
globus p.
pallor
palmar reflex
palm-chin reflex
palmesthesia
palmi (*pl. of* palmus)
palmic
palmist
palmistry
palmodic
palmomental reflex
palmus, pl. **palmi**
palpable liver
palpitant
palpitate
palpitation
palsy
craft p.
creeping p.
lead p.
night p.
posticus p.
pressure p.
Saturday night p.
shaking p.
supranuclear gaze p.
trembling p.
wasting p.
palter
paltry
pamoate
pamper
panacea
Panax ginseng
panchreston
pancreatic
pancreatitis
alcoholic p.
pancuronium
PANDAS
pediatric autoimmune neuropsychiatric disorder associated with streptococcal infection
pandemic epidemiology
pandemonium
pander
pandiculation
pandy
panel
continuous p.
personality p.
panendoscopy
panesthesia
panethnic
pang
hunger p.
pangenesis
panglossia
panhandling
panic
p. attack
p. attack during sleep
p. attack neurotic anxiety
p. attack neurotic anxiety state
p. button
p. delirium
p. diathesis
p. disorder (PD)
p. disorder with agoraphobia
p. disorder without agoraphobia
frequency of p.
homosexual p.
nocturnal p.
primordial p.
situational p.
p. spectrum phenomenon
p. symptom
p. symptomatology
panic-agoraphobic spectrum
panic-disordered patient
panic-free state
panicker
nonsuffocation p.
suffocation p.
panicky
feeling p.
p. voice
panic-like symptom

NOTES

panic-related symptom
panic-stricken
panic-type
p.-t. anxiety
p.-t. anxiety neurosis
Panism
Peter P.
panoramic memory
panphobic melancholia
panplegia
panpotency
panpsychism
pansexualism
pantalgia
pantheism
panthera
Amanita p.
panthodic
panting
pantomime
panum phenomenon
PAP
passive-aggressive personality
Papaver somniferum
paper pica
Papez
P. circle
P. circuit
P. theory of emotion
papilla, pl. **papillae**
papillary dilation
papilledema
papilloma
schneiderian-type p.
papillomatosis
paraballism
parablepsia
parabrachial area
parabulia
paracenesthesia
paracentesis
paracentral
p. gray area
p. scotoma
parachromatopsia
parachute reflex
paracinesia (*var. of* parakinesia)
paracinesis (*var. of* parakinesia)
paracusis, paracousis, paracusia
false p.
localis p.
paracyclic ovulation
parademential
paradigm
attention blink p.
biopsychosocial p.
p. clash
cocktail party p.
diathesis stress p.
dichotic listening p.
learning p.
memory p.
physiologic p.
risk p.
p. shift
Sternberg p.
task-switching p.
transference p.
paradigmatic
p. response
p. shift
p. stress from life experience
paradipsia
PAR admissions testing program
paradox
Sherman p.
paradoxa
obstipatio p.
paradoxic
p. hunger
p. sleep
paradoxica
kinesia p.
paradoxical
p. anxiety
p. cold
p. combination
p. communication
p. depression
p. incontinence
p. injunction
p. intention (PI)
p. intervention
p. orgasm
p. pupil
p. pupillary phenomenon
p. reaction
p. response
p. sleep
p. technique
p. therapy
p. undressing
p. warmth
paraequilibrium
paraeroticism, paraerotism
paraesthesia
paraesthetica
pseudomelia p.
parafunction
paragammacism
paragenital
parageusia
parageusic
paragnomen
paragrammatism
paragraphia
parahippocampal white matter
parahypnosis

parahypophysis
parakinesia, paracinesia, paracinesis, parakinesis
paralalia literalis
paralambdacism
paralanguage
paraldehydism
paraleprosis
paralepsy
paralexia
paralgesia
paralgesic
paralgia
paralimbic region
parallax
parallel
- culturally p.
- p. dream
- p. law
- p. pathways of metabolism
- p. play
- p. processing
- p. subsystem

parallelism
- cultural p.
- psychoneural p.
- psychophysical p.

paralogia
- metamorphic p.
- metaphoric p.
- thematic p.
- themomatic p.

paralogism
paralogistic
paralogy
paralysis, pl. **paralyses**
- acute atrophic p.
- alcoholic p.
- ascending p.
- bilateral abductor p.
- bilateral adductor p.
- catatonic cerebral p.
- central p.
- compression p.
- conjugate p.
- conversion p.
- crossed p.
- exhaustion p.
- facial p.
- familial periodic p.
- faucial p.
- flaccid p.
- gaze p.
- general p.
- ginger p.
- global p.
- histrionic p.
- hysterical p.
- immobilization p.
- immunological p.
- p. of insane
- Jamaica ginger p.
- Kussmaul-Landry p.
- labial p.
- Landry p.
- lead p.
- leaden p.
- mimetic p.
- mixed p.
- musculospiral p.
- myogenic p.
- myopathic p.
- nocturnal p.
- ocular p.
- periodic p.
- postdormital sleep p.
- posticus p.
- predormital sleep p.
- pressure p.
- progressive bulbar p.
- pseudohypertrophic muscular p.
- psychogenic p.
- sensory p.
- sleep p.
- sodium-responsive periodic p.
- spinal p.
- supranuclear p.
- unilateral abductor p.
- unilateral adductor p.
- wasting p.
- work p.

paralytic
- p. abasia
- p. dementia
- p. idiocy
- p. miosis
- p. mydriasis
- p. psychosomatic disorder

paralytica
- p. aphonia
- dementia p.
- Lissauer dementia p.

paralyticus
- ictus p.

paralytique
- folie p.

NOTES

P

paralyzant
paralyze
paralyzer
paralyzing
p. agent
p. depression
p. vertigo
paramania
paramedical
parameter
chance response p.
item discrimination p.
objective sleep p.
pharmacokinetic p.
psychiatric p.
treatment intensity p.
paramethoxyamphetamine (PMA)
parametric
p. study
p. test of significance
paramilitary
paramimia
paramnesia
reduplicative p.
paramour
paramusia
paramyoclonus
paramyotonia
congenital p.
symptomatic p.
paramyotonus
paranalgesia
paranesthesia
paranoia (PA)
acquired p.
acute hallucinatory p.
affect-laden p.
alcoholic p.
amorous p.
classical p.
conjugal p.
p. and delusions psychiatric syndrome
p. dementia gravis
dissociative p.
eccentric p.
erotic p.
exalted p.
p. hallucinatoria
hallucinatory p.
heboid p.
hypochondriac p.
hypochondriacal p.
involutional p.
litigious p.
mystic p.
p. originaria
persecutory p.
projectional p.
p. querulans
p. querulans paranoid state
querulous p.
reformatory p.
rudimentary p.
Seglas-type p.
senile p.
p. senilis
p. simplex
paranoiac
p. character
p. psychosis
reformatory p.
paranoica
aphonia p.
aphrasia p.
metamorphosis sexualis p.
paranoid
p. behavior
p. belief system
p. condition
p. delusion
p. delusional belief
p. dementia
p. eroticism
p. fear
p. feature
floridly p.
p. hostility
p. ideation
p. involutional reaction
p. litigious state
p. look
p. melancholia
p. neurotic personality disorder
p. personality
p. psychoneurosis
p. reaction type
p. schizophrenia
p. schizophrenic psychosis
schizophrenic reaction, acute p. (SR/AP)
schizophrenic reaction, chronic p. (SR/CP)
p. tendency
p. thinking
p. trait
p. transient organic psychosis
p. trend
paranoides
amentia p.
dementia p.
paranoidism
paranoid-schizoid position
paranoid-schizotypal personality disorder
paranoid-type
p.-t. alcoholic psychosis
p.-t. arteriosclerotic dementia
p.-t. arteriosclerotic psychosis

p.-t. presenile dementia
p.-t. psycho-organic syndrome
p.-t. schizophrenia
p.-t. schizophrenic disorder
p.-t. senile dementia
p.-t. senile psychosis

paranomasia
paranomia
paranormal
p. capacity
p. cognition
p. phenomenon
paranosic gain
paranosis
paraparesis
paraparetic
parapathetic proviso
parapathy
paraphasia
extended jargon p.
jargon p.
literal p.
thematic p.
verbal p.
paraphasic error
paraphemia
paraphenomenon
paraphernalia
drug p.
homemade drug p.
paraphiliac p.
paraphia, parapsia
paraphilia
atypical p.
exhibitionism p.
fetishism p.
frotteurism p.
pedophilia p.
transvestism p.
voyeurism p.
paraphiliac, paraphilic
p. behavior
p. coercive disorder
p. fantasy
p. focus
p. imagery
p. object
p. paraphernalia
p. pornography
p. preference
p. stimulus
paraphonia
paraphonic state
paraphora
paraphrasia
literal p.
thematic p.
paraphrenia
climacteric p.
p. confabulans
p. expansiva
p. fantastica
involutional p.
late p.
menopausal p.
p. paranoid state
presenile p.
p. systematica
paraphrenic
p. dementia
p. schizophrenia
paraphronia
paraphysial, paraphyseal
parapithymia
paraplectic
paraplegia
alcoholic p.
congenital spastic p.
infantile spastic p.
painful p.
senile p.
superior p.
tetanoid p.
paraplegic
parapoplexy
parapraxia
paraprofessional
parapsia (*var. of* paraphia)
parapsychology
parapsychosis
parareaction
parareflexia
pararhotacism
parasexuality
parasigmatism
parasite of superego
parasitic
p. superego
p. vampirism
parasitosis
cocaine p.
delusion of p.
parasocial speech
parasomnia

NOTES

P

parasomniac
p. consciousness
p. conscious state
parasomnia-type substance-induced sleep disorder
paraspasm
parasuicidal
p. behavior
p. event
p. incident
parasuicide
parasympathetic
p. epilepsy
p. nervous system (PNS)
parasympathicotonia
parasympatholytic
parasympathomimetic drug
parasympathotonia
paratactic distortion
parataxic
p. distortion
p. mode
parataxis, parataxia
parateresiomania
parathormone
parathymia
parathyreopriva
tetania p.
paratonia progressiva
paratrophy
paratypic
paraverbal therapy
parchment crackling
pardonable
parectropia
pareidolia
parencephalia
parencephalous
parenchymatous
p. neuritis
p. neurosyphilis
parens patriae
parent
absent p.
p. abuse
abusive p.
adoptive p.
adulthood and elderly p.
alcoholic p.
p. at risk
authoritarian rejecting-neglecting p.
battered p.
biologic p.
biological p.
p. burnout
childhood loss of p.
children of transsexual p.
controlling p.
critical p.
custodial p.
p. effectiveness training
p. ego state
p.'s, family, and friends of lesbians and gays (PFLAG)
p. fixation
foster p.
p. image
ineffectual p.
p. neglect
noncustodial p.
overprotective p.
permissive p.
p. perplexity
problem p.
raging p.
refrigerator p.
rejecting p.
rejecting-neglecting p.
search for p.
separation from p.
strict p.
substance-abusing p.
p. subsystem
surrogate p.
surviving p.
p. therapist program
ungiving p.
weak p.
weekend p.
P.'s Without Partners (PWP)
parent-adult-child (PAC)
parental
p. abuse
p. aging
p. alcohol consumption
p. alcohol use
p. attitude toward sex
p. behavior
p. care
p. control
p. control problem
p. criticism
p. custody
p. death
p. denial
p. divorce
p. dysfunction
p. education
p. environment
p. environment characteristic
p. environment item
p. failure to guide
p. feeding practice
p. fit
p. indecisiveness
p. indifference
p. loss
p. marital problem

p. overprotection
p. perplexity
p. rejection
p. right doctrine
p. rights
p. separation
p. socioeconomic class
p. spontaneity
p. value

parent-child
p.-c. bond
p.-c. conflict
p.-c. conflict counseling
p.-c. dyad
p.-c. group therapy
p.-c. model
p.-c. rapport
p.-c. relational problem
p.-c. relationship
p.-c. transmission

parenteral
p. alimentation
p. drug
p. drug administration
p. feeding
p. medication

parenthetical expression

parenthood
Planned P.

parent-infant bonding

parenting
p. ability
disrupted p.
erratic p.
foster p.
high-quality p.
inadequate p.
inept p.
irresponsible p.
limit-setting p.
loving p.
positive p.
reciprocal p.
refrigerator p.
p. skill
p. style
unpredictable p.

parentis
in loco p.

parent-offspring bond

parent's
P. Anonymous
p. marital status

parent-to-child aggression (PTCA)

parent-youth
p.-y. concordance
p.-y. dyad

parepithymia

parerethisis

parergasia

paresis
alcoholic p.
facial p.
general p.
infantile p.
juvenile p.
Lissauer-type p.

paresthesia
laryngeal p.

paresthetica
digitalgia p.

paresthetic conversion reaction

paretic
p. curve
p. dementia
p. impotence
p. melancholia
p. psychosis

Parham decision

parietal
p. cortex
p. lobe
p. lobe dysfunction
p. neocortical association area
p. skull bone
temporal, occipital, p. (TOP)
p. tissue

parietooccipital
p. aphasia
p. hypoperfusion

parietotemporal
p. area
p. perfusion deficit

parimutuel betting

parity

Parkinson disease with dementia (PDD)

parlor
massage p.

parmia

parody in wit

parole
p. condition
condition of p.

NOTES

parole *(continued)*
p. status
p. violation case
parolee
paroniria ambulans
paronomasia
parorexia
parosmia
parosphresia
parousiamania
paroxysm
rapid eye blinking p.
paroxysmal
p. activity
p. convulsion
p. drinking
p. dyskinesia
p. dystonia
p. migraine
p. migraine headache
p. phenomenon
p. psychosis
p. seizure
p. sleep
p. trepidant abasia
parricide
parroting words
parrotlike speech pattern
parry
pars, pl. **partes**
p. pro toto
parsimony
part
p. instinct
p. object
part-brain
partes (*pl. of* pars)
partial
p. adjustment
p. agonist
p. aim
p. amnesia
p. complex seizure
p. correlation
p. cross-dressing
p. delirium
p. delusion
p. epilepsy
p. hallucination
p. hospitalization
p. hospital patient population
p. hospital setting
p. insanity
p. instinct
p. nominal aphasia
p. organic psychosyndrome
p. permanent disability
p. recovery
p. regression
p. reinforcement
p. reinforcement effect (PRE)
p. remission
p. sensory seizure
p. substrate
p. tonic seizure
partialis
psychopathia p.
partialism
persistent p.
partiality
partially disabled
participant
p. modeling
p. observation
p. observer
self-help p.
participated in atrocities
participation
group p.
markedly diminished p.
participative management
particular
bill of p.'s
p. complex
p. task
particularism
particularity
particulate
parting of ways
parti pris
partisan
partitive
part-learning method
partner
abused p.
abusive p.
bed p.
p. bond
compulsive fixation on unobtainable p.
p. conflict
consenting p.
distraught former p.
estranged p.
former p.
lifetime sex p.
multiple sexual p.'s
nonconsenting p.
nongambling p.
Parents Without P.'s (PWP)
phallic p.
p. preference
p. relational problem
sex p.
sexual p.
sleeping p.
p. status

surrogate sexual p.
p. swapping
part-object manner
parturition
party
life of p.
neutral p.
rave p.
paruresis
parviculata
alopecia p.
PAS
personality assessment system
pas
faux p.
PASCET
primary and secondary control enhancement training
PASO
primitive aggressive self-organization
pass
leave on p. (LOP)
weekend p.
passage
bird of p.
p. comprehension
memory p.
rite of p.
Passiflora incarnata
passing stranger effect
passion
crime of p.
passionate attitude
passionelle
attitude p.
psychose p.
passive
p. accommodation
p. aggression
p. algolagnia
p. analysis
p. avoidance
p. behavior
p. castration complex
p. dependence
p. euthanasia
p. immunity
p. immunization therapy
p. incontinence
p. influence
p. introversion
p. learning
p. listening
p. mode of consciousness
p. movement
p. object love
p. opposition
p. parasitic psychopathy
p. personality
p. reaction
p. recreation
p. resistance
p. suicidal thought
p. therapist
p. transport
p. tremor
p. vocabulary
passive-aggressive (PA)
p.-a. acting out
p.-a. behavior
p.-a. feature
p.-a. maneuver
p.-a. neurotic
p.-a. neurotic personality
p.-a. neurotic personality disorder
p.-a. personality (PAP)
p.-a. reaction
passive-avoidance learning
passive-dependent
p.-d. personality (PDP)
p.-d. reaction
p.-d. trait
passively phrased question
passive-receptive longing
passivism
passivity
active p.
p. in anger expression
p. delusion
delusional thought p.
delusion of emotional p.
delusion of somatic p.
motor p.
past
p. alcoholism
p. behavior
criminal p.
p. event
p. experience
p. head injury
p. history (PH)
p. lifetime disorder
p. loss
p. month alcohol use
p. oriented
p. personal history

NOTES

P

past *(continued)*
p. suicidal act
p. suicide attempt
p. tic
violent p.
past-life hypnotic regression
pastoral
p. care
p. counseling
p. counselor
p. help
p. psychiatry
past-pointing
patch
Daytrana transdermal p.
nicotine p.
transdermal nicotine p.
patchy amnesia
patent
p. medicinals
p. medicine
p. medicine abuse
paterfamilias
paternal
p. abuse
p. age
p. attitude
p. behavior
p. care
p. childrearing
p. competency
p. deprivation
p. desertion
p. drive
p. indifference
p. neglect
p. rejection
p. relationship
paternalism
paternity
p. blues
proof of p.
pathema
pathematic aphasia
pathemia
pathergasia
pathetic
pathetism
pathic
pathoclisis
pathocure
pathodixia
pathoformic
pathogen
behavioral p.
p. of violence
pathogenesis
biologic p.
pathogenic, pathogenetic
p. care
p. factor
p. family pattern
pathogenicity
pathogeny
pathognomonic, pathognomic
p. fantasy
p. sign
pathognomy
pathognostic
pathography
psychoanalytic p.
pathohysteria
pathokinesis
patholesia
pathologic, pathological
p. alcoholic intoxication psychosis
p. alcohol intoxication
p. amenorrhea
p. behavior
p. care
p. change
p. character formation
p. communication
p. condition
p. crying
p. defense mechanism
p. diagnosis
p. dissociation
p. drowsiness
p. drug intoxication
p. drug intoxication psychosis
p. drunkenness
p. emotionality
p. fallacy
p. feature
p. finding
p. gambler
p. gambling (PG)
p. gambling disorder (PGD)
p. grief reaction
p. grieving
p. grooming disorder
p. guilt
p. homophobia
p. Internet use
p. intoxication
p. laughter
p. level
p. liar
p. lying
p. mendicancy
p. mood state
p. nature
p. pain
p. personality
p. preoccupation
p. process

p. reaction to alcohol
p. reflex
p. response
p. sexual fantasy
p. sexuality
p. skin picking
p. sleepiness
p. study
p. substance use
p. swindler
p. trait

pathology
association deficit p.
aural p.
borderline p.
brain p.
character p.
cognitive p.
cortical p.
deep white matter p.
focal p.
forensic p.
functional p.
interpersonal p.
ischemic p.
language p.
personality p.
psychosocial p.
structural p.
subcortical p.
white matter p.

pathology-induced memory reconstruction
pathomania
pathomimesis
pathomimia
pathomimicry
pathomiosis
pathomorphism
pathoneurosis
pathophilia
pathophrenesis
pathophysiologic, pathophysiological
p. basis
p. cascade
p. link
p. mechanism
p. pattern
p. process
p. role

pathophysiology
pathopsychology
pathopsychosis
pathos
pathosis
attitudinal p.

pathway
anterior cingulate p.
auditory p.
basic brain p.
biochemical p.
brain dopaminergic p.
cerebellar p.
dopamine p.
dopaminergic p.
dorsolateral p.
heat-loss p.
indirect striatopallidal p.
mesocortical dopamine p.
mesolimbic dopamine p.
neurochemical p.
olfactory p.
orbitofrontal p.
pilomotor p.
psychobiological p.
retrosplenial cingulate p.
serotonergic p.
spinoreticulothalamic p.
p. stimulation
ventral amygdala fugal p.
visceromotor p.

patience
lack of p.

patient (pt)
p. abuse
acutely psychotic schizophrenic p.
p. advocate
agitated p.
akinetic p.
alcohol-dependent p.
American Academy on Physician and P. (AAPP)
amnesic p.
analytic p.
antisocial p.
aphasic p.
at-risk p.
p. authentication
p. autonomy
bipolar p.
borderline p.
catatonic p.
chronically depressed p.
clinic p.
comatose p.
combative p.

NOTES

P

patient *(continued)*
community-residing p.
p. compliance
p. confession
consenting p.
p. contract
criminal justice p.
dangerous p.
p. data bank
p. delay
delirious p.
demented p.
dementia p.
depressed p.
disheveled p.
disoriented p.
p. disquietude
disruptive psychotic p.
dissociative p.
drug-free p.
dual diagnosis p.
dysphoric p.
p. education
elderly depressed p.
p. and family services (PFS)
female p.
p. file
first-episode p.
frail elderly p.
full-dose-treated p.
geriatric p.
p. guide to medication
hallucinating p.
healthy p.
p. hesitancy
high-functioning p.
high-profile p.
high-risk p.
histrionic p.
homeless p.
hypnotic p.
hypnotic-dependent p.
p. illness narrative
incarcerated p.
incoherent p.
insured p.
p. interview
lethargic p.
p. literacy
male p.
manic p.
medicated p.
mood disorder p.
multidimensional scale for rating psychiatric p.'s
multiple-episode p.
mute p.
neuroleptic-free p.
neuroleptic-naive p.
never-medicated p.
nonconsenting p.
nonpsychotic Alzheimer p.
nonsuicidal depressed p.
obese p.
p. obligation
OCD p.
opioid-dependent p.
panic-disordered p.
peregrinating problem p.
person in p.
p. placement criterion
posttraumatic p.
potentially dangerous p.
problem p.
psychiatric p.
psychotic Alzheimer p.
rapid metabolizer p.
p. resistance
p. responsibility
p. rights
sadistic p.
p. safety
p. satisfaction
schizophrenic p.
schizophreniform p.
schizotypal p.
self-destructive p.
slow metabolizer p.
stuporous p.
suicidal depressed p.
symptomatic p.
target p.
traumatized elderly p.
treatment-intolerant p.
treatment-refractory p.
uncooperative p.
uninsured p.
unipolar p.
unmedicated p.
unresponsive p.
violent pediatric p.
young-old p.

patient-care audit

patient-centered
p.-c. approach
p.-c. services

patient-controlled analgesia (PCA)

patient-generated goal

patient-oriented consultation

Patient's Bill of Rights

patriae
parens p.

patriarch

patriarchal family

patricide

patrilineal family

patrilocal family

patrimony

patronize
patronizing manner
patronymic
pattern
abnormal food intake p.
action p.
activation p.
advanced sleep-phase p.
affectomotor p.
p. of aggression
agreed-on p.
p. analysis
anomalous parental vocal p.
p. of antisocial behavior
authoritarian leadership p.
autosomal dominant p.
avoidance p.
behavior p.
beta p.
binge-eating p.
blame-placing communication p.
p. of care
change in sleep p.
changing sleep-wake p.
characteristic p.
checkerboard p.
chronic p.
chronically disabling p.
communication p.
p. of conduct
delusional thought p.
democratic leadership p.
destructive family relationship p.
desynchronized discharge p.
p. of detachment
developmental p.
discharge p.
p. discrimination
disturbed sleep p.
enduring p.
erotic arousal p.
p. of expression
expressive p.
extinction-type p.
familial p.
family p.
fixed action p. (FAP)
food consumption p.
gesturing communication p.
gullwing p.
habit p.
habitual p.
high-risk drinking p.
ineffective communication p.
inflexible perception p.
intellectualization communication p.
intensive habit p.
interpersonal spacing communication p.
irregular sleep p.
irregular sleep-wake p.
Kindling p.
laissez-faire leadership p.
lifelong behavior p.
long-term p.
maladaptive personality p.
manipulation communication p.
mitten p.
monopolization communication p.
mood disorder with seasonal p.
neurodevelopmental p.
noncued memory p.
occupational ability p. (OAP)
parrotlike speech p.
pathogenic family p.
pathophysiologic p.
persistent p.
personality p.
pervasive p.
p. of pervasive unhappiness
phenomenal p.
positive spike p.
power struggle leadership p.
prototypical course p.
rapid-cycling p.
p. recognition
reflex p.
repeating p.
repetitive p.
p. of repetitive behavior
response p.
role p.
scapegoating communication p.
seasonal p.
self-destructive p.
self-disclosure p.
p. of self-injury
semantic argument communication p.
shared thought p.
silence communication p.
sleep p.
specific dynamic p.
speech p.
stable sleep-wake p.
strange behavior p.

NOTES

P

pattern *(continued)*
stress response p.
symptom response p.
syndrome p.
syndromic p.
temporal p.
thought p.
touching communication p.
transactional p.
validation communication p.
patterned interview
pattern-induced epilepsy
patterning
p. exercise
p. psychotherapy
p. vision
pattern-sensitive epilepsy
paucity
p. of data
p. of expressive gestures
p. of movement
p. of reports
p. of speech
p. of speech content
pauperize
pause
apneic p.
fixation p.
respiratory p.
p. in speech
Pausinystalia yohimbe
pauvre
autisme p.
Pavlov
P. method
P. theory of schizophrenia
pavlovian
p. conditioning
p. theory
pavlovianism
pavor
p. diurnus
p. nocturnus
p. scleresis
pay
maladie du p.'s
take-home p.
payer
Paykel classification
PBG
porphobilinogen
PBPD
pediatric bipolar disorder
PC
phrase construction
picture completion
PCA
patient-controlled analgesia
principal-component analysis
PCP
phencyclidine
primary care provider
PCP-induced anxiety disorder
PCP-related disorder, NOS
PD
panic disorder
personality disorder
problem drinker
psychopathic deviant
psychotic depression
PDD
Parkinson disease with dementia
pervasive developmental disorder
primary degenerative dementia
PDD NOS
PDDAT
primary degenerative dementia of Alzheimer type
PDP
passive-dependent personality
PDS
pain dysfunction syndrome
PE
physical examination
probable error
peace
disturb the p.
p. pipe
peaceful coexistence
peacekeeper
peacemaker role
peacetime
peak
p. absorption spike
p. acoustic gain
p. behavioral effect
p. clipping
p. experience
kilovoltage p. (kVp)
p. level of drug activity
p. methadone concentration
Pearson correlation coefficient p.
p. plasma level
p. score
p. and trough levels
Pearson correlation coefficient peak
PEC
politicoeconomic conservatism
peccant
peccavi
pecking order
pectoralgia
pectoris
angor p.
peculiar
p. appearance
p. behavior

p. breathing abnormality
p. personality trait
peculiarity
voluntary movement p.
pedagogy
pedantic
pederast
pederasty
pediatric
American Academy of P.'s (AAP)
p. autoimmune neuropsychiatric disorder associated with streptococcal infection (PANDAS)
p. bipolar disorder (PBPD)
developmental-behavioral p.'s
p. growth chart
p. psychiatry
p. psychologist
p. psychology
p. psychopharmacology
Society for Developmental and Behavioral P.'s
pedication
pedigree
p. data
extended p.
p. method
p. structure
p. study
pedionalgia
pedioneuralgia
pedohebephilia
pedologist
pedology
pedomorphism
pedophile
heterosexual p.
homosexual p.
pedophilia
adolescent p.
bisexual p.
heterosexual p.
homosexual p.
middle age p.
p. paraphilia
senescent p.
pedophilic
p. behavior
p. stimulus
pedotrophy
peduncular hallucinosis
pedunculotomy
peeping Tom
peer
p. abuse
age p.
p. anxiety
p. censure
conflicts with p.'s
p. criticism
p. factor
p. group
p. interaction
p. interactional situation
p. likability
p. mediation
opposite sex p.
p. ostracism
p. play
p. pressure
p. rating
rejection by p.'s
p. rejection
p. relationship
p. review organization (PRO)
same-sex p.
sex play with p.'s
p. smoking
p. support
p. support group
p. support for violence
peer-helping service
peer-to-peer conflict resolution
peeve
peevish
pegboard
Lafayette p.
pejoration
pejorative
p. delusion
p. nature
p. voice
pejorism
pelea
mal de p.
pellagragenic
pellagral
pellagrin
pellagroid
pellagrous
pellucidum
septum p.
pelvic
p. pain
p. thrusting
penal code

NOTES

P

penalize
penalty
p., frustration, anxiety, guilt, hostility (PFAGH)
minor p.
penance
penchant
pendulous
pendulum of diagnosis
penectomy
penes (*pl. of* penis)
penetrable
penetrance
lack of p.
penetrate
penetration
finger p.
oral p.
p. response
vaginal p.
penile
p. arousal
p. erection
p. impotence
p. plethysmograph
p. prosthesis
p. tumescence
penilingus
penis, pl. **penes**
artificial p.
p. captivus
p. envy
erector p.
p. fear
glans p.
immissio p.
p. pride
tenesmus p.
p. wish
penitence
penitent
penitentiare
folie p.
penitentiary
penniless
penology
pense
déjà p.
pensée
echo de la p.
p. opératoire
tic de p.
pension neurosis
pentapeptide
pentazocine
pentetrazol
penurious
penury
peonage
institutional p.
people
aggression toward p.
categorizing p.
kicking p.
recognition of p.
p. skills
street p.
peotillomania
Pepper syndrome
PEP-R
psychoeducational profile-revised
pep talk
peptide
beta amyloid p.
delta sleep-inducing p.
gastrin-inhibiting p.
p. neurotransmitter
opioid p.
sleep-inducing p.
tau protein p.
vasoactive intestinal p. (VIP)
per
p. anum
p. capita
p. rectum
p. vaginam
peracute mania
perazine
perceived
p. danger
p. emotional abandonment
p. interpersonal rejection
p. life dissatisfaction
p. loss
p. maternal dysfunction
p. neglect
p. parental dysfunction
p. power
p. reality
p. sin
p. stress
p. trauma characteristic
percentile
p. norm
p. rank
p. score
percept
p. analysis
body p.
delusional p.
p. image
perceptible
perception
aberration of p.
abnormal p.
abstract p.
alteration in time p.

altered mind-body p.
altered sensory p.
altered time p.
p. analysis
applied extrasensory p. (AESP)
p. asymmetry
auditory space p.
automorphic p.
binocular p.
p. of body image
body image p.
clerical p. (Q)
color p.
concept-driven p.
conscious p.
cross-modality p.
p. of dangerousness
p. deficit
depth p.
p. disorder
distance p.
distorted p.
p. disturbance
ecological p.
p. ego
p. of environment
exaggerated p.
extrasensory p. (ESP)
facial p.
false sensory p.
family p.
figure-ground p.
fingertip number-writing p.
form p.
gravity p.
hallucination of p.
haptic p.
heightened sensory p.
hypnagogic p.
hypnopompic p.
inferential p.
internal world of p.
kinesthetic p.
p. localized within body
LSD-type p.
motion p.
narrative speech p.
object p.
obligatory p.
olfactory p.
pain p.
person p.
physiognomic p.
posthallucinogen p.
proprioceptive p.
p. of reality
sensory p.
situational p.
size p.
social p.
p. of sound
p. of sound inside head
p. of sound outside head
space p.
p. of spatial relations
speech p.
stereognostic p.
subconscious p.
subliminal p.
substance-induced p.
tactile p.
time p.
touch p.
transactional theory of p.
true p.
visual p.
weight p.

perception-hallucination

perceptive
p. deafness
p. epilepsy

perceptivity

perceptorium

perceptual
p. abnormality
p. analysis
p. anchoring
p. aspect
p. asymmetry
p. closure
p. cognitive mechanism
p. consciousness
p. consistency
p. constancy
p. cue
p. cycle
p. defect
p. defense
p. deficit
p. deprivation
p. disability
p. disorder
p. distortion
p. disturbance
p. emotive stimulus
p. error

NOTES

P

perceptual *(continued)*
p. expansion
p. experience
p. extinction
p. field
p. filter
p. immaturity
p. induction
p. learning
p. level
p. maintenance
p. masking
p. motor ability
p. motor dysfunction
p. organization
p. organizational index
p. process
p. psychology
p. restructuring
p. retardation
p. rivalry
p. schema
p. segregation
p. sensitization
p. set
p. skill
p. sociogram
p. speed
p. structure
p. style
p. symptom
p. synthesis
p. training
p. transformation
p. vigilance
perceptually handicapped
perceptual-motor
p.-m. behavior
p.-m. disability
p.-m. impairment
p.-m. learning
p.-m. match
p.-m. region
perceptus motor skill
percipient
percussion
percutaneous stimulation
perdida del alma
peregrinating problem patient
peregrination
perencephaly
perennial dream
perfect
p. negative relationship
p. performance
p. positive relationship
perfectible
perfection
manie de p.
p. preoccupation
p. state
perfectionism preoccupation
perfectionist
perfectionistic personality
perfervid
perfidious
perfidy
perforate
perforation
perforator
perforatum
Hypericum p.
performance
p. abnormality
academic p.
p. anxiety
as-if p.
p. assessment
attentional p.
automaticity of p.
baseline p.
p. characteristic
cognitive p.
decreased work p.
p. fear
impaired p.
impaired sexual p.
p. intensity function
job p.
p. level
memory p.
memory-continuous p.
motor p.
neuropsychologic p.
p. neurosis
novel task p.
p. objective
perfect p.
poor academic p.
poor school p.
psychometric p.
psychomotor p.
quality of p.
recall p.
p. requirement
school p.
p. score
sexual p.
p. situation
social p.
standard of p.
task p.
vocational p.
work p.
performative speech
performer
performing symbolically
perfunctory

Periactin
periamygdaloid cortex
perianal
periaqueductal gray matter
periarterial sympathectomy
periblepsis
perichareia
pericranitis
periencephalitis
perikaryal
peril
perilous
p. activity
p. course
periluteal phase dysphoric disorder
perimeningitis
perineometer
perineural
p. anesthesia
p. infiltration
perineuritis
period
adaptation p.
apneic p.
apneustic p.
child-raising p.
chum p.
commitment p.
concrete operation p.
crisis p.
critical p.
depression p.
developmental p.
discrete p.
drug-free p.
emotional recovery p.
enactive p.
endogenous circadian p.
evaluation p.
fantasy p.
followup p.
formal operations p.
growth p.
honeymoon p.
ictal p.
interictal p.
involutional p.
latency p. (LP)
latent p.
major risk p.
observation p.
oedipal p.
Oedipus p.
p. of optimism
oral biting p.
practicing p.
prenatal p.
preoperational thought p.
p. prevalence
prodromal p.
psychological refractory p.
refractory p.
REM p.
p. of remission
sadness p.
sensorimotor intelligence p.
silent p.
sleep-onset REM p.
storm-and-stress p.
thought p.
treatment p.
periodic
p. catatonia
p. drinker
p. drinking
p. insanity
p. jactitation
p. limb movement disorder
p. mania
p. migrainous neuralgia
p. paralysis
p. psychosis of puberty
p. reinforcement
p. reinforcement relationship
p. screening
periodical mania
periodicity theory
periontogenic
perioral tremor
peripatetic
peripheral
p. anesthesia
p. autonomic neuropathy
p. catecholamine
p. catecholamine receptor
p. cholinergic activity
p. dysautonomia
p. epilepsy
p. examination
p. field image
p. lymphocyte
p. masking
p. nervous system (PNS)
p. neuritis
p. norepinephrine
p. sensation

NOTES

peripheral *(continued)*
p. sensory loss
p. sympathomimetic effect
p. tabes
peripheralism
peripheralist psychology
peripherally acting anticholinergic medication
periphery
periphrastic
peripolar zone
periproctic
perirectal
perirectitis
perish
perispondylitis
peristasis
peritonism
peritraumatic
p. dissociation
p. predictor
periurethral
perivaginal
periventricular
p. gray matter area
p. gray region
p. hyperintensity
p. white matter
periwinkle
perjury
perky
permanence
p. concept
object p.
Permanency Planning: Service Use and Child Outcomes
permanent
p. disability
p. dominant idea
p. epilation
p. memory
p. planning
p. residual impairment
permeable
permeation
permissible
p. dose
ethically p.
permission, limited information, specific suggestions, intensive therapy (PLISSIT)
permissive
p. environment
p. hypothesis of affective disorder
p. parent
permissiveness
permit
permutation
perneoscrotal
perneovaginal
pernicious trend
peroneal phenomenon
peroral
peroration
peroxisomal proliferator acting receptor (PPAR)
perpend
perpetrate
perpetrator
p. of abuse
p. of violence
perpetual
perpetuate
perpetuating factor
perpetuity
perplexed manic-depressive psychosis
perplexed-type
p.-t. manic-depressive
p.-t. manic-depressive psychosis
perplexing behavior
perplexity
morbid p.
parent p.
parental p.
p. psychosis
p. state
vague p.
persecute
persecution
p. complex
delirium of p.
delusion of p.
p. delusion
folie des p.'s
p. ideation
social p.
p. syndrome
p. theme
persecutor
persecutory
p. anxiety
p. belief
p. delusion
p. delusional disorder
p. delusional system
p. delusional theme
p. idea
p. paranoia
p. subtype
p. type
persecutory-type
p.-t. delusional disorder
p.-t. paranoid disorder
p.-t. schizophrenia
perseverance
lack of p.
perseverate
perseveration
p. deficit

infantile p.
motor p.
p. set
verbal p.
perseverative
p. error
p. functional autonomy
p. movement
p. response
p. speech
p. trace
persevere
Persian Gulf War syndrome
persistence
motor p.
p. task
persistent
p. delusion
p. discomfort
p. emotional condition
p. episodic anxiety
p. fatigue
p. hypersomnia
p. inappropriate idea
p. inappropriate image
p. inappropriate impulse
p. insomnia
p. intrusive idea
p. intrusive image
p. intrusive impulse
p. morbidity
p. motor activity
p. partialism
p. pattern
p. pattern of conduct
p. puberism
p. risk
p. rumination
p. thought
p. tremor
p. vegetative state (PVS)
p. vegetative state disorder
persistently expansive mood
persisting
p. dementia
p. mental symptom
p. perception disorder
person
aged p.
composite p.
p. deixis
displaced p.
disturbed p.
dominant p.
evil p.
exposure of p.
homeless p.
inflated relationship to famous p.
inhibited p.
inner-directed p.
p. in need of supervision
other-directed p.
p. in patient
p. perception
religious p.
significant supporting p.
spectral relationship to famous p.
spiritual p.
street p.
time, place, and p. (TP&P)
p. with AIDS (PWA)
persona
p. non grata
organic p.
in propria p.
symbolic p.
personable
personal
p. adjustment
p. agenda
p. agony
p. anguish
p. assault
p. attribution
p. audit
p. belief
p. care
p. care home
p. communication
p. consequences
p. construct
p. construct theory
p. counselor
p. data sheet
p. demoralization
p. development
p. diary
p. disposition
p. distance zone
p. document analysis
p. dysjunction
p. effects
p. episode
p. equation
p. event
p. experience

NOTES

P

personal *(continued)*
p. factor
p. followup data
p. function
p. growth
p. growth group
p. growth laboratory
p. history (PH)
p. honor
p. hygiene
p. identity
p. identity confusion
p. idiom
p. image
p. import
p. inadequacy
p. inadequacy theme
p. information
p. involvement
p. issue
p. judgment
p. locus of control (PLC)
p. loss
p. man
p. memory
p. memory score
p. motivation
p. myth
p. need
p. neglect
p. opinion
p. psychiatric history
p. recovery
p. relationship
p. relevance
p. response
p. responsibility
p. satisfaction
p. skills gambling
p. skills map
p. and social history (P&SH)
p. social motive
p. space
p. space invasion
p. spirituality
p. strength
p. unconscious
p. value
personalism
personality
abnormal p.
p. abnormality
acromegaloid p.
action-oriented p.
addiction-prone p. (APP)
addictive p.
affective p.
aggressive p.
alexithymic p.
allotropic p.
altered p.
alternating p.'s
altruistic p.
amoral psychopathic p.
anal p.
anal-retentive p.
anancastic p.
antisocial p. (ASP)
antisocial neurotic p.
antisocial trends psychopathic p.
as-if p.
asocial trend psychopathic p.
p. assessment
p. assessment system (PAS)
asthenic p.
authoritarian p.
avoidant p.
basic p.
borderline p.
brooding p.
p. change
p. change disorder
p. change due to general medical condition
p. change due to general medical condition, aggressive type
p. change due to general medical condition, aphasic type
p. change due to general medical condition, disinhibited type
p. change due to general medical condition, labile type
p. change due to general medical condition, paranoid type
p. characteristic
charismatic p.
chronic depressive p.
chronic hypomanic p.
p. clash
coarctated p.
coconscious p.
codependent p.
composite p.
compulsive p.
p. configuration
controlling p.
p. cult
cycloid p.
cyclothymic p.
dependent p.
depressive p.
p. deterioration
p. development
p. deviance
p. deviation
diehard p.
p. dimension
p. disintegration

p. disorder (PD)
p. disorder diagnosis
p. disorder NOS
p. disorder profile
p. disorder score
p. disorder taxonomy
p. disorder typology
distressed p.
disturbed p.
dominant p.
double p.
dual p.
dynamic p.
p. dynamics
p. dysfunction
dyssocial p.
eccentric p.
emotional p.
emotionally unstable p.
epileptic p.
exploitative p.
explosive p.
extroverted p.
Eysenck and Gray biological theories of p.
factor theory of p.
fanatic p.
p. feature
p. formation
freudian theory of p.
p. functioning
p. and gender
haltlose-type p.
histrionic p.
hoarding p.
hostile p.
hyperesthetic p.
hypomanic p.
hysterical p.
hysteroid p.
ideal p.
immature p.
p. impoverishment
impulsive trait of p.
inadequate p.
inmate p.
p. integration
interactional theory of p.
intraconscious p.
introverted schizoid p.
Jekyll and Hyde p.
lifetime p.
magnetic p.
maladaptive p.
marketing p.
masochistic p.
melancholic p.
migraine p.
mixed psychopathic p.
mixed-type psychopathic p.
model of p.
multiple p.
multiplication of p.
narcissistic p.
neurasthenic p.
neurotic p.
p. neurotic disorder
normal p.
obsessional p.
obsessive p.
obsessive-compulsive p.
oral p.
p. organization
p. panel
paranoid p.
passive p.
passive-aggressive p. (PAP)
passive-aggressive neurotic p.
passive-dependent p. (PDP)
pathologic p.
p. pathology
p. pattern
p. pattern disturbance
perfectionistic p.
physiologic basis of p.
posttraumatic p.
premorbid p.
prepsychotic p.
presenting p.
p. problem
p. process
productive p.
psychoinfantile p.
p. psychologist
p. psychology
p. psychoneurosis
psychoneurotic p.
psychopathic p.
p. reaction
receptive p.
repressive p.
p. research
p. researcher
role theory of p.
sadistic p.
schizoid p.

NOTES

P

personality *(continued)*
schizophrenic p.
schizothymic p.
schizotypal schizoid p.
Schneider definition of p.
schneiderian criteria for depressive p.
seclusive p.
secondary p.
seductive p.
self-defeating p.
shut-in p.
sociopathic p.
p. sphere
split p.
stable p.
stormy p.
p. structure
p. syndrome
syntonic p.
p. trait
p. trait disturbance
p. trait stability
p. trait theory
type A, B p.
ulcer p.
unstable p.
unusual p.
viscosity p.
volatile p.
von Zerssen circumplex model of premorbid p.

personality-descriptive
p.-d. item
p.-d. statement

personalization

personalized interpretation

personalizing violence

personally
p. saddening experience
p. significant anniversary

personate

person-centered theory

person-environment interaction

personification
eidetic p.

personified self

personify

2-person interview team

personnel
p. date
nonmedical p.
p. placement
p. psychology
p. selection
p. training

personology

person-situation-interaction approach

perspective
alternating p.
alternative p.
atmospheric p.
behavioral p.
biological p.
categorical p.
clinical p.
developmental p.
extraspective p.
humanistic p.
linear p.
neurobiological p.
psychoanalytic p.
psychosocial p.
religious p.
symptomatic p.
temporal p.

perspective-taking skills

perspicacious

perspiration

persuade

persuasion
coercive p.
p. therapy

persuasive communication

pertinacious

pertinence

pertinent

Pertofrane

perturb

perturbation magnitude

pervasive
p. affect
p. anger disorder
p. anhedonia
p. anxiety
p. desire for death
p. developmental disorder (PDD)
p. disinhibited type developmental disorder
p. distrust
p. emotion
p. impairment of development
p. inhibition
p. pattern
p. pattern of disregard
p. and persistent maladaptive personality traits
p. pessimism
p. problem
p. proneness to guilt
p. self-criticism
p. unhappiness

perverse

perversion
excretory p.
polymorphous p.

sex p.
sexual p.

pervert
sexual p.

perverted
p. appetite
p. logic
p. sexuality
p. thinking

pervigilium

PES
psychiatric emergency service

pessimism
chronic p.
oral p.
pervasive p.
self-reported p.
therapeutic p.

pessimist

pessimistic
p. attitude
p. outlook
p. relapser

pesticide
organophosphate p.

PET
psychiatric emergency team

petechial

Peter
P. Panism
P. principle

pethidine

petit
p. mal
p. mal epilepsy
p. mal status
p. mal variant seizure

petition of mental illness (PMI)

petrification

pettifog

petting behavior

petty
p. punishment
p. theft

petulance

petulant

peyote
p. cactus
p. dependence

peyotism

PFAGH
penalty, frustration, anxiety, guilt, hostility

PFAMC
psychological factor affecting medical condition

PFLAG
parents, family, and friends of lesbians and gays

pfropfhebephrenia

pfropfschizophrenia

PFS
patient and family services
picture frustration study

PG
pathological gambling
pathologic gambling

PGD
pathologic gambling disorder

PGR
psychogalvanic reflex
psychogalvanic response

PGSR
psychogalvanic skin resistance

PGT
play group therapy

PH
past history
personal history

Phaedra complex

phagomania

phagotherapy

phalli (*pl. of* phallus)

phallic
p. character
p. level
p. love
p. mother
p. overbearance
p. partner
p. phase
p. pride
p. primacy
p. sadism
p. stage
p. stage psychosexual development
p. symbol
p. woman

phallicism, phallism

phallic-narcissistic character

phallic-oedipal phase

phalliform

phallism (*var. of* phallicism)

phallocentric culture

phalloid

NOTES

P

phalloides
Amanita p.
phallometry
phallus, pl. **phalli**
p. envy
p. girl
phaneromania
phanerothyme
phantasia
phantasm
phantasmagoria
phantasmatomoria
phantasmology
phantasmoscopia, phantasmoscopy
phantastica (*var. of* fantastica)
phantasy (*var. of* fantasy)
phantogeusia
phantom
p. boarder
p. extremity
p. limb
p. limb pain
p. lover syndrome
p. reaction
p. sensation
sensory p.
p. speech
p. vision
phantomize
pharmaceutical
p. alternative
p. analgesic
p. equivalent
pharmacist
pharmacodynamic
p. change
p. tolerance
pharmacodynamics
age-related p.
pharmacoeconomics
pharmacogenetics
pharmacogenic orgasm
pharmacogenomics
pharmacogeriatrics
pharmacokinetic
p. change
p. parameter
p. reason
pharmacologic, pharmacological
p. agent
p. approach
p. armamentarium
p. difference
p. experimentation
p. factor
p. impact
p. intervention
p. management
p. mechanism
p. predictor
p. property
p. prophylaxis
p. provocation
p. sensitivity
p. stimulus
p. treatment
pharmacologically induced penile erection (PIPE)
pharmacology
p. of abuse
p. of abuse and dependence
nicotine p.
serotonergic p.
pharmacomania
pharmacopedia
Pharmacopeia
United States P. (USP)
pharmacophilia
pharmacopsychosis
pharmacotherapeutic intervention
pharmacotherapy
adolescent p.
antipsychotic p.
chemical aversion p.
conventional p.
p. regimen
pharmacothymia
pharmacy
online p.
pharyngeal psychophysiologic reaction
pharyngismus
pharyngoplegia
pharyngospasm
phase
active p.
acute p.
p. advance
anal p.
appetitive p.
ascension p.
autistic p.
Band-Aid p.
circadian rhythm sleep disorder, delayed sleep p.
p. cue
p. delay
delayed sleep p.
dementia p.
depressive p.
developmental p.
p. difference
p. disparity
endogenous circadian rhythm p.
equatorial p.
excitement p.
follicular p.
genital p.
group p.

hypomanic p.
illness p.
insomnia p.
p. lag on EEG
latency p.
libidinal p.
p. of life
p. locking
luteal p.
magic p.
manic p.
moon p.
normal autistic p.
oedipal p.
opposite p.
oral eroticism p.
oral incorporative p.
orgasmic p.
phallic p.
phallic-oedipal p.
plateau p.
p. position
postcontraction recovery p.
preambivalent p.
pregenital p.
preoedipal p.
preoperational p.
presuperego p.
prodromal p.
recovery p.
reference p.
relaxation p.
residual p.
resolution p.
p. reversal
rhythm p.
schizophrenia p.
second negative p.
p. of seizure
sensorimotor p.
separation-individuation p.
p. sequence
p. shift
p. shift of sleep-wake cycle
sleep p.
p. spike on EEG
symbiotic p.
treatment p.
urethral p.

phase-of-life problem

phasic
p. activation
p. function
p. reflex

phasophrenia

phencyclidine (PCP)

phencyclidine-associated psychosis

phencyclidine-induced
p.-i. disorder
p.-i. psychosis
p.-i. psychotic disorder with delusions
p.-i. psychotic disorder with hallucinations

phencyclidine-related
p.-r. disorder
p.-r. disorder NOS

phenocopy

phenogenetic

phenology

phenomena (*pl. of* phenomenon)

phenomenal
p. absolutism
p. field
p. motion
p. pattern
p. regression
p. report
p. self

phenomenalism

phenomenalistic
p. introspection
p. thought

phenomenistic
p. causality
p. thought

phenomenological
p. analysis
p. characteristic
p. feature
p. measure
p. reality
p. subgroup

phenomenology
clinical p.
existential p.
intoxication-related p.

phenomenon, pl. **phenomena**
abrupt withdrawal p.
abstinence p.
arm p.
autoscopic p.
Bezold-Brucke p.
boundary p.
breakaway p.

NOTES

P

phenomenon *(continued)*
breakoff p.
breast phantom p.
Capgras p.
choo-choo p.
clasp-knife p.
clinical p.
cogwheel p.
complex p.
constancy p.
conversion p.
crossed phrenic p.
cultural p.
déjà vu p.
dissociative p.
disturbance associated with conversion p.
Doppelganger p.
duplication p.
echo p.
escape p.
facialis p.
Fere p.
finger p.
freezing p.
Fregoli p.
gestalt p.
Grasset-Gaussel p.
hesitation p.
hidden observer p.
Hoffmann p.
hypofrontality p.
p. identification
identification p.
implausible p.
interactive p.
intoxication p.
Isakower p.
jamais p.
jet lag p.
knee p.
Kohnstamm p.
la belle indifferénce p.
leg p.
Leichtenstern p.
mental p.
misdirection p.
motor p.
napping p.
normal voluntary napping p.
panic spectrum p.
panum p.
paradoxical pupillary p.
paranormal p.
paroxysmal p.
peroneal p.
phi p.
Pool p.
postattack p.
psi p.
psychic p.
psychomotor p.
psychotic-like p.
radical p.
rebound p.
release p.
riddance p.
Ritter-Rollet p.
Schüller p.
sensory p.
soft psychotic-like p.
split-screen p.
Tarchanoff p.
thought transfer p.
tip-of-the-tongue p.
toe p.
tongue p.
trailing p.
transference p.
transient p.
transvestic p.
voluntary napping p.
Westphal p.
Westphal-Piltz p.
Wever-Bray p.
Zeigarnik effect p.

phenomotive

phenoplegia

phenotype
alcohol-related p.
clinical p.
membrane p.
polymorphous p.

phenotypic
p. factor
p. marker
p. study

phentermine

phenylpyruvic
p. amentia
p. oligophrenia

Phenytek

pheromone

PHI
physiologic hyaluronidase inhibitor

philandering

philanthropy

Philippines
The P.

philobat

philology

philomimesia

philoneism

philopatridomania

philoprogenitive

philosophical
p. analysis
p. decision

p. discussion
p. inclination
p. problem
p. psychology

philosophize

philosophy
analytical p.
anthropological p.
coercive p.
humanistic p.
p. of life
moral p.
place-then-train p.
train-then-place p.
treatment p.

philter, philtre

philtrum

phi phenomenon

phlegm

phlegmatic constitutional type

phobanthropy

phobia
childhood-onset p.
lifetime social p.
school p.
simple p.
social p.
specific p.

phobia-induced migraine headache

phobic
p. anxiety
p. attitude
p. avoidance
p. avoidance behavior
p. avoidant behavior
p. character
p. companion
p. desensitization
p. neurotic disorder
p. obsessional neurosis
p. psychogenic disorder
p. psychoneurotic reaction
p. situation
p. state
p. stimulus
p. syndrome
p. trend

phobic-anxiety-depersonalization neurosis

phoesthesia

pholcodine

phonasthenia

phonation

phonatory theory

phoneme
anterior feature English p.
diffuse p.

phoneme-grapheme association

phonemic
p. analysis
p. awareness

phonetic
acoustic p.'s
p. analysis
p. babble
p. clarity
p. information
p. input
p. noise

phonetically balanced words

phoniatrics

phonic spasm

phonism

phonogram

phonological, phonologic
p. agraphia
p. analysis
p. assembly impairment
p. disorder
p. processing

phonologically
p. irregular words
p. regular words

phonomania

phonomyoclonus

phonomyography

phonopathy

phonopsia

phosphatase
alkaline p.

phosphorus

phosphorylation

photalgia

photesthesia

photic
p. driving
p. epilepsy
p. stimulation

photism

photoaxis

photodynia

photodysphoria

photoesthetic

photogenic
p. epilepsy
p. seizure

photographic memory

NOTES

photography
pornographic p.
photokinetic
photolabile
photoma
photomania
photomyoclonus
photon
photopathy
photophilic
photophobic
photopic vision
photoptarmosis
photoreceptor cell
photosensitive epilepsy
photosensitivity
phototherapy
phrase
coin new p.
p. construction (PC)
phren
phrenalgia
phrenectomy
phrenemphraxis
phrenetic
phrenic
phrenicectomy
phreniclasia
phrenicoexeresis
phreniconeurectomy
phrenicotomy
phrenicotripsy
phrenitica
aphrodisia p.
phrenitis
phrenocardia
phrenoglottic
phrenologist
phrenology
phrenoplegia
phrenopraxic
phrenospasm
phrenotropic
phrictopathia
phrictopathic
phronemomania
phronesis
phthinoid
phthisica
spes p.
phthisicus
habitus p.
phyloanalysis
phylobiology
phylogenesis
phylogenetic
p. mneme
p. predecessor
p. principle
p. symptom
phylogenetically
phylogeny
physaliformis
ecchordosis p.
physiatrics
physiatry
physic
physical
p. abuse
p. activity
p. aggression
p. aggression against objects
p. aggression against others
p. aggression against self
p. agitation
p. anergy
p. anthropology
p. appearance
p. assault
p. attack
p. bondage
p. capacity
p. change
p. comorbid disorder
p. concern
p. condition organic psychosis
p. danger
p. defect
p. dependence
p. discipline
p. discomfort
p. disturbance
p. education
p. environment
p. examination (PE)
p. exercise
p. experience
p. fight
p. fitness
p. harm
history and p. (H&P)
p. impairment
p. inactivity
p. independence
p. injury
p. integrity
p. intersex condition
p. intimacy
p. manifestation of pain
p. medicine
p. posturing
p. problem
p. psychogenic disorder
p. restraint
p. sensation
p. sign
p. signs and symptoms

p. skill
p. strain
p. stress
p. support
p. symptom distress
p. symptoms adjustment reaction
p. tension
p. therapist
p. therapy
p. trauma
p. withdrawal

physically aggressive behavior

physician
American Society of Psychoanalytic P.'s (ASPP)
attending p.
p. expert
family p.
general medical p.
house p.
National Association of Inpatient P.'s (NAIP)
primary care p.
resident p.

physician-assisted suicide

physician-patient
p.-p. communication
p.-p. encounter
p.-p. relationship
p.-p. scenario

physician's assistant (PA)

physiodrama

physiogenesis

physiogenetic depression

physiogenic

physiognomic
p. perception
p. thinking

physiognomy

physiognosis

physiologica
alalia p.

physiologic, physiological
p. age
p. amenorrhea
p. arousal
p. aspect
p. basis
p. basis of personality
p. component
p. dependence
p. drive
p. effect
p. feedback
p. functional variation
p. hyaluronidase inhibitor (PHI)
p. hyperarousal
p. intoxication
p. limit
p. maintenance
p. manifestation
p. measure
p. mechanism
p. memory
p. motive
p. need
p. norm
p. paradigm
p. process
p. psychology
p. reactivity
p. reflex
p. response
p. response specificity
p. risk factor
p. sleepiness
p. sleepiness index
p. tremor

physiology
ejaculation p.
sexual p.
p. of women

physiomedical

physioneurosis

physiopathologic

physiopathology

physioplastic stage

physiopsychic

physiotherapy

physique type

physocephaly

physostigmine

phytochemicals

phytogenous

PI
paradoxical intention
present illness
proactive inhibition

Piaget cognitive development stage

pianist's cramp

piano player's cramp

PIAPACS
psychological information, acquisition, processing, and control system

piblokto, pibloktog
p. syndrome

NOTES

P

pica
p. disorder
paper p.
Pick
P. atrophy
P. cell
P. disease dementia
P. syndrome
picking
p. at face
p. movement
orifice p.
pathologic skin p.
skin p.
pickwickian syndrome
picky eater
picolinate
chromium p.
picrotoxin
PICSYMS
picture symbols
pictogram
pictophilia
pictorial
p. aphasia
p. imagery
picture
p. arrangement
p. assembly
clinical p.
p. completion (PC)
concrete p.
cookie theft p.
p. frustration study (PFS)
inward p.
p. symbols (PICSYMS)
picture-caption pair
picture-in-picture technique
PICU
psychiatric intensive care unit
piercing
body p.
Pierre Robin complex
piesesthesia
piety
filial p.
PIF
premorbid inferiority feeling
Pigem question
PIL
purpose in life
pilfer
pilgrimage
spiritual p.
pill
birth control p. (BCP)
p. ingestion
morning-after p.
pop p.'s
sleeping p.
pillage
pillow
psychological p.
pill-rolling tremor
piloerection
piloid
pilojection
pilomotor
p. pathway
p. reflex
p. response
pilot
p. interview
p. program
p. study
pimozide
pimp
pimping
pineal
p. body
p. substance
p. therapy
pinealopathy
Pinel-Haslam syndrome
Pinel system
ping-pong gaze
pinheaded
pining
pink
p. noise
p. spot
pink-collar worker
pinpoint pupil
pins-and-needles sensation
pin-sticking sensation
pious
PIPE
pharmacologically induced penile erection
pipe
p. dream
peace p.
Piportil Depot
pipotiazine
pique
Pisa syndrome
pistol
snub-nose p.
pitch
absolute p.
basal p.
p. discrimination
pithecoid idiot
pithiatism
pithiatric
pitiable
pitiful

Pitres
P. law
P. rule
P. sign
pitting edema
pituitary
p. basophilia
p. cachexia
p. eunuchism
p. prolactin release
p. stalk section
pityrodes
alopecia p.
piuturi
pivotal role
pixelated parietotemporal perfusion deficit
pixieish
pixilated
PK
psychokinesis
psychokinetic
PKC
protein kinase C
PL
psychosocial-labile
placate
place
p. blame
closed p.
p. conditioning
crowded p.
deep p.
p. deixis
deserted p.
p. identity
open p.
oriented to time and p.
p. of respite
safe p.
sense of p.
p. theory
unfamiliar p.
placebo
active p.
balanced p.
p. effect
p. medication trial
p. reactor
p. response rate
placebo-controlled
p.-c. drug study
p.-c. trial
placement
community p.
p. counseling
electrode p.
foster care p.
home p.
job p.
long-term care p.
nursing home p.
personnel p.
residential p.
sheltered workshop p.
skilled nursing facility p.
therapeutic school p.
therapeutic vocational p.
unavoidable p.
place-specific event
place-then-train philosophy
placid disposition
placidity
plagiocephalic idiocy
plain-folks technique
plaintive
plaisir
maitre de p.
plan
absence of eating p.
acceptable treatment p.
behavioral p.
complete treatment p.
cottage p.
electronic disaster recovery p.
exercise p.
family health insurance p. (FHIP)
game p.
homicidal p.
life p.
multidisciplinary treatment p. (MTP)
organizational p.
overcontrolled eating p.
realistic p.
rigid eating p.
subjective, objective, assessment, p.
suicidal p.
suicide p.
treatment p. (TRPL)
plane
coronal p.
median sagittal p.
sagittal p.
subjective p.
planigraphy

NOTES

P

planned
p. after-school activity
p. behavioral therapy
p. course
p. learning environment
P. Parenthood
p. pregnancy
planning
career p.
comprehensive treatment p.
conceptual p.
p. disturbance
family p.
forward p.
lack of future p.
motor p.
operational p.
permanent p.
poor motor p.
retirement p.
social policy p.
strategic p.
treatment p.
uninhibited motor p.
planomania
planophrasia
planotopokinesia
plant
loco p.
plantalgia
plantar response
planum
p. temporale
p. temporale morphology
plaque
amyloid p.
argentophilic p.
neuritic p.
senile p.
plasma
p. cortisol
p. C-peptide level
p. leptin level
p. R-methadone concentration
plastic
p. arts therapy
p. compensatory mechanism
p. reorganization
p. surgery
p. tonus
plasticity
decerebrate p.
functional p.
hippocampal synaptic p.
p. of libido
neural p.
neuronal p.
synaptic p.
plat
plateau
p. in improvement
p. masking technique
p. method
p. phase
p. speech
platelet
p. membrane fluidity
p. monoamine oxidase
platform
orgasmic p.
platitude
platonic
p. friendship
p. love
p. nymphomania
p. relationship
platonism
platonization
platybasia
plausible
plausive
play
p. acting
associative p.
p. both ends against middle
breath control p.
dramatic p.
extended p.
fantasy p.
p. the field
foul p.
free p.
p. the game
games people p.
group p.
p. group psychotherapy
p. group therapy (PGT)
imaginative p.
independent p.
joint p.
make-believe p.
p. on words
organized p.
parallel p.
peer p.
repetitive p.
rough-and-tumble p.
p. session
sex p.
shadow p.
symbolic p.
p. technique
p. therapy
p. therapy activity
verbal p.
p. with oneself
play-based assessment

player
game p.
team p.
war game p.
playfulness
playing
card p.
compulsive computer game p.
p. dead
game p.
role p.
playroom
PLC
personal locus of control
plea
p. bargain
p. for help
p. of insanity
plead
pleasant
p. memory
p. stimulus
pleasantness rating
pleasurable
p. affect
p. distraction
p. emotion
p. stimuli
pleasure
activity p.
aesthetic p.
autoerotic p.
p. center
p. ego
p. experience
p. fear
function p.
loss of p.
muscle p.
organ p.
organic p.
p. principle
p. seeking
sensual p.
sexual p.
pleasure-oriented behavior
pleasure-pain principle
pleasuring
pledge
plenary indulgence
pleniloquence
plentitude
pleonasm
pleonexia
plethysmograph
penile p.
vaginal p.
plethysmography
pleurothotonos, pleurothotonus
plexectomy
plexiform
plexitis
pliable
plight
PLISSIT
permission, limited information, specific suggestions, intensive therapy
PLISSIT model
plod
plot
funnel p.
ploy
plucking
p. at clothes
hair p.
plucky
plumbism
plunder
plunge
postpartum psychological p.
pluralistic utilitarianism
plusieurs
folie á p.
plutocracy
plutomania
PM
Legatrin P.
PMA
paramethoxyamphetamine
positive mental attitude
PMDD
premenstrual dysphoric disorder
PMI
petition of mental illness
PMS
premenstrual syndrome
PMTS
premenstrual tension syndrome
PN
pontine nucleus
psychoneurotic
PNAvQ
positive-negative ambivalent quotient
PND
postnatal depression
pneumatocele

NOTES

pneumocele
pneumocephalus
pneumonitis
chemical p.
pneumophonia
pneumorhachis
PNI
psychoneuroimmunology
PNP
psychogenic nocturnal polydipsia
PNS
parasympathetic nervous system
peripheral nervous system
pococurante
podismus
Poggendorf illusion
poiesis
poignancy
poignant
poikilothymia
point
apophysary p.
beside the p.
case in p.
change p.
choice p.
critical p.
end p.
p. fear
fixation p.
flicker-fusion p.
p. of honor
indifference p.
p. localization
moot p.
motor p.
p. of no return
painful p.
4-p. restraint
pressure p.
p. prevalence
racial saturation p.
p. of regard
p. of subjective equality (PSE)
tender p.
time p.
to the p.
trigger p.
Trousseau p.
Valleix p.
p. of view
point-and-shoot video game
pointed object
pointes
point-for-point correspondence
pointing
bone p.
p. of bone
finger p.
pointless
point-resolved spectroscopy (PRESS)
poise
tough p.
poison
cultural p.
p. hemlock
social p.
poisoning
acetaminophen p.
acute amphetamine p.
acute lead p.
alcohol p.
alcoholic p.
amphetamine p.
aspirin p.
blood p.
bromide p.
carbon dioxide p.
carbon monoxide p.
chronic lead p.
copper p.
deadly nightshade p.
food p.
gas p.
lead p.
narcotic p.
nicotine p.
nightshade p.
opiate p.
opioid p.
paregoric p.
thallium p.
poisonous
Poisson distribution
poker
p. face
p. spine
polacrilex
polar
p. opposite
p. zone
polarity
p. response
sorting p.'s
polarization
mass p.
principle of dynamic p.
sexual p.
polemic
polemicize
police power
policy
p. analysis
health p.
p. implication
Office of National Drug Control P.

open-door p.
social p.
polioclastic
politeness
politesse
politic
political
p. affiliation
p. genetics
p. group
p. mania
p. psychiatry
p. value
politically incorrect
politicoeconomic conservatism (PEC)
politicomania
politikon
zoon p.
poll
opinion p.
pollodic
pollution
Pollyanna-like view
Pollyanna mechanism
poltergeist
polyandry
polyarteritis nodosa dementia
Polybus love
polyclonia
Polycrates complex
polycratism
polydipsia
hysterical p.
psychogenic p.
psychogenic nocturnal p. (PNP)
psychosis-induced p.
polydrug
p. abuse
p. addiction
polydystrophic oligophrenia
polyesthesia
polyethic criteria set
polygamist
polygamous strategy
polygamy
polygenic
p. inheritance
p. trait
polyglot
p. amnesia
p. neophasia
polygraph
Keeler p.
polygynous
polygyny
polygyria
polyideic somnambulism
polyleptic
polylogia
polymatric
polymorphism
DRD4 Exon II p.
gene p.
insertion-deletion p.
restriction fragment length p. (RFLP)
p. screening
single nucleotide p.
polymorphous
p. perverse disposition
p. perverse sexuality
p. perversion
p. phenotype
polyneuritica
psychosis p.
polyneuritic alcoholic psychosis
polyneuritiformis
heredopathia atactica p.
polyneuritis
acute idiopathic p.
chronic familial p.
polyneuronitis
polyneuropathy
buckthorn p.
critical illness p. (CIP)
nutritional p.
polyopia
polyparesis
polyphagia
polyphallic
polypharmacy
polyphasic
p. activity
p. potential
p. sleep rhythm
polyphrasia
polyphyria
polyplegia
polypnea
polyposia
polypsychism
polysemous
polysemy
polysensory unit

NOTES

P

polyserositis
polysomnogram (PSG)
polysomnograph (PSG)
polysomnographic abnormality
polysomnography
polysteraxic
polysubstance
p. abuse
p. addiction
p. dependence
p. use disorder
polysubstance-related disorder
polysurgical addiction
polysymptomatic
p. case
p. syndrome
polytheism
polythetic
polytomography
polytomous regression
polytoxicomanic
polytrophic defect
polyvalent
POM
prescription-only medicine
Pompadour fantasy
pompous, pomposity, pompousness
POMS
profile of mood states
ponderous
ponopathy
pons, pl. **pontes**
pontifical
pontificate
pontine
p. nucleus (PN)
p. sleep
pontocerebellar angle syndrome
pool
autonomic motor p.
dirty p.
gene p.
P. phenomenon
pooling
poor
p. academic performance
p. academic preparation
p. appetite
p. attachment
p. awareness of danger
p. body image
p. eating habit
p. eye contact
p. family relationship
p. form response (F-)
p. genital response
p. historian
p. hygiene
p. impulse control
p. insight
p. job history
p. judgment
p. language skills
p. law
p. motor planning
p. mouth
p. peer relationship
p. performance evaluation
p. prognosis
p. reasoning ability
p. response to medication
p. schooling
p. school performance
p. self-care
p. self-confidence
p. sleep quality
p. vocabulary
p. work outcome
poorly
p. developed
p. educated
p. groomed
p. systematized delusion
pop
p. culture
p. pills
p. psychology
popper
poppy
opiate p.
popular
p. culture
p. response
population
adolescence in special p.
adolescent p.
p. cage
clinical p.
clinic patient p.
community p.
criminal p.
culturally diverse p.
p. density
gay p.
general p.
p. genetics
geriatric p.
high-risk p.
lesbian p.
outpatient patient p.
partial hospital patient p.
primary care patient p.
prison p.
p. research
p. setting
p. standard deviation
p. stratification
target p.

POR
problem-oriented record
porencephalia (*var. of* porencephaly)
porencephalic, porencephalous
porencephalitis
porencephalopathy
porencephalous (*var. of* porencephalic)
porencephaly, porencephalia
poriomania
poriomanic fugue
porn
kiddie p.
pornerastic
pornographic
p. illustration
p. mania
p. photography
p. writing
pornography
child p.
p. dependence
Internet child p.
online p.
paraphiliac p.
pornolagnia
porosis, pl. **poroses**
cerebral p.
porphobilinogen (PBG)
porphyria
hepatic p.
porphyrismus
porropsia
portend
portent
portentous
portosystemic encephalopathy (PSE)
Posey restraint
posiomania
position
p. agnosia
p. of attack
body p.
coital p.
cortical thumb p.
depressive p.
information optimization p.
observer p.
ordinal p.
paranoid-schizoid p.
phase p.
p. response
p. of responsibility
rigid body p.
schizoid p.
p. sense
sexual p.
sociopolitical p.
subordinate p.
sustained p.
positional tremor
positive
p. acceleration
p. adaptation
p. afterimage
p. attention behavior (PAB)
p. attitude change
p. cathexis
chromatin p.
p. communication skills
p. comparison
p. conditioned reflex
p. correlation
p. effect
p. emotion
p. emotionality
p. eugenics
p. event
false p.
p. family relationship
p. feedback
p. feeling
p. frontal release sign
guaiac p.
p. image
p. incentive
p. induction
p. mental attitude (PMA)
p. motivation
p. and negative affect schedule
p. parenting
p. picture-caption pair
p. predictive power
p. recency
p. regard
p. reinforcement
p. reinforcement therapy
p. reinforcer
p. response
p. result
p. schizophrenia
p. schizophrenic symptoms
p. score
p. speech content
p. spike pattern
p. symptom dimension
p. symptom distress index

NOTES

P

positive *(continued)*
p. symptoms psychosis
p. thought disorder
p. transfer
p. transference
true p.
p. valence
p. word
positively
p. bathmotropic
p. correlated region
positive-negative ambivalent quotient (PNAvQ)
positivism
logical p.
positivity
positron emission tomography technique
possessed by spirit
possessing agent
possession
demonic p.
drug p.
handgun p.
spirit p.
spiritual p.
p. trance
p. trance disorder
p. trance state
p. trance symptom
p. of weapon
possessor-possession
possibility
causal p.
noncausal p.
possible
as soon as p. (ASAP)
possumus
non p.
post
p. ambivalent phase stage
p. concentration camp syndrome
p. hoc analysis
p. hoc comparison
p. hoc explanation
p. hoc stratification
postabortion syndrome
postadrenalectomy syndrome
postambivalence
postanalytic supervision
postanoxic
p. dementia
p. encephalopathy
p. epilepsy
p. state
postapoplectic
postattack phenomenon
postbaseline visit
postbasic stare
postbinge anguish
postcentral sulcus
postcoital
p. contraceptive
p. dysphoria
p. euphoria
p. headache
postcoitum triste
postconcussion
p. amnesia
p. disorder
p. headache
p. neurosis
postconflict society
postcontraction recovery phase
postcontusion
p. syndrome
p. syndrome encephalopathy
postconvulsive stupor
postdisaster
p. psychosocial intervention
p. stress
postdischarge
postdivorce depression
postdormital
p. chalastic fit
p. depression
p. sleep paralysis
postdormitum
post-ECT
p.-ECT amnesia
p.-ECT seizure
postelectroconvulsive
p. amnesia
p. therapy
postencephalitic
p. oculogyric crisis
p. syndrome
post-9/11 environment
postepileptic twilight state
posterior
p. alexia
p. cingulate
p. cingulate region
p. frontal hypoperfusion
p. hypothalamus
p. language zone
posteriori
a p.
posterodorsal temporal lobe
posteroinferior cerebellar artery syndrome
postexertional malaise
postfebrile dementia
postgraduate education
posthallucinogen
p. perception
p. perception disorder
posthemiplegic
posthion

posthypnotic
p. amnesia
p. psychosis
p. suggestion
posthysterectomy depression
postictal
p. confusion
p. depression
p. depression phase of seizure
p. psychosis
p. state
postinfection depression
postleukotomy syndrome
postlobotomy syndrome
posticus
p. palsy
p. paralysis
tetanus p.
postinfectious psychosis
postketamine
postmature
postmigration stressor
postmortem
p. brain tissue
p. data
p. finding
p. investigation
p. study
p. technique
postnatal
p. depression (PND)
p. development
postoperative
p. confusional state
p. dementia
p. depression
p. pressure alopecia
p. psychosis
p. status
p. tetany
postparalytic
postpartum
p. alopecia
p. blues
p. depression (PPD)
p. mania
p. psychiatric problem
p. psychological plunge
p. psychosis (PPP)
p. syndrome
postpsychotic
p. depression
p. depressive disorder
postpubertal social decline
postpuberty
postpubescence
postpubescent
postrape syndrome
postreceptor
heterotrimeric p.
p. information transduction
postrecovery
postrelevant history (PRH)
postrema
postsaccadic neuronal response
postschizophrenic depression
post-September 11 consciousness
poststroke
p. depression
p. mania
postsurgical loss
postsynaptic
p. compensatory mechanism
p. 5-HT-2 receptor
p. 5-HT-3 receptor
p. potential (PSP)
p. stimulation
posttermination boundary
posttest level
post-TIA depression
posttranslational modification
posttraumatic
p. amnesia (PTA)
p. amnestic syndrome
p. brain syndrome
p. chronic disability
p. cortical dysfunction
p. delirium
p. dementia
p. deterioration
p. disorientation
p. dissociative disorder
p. distress
p. disturbance
p. encephalopathy
p. hallucination
p. headache
p. neurosis
p. osteoporosis
p. pain
p. patient
p. personality
p. personality disorder
p. psychopathic constitution
p. psychosis
p. seizure

NOTES

P

posttraumatic *(continued)*
p. stress disorder (PTSD)
p. stress disorder complex
p. stress disorder by proxy
p. stress disorder reaction index
p. stress symptom
p. stress syndrome
p. symptom formation
posttreatment
postural
p. awareness
p. change
p. hypotension
p. instability
p. myoneuralgia
p. reflex
p. seizure
p. set
p. syncope
p. tremor
p. unsteadiness
p. vertigo
posture
bent p.
bizarre p.
body p.
combative p.
curled-into-fetal-position p.
decerebrate p.
hunched p.
inappropriate p.
open p.
rigid p.
sagging p.
p. sense
sleep p.
slumped p.
unusual sleep p.
posturing
bizarre p.
catatonic p.
cerebrate p.
decorticate p.
dystonic p.
odd p.
physical p.
psychotic p.
sexual p.
post-Vietnam psychiatric syndrome (PVNPS)
potassium
potatorum
potency
hallucinogenic p.
orgastic p.
sexual p.
potent
p. pleasure source
p. risk factor
potential
abuse p.
acoustic evoked p.
acting-out p.
action p.
addiction p.
p. adverse effect
auditory evoked p. (AEP)
bioelectric p.
biotic p.
brain evoked p. (BEP)
brainstem auditory evoked p.
cerebral p.
p. correlation
cortical evoked p.
demarcation p.
early latency p.
effective reaction p.
electrical p.
p. energy
estimated learning p. (ELP)
event-related p. (ERP)
evoked p. (EP)
excitatory postsynaptic p. (EPSP)
p. external reward
extrapyramidal symptom p.
extreme somatosensory evoked p. (ESEP)
far-field evoked p.
glossokinetic p.
graded p.
high tolerance p.
human p.
p. impact
inhibitory postsynaptic p. (IPSP)
injury p.
p. intellectual capacity
lack of performing to p.
leadership p.
local p.
low tolerance p.
motor evoked p. (MEP)
multimodality evoked p. (MEP)
polyphasic p.
p. positive event
postsynaptic p. (PSP)
p. predisposing factor
pretreatment binding p.
resource holding p.
resting p.
sensory evoked p. (SEP)
somatosensory evoked p. (SEP)
specific action p.
suicidal p.
suicide p.
p. suicide victim
p. target
tolerance p.
violence p.

visual evoked p. (VEP)
weight gain p.

potentially
p. dangerous patient
p. fatal complications of illicit drug use

potentiate

potentiation
long-term p. (LTP)

potentiometer

potlatch

potomania

potu
mania á p.

potus
fastidium p.

pounding
p. heart
p. pain

pourquoi
folie du p.

pout reflex

poverty
clinical p.
p. of content
p. of content of speech
delusion of p.
p. of ideas
Liddle psychomotor p.
p. of movement
psychomotor p.
speech p.
p. of thought

POW
prisoner of war
POW syndrome

powder
crystalline p.

powdered opium

power
combined predictive p.
delusion of p.
distribution of p.
p. dynamic
higher p.
illusion of p.
inflated p.
instantaneous p.
mind p.
negative predictive p.
perceived p.
police p.
positive predictive p.
predictive p.
special p.
p. struggle
p. struggle leadership pattern
p. theme
war p.
will to p.

powerless

powerlessness
overt sign of p.

PPAR
peroxisomal proliferator acting receptor

PPD
packs per day
postpartum depression

PPP
postpartum psychosis

PR
psychotherapy responder

practical
p. counseling
p. difficulty
p. reasoning
p. social judgment score

practice
autoerotic p.
clinical diagnostic p.
contemporary p.
contraceptive p.
p. effect
p. experience
group p.
p. guideline
massed negative p.
negative p.
parental feeding p.
programmed p.
reinforced p.
religious p.
P. Research Network
rigid sleep p.
spiritual p.
standard p.
traditional p.

practice-based learning and improvement

practiced task

practicing period

practitioner
p. data bank
general psychiatric p.
mental health p.
nurse p.

NOTES

P

practitioner *(continued)*
primary care p.
psychiatric p.
psychodynamic p.
praecocissima
dementia p.
praecox
dementia p.
ejaculatio p.
heboid p.
neurasthenia p.
predementia p.
pubertas p.
senium p.
pragmatagnosia
pragmatamnesia
pragmatic
p. aphasia
p. level
p. structure
p. text
pragmatism
prameha
sukra p.
pranayama
praxiology
praxis
ideokinetic p.
prayer
healing p.
prayerful life
PRE
partial reinforcement effect
preadaptive attitude
preadolescence
preambivalence
preambivalent phase
prearchaic thinking
preataxic
preattachment stage
precausal thinking
precaution
assault p.
elopement p.
suicide p.
preceding association
precentral
p. seizure
p. sulcus
precept
moral p.
precipice
precipitant
precipitate
precipitating
p. crisis
p. of epilepsy
p. event
p. factor
p. stress
p. tremor
precipitous
p. cognitive decline
p. mood shift
precision
law of p.
p. therapy
preclinical
p. medicine
p. observation
p. stage
precocious
p. aging
p. puberty
p. sexual interest
precocity
islet of p.
precognition
preconcept
preconceptual stage
precondition
preconscious
p. level
p. thinking
preconsciousness
precontemplation
preconvulsive
precuneus
precursor load strategy
predation
predator
sexual p.
sexually violent p.
predatory
p. delinquent
p. violence
predecessor
phylogenetic p.
predelay reinforcement
predementia praecox
predestination
predeterminism
predicate thinking
predictability
establish p.
predictable
predictably
prediction
clinical p.
p. of dangerousness
p. of mortality
p. study
violence p.
predictive
p. characteristic
p. factor
p. power
p. property

p. relationship
p. validity
p. value

predictor
early p.
independent p.
peritraumatic p.
pharmacological p.
psychometric p.
suicide p.
symptom-related p.
p. variable

predispose

predisposed
p. individual
situationally p.

predisposing
p. factor
p. socioculture factors for violence
p. vulnerability

predisposition
p. to attachment
biologic p.
fundamental p.
genetic p.
p. to suicidal act
suicide p.

predominant
p. affect
p. current defense level
p. feature
p. mood disturbance
p. symptom presentation

predominate

predormital sleep paralysis

predormitum

preemployment drug screening

preemptive violence

preepisode status

preexisting
p. condition
p. dementia
p. emotional problem
p. illness
p. mental disorder
p. mental disorder symptom
p. representation
p. seizure disorder
p. symptom
p. tremor
p. underlying emotional issue

preference
color p.
conditioned place p. (CPP)
delayed-phase p.
eye p.
food p.
hand p.
paraphiliac p.
partner p.
risk p.
sexual p.

preferential occupancy

preferred
least p.
p. method
p. provider organization
p. representational system

prefrontal
p. cortex
p. cortex activation
p. cortex of brain
p. cortical activity dysregulation
p. cortical area
p. cortical volume
p. flow
p. hyperactivity
p. hypermetabolism
p. hypofunction
p. lobe
p. lobotomy
p. metabolism
p. region
p. sonic treatment (PST)

pregabalin

pregenital
p. factor
p. love
p. organization
p. phase
p. stage

pregnancy
accidental p.
adolescent p.
anxiety during p.
p. and birth complication
depression during p.
false p.
p. fear
hysterical p.
p. loss
planned p.
psychosis in p.
psychosis during p.
termination of p.
unplanned p.

NOTES

P

pregnancy *(continued)*
untimely p.
unwanted p.
voluntary interruption of p. (VIP)
pregnant smoker
preindustrial
prejudice
age p.
ethnic p.
expression of p.
lifestyle p.
radical p.
roots of p.
preliminary analysis
prelingual deafness
preliterate
prelogical
p. mind
p. thinking
Premack principle
premaniacal
premarital
p. counseling
p. sex
prematura
alopecia p.
premature
p. alopecia
p. birth
p. confrontation
p. death
p. discharge
p. ejaculation
p. ejaculation psychosexual dysfunction
p. female orgasm
p. male orgasm
prematurity
premeditated violent behavior
premeditation
lack of p.
level of p.
premenopausal amenorrhea
premenstrual
p. dysphoria
p. dysphoric disorder (PMDD)
p. syndrome (PMS)
p. tension
p. tension state
p. tension syndrome (PMTS)
premigration stressor
premise
premium
incitement p.
premonition of seizure
premonitory
p. feeling
p. sigh
p. sign
p. symptom
p. urge
premorality
premorbid
p. ability
p. adjustment
p. asociality
p. inferiority feeling (PIF)
p. intellectual function
p. level of functioning
p. personality
p. personality trait
p. psychiatric history
p. state
p. trauma
premotor
p. area
p. syndrome
prenatal
p. alcoholism
p. anxiety
P. Determinants of Schizophrenia Study
p. exposure to alcohol
p. history
p. illicit drug use
p. period
p. smoking
prenubile
preoccupation
appearance p.
p. of bodily functions
control p.
death p.
defect p.
delusion-like p.
gambling p.
homicidal p.
hypochondriacal p.
intense p.
list p.
obsessive p.
orderliness p.
organization p.
pathologic p.
perfection p.
perfectionism p.
rule p.
schedule p.
sexual p.
stalker p.
suicidal p.
p. of thought
unshakable p.
p. with appearance
p. with death
p. with defect
p. with detail
p. with guilt

p. with sameness
p. with worthlessness
preoccupied
excessively p.
preoedipal
p. factor
p. level
p. phase
p. stage
preoperational
p. development
p. phase
p. thinking
p. thought
p. thought period
p. thought stage
preorgasmic
preparalytic
preparation
academic p.
antipsychotic p.
atypical antipsychotic p.
depot antipsychotic p.
drug p.
herbal p.
marijuana p.
poor academic p.
split-brain p.
preparedness
anxiety p.
principle of p.
prephallic
preponderance of evidence
prepotent
prepsychotic
p. pain
p. personality
p. psychosis
p. schizophrenia
prepubertal
p. borderline psychosis
p. child
p. children
p. mania
p. psychopathology
prepuberty
prepubescent
prepulse inhibition
preputial sensation
presbyophrenia
presbyophrenic psychosis
presbyosmia
preschizophrenic ego
preschool child
preschooler
depressed p.
prescience
prescribed treatment
prescribing
p. consultant
p. privilege
prescription (Rx)
p. drug
p. drug abuse
p. drug addiction
p. drug dependence
p. drug-related disorder
p. forgery
p. medication
prescription-only medicine (POM)
prescriptive authority
preselection
sex p.
presence of frenzy
presenile
p. dementia
p. dementia confusional state
p. mental disorder
p. organic psychotic state
p. paraphrenia
p. psychosis
presenilis
alopecia p.
anxietas p.
dementia p.
presenility
presenium
present
p. distress
p. illness (PI)
p. oriented
present-absent dichotomy
presentation
atypical p.
catatonic p.
clinical p.
conversion disorder with mixed p.
depressed p.
distinct depressed p.
distinct dysphoric p.
distinct euphoric p.
dysphoric p.
equivalent symptomatic p.
euphoric p.
general p.
heterogeneous clinical p.

NOTES

presentation *(continued)*
historical p.
histrionic p.
mixed p.
pain p.
predominant symptom p.
psychotic p.
substance-induced p.
subthreshold p.
symptom p.
symptomatic p.
typical p.
presentational ritual
presenting
p. characteristic
p. personality
p. psychopathology
p. symptom
preservation of affect
President's New Freedom Commission on Mental Health
PRESS
point-resolved spectroscopy
press
environmental p.
pressing thought
pressure
acoustic p.
ambient air p.
p. anesthesia
blood p.
cerebral perfusion p. (CPP)
cerebrospinal p.
cranial perfusion p. (CPP)
environmental p.
group p.
p. of ideas
intracranial p. (ICP)
job p.
mental p.
minimal audible p.
p. palsy
p. paralysis
peer p.
p. point
p. sense
social p.
p. of speech
systolic p. (SP)
thought p.
time p.
pressured
p. behavior
p. speech
pressure-volume index
prestige suggestion
presumed
p. causality
p. etiology
presumption
p. of competence
tender years p.
presumptive basis
presuperego phase
presupposition
presynaptic
p. functional deficit
p. neuron
pretense
false p.
pretraumatic
p. risk factor
p. vulnerability
pretreatment
p. binding potential
p. measure
prevalence
cross-sectional p.
differential p.
gambling p.
lifetime p.
period p.
point p.
p. rate
suicide p.
prevalent
prevention
accident p.
alcohol relapse p.
American Foundation for Suicide P.
anxiety p.
Centers for Disease Control and P.
cognitive response p.
disease p.
dropout prediction and p. (DPP)
p. and early intervention program for psychosis
exposure and response p. (ERP)
new age suicide p.
Office of Juvenile Justice and Delinquency P.
primary p.
relapse p.
response p.
ritual p.
secondary p.
stress p.
suicide p.
P. of Suicide in Primary Care Elderly: Collaborative Study (PROSPECT)
tertiary p.
p. and treatment of depression (PTD)
violence p.
preventive
p. intervention

p. medicine
p. psychiatry

preverbal attentional processing

previous
p. attempt
p. detoxification
p. history
p. suicide behavior
p. treatment

previously stabilizing social situation

prewiring

PRH
postrelevant history

priapism

pride
brute p.
domesticated p.
excessive p.
moral p.
penis p.
phallic p.
p. in self
p. system

priest

primacy
complete genital p.
early genital p.
genital p.
oral p.
phallic p.

prima donna

primal
p. anxiety
p. fantasy
p. father
p. libido
p. repression
p. sadism
p. scene
p. scream
p. scream therapy
p. trauma

primary
p. active compound
p. affective disorder (PAD)
p. affective witzelsucht
p. afferent neuron
p. amentia
p. anesthesia
p. anxiety
p. anxiety disorder
p. auditory cortex
p. autism
p. autonomous function
p. behavior
p. behavior disorder
p. care
p. care evaluation of mental disorder (PRIME-MD)
p. caregiver
p. care patient population
p. care physician
p. care practitioner
p. care provider (PCP)
p. care setting
p. caretaker
p. circular reaction
p. color
p. complaint
p. defense symptom
p. degenerative dementia (PDD)
p. degenerative dementia of Alzheimer type (PDDAT)
p. diagnosis
p. disorder of sleep
p. disorder of wakefulness
p. drive
p. dysthymia
p. effect
p. efficacy outcome
p. encopresis
p. enduring negative symptom
p. feeble-mindedness
p. gain
p. generalized epilepsy
p. hue
p. hypersomnia
p. hypersomnia, recurrent type
p. ictal automatism
p. identification
p. identity
p. impotence
p. insomnia
p. integration
p. language
p. mechanism
p. memory
p. mental ability
p. mental image
p. mood disorder
p. motivation
p. motor deficit
p. narcissism
p. need
p. neurasthenia
p. nocturnal enuresis

NOTES

primary *(continued)*
p. nonenduring negative symptom
p. object-love
p. oppositional attitude
p. orgasmic dysfunction
p. personality trait
p. pharmacological approach
p. prevention
p. process thinking
p. progressive aphasia
p. psychiatric disorder
p. psychiatrist
p. psychic process
p. purpose
p. quality
p. reinforcement
p. reinforcer
p. repression
p. responsibility
p. retarded ejaculation
p. reward conditioning
p. risk factor
p. schizophrenia
p. and secondary control enhancement training (PASCET)
p. seizure
p. senile dementia
p. sensation
p. sensory cortex
p. sex characteristic
p. sexual deviation
p. sexual relationship
p. shock
p. sleep disorder
p. somatic problem
p. stress
p. support group
p. syphilis
p. task
p. thought disorder
p. tic
p. transitional object
p. victim
p. zone
primary-secondary distinction
prime of life
PRIME-MD
primary care evaluation of mental disorder
priming
p. dose
p. memory
primitive
p. aggressive self-organization (PASO)
p. drive
p. emotional level
p. idealization
p. narcissism
p. psychosomatic language
p. reflex
p. superego
primitivization
primordial
p. delusion
p. panic
primrose
evening p.
evening p.
primum non nocere
principal
p. diagnosis
p. focus
p. investigation
p. objective
p. symptom
p. trauma
principal-component analysis (PCA)
principle
anticipatory maturation p.
p. of anticipatory maturation
authority p.
binary p.
Bolam p.
p. of Buddhist meditation
closure p.
communion p.
consistency p.
disuse p.
dynamic p.
p. of dynamic polarization
echo p.
economic p.
epigenetic p.
ethical p.
homeopathic p.
homeostatic p.
p. of inertia
intimacy p.
isopathic p.
least-effort p.
moral p.
morality of self-accepted moral p.
nirvana p.
normalization p.
optimal stimulation p.
organizing p.
pain p.
pain-pleasure p.
Peter p.
phylogenetic p.
pleasure p.
pleasure-pain p.
Premack p.
p. of preparedness
psychophysiologic p.
reality p.
rebus p.

repetition-compulsion p.
self-chosen ethical p.
talion p.
Tarasoff p.
transfer of p.'s
treble safeguard p.
p. of truth telling
utilitarian p.
von Domarus p.
weighted-harm p.
wellness p.

principlism

prion
p. analog
p. disease

prior
p. to admission (PTA)
p. violence

priori
p. approach
p. expectation of gratitude

prioritize

pris
parti p.

prison
p. confinement
p. disciplinary infraction
Federal Bureau of P.'s
p. history
in p.
p. inmate
maximum-security p.
p. neurosis
p. population
p. psychiatry
p. psychologist
p. psychosis
p. sentence

prisoner
maximum-security p.
medium-security p.
minimum-security p.
p. privileges
p. of war (POW)

prisoner-of-war
p.-o.-w. experience
p.-o.-w. syndrome

Pritikin diet

privacy
p. clearinghouse
p. compliance
erosion of p.
invasion of p.
p. right

private
p. agony
p. belief system
p. psychiatric hospital
p. psychosis

privilege
bathroom p.
lost p.'s (LP)
prescribing p.
prisoner p.'s
psychotherapist-patient p.
testimonial p.

privileged
p. communication
p. information

p.r.n., PRN
as needed

PRO
peer review organization

proactive
p. coping
p. inhibition (PI)

proapoptotic gene expression

probabilistic fashion

probability
conditional p.
p. curve
p. learning
transitional p.

probable error (PE)

proband
adult-onset p.
autistic p.
p. condition
p. diagnosis
p. method
p. status

probation
p. officer
special needs p.
standard p.
p. status
supervised p.
p. violation

probe
indirect p.
radiolabeled p.

problem
academic p.
acculturation p.
acute sleep p.

NOTES

P

problem *(continued)*
addiction-related p.
affect intensity p.
aggregation p.
alcohol p.
alcohol-related physical p.
alcohol-related psychiatric p.
arithmetic p.
p. at home
attention p.
attentional p.
behavior p.
p. behavior cluster
boundary p.
p. child
p. of childhood
communication p.
concentration-related p.
conceptual p.
concurrent psychiatric p.'s
conduct p.
core p.
court-related p.
daily record of severity of p.'s (DRSP)
developmental learning p. (DLP)
Diagnosis and Remediation of Handwriting P.'s
disciplinary p.
p. drinker (PD)
p. drinking
emotional p.
employment p.
enduring p.
environmental p.
faith conversion p.
familial aggregation p.
feeding p.
fundamental conceptual p.
fundamental psychometric p.
gait p.
p. gambler
human p.
hyperactivity p.
identity p.
impulse control p.
p. initiating sleep
International Statistical Classification of Diseases and Related Health P.'s
interpersonal cognitive p.
interpersonal relationship p.
language p.
learning p.
legal p.
life circumstance p.
p. maintaining sleep
marital p.
medical p.
mind-body p.
nuclear p.
occupational p.
orgasmic p.
other interpersonal p.'s
p. parent
parental control p.
parental marital p.
parent-child relational p.
partner relational p.
p. patient
personality p.
pervasive p.
phase-of-life p.
philosophical p.
physical p.
postpartum psychiatric p.
preexisting emotional p.
primary somatic p.
psychiatric p.
psychological p.
psychometric p.
psychophysiological p.
psychosexual p.
psychosocial p.
questioning faith p.
real-life p.
p. related to abuse
p. related to neglect
relational p.
relationship p.
religious or spiritual p.
retrieval p.
p. in school
school discipline p.
school entering p.
secondary emotional p.
sibling relational p.
sleep p.
social p.
p. solving
somatic p.
stress-related psychophysiological p.
substance-related legal p.
subtle memory p.
unemployment p.
word-finding p.
workplace p.

problematic
p. Internet use
p. sexual behavior

problem-based learning

problem-focused coping

problem-oriented record (POR)

problem-solving
p.-s. communication
failure of p.-s.
group p.-s.
inductive p.-s.

interpersonal cognitive p.-s. (ICPS)
p.-s. negotiation
rational p.-s.
p.-s. skills
p.-s. skills training
p.-s. strategy
p.-s. style
p.-s. task
visuospatial problem p.-s.

procedural
p. learning task
p. memory

procedure
acquaintanceship p.
age correction p.
analysis p.
assessment p.
attention focusing p.
aversive smoking p.
blocking p.
carotid Amytal p. (CAP)
civil commitment p.
clinical p.
commitment p.
Committee on Standards and Survey P.'s
decremental p.
diagnostic p.
Dunnett-Hsu p.
functional pragmatic p.
Mitofsky-Waksberg random digit dialing p.
prototype matching p.
psychological p.
Q-Sort p.
rating p.
recording p.
response-driven p.
Shedler-Western Assessment P.-200 (SWAP-200)
standard rating p.
surgical p.
SWAP-200 assessment p.
test orientation p. (TOP)
time-out p.

proceeding
care and protection p.
incompetency p.
protection p.

process
action group p.
active pathophysiologic p.
adaptive p.
adjustment p.
affective p.
age-related developmental p.
analytical p.
automatic psychological p.
biologic p.
bizarre thought p.
brain p.
central timing p.
children's language p.'s
circumstantial thought p.
closure p.
cognitive p.
collaborative treatment p.
common central p.
complex learning p.
comprehensive identification p. (CIP)
computational p.
concrete thought p.
conscious p.
consciously accessible p.
consciously inaccessible p.
counseling p.
cultural p.
decision-making p.
declarative memory p.
defensive p.
dementia p.
dementing p.
deterioration p.
developmental p.
diagnostic p.
disease p.
disorganized thought p.
disruption of thought p.
due p.
egocentric thought p.
elementary p.
p. of elimination
emotional memory p.
emotive p.
empirical p.
environmental p.
ergotropic p.
evidence-based p.
excitatory-inhibitory p.
executive p.
explicit p.
family p.
fantasy p.
feature contrast p.

NOTES

P

process *(continued)*
feeling of being detached from one's mental p.'s
free access to p.'s
fundamental cognitive p.
fundamental response p.
goal-oriented p.
group p.
harmony p.
healing p.
higher mental p.
identification p.
idiosyncratic p.
imaginable p.
imaginal p.
implicit p.
information input p.
intentional p.
interpersonal p.
intracellular metabolic p.
p. issue
judicial p.
linear thought p.
p. mania
memory p.
mental p.
metabolic p.
motivational p.
motoric reproduction p.
neurocognitive p.
neurodegenerative p.
neurodevelopmental telencephalic ontogenic p.
neuronal p.
neurotic p.
nicotine reinforcement p.
normative aging p.
ongoing cognitive p.
ontogenic p.
pathologic p.
pathophysiologic p.
perceptual p.
personality p.
physiologic p.
primary psychic p.
psychobiological p.
psychological p.
p. psychosis
psychosocial p.
psychotic p.
reactivation p.
revision p.
p. schizophrenia
schizophrenic p.
secondary p.
secondary psychic p.
self-limited p.
semantic p.
sensory p.
separation-individuation p.
social p.
stress-illness p.
switch p.
systematic p.
therapeutic p.
p. thinking
thought p.
transition p.
unconscious p.
withdrawal p.
processed cocaine
processing
affective p.
affect-related p.
altered tau p.
p. area
attentional p.
attention-information p.
auditory p.
cognitive p.
context p.
declarative emotional memory p.
p. disorder
distributed p.
emotional information p.
emotional memory p.
higher integrative language p.
information p.
language p.
lexical p.
lexicosemantic p.
memory p.
normal affective p.
parallel p.
phonological p.
preverbal attentional p.
psycholinguistic p.
receptive language p.
semantic p.
serial p.
speech p.
speed of p.
tau p.
p. time
unconscious p.
visual p.
visuospatial p.
word p.
procognitive
procrastination
proctoparalysis
proctoplegia
proctospasm
procursiva
aura p.
procursive
p. chorea
p. epilepsy

procyclidine
prodigy
child p.
idiot p.
prodromal
p. condition
p. episode
p. period
p. phase
p. phase of schizophrenia
p. psychotic symptom
p. sign
prodrome, pl. **prodromata, prodromes**
dementia p.
p. of psychosis
visual p.
product
end p.
nicotine replacement p.
nutriceutical p.
production
divergent p.
emotion p.
language comprehension and p.
word p.
productive
p. love
p. personality
p. symptoms
p. thinking
productivity of thought
product-moment correlation
proenkephalin
profanity
profession
medical p.
professional
allied health p.
p. burnout
child mental health p.
p. code
p. counselor
p. criticism
p. dishonesty
p. distance
p. ethics
p. exploiter
p. gambler
p. gambling
health p.
p. help
medical p.
mental health p.
mental healthcare p.
p. negligence
p. neurasthenia
p. neurosis
p. patient syndrome
P. Standards Review Organization (PSRO)
professional-family relation
proficiency
profile
adaptability p.
anxiety p.
behavioral deviancy p.
clinical p.
criminal p.
development p.
diagnostic p.
employment p.
high p.
inhibition p.
left-out sibling p.
low p.
metapsychological p.
mood p.
p. of mood states (POMS)
neurotic direction p.
personality disorder p.
psychodiagnostic p.
psychotic direction p.
Q-score p.
risk p.
risk-benefit p.
sibling p.
side effect drug p.
spiked p.
structural p.
symptom p.
terrorist p.
therapeutic p.
trait p.
validity indicator p.
Wheatley stress p.
work personality p.
profile-revised
psychoeducational p.-r. (PEP-R)
profiling
ethnic p.
racial p.
terrorist p.
profound
p. amnesia
p. anxiety
p. dementia

NOTES

profound *(continued)*
p. idiocy
p. lethargy
p. mental subnormality
p. sadness
p. shame
profoundly retarded
prognosis (Px, px)
direction p.
extent p.
poor p.
prognostic
p. status
p. value
program
alcohol treatment p.
p. of assertive community treatment (PACT)
behavior modification p.
career planning p. (CPP)
chemical dependency p.
child and adolescent fear and anxiety treatment p.
clinical intervention p.
coercion p.
College Outcome Measures P.
community-based psychiatric p.
community outreach p.
community psychiatry p. (CPP)
community treatment and reintegration p.
comparative guidance and placement p. (CGPP)
cooperative institutional research p. (CIRP)
daycare p.
day treatment p.
detoxification p.
development p.
Dole-Nyswauder p.
drug abuse rehabilitation p.
drug court p.
drug-free p.
dual diagnosis p.
DUF p.
educational p.
enhanced standard methadone maintenance treatment p.
enrichment p.
entitlement p.
fast-track p.
Frostig-Horne training p.
GROW The Marriage Enrichment P.
Head Start p.
individual p.
individualized education p.
infant stimulation p.
intensive day treatment p.
jail-based treatment p.
jail diversion p.
long-term detoxification p.
long-term mental health p.
maintenance treatment p.
mentoring p.
methadone maintenance treatment p.
multicomponent p.
outpatient p.
outreach p.
PAR admissions testing p.
parent therapist p.
pilot p.
research p.
residential OCD p.
reward-and-punishment p.
standard methadone maintenance treatment p.
12-step p.
supported employment p.
tertiary intervention p.
therapeutic p.
Transformational Leadership Development P.
transitional p.
treatment p.
Treatment of Depression Collaborative Research P.
weight-control p.
weight-loss p.
work-study p.
programmed
p. practice
p. therapy
programming
genotypic p.
neurolinguistic p.
progredient neurosis
progress
p. chart
treatment p.
progression
behavioral characteristics p.
dementia p.
obstinate p.
symptom p.
symptomatic p.
progressiva
dementia paratonia p.
dysbasia lordotica p.
dyssynergia cerebellaris p.
paratonia p.
progressive
p. assimilation
p. bulbar paralysis
p. cerebellar tremor
p. degenerative subcortical encephalopathy
p. dementia

p. dementing illness
p. deterioration
p. disability
p. disease
p. education
p. hepatolenticular degeneration
p. lingual hemiatrophy
p. muscular relaxation
p. paratonia
p. paratonia dementia
p. psychosis
p. teleologic regression
p. torsion spasm
p. traumatic encephalopathy

prohormone

project
adolescent diversion p.
Aptitude Research P. (ARP)
Harvard-Brown Anxiety Disorders Research P. (HARP)
Healthy Lesbian, Gay, and Bisexual Students P. (HLGBSP)
Human Genome P.
Iowa Case Management P.
live in the p.
Manchester and Salford self-harm p.
Menninger Clinic Treatment Intervention P.
methamphetamine treatment p.
National Mental Illness Screening P.
Oregon Adolescent Depression P.
Stony Brook High Risk P.

projected jealousy

projection
applied extrasensory p.
astral p.
p. defense mechanism
delusional p.
dopamine p.
eccentric p.
extrasensory p. (ESP)
impersonal p.
maximum-intensity p.
minimum-intensity p.
p. neuron
optical p.
retrospective p.
ventral amygdaloid fugal p.

projectional paranoia

projective
p. identification
p. personality assessment
p. technique

prolactin
p. elevation
p. release

proliferation
T-cell p.

Prolixin decanoate

prolongata
alalia p.

prolongation

prolongatus
coitus p.

prolonged
p. depressive reaction
p. exposure
p. grief
p. grief reaction
p. nocturnal sleep
p. nocturnal sleep episode
p. posttraumatic stress disorder
p. prodrome of schizophrenia
p. sadness
p. sedation
p. separation
p. situational depression
p. sleep latency
p. sleep therapy
p. sleep treatment
p. transition to fully awake state

prominent
p. anxiety
p. aspect
p. deterioration
p. grimacing
p. hallucination
p. irritable mood
p. mood symptom
p. narcissistic dynamic
p. phobic anxiety component

promiscuity
conjugal consequence of p.
ego-dystonic p.
protracted p.
sexual p.

promiscuous
p. act
p. sex
p. sexual behavior

promise
broken p.
false p.

promotion neurosis

NOTES

P

proneness to addiction
prone to relapse
pronoun
anaphoric p.
pronounced improvement
proof
forensic p.
incontrovertible p.
obvious p.
p. of paternity
scientific p.
proopiomelanocortin
propaganda
propellant
aerosol p.
propensity for depression
proper
p. burial
ego p.
p. repression
property
affective p.
aggression against p.
anticholinergic p.
p. damage
destruction of p.
p. destruction
field p.
hebbian p.
pharmacological p.
predictive p.
psychometric p.
receptor-binding p.
reinforcing p.
sedative p.
social p.
thermoregulatory p.
thermosensory p.
prophase
prophecy
self-fulfilling p.
prophetic dream
prophylactic treatment
prophylaxis
pharmacologic p.
propionic acidemia
propizepine
proportion
delusional p.
p. of survivors affected (PSA)
proposition
intrusive sexual p.
propositional learning
propositus
propriem
proprioception
proprioceptive
p. feedback
p. perception
p. sensation
p. sensibility
propulsion
proscription
religious p.
prosocial
p. behavior
p. motivation
prosodic feature
prosody
prosopagnosia
prosopalgia
prosopodiplegia
prosoponeuralgia
prosopoplegia
prosopospasm
PROSPECT
Prevention of Suicide in Primary Care Elderly: Collaborative Study
prospective
p. experimental study design
p. memory
p. study
prospermia
ProStep
prosternation
prosthesis, pl. **prostheses**
behavioral p.
NeuroCybernetics P. (NCP)
penile p.
prosthetic device
prostrate
prostration
protagonist
protanope
protease
protected file
protection
p. factor
p. proceeding
protective
p. barrier
p. effect
p. survival strategy
protector
p. identity
p. role
protein
agouti-related p.
alpha synuclein p.
amyloid precursor p.
beta amyloid p.
cAMP response element binding p.
cholesteryl ester transfer p.
growth-associated p. (GAP)
heat shock p. 90 (hsp90)
heterotrimeric G p.
human cell death p.
hyperphosphorylated tau p.

p. kinase C (PKC)
N p.
signal-transducing guanine-nucleotide binding p.
tau p.
ubiquitin p.
protensity
proteome image
protest
body p.
masculine p.
p. psychosis
Protestant
P. Christian religion
white Anglo-Saxon P. (WASP)
proteus maze
prothipendyl
prothymia
protocol
close observation p.
elopement p.
interview p.
Managed Care Appropriateness P.
surveillance p.
test p.
treatment p.
protomasochism
protopathic sensibility
protophallic
protoplasmic
protospasm
prototaxic mode
prototype
borderline diagnosis p.
diagnostic p.
p. matching
p. matching procedure
schizoid diagnostic p.
prototypical
p. course pattern
p. schizophrenia
protracta
catatonia p.
protracted
p. detoxification
p. difficulty
p. promiscuity
p. reactive paranoid psychosis
p. withdrawal syndrome
protrusion
tongue p.
proverb interpretation
provider
general medical p.
medical p.
mental health p.
primary care p. (PCP)
Provigil
provisional diagnosis
proviso
parapathetic p.
provocation
aggression without p.
minimal p.
pharmacological p.
sexual p.
provocative
p. behavior
p. clowning
p. diagnosis
p. stimulus
provoked
p. anxiety
easily p.
provoking
p. stimulus
thought p.
prowess
sexual p.
proxemic
proxibarbal
proximal receptor
proximity
mother-infant p.
proximoataxia
proxy
p. directive
factitious disorder by p.
factitious illness by p.
healthcare p.
Munchausen disease by p.
Munchausen syndrome by p.
posttraumatic stress disorder by p.
p. symptom
proxy-for-deficit syndrome
Prozac Weekly
prude
prudery
prudish
pruritic psychosomatic disorder
pruritus
generalized p.
psychogenic p.
PS
psychiatric

NOTES

PSA
proportion of survivors affected
PSAN, PSAn, PsAn
psychoanalysis
psychoanalyst
PSE
point of subjective equality
portosystemic encephalopathy
psellism
pseudagraphia, pseudoagraphia
pseudaphia
pseudesthesia, pseudoesthesia
pseudoaddiction
pseudoaggression
pseudoagrammatism
pseudoagraphia (*var. of* pseudagraphia)
pseudoaltruism
pseudoamnesia
pseudoapoplexy
pseudoapraxia
pseudo as-if
pseudoataxia
pseudoathetosis
pseudoauthenticity
pseudoautosomal locus for schizophrenia
pseudocatatonia
traumatic p.
pseudochorea
pseudochromesthesia
pseudoclonus
pseudocollusion
pseudocoma
pseudocombat fatigue
pseudocommunity
pseudoconvulsion
pseudocyesis syndrome
pseudodebility
pseudodelirium
pseudodementia
depressive p.
hysterical p.
pseudodepression
pseudoesthesia (*var. of* pseudesthesia)
pseudofeeblemindedness
pseudoflexibilitas
pseudogeusesthesia
pseudogeusia
pseudogiftedness
pseudo-Graefe sign
pseudographia
pseudohallucination
ego-dystonic p.
image p.
manipulative p.
pseudohermaphrodite
pseudohermaphroditism
pseudohomosexual
pseudohypersexuality
pseudohypertrophic muscular paralysis
pseudohypnotics
pseudoidentification
pseudoillusion
pseudoimbecility
pseudoinsomnia
pseudointoxication
pseudolalia
pseudolobulated
pseudologia fantastica
pseudologue
pseudomalignancy
pseudomania
pseudomasturbation
pseudomelancholia
pseudomelia paraesthetica
pseudomeningitis
pseudomnesia
pseudomotivation
pseudonarcotic
pseudonarcotism
pseudonecrophilia
pseudoneurogenic bladder
pseudoneuroma
pseudoneurotic schizophrenia
pseudonomania
pseudonym
pseudonymity
pseudonymous
pseudoparalysis
congenital atonic p.
pseudoparameter
pseudoparanoia
pseudoparaplegia
pseudoparesis
alcoholic p.
pseudoparkinsonism
pseudopellagra
pseudoperitonitis
pseudopersonality
pseudophotesthesia
pseudoplegia
pseudopsia
pseudopsychopathic schizophrenia
pseudopsychosis
pseudoquerulant
pseudoreminiscence
pseudorosette
pseudosauthenticity
pseudoschizophrenia
pseudoscience
pseudosclerosis
Westphal p.
pseudoseizure
pseudosenility
pseudosexuality
pseudosmia
pseudosocial personality disorder
pseudosphresia

pseudotabes
pupillotonic p.
pseudothrill
pseudotransference
pseudotumor
pseudoventricle
pseudovomiting
PSG
polysomnogram
polysomnograph
P&SH
personal and social history
PSI
psychosomatic inventory
psi
p. phenomenon
p. system
psilocybin dependence
PsiTri registry
psittacism
PSMed
psychosomatic medicine
psopholalia
PSP
postsynaptic potential
PSRO
Professional Standards Review Organization
PSS
psychiatric services section
PST
prefrontal sonic treatment
PSUD
psychoactive substance use disorder
PSV
psychological, social, and vocational
Psy, psy
psychiatry
psychology
psych
psychiatry
psychagogy
psychalgia, psychalgalia
psychalgic
psychalia
psychanopsia
psychasthene
psychasthenia
compulsive p.
mixed compulsive states p.
obsession p.
psychasthenic
p. delirium
p. neurosis
psychataxia
psyche
contrasexual component of p.
national p.
psycheclampsia
psychedelia
psychedelic
p. agent
p. agent dependence
p. therapy
psychehormic
psycheism
psychelytic
psychentonia
psychephoric
psycheplastic
psycherhexic
psychezymic
psychiatric, psychiatrics (PS)
p. admission
p. anaphylaxis
p. assessment
p. assistant
p. care
p. case register
p. chemistry
p. clinician
p. comorbid disorder
p. comorbidity
p. complication
p. condition
p. conflict
p. consequence
p. consult
p. consultation
p. CPT code
p. criterion
p. data
p. deviance
p. diagnosis
p. disability
p. disease
p. disorder associated with alcoholism
p. disorders in elderly
p. disturbance
p. education
p. effect
p. emergency
p. emergency department

NOTES

P

psychiatric *(continued)*
p. emergency service (PES)
p. emergency team (PET)
p. epidemiologist
p. epidemiology
p. evaluation
p. evidence
p. examination
p. facility
p. family history
p. genetics
p. ghetto
p. help
p. hospital
p. hospitalization
p. illness
p. inpatient
p. intensive care unit (PICU)
p. intervention
p. interview
p. manifestation
p. medication
p. morbidity
p. nomenclature
p. nosology
p. nurse
p. parameter
p. patient
p. patient assault
p. practitioner
p. problem
p. rationale
p. referral
p. research
p. researcher
p. risk
p. risk factor
p. sequela of terrorism
p. services section (PSS)
p. setting
p. severity
p. severity rating
p. social work
p. social worker
P. Society for Informatics
p. somatic therapy
p. statistic
p. symptom
p. syndrome
p. system interface disorder
p. technician
p. testimony
p. treatment
p. trend
p. unit
p. variable
p. ward

psychiatrically disabled

psychiatrism

psychiatrist
academic p.
American Academy of Clinical P.'s (AACP)
American Association of Community P.'s
American Association of General Hospital P.'s
American Board of Forensic P.'s (ABFP)
American College of P.'s (ACP)
Arab Federation of P.'s
Association for Child P.'s
Barbados Association of P.'s
biologic p.
board certified p.
board eligible p.
child p.
clinical p.
Commission on Psychotherapy by P.'s
consulting p.
court-appointed p.
forensic p.
geriatric p.
liaison p.
National Guild of Catholic P.'s (NGCP)
primary p.
psychodynamic p.
Royal College of P.'s (RCP)

psychiatrize

psychiatry (Psy, psy, psych)
academic p.
Academy of Organizational and Occupational P. (AOOP)
addiction p.
administrative p.
Administrators in Academic P. (AAP)
adolescent p.
adulthood p.
American Academy of Addiction P. (AAAP)
American Academy of Child and Adolescent P. (AACAP)
American Academy of Psychoanalysis and Dynamic P. (AAPDP)
American Association of Chairmen of Departments of P.
American Association of Emergency P.
American Association of Emergency P.
American Association for Geriatric P. (AAGP)
American Board of P. (ABP)
American Board of Forensic P.

American College of Forensic P.
American Society for Adolescent P.
analytic p.
Archives of General P.
Association for Academic P.
Association of Directors of Medical Student Education in P. (ADMSEP)
behavioral p.
biologic p.
biological p.
Bolivian Society of P.
British Journal of P.
Canadian Academy of Child P.
child p. (CHP, CP)
child and adolescent p.
clinical p.
Clunis inquiry forensic p.
common sense p.
community p.
comparative p.
consultation p.
consultation-liaison p.
contractual p.
correctional p.
criminal p.
cross-cultural p.
cross-culture p.
Cuban glossary of p.
cultural p.
descriptive p.
disaster p.
dynamic p.
ecological p.
emergency p.
p. emergency team
evidence-based p.
existential p.
experimental p.
folk p.
forensic p.
genetic-dynamic p.
geriatric p.
gerontologic p.
gerontological p.
gestalt p.
Group for Advancement of P. (GAP)
hospital-based p.
hospital and community p.
industrial p.
infant p.
p. inpatient service
International Society for Adolescent P.
interpersonal p.
legal p.
liaison p.
military forensic p.
minority group p.
modern p.
molecular p.
multidisciplinary group p.
National Association of Veterans Affairs Chiefs of P. (NAVACP)
neuropsychiatric p.
North Pacific Society of Neurology, Neurosurgery and P.
occupational p.
old-age p.
organic p.
organized care p.
orthomolecular p.
outpatient-based p.
pastoral p.
pediatric p.
political p.
preventive p.
prison p.
psychoanalytic p.
psychopharmacological p.
public p.
rehabilitation p.
rural p.
social p.
Society of Biological P.
spiritual dimension in p.
Standard System of P. (SSOP)
transcultural p.
urban p.
World Association for Social P. (WASP)
World Congress of P.
World Federation of Biological P.
young adult p.

psychic, psychical
p. ability
p. aftershock
p. akinesia
p. anaphylaxis
p. anxiety
p. apparatus
p. blindness
p. causality
p. censor

NOTES

psychic *(continued)*
p. contagion
p. deafness
p. dependence
p. determinism
p. disorder
p. distress
p. disturbance
p. divorce
p. dualism
p. dysuria
p. energizer
p. energy
p. epilepsy
p. equivalent
p. experience
p. factor
p. force
p. helplessness
p. impotence
p. inertia
p. masturbation
p. numbing
p. numbness
p. ontogeny
p. organization
p. overtone
p. pain
p. paralysis of fixation of gaze
p. phenomenon
p. reality
p. reflex
p. reward
p. scar
p. seizure
p. shock
p. shock syndrome
p. suicide
p. tic
p. trauma
p. vaginismus
p. wound
psychism, psychicism
psychoacoustics
psychoactive
p. chemical
p. drug
p. drug abuse
p. effect
p. ingredient
p. medication
p. substance
p. substance abuse
p. substance abuse disorder
p. substance delirium
p. substance dementia
p. substance dependence
p. substance hallucinosis
p. substance-induced organic mental disorder
p. substance-induced organic syndrome
p. substance intoxication
p. substance use
p. substance use disorder (PSUD)
p. substance withdrawal
psychoaffective disorder (PAD)
psychoalgalia
psychoallergy
psychoanaleptic
psychoanalysis (PA, PSAN, PSAn, PsAn)
active p.
adlerian p.
American Academy of P. (AAP)
applied p.
Association for the Advancement of P. (AAP)
boundaries in p.
classic p.
existential p.
freudian p.
fundamental rule of p.
jungian p.
National Psychological Association for P.
The American Academy of P.
wild p.
psychoanalyst (PA, PSAN, PSAn, PsAn)
medical p.
psychoanalytic, psychoanalytical
p. concept
p. group
p. group psychotherapy
p. interpretation
p. investigation
p. neurosis
p. pathography
p. perspective
p. psychiatry
p. situation
p. technique
p. theory
p. therapy
psychoanalyze
psychoasthenics
psychoauditory
psychobabble
psychobacillosis
psychobioanalysis
psychobiogram
psychobiological, psychobiologic
p. pathway
p. process
p. process of dementia
psychobiology
clinical p.

development p.
objective p.
psychocardiac reflex
psychocatharsis
psychocentric
psychochemistry
psychochrome
psychochromesthesia
psychocoma
psychocortical center
psychocutaneous
psychodiagnosis
psychodiagnostic profile
psychodietetics
psychodometer
psychodometry
psychodrama
American Society of Group Psychotherapy and P. (ASGPP)
form of p.
p. group therapy
psychodramatic
p. catharsis
p. shock
psychodynamic
adaptational p.
p. approach
p. cerebral system
p. clinician
cognitive p.'s
p. concept
p. conflict
p. denial
p. effect
p. formulation
p. group psychotherapy
p. interpretation
p. interpretation and treatment
p. interview
p. origin
p. practitioner
p. psychiatrist
p. research orientation
p. theory
psychodynamic-experiential model
psychodysleptic drug
psychoeducational, psychoeducation
p. evaluation
p. group
p. group therapy
p. profile-revised (PEP-R)
psychoendocrinology
psychoepilepsy
psychoexploration
psychogalvanic
p. reaction
p. reflex (PGR)
p. response (PGR)
p. skin resistance (PGSR)
psychogalvanometer
psychogender
psychogenesis
psychogenetic
psychogenia
psychogenic
p. air hunger
p. alopecia
p. amnesia
p. anxiety
p. aphagia
p. aphasia
p. aspermia (PA)
p. asthenia
p. ataxia
p. backache
p. cardiac nondisease
p. cardiospasm
p. chest pain
p. confusion
p. constipation
p. convulsion
p. cough
p. cyclical vomiting
p. deafness
p. depression
p. depressive psychosis
p. dermatitis
p. diarrhea
p. drug
p. duodenal ulcer
p. dysmenorrhea
p. dyspareunia
p. dyspepsia
p. dystonia
p. dysuria
p. eczema
p. effort syndrome
p. enuresis
p. excitation
p. excoriation
p. fatigue
p. fugue
p. gastric ulcer
p. headache
p. hearing impairment
p. hearing loss

NOTES

psychogenic *(continued)*
- p. hiccup
- p. hyperventilation
- p. illness
- p. impotence
- p. learning disorder
- p. limb disorder
- p. megacolon
- p. motor disorder
- p. muscle disorder
- p. musculoskeletal disorder
- p. neurocirculatory disorder
- p. nocturnal polydipsia (PNP)
- p. nocturnal polydipsia syndrome
- p. obesity
- p. obsessional disorder
- p. oculogyric crisis
- p. origin
- p. overlay
- p. pain disorder
- p. painful coitus
- p. painful erection
- p. painful menstruation
- p. paralysis
- p. paranoid nonorganic psychosis
- p. paranoid psychosis, nonorganic
- p. paroxysmal tachycardia
- p. pelvic pain
- p. penis pain
- p. peptic ulcer
- p. phobic disorder
- p. physical symptom
- p. physiological manifestation
- p. polydipsia
- p. precordial pain
- p. pruritus
- p. purpura syndrome
- p. reaction
- p. respiratory disorder
- p. retention
- p. rheumatic disorder
- p. rumination
- p. seizure
- p. sexual disorder
- p. skin disorder
- p. sleep disorder
- p. stomach disorder
- p. stupor
- p. testicular pain
- p. testis pain
- p. tic
- p. torticollis
- p. tremor
- p. twilight state
- p. urticaria
- p. uterus pain
- p. vertigo
- p. yawning

psychogenous
psychogeny
psychogeriatrics
psychogerontology
psychogeusic
psychognosis, psychognosia
psychognostic
psychogogic
psychogonical
psychogony
psychogram
psychograph
psychographic disturbance
psychography
psychohistory
psychohormonal therapy
psychoimmunology
psychoinfantile personality
psychoinfantilism
psychokinesis, psychokinesia (PK)
psychokinetic (PK)
psychokyme
psycholagny
psycholepsy
psycholeptic episode
psycholinguistic, psycholinguistics
- p. ability
- p. processing
- p. theory

psychological, psychologic
- p. abuse
- p. acculturation
- p. addiction
- p. adjustment
- p. aspect of war
- p. autopsy
- p. autopsy study
- p. basis
- p. birth of human infant
- p. burden
- p. capacity
- p. cause
- p. change
- p. characteristic
- p. concern
- p. consequence
- p. construct
- p. debriefing
- p. defense system
- p. defensiveness
- p. deprivation
- p. description
- p. desensitization
- p. determinant
- p. dissociation
- p. distortion
- p. distress
- p. disturbance
- p. dysfunction
- p. dysfunction symptom

p. effect
p. evaluation
p. examination
p. factor affecting medical condition (PFAMC)
p. factor affecting a mental condition
p. factor affecting physical condition
p. feature
p. field
p. foundation
p. game
p. health
p. impact
p. information, acquisition, processing, and control system (PIAPACS)
p. intervention
p. interview
p. issue
p. loner
p. management
p. marker
p. maturation
p. maturity
p. meaning
p. medicine
p. mindedness
p. model
p. motivation
p. need
p. pain
p. pillow
p. problem
p. procedure
p. process
p. programming therapy
p. rapport
p. reaction
p. refractory period
p. research
p. resource
p. response
p. scar
p. sequela of torture
p. signs and symptoms
p., social, and vocational (PSV)
p. state
p. strain
p. strength
p. stress
p. stress factor
p. suicide
p. syndrome
p. technique
p. testing
p. theory
p. toll
p. toner
p. trait
p. trauma
p. tremor
p. warfare (PW)
p. weakness

psychologically
p. insightful
p. mediated response
p. overwhelming experience
p. stressful

psychological-physiological arousal

psychological-related symptoms

psychologist
Association of Correctional P.'s
child p.
clinical p.
consulting p.
counseling p.
engineering p.
environmental p.
geriatric p.
industrial organizational p.
licensed p.
pediatric p.
personality p.
prison p.
social p.

psychology (Psy, psy)
abnormal p.
p. act
adlerian p.
adolescent p.
advertising p.
American Board of Professional P.
analytic p.
analytical p.
applied p.
atomistic p.
behavioral p.
behaviorism school of p.
behavioristic p.
blame p.
centralist p.
child p. (CP)
clinical p.
cognitive p.

NOTES

P

psychology *(continued)*
community p.
comparative p.
constitutional p.
consumer p.
content p.
correctional p.
counseling p.
courtroom p.
criminal p.
depth p.
developmental p.
dynamic p.
educational p.
ego p.
engineering p.
environmental p.
existential p.
experimental p.
faculty p.
folk p.
forensic p.
functional p.
general p.
genetic p.
geriatric p.
gestalt p.
health p.
health-related p.
holistic p.
human factor p.
humanistic p.
id p.
individual p.
industrial p.
jungian p.
legal p.
mass p.
medical p.
military p.
mob p.
objective p.
organismic p.
organizational p.
pediatric p.
perceptual p.
peripheralist p.
personality p.
personnel p.
philosophical p.
physiologic p.
pop p.
rational p.
p. of scent
social p.
Society for Industrial and Organizational P.
subjective p.
topographical p.
topological p.
transpersonal p.
uprooted p.
victim p.
p. of women

psychomathematics

psychometer

psychometric, psychometrics
p. advantage
p. evaluation
p. measure
p. performance
p. performance characteristic
p. predictor
p. problem
p. property
p. setting
p. standard
p. term
p. testing
p. validity

psychometrically established measure

psychometrician

psychometrics (*var. of* psychometric)

psychometry

psychomimetic

psychomimic syndrome

psychomotility

psychomotor
p. abnormality
p. activity
p. agitation
p. attack
p. behavior
p. change
p. convulsion
p. development
p. disorder
p. disturbance
p. disturbance stress reaction
p. epilepsy
p. excitement
p. fit
p. intelligence
p. measurement
p. overactivity
p. performance
p. phenomenon
p. poverty
p. rehabilitation
p. restlessness
p. retardation
p. seizure
p. slowing
p. speed
p. stimulant
p. stupor
p. symptom

psychoneural parallelism
psychoneuroimmunology (PNI)
psychoneurologist
psychoneurology
psychoneurosis, pl. **psychoneuroses**
- anxiety p.
- battle p.
- climacteric p.
- compensation p.
- compulsion p.
- conversion hysteria p.
- defense p.
- depersonalization p.
- depressive-type p.
- dissociative p.
- dissociative hysteria p.
- hypochondriac p.
- hypochondriacal p.
- hysteria p.
- p. maidica
- mixed p.
- neurasthenic p.
- obsessional p.
- obsessive-compulsive p.
- occupational p.
- paranoid p.
- personality p.
- senile p.

psychoneurotic (PN)
- p. depression
- p. depressive reaction
- p. mental disorder
- p. personality

psychonoetism
psychonomic
psychonomy
psychonosis
psychonosology
psychonoxious
psychooncology
psychooptical reflex control
psychoorganic brain syndrome
psychoparesis
psychopath
- criminal sexual p. (CSP)
- industrial p.
- sexual p.
- workplace p.

psychopathia
- p. partialis
- p. sexualis

psychopathic
- p. constitution
- p. deviance
- p. deviant (PD)
- p. diathesis
- p. inferiority
- p. personality
- p. state
- p. trait

psychopathist
psychopathologic, psychopathological
- p. accompaniment
- p. deterioration
- p. thought

psychopathologist
psychopathology
- acute p.
- adult p.
- child p.
- coexisting p.
- comorbid p.
- disinhibitory p.
- p. of epilepsy
- general adult p.
- global p.
- impulsive-compulsive p.
- p. level
- p. measure
- overall p.
- prepubertal p.
- presenting p.
- related p.
- retardation p.
- p. of retardation
- scientific p.
- stress-related p.
- p. symptom

psychopathosis
psychopathy
- autistic p.
- benign p.
- passive parasitic p.
- sexual p.
- workplace p.

psychopedagogy
psychopetal
psychopharmaceutical intervention
psychopharmacological, psychopharmacologic
- p. agent
- p. intervention
- p. psychiatry
- p. therapy
- p. treatment

psychopharmacologist

NOTES

psychopharmacology
adolescent p.
P. Bulletin
child p.
clinical p.
p. consultation
essential p.
gender-sensitive p.
geriatric p.
pediatric p.
psychophonasthenia
psychophylaxis
psychophysical
p. function
p. parallelism
psychophysics
psychophysiologic
p. correlate
p. disorder
p. manifestation
p. principle
p. reaction
p. response
psychophysiological
p. change
p. insomnia
p. problem
psychophysiology
psychoplegia
psychoplegic
psychopneumatology
psychoprophylactic treatment
psychoprophylaxis
psychoreaction
psychorelaxation
psychorhythm
psychorhythmia
psychormic
psychosedation
psychosedative
psychosensorial
psychosensory
p. aphasia
p. epilepsy
p. stimulus
p. symptom
psychose passionelle
psychoses (*pl. of* psychosis)
psychosexual
p. development
p. dysfunction
p. factor
p. gender identity disorder
p. history
p. identity
p. identity crisis
p. intercourse
p. moratorium
p. problem
p. sphere
p. stage
p. symptom
psychosexuality
psychosis, pl. **psychoses**
accidental p.
active p.
acute delusional p.
acute hysterical p.
acute infective p.
acute posttraumatic organic p.
acute psychogenic paranoid p.
acute shock p.
addiction organic p.
addiction-type organic p.
affective alcoholic p.
affective paranoid organic p.
affective schizophreniform p.
akinetic p.
alcoholic Korsakoff p.
alcoholic liver disease-type organic p.
alcoholic paranoid p.
alcoholic polyneuritic p.
alternating p.
alternative p.
Alzheimer p.
amnestic confabulatory alcoholic p.
amphetamine p.
anergastic organic p.
anxiety-blissfulness p.
arteriosclerotic brain disease-type organic p.
p. of association
atropine p.
atypical childhood p.
autistic p.
autoscopic p.
barbed-wire p.
biogenic p.
bipolar affective p.
birth brain trauma organic p.
black patch p.
borderline p.
brain disease organic p.
brain infection organic p.
brain trauma organic p.
brief reactive p.
buffoonery p.
cannabis p.
cardiac p.
cerebral glucose metabolic-type organic p.
cerebrovascular disease organic p.
Cheyne-Stokes p.
child p.
p. in childbirth
childbirth organic p.
childhood p.

p. of childhood
childhood-onset p.
chronic paranoid p.
circular p.
circulatory p.
climacteric paranoid p.
cocaine p.
collective p.
confusional schizophreniform p.
confusion reactive p.
conjugal p.
constitutional p.
cycloid p.
degeneration p.
degenerative p.
delirious transient organic p.
delirium state drug p.
delirium transient organic p.
delirium tremens alcoholic p.
delusional syndrome drug p.
delusional transient organic p.
dementia-state drug p.
dependence-type organic p.
depressed bipolar affective p.
depressive transient organic p.
depressive-type nonorganic p.
disintegrative childhood p.
drug p.
drug-induced p.
p. due to physical condition
p. during pregnancy
dysmnesic p.
p. in elderly
electrical current brain trauma organic p.
electroshock-induced p.
embarrassment p.
emotional stress depressive p.
endocrine-type organic p.
epilepsy organic p.
epileptic transient organic p.
excitation p.
excitative p.
excitative-type nonorganic p.
exhaustion p.
exhaustive p.
exogenous p.
exotic p.
p. factor
familial p.
febrile p.
first-episode p.
florid p.
frank p.
full-blown p.
functional p.
furlough p.
gender ambiguity p.
gestational p.
governess p.
group p.
hallucinatory-state drug p.
hallucinatory transient organic p.
hallucinosis alcoholic p.
heredofamilial p.
housewife p.
Huntington chorea organic p.
hypochondriacal p.
hypomanic p.
hyposomnia associated with p.
hysteria p.
hysterical p.
iatrogenic p.
ICU p.
idiopathic p.
idiophrenic p.
incipient schizophrenic p.
induced p.
infantile p.
infection-exhaustion p.
infection-organic p.
infectious-exhaustive p.
infective p.
influenced p.
insomnia associated with p.
interactional childhood p.
interictal p.
intermittent p.
interval p.
intoxication organic p.
intoxication-type organic p.
intracranial infection organic p.
invocational p.
involutional paranoid p.
ischemia organic p.
Jakob-Creutzfeldt disease organic p.
juvenile p.
koro p.
Korsakoff alcoholic p.
Korsakoff nonalcoholic p.
kraepelinian view of p.
latent p.
liver disease organic p.
major depressive affective p.
malignant p.
manic p.

NOTES

psychosis *(continued)*
manic-depressive affective p.
marijuana p.
melancholia affective p.
meningismus p.
menopausal paranoid p.
metabolic disease organic p.
migration p.
mixed bipolar affective p.
mixed manic-depressive p.
mixed schizophrenic-affective p.
model p.
monosymptomatic hypochondriacal p.
mood-congruent p.
mood-incongruent p.
mood swing affective p.
motility p.
motor p.
multiinfarct p.
multiple sclerosis-type organic p.
nonaffective p.
nonorganic p.
organic p.
paranoiac p.
paranoid schizophrenic p.
paranoid transient organic p.
paranoid-type alcoholic p.
paranoid-type arteriosclerotic p.
paranoid-type senile p.
paretic p.
paroxysmal p.
pathologic alcoholic intoxication p.
pathologic drug intoxication p.
perplexed manic-depressive p.
perplexed-type manic-depressive p.
perplexity p.
phencyclidine-associated p.
phencyclidine-induced p.
physical condition organic p.
p. polyneuritica
polyneuritic alcoholic p.
positive symptoms p.
posthypnotic p.
postictal p.
postinfectious p.
postoperative p.
postpartum p. (PPP)
posttraumatic p.
p. in pregnancy
prepsychotic p.
prepubertal borderline p.
presbyophrenic p.
presenile p.
prevention and early intervention program for p.
prison p.
private p.
process p.
prodrome of p.
progressive p.
protest p.
protracted reactive paranoid p.
psychogenic depressive p.
psychogenic paranoid nonorganic p.
puerperal p.
p. in puerperium
purpose p.
reactive confusion nonorganic p.
reactive depressive p.
reactive paranoid p.
recurrent episode depressive p.
refractory p.
scale of p. (SP)
schizoaffective p.
schizophrenia p.
schizophrenic-affective p.
schizophrenic paranoid p.
schizophreniform p.
semantic p.
senile paranoid p.
senile paroxysmal p.
sensory p.
septicemia p.
shock p.
simple deterioration senile p.
simple-type arteriosclerotic p.
single-episode depressive p.
situational p.
sleeplessness associated with p.
somatic p.
status epilepticus organic p.
steroid p.
stigma of p.
stress p.
stuporous manic-depressive p.
stuporous-type manic-depressive p.
subacute posttraumatic organic p.
substance-induced chronic p.
surgical brain trauma organic p.
symbiotic infantile p.
symptomatic p.
p. of syphilis
tabetic p.
toxic p.
toxic-infectious p.
transient organic p.
transitory p.
traumatic p.
uncomplicated arteriosclerotic p.
unipolar manic-depressive p.
untreated p.
voluntary social withdrawal without p.
Windigo p.
withdrawal syndrome alcoholic p.
withdrawal syndrome drug p.
p. with mental retardation

Wittigo p.
zoophile p.
psychosis-induced polydipsia
psychosocial
p. assessment (PA)
p. complication
p. deprivation
p. development
p. dwarfism
p. event
p. factor
p. factor evaluation
p. functioning
p. history
p. intervention
p. issue
p. management
p. moratorium
p. morbidity
p. neglect
p. pain
p. pathology
p. perspective
p. problem
p. process
p. rehabilitation
p. residential care
p. retardation
p. service
p. setting
p. skill acquisition
p. stigma
p. stress
p. stressor
p. symptom outcome
p. treatment
p. turbulence
psychosocial-environmental
psychosocial-labile (PL)
psychosocially determined short stature
psychosolytic
psychosoma
psychosomatic
p. illness
p. inventory (PSI)
p. medicine (PSMed)
p. paralytic disorder
p. pruritic disorder
p. reaction
p. skin disorder
p. symptom
psychosomaticist
psychosomimetic
psychostimulant
p. dependence
p. drug
p. effect
psychostimulant-induced hyperthermia
psychostimulation
subjective p.
psychosuggestive
psychosuggestivity
psychosurgeon
psychosurgery
seed p.
psychosyndrome
algogenic p.
focal organic p.
organic p.
partial organic p.
psychosynthesis
psychotaxis
psychotechnic
psychotherapeusis
psychotherapeutic
p. approach
p. background
p. drug
p. intervention
p. measure
p. neuroscience
p. spectrum
p. therapy
p. treatment
psychotherapist
American Academy of P.'s (AAP)
American Association of P.'s
psychotherapist-patient privilege
psychotherapy
active analytic p.
activity group p.
activity-interview group p. (A-IGP)
adlerian p.
adolescent p.
p. alternative
anaclitic p.
analytic group p.
Association for the Advancement of P. (AAP)
autonomous p.
behavioral p.
bioenergetic p.
brief dynamic p.
child p.
client-centered p.
cognitive p.

NOTES

P

psychotherapy *(continued)*
cognitive-behavioral p.
cognitive-behavioral analysis system of p. (CBASP)
contractual p.
cooperative p.
crisis intervention group p.
didactic group p.
directive p.
dyadic p.
dynamic p.
educational p.
ego p.
emergency p.
existential p.
experiential p.
exploratory insight-oriented p. (EIO)
expressive p.
family p.
focal p.
freudian p.
gestalt p.
group p.
heteronomous p.
hypnotic p.
individual p.
insight-oriented p.
intensive p.
interactional group p.
International Association of Group P.
Internet p.
interpersonal p. (IPT)
interview group p.
long-term p.
manual-based interpersonal p.
marathon group p.
medical p.
Morita p.
multiple p.'s
nondirective p.
objective p.
outpatient p.
patterning p.
play group p.
psychoanalytic group p.
psychodynamic group p.
rational p.
rational-emotive p.
reciprocal inhibition p.
reconstructive p.
regressive inspirational group p.
relationship p.
remedial p.
repressive inspirational group p.
p. responder (PR)
p. session
short-contact p.
short-term anxiety-provoking p. (STAPP)
short-term dynamic p.
specific p.
structured interactional group p.
suggestive p.
superficial p.
supportive p.
supportive-expressive p.
terminal reinforcement p.
time-limited p. (TLP)
traditional p.
transactional p.

psychothymia

psychotic
p. aggressive behavior
p. agitation
p. Alzheimer patient
p. attack
p. break
p. catatonia
p. decompensation
p. denial
p. depression (PD)
p. depressive reaction
p. depressive subtype
p. dimension of schizophrenia
p. direction
p. direction profile
p. disease
p. disorder due to general medical condition
p. disorder, NOS
p. disorder with delusions
p. disorder with hallucinations
p. disorganization
p. disorganization in schizophrenia
p. disruptive behavior
p. distortion
p. disturbance
p. exacerbation
p. factor
p. feature
p. fugue
p. illness
p. inpatient
p. manifestation
p. posttraumatic brain syndrome
p. posturing
p. presenile disorder
p. presentation
p. process
p. relapse
p. schizophrenic episode
p. sign
p. signs and symptoms
p. speech
p. state
p. symptomatology

p. thinking
p. trigger reaction (PTR)
p. veteran
psychoticism
psychotic-like
p.-l. idea
p.-l. phenomenon
psychotogen
psychotogenic
psychotoid
psychotomimetic
p. agent dependence
p. drug
psychotonic
psychotoxicomania
psychotropic
p. agent
p. drug (PTD)
p. effect
p. medication
p. metabolism
psychroalgia
psychroesthesia
pt
patient
PTA
posttraumatic amnesia
prior to admission
PTCA
parent-to-child aggression
PTD
prevention and treatment of depression
psychotropic drug
ptosis sympathetica
PTR
psychotic trigger reaction
PTSD
posttraumatic stress disorder
comorbid schizophrenia and PTSD
complex PTSD
puberal
puberism
persistent p.
pubertal
p. sexual recapitulation
p. stage
pubertas praecox
puberty
atypical p.
p. melancholia
periodic psychosis of p.
precocious p.
p. rite
pubescence, pubescency
pubescent
public
p. display of emotion
p. disrobing
p. drunkenness
p. health
p. health issue
p. health model
p. health mood
p. image
p. masturbation
p. nudity
p. opprobrium
p. psychiatry
p. residential treatment center
p. sentiment
use of profanity in p.
puckering
lip p.
pudding opium
pudendum, pl. **pudenda**
puer
p. aeternus
p. externus
Pueraria lobata
puericulture
puerile
puerilism
hysterical p.
puerperal
p. convulsion
p. delirium
p. dementia
p. mania
p. melancholia
p. psychosis
p. seizure
puerperium
psychosis in p.
Puerto Rican
puesto
mal p.
puffy eye
pugilistica
dementia p.
pulling
p. of clothes
ear p.
hair p.
skin p.
pulsating
p. headache

NOTES

P

pulsating *(continued)*
p. neurasthenia
p. pain
pulsation
pulse
alternating p.
chest p.
p. rate
p. waveform
pulveratum
pulvinar
p. nucleus
p. nucleus of thalamus
pump
punch-drunk
p.-d. encephalopathy
p.-d. syndrome
punch-drunkenness
puncture
cisternal p.
Quincke p.
suboccipital p.
punishing spouse behavior
punishment
contingent p.
corporal p.
cruel p.
deserved p.
p. dream
expiatory p.
legal p.
Midas p.
need for p.
petty p.
reciprocal p.
unconscious need for p.
unusual p.
punitive psychologic attitude
punk music
punning
pupil
constricted p.
dilated p.
fixed p.
Hutchinson p.
paradoxical p.
pinpoint p.
reactive p.
rigid p.
Robertson p.
tonic p.
pupillary
p. constriction
p. reaction
p. skin reflex
pupillomotor
pupilloplegia
pupillotonia
pupillotonic pseudotabes
pupil-teacher fit
puppy love
pure
p. absence
p. agraphia
p. alexia
p. aphasia
p. aphemia
p. depressive disease
p. line
p. mania
p. mood
p. obsession
purgation
purge
binge and p.
bulimic p.
p. episode
purging
p. behavior
binge eating and p.
eating and p.
p. method
purging-type bulimia
purified pleasure ego
purine metabolism
purist
language p.
puritanical aversion to intercourse
Purkinje afterimage
Purmann method
purple
p. heart
p. people syndrome
purpose
clinical p.
dual p.
p. in life (PIL)
primary p.
p. psychosis
purposeful
p. behavior
p. contamination
p. movement
purposeless
p. activity
p. agitation
p. movement
purposive movement
purpura simplex
purse snatcher
pursing
lip p.
pursuit
p. abnormality
family p.
purveyor of mysticism
pusher
putamen

putative
p. adoptee
p. adoptee vulnerability
p. effect
p. index
p. influence
p. insult
p. neurotransmitter
putting affairs in order
puzzle
Tower of Hanoi p.
p value
PVNPS
post-Vietnam psychiatric syndrome
PVS
persistent vegetative state
PW
psychological warfare
PWA
person with AIDS
PWP
Parents Without Partners
Px, px
prognosis
pyencephalus
Pygmalion effect
pygmalionism
pyknic constitutional type
pyknophrasia
pylorospasm
pyocephalus
circumscribed p.
pyogenic pachymeningitis
pyramidal decussation
pyramidotomy
spinal p.
pyrimidine metabolism
pyrolagnia
pyromania
p. disorder
erotic p.
pyromaniac
pyroptothymia
pyrosis
pyruvate

NOTES

Q

Q
clerical perception
Q data
Q factor
Q method
Q methodology
Q score
Q technique
QALY
quality-adjusted life year
QEEG
quantitative electroencephalogram
quantitative electroencephalography
qi
qi gong movement-based meditation
qi gong psychotic reaction
QIAamp blood kit
Q-score profile
Q-Sort
Q-S. description
Q-S. method
Q-S. procedure
Q-S. technique
qt
quiet
QTL
quantitative trait loci
quadrangular therapy
quadrantanopia, quadrantanopsia
quadrigemina
corpora q.
quadriparesis
quadriplegia
qualitative
q. approach
q. difference
q. impairment in communication
q. judgment
quality
Agency for Healthcare Research and Q.
American Institute for Healthcare Q. (AIHQ)
q. of caring
compulsive q.
determining q.
exaggerated negative q.
exaggerated positive q.
histrionic q.
hypomanic q.
q. of life
Q. of Life, Effectiveness, Safety, and Tolerability Study (Q.U.E.S.T.)
q. of life measure
q. of life rehabilitation assessment
q. of mood
narcissistic q.
negative q.
q. of obsession
q. of performance
poor sleep q.
primary q.
semiautomatic q.
q. of sexual functioning
q. of sleep
q. of speech
q. time
uncontrollable q.
quality-adjusted life year (QALY)
quandary
ethical q.
quanta (*pl. of* quantum)
quantal hypothesis
quantification
quantified
q. clinical observation
q. cognitive assessment
quantitative
q. approach
q. data
q. electroencephalogram (QEEG)
q. electroencephalography (QEEG)
q. judgment
q. measure
q. morphometric technique
q. score
q. semantics
q. trait loci (QTL)
q. variable
quantity
absolute q.
q. of speech
sufficient q.
quantum, pl. **quanta**
libido q.
q. theory
quarrel
domestic q.
quarrelsomeness
quarter-way house
quartile deviation (q)
quasi-action
quasi-contract
quasi-experimental
q.-e. design
q.-e. research
quasi-expert
Quasimodo complex
quasi-need

quasi-purposive movement
quasi-representative
quasi-rhythmic
quaternity
quatre
folie á q.
quavering voice
querulans
paranoia q.
querulent
querulous paranoia
query
closed-ended q.
Q.U.E.S.T.
Quality of Life, Effectiveness, Safety, and Tolerability Study
quest for attention
question
actively phrased q.
closed-ended q.
direct q.
empirical q.
end-of-life q.
exception q.
generic q.
key q.
open-ended q.
passively phrased q.
Pigem q.
repetitive q.
screening q.
self-help q.
q. stage
unanswered q.
yes-no q.
questioning
circular q.
q. faith problem
socratic q.
q. under hypnosis
quick
q. to anger
q. and dirty
quick-tempered
quick-witted
quick-wittedness
quid pro quo harassment
quiescent
quiet (qt)
q. biting attack
q. environment
q. niche
q. room
q. sleep
q. wakefulness
q. wakefulness mode
quieting
quietism
quietude
Quincke puncture
quintessential
quiver
muscular q.
Quixote
Don Q.
quixotic
quixotism
quo
status q. (SQ)
quoque
quota system
quotient
accomplishment q. (AQ)
achievement q. (AQ)
activity q.
adolescent language q.
ambivalent q.
aphasia q. (AQ)
brain age q. (BAQ)
circadian q. (CQ)
conceptual q. (CQ)
custody q.
deterioration q.
deviation q.
education q. (EQ)
educational q. (EQ)
expressive language q.
full-scale intelligence q. (FIQ, FSIQ)
intelligence q. (IQ)
language q.
listening language q.
memory q. (MQ)
open q.
positive-negative ambivalent q. (PNAvQ)
reading language q.
receptive language-processing q.
social q. (SQ)
speed q.
spoken language q.
verbal language q.
vocabulary language q.
written language q.

R
relapse
relation
remission
90-R
rabbi
rabid
raccoon eye
race
mixed r.
race-ethnicity
racemic
r. amphetamine
r. mirtazapine
race-related
r.-r. stressor
r.-r. trauma
rachicentesis
rachigraph
rachitome
racial
r. bias
r. discrimination
r. memory
r. minority
r. profiling
r. saturation point
r. slur
racing thoughts
racism
aversive r.
racist
racket
racketeer
raconté
déjà r.
racy
radar
interpersonal r.
radiant
radiation
acoustic r.
auditory r.
visual r.
radiation-induced mental deterioration
radical
r. behaviorism
free r.
r. fringe
r. phenomenon
r. prejudice
r. therapy
radiculalgia
radiculopathy
radioactive count
radioimmunoassay
radioisotope brain scanning
radiolabeled probe
radioligand
radiological
chemical, biological, and r. (CBR)
R. Society of North America
radionuclide
radioreceptor
Rado view of depressive disorder
raffish
rage
r. attack
r. behavior
defiant r.
driver's r.
explosive r.
feeling of r.
hidden r.
jealous r.
narcissistic r.
overt r.
retributive r.
retroflexed r.
road r.
sham r.
unconscious r.
rageful feeling
raging parent
railroad neurosis
rain
raise
r. Cain
r. hell
raising
consciousness r.
raison d'etre
raisonnante
folie r.
RAM
rapid alternating movements
ramble
rambling
r. flow of speech
r. flow of thought
rambunctious
ramification
ramisection
rampage
murder r.
shooting r.
rampant
rancorous
random
r. activity

random *(continued)*
r. act of violence
r. assignment
r. digital dialing (RDD)
r. mating
r. model
r. movement
r. noise
r. observation
r. regression
r. sample
r. urine testing
r. variable
r. wave
randomization
randomized
r. clinical trial (RCT)
r. controlled trial (RCT)
r. group design
range
r. of affect
affect within normal r.
borderline r.
bright normal r.
dose r.
dull normal r.
dynamic r.
emotional r.
extreme r.
r. of feelings
r. of interests
normal r.
significant r.
some degree of r.
subclinical r.
therapeutic r.
tolerance r.
wide r.
rank
r. correlation
r. and file
military r.
r. order
r. in peer group
percentile r.
rank-difference correlation
rankian theory
ranking
merit r.
rankle
ransom
rant
rap
r. group
r. music
r. session
r. song
rape
r. act
anal r.
r. crisis center
date r.
drug-facilitated r.
r. fantasy
gang r.
heterosexual r.
male r.
sadistic act of r.
spousal r.
spouse r.
statutory r.
r. trauma syndrome
r. victim
rapid
r. alternating movements (RAM)
r. change in activity
r. cycler
r. cycling
r. cycling bipolar disorder
r. eye blinking paroxysm
r. eye movement (REM)
r. eye movement latency
r. eye movement sleep
r. eye movement state
r. fine movement
r. metabolizer patient
r. motor movement
r. neuroleptization
r. repetitive movement
r. shift in affective expression
r. smoking
r. speech
r. time zone change syndrome
r. tranquilization
r. tremor
r. vocalization
rapid-change theory
rapid-cycling
r.-c. course
r.-c. pattern
rapidity
r. of analyzing information
r. of assimilating information
r. of reinforcement
rapidly progressive dementia
rapid-smoking theory
rapist
adolescent r.
rapper
rapport
en r.
inadequate r.
interpersonal r.
parent-child r.
psychological r.
rapprochement
r. crisis
r. subphase

rapture-of-the-deep syndrome
raptus
r. action
r. of attention
impulsive r.
r. melancholicus
status r.
Rapunzel syndrome
rare detail response
rarefaction
RAS
reticular activating system
rasa
tabula r.
rash
acne-like r.
r. decision-making
glue sniffer's r.
ratchet rigidity
rate
accelerated heart r.
age-specific cumulative incidence r.
alternate motion r. (AMR)
attrition r.
basal metabolic r. (BMR)
base r.
birth r.
case fatality r.
compliance r.
concordance r.
r. control
cumulative incidence r.
cure r.
death r.
decline r.
decreased respiratory r.
divorce r.
dropout r.
drug response r.
exacerbation r.
r. of fluency disturbance
heart r.
homicide-suicide r.
hospital mortality r.
incidence r.
long-term mortality r.
maturation r.
mentation r.
metabolic r.
mortality r.
mutation r.
nonspecific response r.
placebo response r.
prevalence r.
r. of production of speech
pulse r.
r. of recovery
r. of recovery at discharge
relapse r.
response r.
sex-specific r.
suicide attempt r.
treatment completion r.
treatment response r.
rate-limiting enzyme
ratification theory
rating
baseline r.
behavior r.
Bunney-Hamburg global psychosis r.
Bunney-Hamburg nurse r.
clinician r.
daily symptom r.
desire-for-death r.
dimensional r.
employment problem r.
evaluative r.
3-factor model of global r.
global clinician r.
grade r.
hyperintensity r.
intent r.
internalized-state r.
lethality r.
maturity r.
maximum intent r.
maximum lethality r.
merit r.
r. method
nonrandom r.
peer r.
pleasantness r.
r. procedure
psychiatric severity r.
risk rescue r. (RRR)
sexual maturity r.
social impairment r.
subjective unit of distress r.
symptom r.
trait r.
ratio
achievement r. (AR)
affective r.
affectivity r.
age r.

NOTES

ratio *(continued)*
association-sensation r.
brain-to-plasma r.
correlation r.
critical r.
dopamine r.
extinction r.
fixed r. (FR)
high affectivity r.
male-to-female r.
odds r. (OR)
oral-nasal acoustic r.
risk r. (RR)
risk-benefit r.
sex r.
stimulation r.
T r.
variable r. (VR)
ventricle-to-brain r. (VBR)
rational
r. cognitive coping
r. emotive therapy (RET)
r. medicine
r. problem-solving
r. psychology
r. psychotherapy
r. suicide
r. therapy (RT)
rationale
psychiatric r.
rational-emotive
r.-e. behavior
r.-e. psychotherapy
rationality
rationalization defense mechanism
rationalize
rattle
death r.
raucous
raunchy
Rauwolfia serpentina
ravage
rave
r. drug
r. gathering
r. party
ravenous
Raven progressive matrices-R (RPM-R)
raver
raving madness
ravish
raw
r. score
r. volume
razor
RBD
REM behavior disorder
rCBF
regional cerebral blood flow
RCP
Royal College of Psychiatrists
RCT
randomized clinical trial
randomized controlled trial
RD
reaction of degeneration
reward dependence
RDA
recommended daily allowance
RDD
random digital dialing
rea
mens r.
reach
grasp and r.
reacquaint
reactance
inductive r.
reaction
Abderhalden-Fauser r.
abnormal r.
accelerated r.
acute anxiety r.
acute organic r.
acute paranoid r.
acute paranoid schizophrenic r. (APSR)
acute situational maladjustment r.
acute situational stress r.
acute stress r.
acute undifferentiated schizophrenic r. (AUSR)
adaptation r.
adjustment situational r.
r. of adolescence
adolescent turmoil r.
adult situational stress r. (ASSR)
adverse drug r. (ADR)
affective depressive r.
aggressive undersocialized r.
agitated r.
alarm r. (AR)
alcohol-Antabuse r.
allele-specific polymerase chain r.
allergic r.
all-or-none r.
anergastic r.
anesthetic conversion r.
anger r.
angry r.
anniversary r.
antigen-antibody r.
antisocial r.
anxiety panic r.
anxiety psychoneurotic r.
anxious mood adjustment r.
arousal r.
arrest r.

Asian alcohol flush r.
associative r.
asthenic r.
autonomic conversion r.
aversion r.
behavior r.
brief depressive r.
brief psychotic r.
cancer r.
cardiac r.
catastrophic r.
r. of childhood
choice r.
chronic paranoid r.
chronic paranoid schizophrenic r. (CPSR)
chronic stress r.
chronic undifferentiated schizophrenic r.
circular r.
civilian catastrophe r.
climacteric paranoid r.
combat r.
compulsive psychoneurotic r.
conduct disturbance adjustment r.
confusional psychotic r.
consciousness disturbance stress r.
consensual r.
conversion psychoneurotic r.
countertransferential r.
cutaneous r.
dangerous behavior r.
r. to death
defense r.
defensive r.
deferred r.
r. of degeneration (RD)
dehydration r.
delayed r.
delirious r.
dental patient r.
depersonalization psychoneurotic r.
depressed mood adjustment r.
depressive psychoneurotic r.
depressive psychotic r.
depressive situational r.
dissociate-dysmnesic substitution r.
dissociative psychoneurotic r.
doll's eye r.
duplicative r.
dysergastic r.
dyssocial r.
dysthymic adjustment r.
dystonic r.
echo r.
elective mutism adjustment r.
emotional disturbance adjustment r.
emotional disturbance stress r.
emotionally unstable immaturity r.
emotional stress r.
emotion-conduct adjustment r.
escape r.
excitation psychotic r.
fear r.
fight-or-flight r.
fixation r.
r. formation
r. formation defense mechanism
galvanic skin r.
gemistocytic r.
general adaptation r.
grief r.
gross stress r.
group delinquent r.
group stress r.
hand-to-mouth r.
harsh r.
heeltap r.
hyperkinetic conversion r.
hypochondriacal psychoneurotic r.
hypochondriac psychoneurotic r.
hypomanic-depressive r.
hypomanic manic-depressive r.
hysterical conversion r. (HCR)
hysterical psychoneurotic r.
idiosyncratic r.
immaturity r.
indifference r.
initial stress r.
instinctive r.
intensity of r.
intermittent emotional conflicts or r.'s
involutional paranoid r.
involutional psychotic r.
Jolly r.
justifiable r.
laryngeal psychophysiologic r.
late r.
latent schizophrenic r.
lengthening r.
r. to life stress
LSD r.
magnet r.
maladaptive r.
maniacal grief r.

NOTES

reaction *(continued)*

manic r.
manic-depressive r.
melancholic involutional r.
menopausal paranoid r.
r. to minor stimulus
mixed disturbance stress r.
mixed paralytic conversion r.
mobilization r.
myasthenic r.
negative therapeutic r.
neurasthenic psychoneurosis r.
neurasthenic psychoneurotic r.
neurogenic r.
neurotic r.
neurotic-depressive r.
nonpathological r.
normal grief r.
obsessional psychoneurotic r.
obsessive-compulsive r.
obsessive psychoneurotic r.
organic r.
overanxious r.
pain r.
paradoxical r.
paranoid involutional r.
paresthetic conversion r.
passive r.
passive-aggressive r.
passive-dependent r.
pathologic grief r.
personality r.
phantom r.
pharyngeal psychophysiologic r.
phobic psychoneurotic r.
physical symptoms adjustment r.
primary circular r.
prolonged depressive r.
prolonged grief r.
psychogalvanic r.
psychogenic r.
psychological r.
psychomotor disturbance stress r.
psychoneurotic depressive r.
psychophysiologic r.
psychosomatic r.
psychotic depressive r.
psychotic trigger r. (PTR)
pupillary r.
qi gong psychotic r.
recurrent psychotic r.
repetition r.
runaway r.
schizophrenic r.
senile paranoid r.
shock r.
shortening r.
simple paranoid r.
single psychotic r.
situational stress r.
sleeplessness associated with acute emotional conflicts or r.'s
sleeplessness associated with intermittent emotional conflicts or r.'s
socialized runaway r.
somatization r.
spite r.
spoiled child r.
startle r.
stress r.
subacute organic r.
suspected adverse drug r. (SADR)
sympathetic stress r.
symptomatic r.
task-oriented r.
tension state psychoneurotic r.
tertiary circular r.
therapeutic r. (TR)
thymonoic r.
r. time (RT)
toxic r.
transference r.
transient depressive r.
transplantation r.
trigger r.
r. type
unaggressive undersocialized r.
undersocialized aggressive r.
undersocialized nonaggressive r.
undersocialized runaway r.
unexpected r.
unsocialized aggressive r.
visual disorientation r.
Wernicke r.
withdrawal adjustment r.

reactional biography

reaction-type deterioration

reactivation process

reactive

r. alcoholism
r. attachment disorder
r. attachment disorder of infancy or early childhood
r. attachment disorder of infancy or early childhood, disinhibited type
r. attachment disorder of infancy or early childhood, inhibited type
r. bowel
r. cell
r. clinical depression
r. confusion
r. confusional state
r. confusion nonorganic psychosis
r. depression and anxiety
r. depressive psychosis
r. ego alteration

r. epilepsy
r. exaltation
r. excitation
r. inhibition
r. mania
r. measure
r. melancholia
r. mental excitement
r. paranoid psychosis
r. psychotic depression
r. pupil
r. reinforcement
r. response
r. schizophrenia
symptomatically r.
r. thought

reactivity
affective r.
automatic r.
autonomic r.
emotional r.
lack of r.
mood r.
physiologic r.

reactor
placebo r.

ReaCTor system

readaptation
neurobehavioral r.

reader
mind r.

readiness
complex r.
explosion r.
reading r.

reading
r. achievement
r. activities in life
r. backwards
r. comprehension impairment
delusion of mind r.
r. developmental delay disorder
r. disability
r. epilepsy
r. grade equivalent
r. language quotient
lip r.
mind r.
mirror r.
r. readiness
r. skill acquisition
r. skills learning retardation
thought r.

readjust

readjustment
business r.
social r.

readmission

readout

reaffirm

real
r. abandonment
r. anxiety
r. external stimulus
feeling that self is not r.
feeling that things are not r.
r. image
r. life
r. loss
r. self

realignment
circadian r.

realism
experimental r.
moral r.
mundane r.

realistic
r. attitude
r. expectation
r. fear
r. guilt
r. plan
r. thinking

reality
r. ability testing
r. adaptation
r. anxiety
r. assumption
r. awareness
break with r.
r. confrontation
contact with r.
deficient sense of r.
r. denial
denial of external r.
disconnection with r.
distorted perception of r.
r. distortion
escape from r.
external r.
flight from r.
independent physical r.
r. issue
r. life of ego
loss of touch with r.
objective r.

NOTES

reality *(continued)*
r. orientation (RO)
r. oriented (RO)
out of touch with r.
perceived r.
perception of r.
phenomenological r.
r. principle
psychic r.
relativity of r.
retreat from r.
sense of r.
sociopolitical r.
r. system
r. testing
r. testing ability
r. ties
ties with r.
transcendent r.
unseen r.
reality-adaptive supportive
reality-oriented
r.-o. supportive strategy
r.-o. therapy
realization
symbolic r.
real-life
r.-l. behavior
r.-l. circumstance
r.-l. decision-making
r.-l. emotional episode
r.-l. problem
r.-l. stimulus
realm
interpersonal r.
real-world
r.-w. setting
r.-w. situation
reanalysis strategy
reanalyzed data
reappear
rearing
child r.
r. environment
violent r.
reason
r. for living
medical r.
pharmacokinetic r.
r. for visit
reasonable
r. ego
r. fear
r. willingness
r. zest
reasoning
r. ability
abstract r.
age of r.
arithmetical r.
clinical r.
conceptual r.
deductive r.
r. disturbance
dynamic r.
ethical r.
evaluative r.
exonerative moral r.
hypothetical deductive r.
idiosyncratic r.
illogical r.
inductive r.
r. mania
r. and memory skills
nonverbal r.
practical r.
syllogistic r.
verbal r.
verbal, numerical, and r. (VNR)
reassessment
attitude r.
sexual attitude r. (SAR)
reassignment
gender r.
hormonal sex r.
sex r.
sexual r.
surgical sex r.
reassociation
reassurance
r. seeking
r. sensitivity
reassure
reassuring explanation
reattribution technique
rebel against authority
rebellion
adolescent r.
rebellious
r. teen
r. youngster
rebelliousness
rebirth fantasy
reborn
rebound
r. effect
r. headache
r. hyperthermia
r. insomnia
r. mood swing
r. phenomenon
REM sleep r.
r. suppression
reboxetine
rebreathe
rebreathing
rebuild
rebuke

rebus principle
rebuttal
recalcitrant pain
recall
body-image r.
delayed r.
digit r.
diminished r.
dream r.
event r.
r. failure
free r.
immediate r.
inconsistent r.
memory r.
r. method
r. performance
recognition vs r.
recollection and r.
remote r.
retention and r.
rote r.
short-term r.
total r.
verbatim r.
vivid dream r.
recall-generated
r.-g. emotion
r.-g. sadness
recalling new information disturbance
recant
recap
recapitulation
pubertal sexual r.
recapture
recathexis
recede
receiver operating characteristic (ROC)
receiving type
recency
positive r.
recent
r. life event (RLE)
r. loss
r. memory
r. violence
recent-onset schizophrenia
receptive
r. aphasia
r. character
r. dysphasia
r. function
r. language development
r. language disorder
r. language processing
r. language-processing quotient
r. orientation
r. personality
receptive-expressive observation (REO)
receptor
acetylcholine cholinergic r.
adenosine r.
r. affinity
alpha adrenergic r.
alpha-2 adrenergic r.
r. alteration
beta adrenergic r.
catecholamine r.
cholinergic r.
9-*cis* retinoic acid r. (RXR)
r. D4
delta opiate r.
distance r.
dopamine D_2 r.
r. functioning
5-HT-1 r.
5-HT-2 r.
insulin r. (IR)
kappa opiate r.
kappa opioid r.
limbic dopamine r.
mu opiate r.
muscarinic cholinergic r.
neurotransmitter r.
nicotinic cholinergic r.
noradrenergic r.
r. occupancy
opiate r.
opioid r.
pain r.
peripheral catecholamine r.
peroxisomal proliferator acting r. (PPAR)
postsynaptic 5-HT-2 r.
postsynaptic 5-HT-3 r.
proximal r.
resiniferatoxin r.
sensory r.
serotonergic r.
serotonin 5-HT-2 r.
sigma r.
unencapsulated joint r.
r. up-regulation
vitamin D r. (VDR)
receptor-binding property

NOTES

recessive
autosomal r.
r. gene
r. trait
recessiveness
recidivation
recidivism, recidivity
r. in schizophrenia
victim r.
recidivist
recipient
action r.
recipiomotor
reciprocal
r. agreement
r. assimilation
r. circuitry
r. communication
r. connection
r. deference
r. determinism
r. inhibition
r. inhibition and desensitization
r. inhibition psychotherapy
r. parenting
r. punishment
r. regulation
r. relationship
r. social interaction
reciprocate
reciprocity
behavioral r.
emotional r.
overadequate-inadequate r.
recitation
recitative
recite
reckless
r. behavior
r. disregard for safety of self
r. driving
recluse
recognition
disturbance of r.
face r.
facial r.
impaired r.
r. memory
pattern r.
r. of people
r. site
r. time
visual pattern r.
r. vs recall
r. in wit
recognizable
recognizance
recognize, empathize, think, hear, integrate, notice, keep (RETHINK)
recoil
recollection
explicit r.
intrusive r.
r. and recall
r. of trauma
recommencement mania
recommendation
recommended
r. daily allowance (RDA)
r. diet
r. dose
recommission
recommit
recompensation
reconcile
reconciliation
r. attempt
attempt at r.
reconditioning
orgasmic r.
r. therapy
reconnaissance
fausse r.
reconnoiter
reconstituted family
reconstruct
reconstruction
cosmetic r.
r. dream
memory r.
r. method
pathology-induced memory r.
reconstructive
r. psychotherapy
r. therapy
record
activity r.
automated clinical r.
Bayley behavior r.
behavior r.
chronological drinking r.
confidential r.
criminal r.
cumulative r.
dysfunctional thought r.
electronic health r.
electronic medical r. (EMR)
hospital r.
infant behavior r.
medical r.
mental status examination r.
problem-oriented r. (POR)
r. review
recording
behavior specimen r.
depth r.
r. procedure
recount

recoup
recourse
recovered memory
recovery
adolescent r.
r. from delinquency
full r.
r. of function
r. issue
language r.
long-term r.
partial r.
personal r.
r. phase
post r.
rate of r.
r. and reorganization
social r.
spontaneous r.
r. stage
uncomplicated r.
r. wish
recreate
recreation
active r.
passive r.
therapeutic r.
recreational
r. drinking
r. drug
r. drug use
r. gambler
r. service
r. therapy (RT)
recriminate
recruit
recruiting response
recta (*pl. of* rectum)
rectifier
delayed r.
rectify
rectitude
rectum, pl. **recta, rectums**
per r.
recur
recurred
recurrence
likelihood of r.
r. risk
recurrent
r. abuse
r. brief depressive disorder
r. catatonia
r. course
r. depersonalization
r. distressing dream
r. encephalopathy
r. episode
r. episode chronic mania
r. episode depressive psychosis
r. episode psychotic reaction
r. illusion
r. image
major depressive disorder, r.
r. melancholia
r. memory
r. migraine headache
r. mood disorder
r. motor movement
r. nightmare
r. panic attacks
r. physical fights
r. psychotic depression
r. seizure
r. suicidal ideation
r. thought
r. urinary tract infection
r. vocalization
recurring
r. dream
r. idea
r. symptom
r. theme
r. trauma memory
recursion
recursive autoassociative memory
recutita
Matricaria r.
recycled air
recycling
synaptic vesicle r.
redescribe
red-handed
redintegration
redirect
redirecting anger
redirection
verbal r.
red-light district
reduced
r. aggression level
r. agitation
r. anxiety
r. attention ability
r. awareness of surroundings
r. body tone

NOTES

reduced *(continued)*
r. gratification
r. intellectual function
r. level of consciousness
r. motivation
r. rapid eye movement latency
r. responsiveness
r. sexual desire
r. verbal output
reduced-sodium diet
reducer
craving r.
reduction
accident r.
anxiety r.
cluster r.
cue r.
cumulative medication r.
dose r.
drive r.
gambling r.
medication r.
meditation-based stress r.
mindfulness-based stress r.
risk r.
ritual r.
smoking-related r.
stress r.
symptom r.
tension r.
tobacco use r.
reductionism
biologic r.
reductive
redundancy
correlation r.
genetic r.
r. rule
redundant
reduplicated babbling
reduplicative paramnesia
reeducation
emotional r.
reeducative therapy
reemergence
reemploy
reenactment
emotional r.
trauma-specific r.
reenforce
reentry
reestablish
reevaluation counseling
reexperienced
r. trauma
r. traumatic event
reexperiencing
r. category
r. perceptual symptom
referee
reference
cultural frame of r.
r. delusion
distorted ideas of r.
r. electrode
frame of r.
r. group
idea of r.
memory r.
r. phase
r. picture-caption pair
standard r.
transient ideas of r.
r. zero level
referential
r. attitude
r. delusion
r. function
r. idea
r. index
r. semantics
referral
psychiatric r.
referred
r. pain
r. sensation
refined
reflection
factor r.
r. of feeling
reflective
reflex, pl. **reflexes**
acquired r.
acromial r.
r. act
acute affective r.
allied r.
antagonistic r.
r. arc
r. asymmetry
attention r.
attitudinal r.
bar r.
behavior r.
blink r.
brisk r.
r. center
chain r.
r. change
conditioned r. (CR)
consensual r.
contralateral r.
r. control
r. convulsion
convulsive r.
coordinated r.
cry r.
darwinian r.

r. decay
deep tendon r. (DTR)
defecation r.
defense r.
delayed r.
depressed r.
diffused r.
diminished r.
diving r.
doll's eye r.
dorsal r.
ejaculatory r.
emptying r.
extensor plantar r.
eye closure r.
foot r.
gag r.
galvanic skin r.
grasp r.
grasping and groping r.
gustatory-sudorific r.
r. hallucination
r. headache
inborn r.
r. incontinence
r. inhibition of epilepsy
innate r.
intrinsic r.
inverted radial r.
investigatory r.
ipsilateral r.
jaw r.
jaw-jerk r.
jaw-working r.
labyrinthine righting r.
r. latency
latent r.
laughter r.
lip r.
magnet r.
mass r.
Mendel instep r.
milk ejection r.
r. movement
muscle r.
muscular r.
neck r.
r. neurogenic bladder
orienting r.
palmar r.
palm-chin r.
palmomental r.
parachute r.
pathologic r.
r. pattern
phasic r.
physiologic r.
pilomotor r.
positive conditioned r.
postural r.
pout r.
primitive r.
psychic r.
psychocardiac r.
psychogalvanic r. (PGR)
pupillary skin r.
r. seizure
r. sensation
snout r.
startle r.
stress-altered startle r.
sucking r.
r. therapy
r. threshold
r. time
trace conditioned r.
trained r.
unconditioned r. (UCR)
upper abdominal periosteal r.
urogenital r.
utricular r.
vomiting r.
withdrawal r.

reflexive movement

reflexogenic, reflexogenous
reflexogenic zone

reflexograph

reflexometer

reflexotherapy

reflux
ejaculation r.
r. management

reform
mental health r.
thought r.

reformation

reformatory
r. paranoia
r. paranoiac

reformist delusion

reformulation
sequential diagrammatic r. (SDR)

refractoriness
medication r.

refractory
r. depression

NOTES

refractory *(continued)*
r. erectile dysfunction
r. mental illness
r. period
r. psychosis
r. schizophrenia
r. state
treatment r.
refraining
reframing
context r.
meaning r.
refreshing sleep attack
refrigerant
refrigerator
r. parent
r. parenting
refuge
refugee
Bosnian r.
Cambodian r.
r. camp
Chilean r.
Guatemalan r.
Hmong r.
Indochinese r.
Laotian r.
Southeast Asian r.
Tamil r.
tortured r.
r. trauma
traumatized r.
Vietnamese r.
war-wounded r.
Yugoslavian r.
refusal
r. to eat
medication r.
school r.
treatment r.
regard
field of r.
mutual r.
point of r.
positive r.
unconditional positive r.
regardant
regenerate
regeneration
aberrant r.
regime
regimen
birth control r.
drug r.
holistic r.
medication r.
multiple-dose r.
pharmacotherapy r.
steady-state r.
treatment r.
region
anterior insula r.
auditory r.
bilateral r.'s
brain r.
central gray matter r.
cerebellar r.
cerebral r.
circumscribed r.
comparison r.
cortical r.
critical r.
deep white matter r.
dorsal anterior cingulate r.
dorsal limbic r.
dorsal neocortical r.
frontal brain r.
gray matter r.
inferior parietal r.
interconnected cerebral r.
limbic brain r.
limbic-related r.
motor r.
negatively correlated r.
neocortical r.
orbitofrontal r.
paralimbic r.
perceptual-motor r.
periventricular gray r.
positively correlated r.
posterior cingulate r.
prefrontal r.
septal r.
speech perception r.
subcortical gray r.
subgenual cingulate r.
temporal speech r.
terminal r.
thalamic r.
ventral paralimbic r.
visual r.
white matter r.
regional
r. background
r. blood flow
r. brain glucose metabolism
r. brain lactate
r. cerebral blood flow (rCBF)
r. differentiation
r. distribution
r. epilepsy
r. glucose metabolism at rest
register
case r.
National Population R.
psychiatric case r.

registered
Music Therapist, R. (MTR)
r. recreation therapist (RRT)
r. sex offender
registration
image r.
imperfect image r.
registry
Clozaril National R.
PsiTri r.
regnancy
regress
regressed
regression
age r.
age-adjusted logistics r.
r. analysis
atavistic r.
r. defense mechanism
dream r.
r. equation
Galton law of r.
hierarchical r.
logistic r.
r. of mean
multiple r.'s
r. neurosis
partial r.
past-life hypnotic r.
phenomenal r.
polytomous r.
progressive teleologic r.
random r.
Ribot law of r.
teleologic r.
verbal r.
regressive
r. alcoholism
r. assimilation
r. behavior
r. electroshock treatment (REST)
r. infantilism
r. inspirational group
r. inspirational group psychotherapy
r. substitute
r. symptoms of schizophrenia
r. transference neurosis
regressive-reconstructive approach
regret
regrettable
regrettably
regroup
regular
r. caffeine consumption
r. caffeine user
r. diet
r. drug user
r. eating schedule
r. gambler
r. sleeping schedule
r. waking schedule
regularity
regularly
regulation
emotion r.
emotional r.
immune system r.
impulse r.
mood r.
occupational safety r.
reciprocal r.
self-esteem r.
sexual r.
temperature r.
top-down r.
weight r.
regulator
mood r.
regulatory
r. center
r. input
r. role
regurgitation
rehab
rehabilitation
rehabilitate
rehabilitation (rehab)
acoupedic r.
alcoholic r.
r. assessment
r. behavior
Boston University Model of Psychiatric R.
cognitive r.
r. counselor
r. evaluation
r. facility
geriatric r.
neuromuscular r.
occupational r.
r. psychiatry
psychomotor r.
psychosocial r.
sexual r.
social r.

NOTES

rehabilitation *(continued)*
r. stage
testing, orientation, and work evaluation for r. (TOWER)
r. treatment
vocational r. (VR)
work r.
rehabilitative issue
rehashing
rehearsal
behavior r.
behavioral r.
cognitive r.
obsessional r.
thought r.
reification
reign of terror
reimbursement
ICD-9 diagnostic codes for Medicare r.
r. issue
rein
free r.
reincarnation
reindoctrination
reinforced
r. practice
r. thought
reinforcement
adventitious r.
aperiodic r.
chained r.
concurrent r.
conjunctive r.
contingency r.
continuous r.
r. counseling
covert r.
delayed r.
differential r.
drug r.
fixed r.
homogeneous r.
homogenous r.
intermittent r.
interval r.
mixed r.
multiple r.'s
negative r.
partial r.
periodic r.
positive r.
predelay r.
primary r.
rapidity of r.
reactive r.
schedule of r.
r. schedule
secondary r.
self-managed r.
social r.
systematic r.
tandem r.
terminal r.
time out from r.
variable r.
verbal r.
reinforcer
conditioned r.
negative r.
positive r.
primary r.
secondary r.
reinforcing
r. agent
r. drug response
r. effect
r. property
r. stimulus
reinsert
reinstatement
job r.
reinstinctualization
reintegrate
reintegration
community r.
reinterpret
reinterpretation
reintroduction
reintrojection
Reitan rules to assess learning disorders
reiterate
reject
rejecting-neglecting parent
rejecting parent
rejection
r. of authority
explicit r.
fear of r.
r. fear
feeling of r.
interpersonal r.
r. of intimacy
maternal r.
parental r.
paternal r.
peer r.
r. by peers
perceived interpersonal r.
r. sensitivity
rejoice
rejuvenate
rejuvenation fantasy
relabeling
relapse (R)
full r.
impending r.

r. mechanism
r. prevention
r. prevention counseling
r. prevention technique
prone to r.
psychotic r.
r. rate
smoking r.

relapser
optimistic r.
pessimistic r.

relapsing

related
alcohol r. (AR)
drug r.
r. psychopathology
r. sleep disorder
transformationally r.

relatedness
developmentally inappropriate social r.
disturbed social r.
failure to develop r.
functional r.
inappropriate social r.
semantic r.
social r.
symbiotic r.

relating
disordered r.
form of satisfactory r.
r. to others
time period of satisfactory r.

relation (R)
afferent r.
r. to age
community-institutional r.'s
court of domestic r.'s
dose-response r.
efferent r.
extramarital r.
family r.
human r.'s
intergenerational r.
interpersonal r.
intimate human r.'s
negative r.
object r.
perception of spatial r.'s
professional-family r.
sexual r.
sibling r.

relational
r. alliance
r. behavior
r. efficacy
r. opposite
r. problem
r. threshold
r. unit

relationship
addiction r.
r. addiction
adversarial r.
anaclitic r.
appropriate r.
attachment r.
r. behavior
bisexual r.
brain-behavior r.
causal r.
cause-effect r.
chewing-speech r.
chronological r.
clearly demarcated r.
clinician-client r.
collaborative r.
competent r.
complainant-listener r.
complex r.
complicated r.
conflictual r.
consistent r.
consultative r.
counseling r.
dating r.
demarcated r.
dependent r.
dependent-protective r.
depression-hyperglycemia r.
destructive r.
detachment from social r.
disrupted r.
disturbed attachment r.
disturbed interpersonal r. (DIR)
doctor-patient r.
dose-response r.
dramatic interpersonal r.
dual r.
dysfunctional r.
early r.
email r.
etiological r.
failed r.
failure to sustain a monogamous r.

NOTES

R

relationship *(continued)*
family r.
family-of-origin r.
fantasy-based element of the doctor-patient r.
forced r.
former r.
genetic r.
harmful sexual r.
helping r.
heterosexual r.
r. history
homosexual r.
human r.
hypnotic r.
I-it r.
imaginary r.
impaired r.
impersonal r.
inappropriate r.
incestuous r.
independent r.
initiate r.
instability in interpersonal r.'s
intense interpersonal r.
Internet r.
interpersonal r.
r. intimacy
intimate r.
intrafamilial r.
intrinsic r.
inverse r.
inversion r.
I-thou r.
live-in r.
loss of r.
love r.
love-hate r.
maternal r.
meaningful interpersonal r.
monogamous r.
mother-child r. (MCR)
mother-infant r.
multiple r.'s
negative r.
no-win r.
nurturing r.
object r.
online r.
optimal r.
parent-child r.
paternal r.
peer r.
perfect negative r.
perfect positive r.
periodic reinforcement r.
personal r.
physician-patient r.
platonic r.
poor family r.
poor peer r.
positive family r.
predictive r.
primary sexual r.
r. problem
r. problem of childhood
r. psychotherapy
reciprocal r.
replacement r.
required r.
romantic r.
sadomasochistic r.
r. satisfaction
semantic r.
sexual r.
shared r.
social r.
spectral r.
stable therapeutic r.
stress-strain r.
supervisory r.
supportive r.
teacher-student r.
temporal r.
terminate r.
therapeutic r.
therapist-patient r.
r. therapy
r. tool
transference r.
troubled r.
trusting physician-patient r.
unsatisfactory r.
unstable interpersonal r.
r. with God
working r.

relative
death of r.
r. dementia
r. elective mutism
first-degree biological r.
r. frequency
r. hypoxia
r. impotence
r. risk
r. scotoma
r. slow-wave sleep stability
r. unpleasantness

relatively stable

relativism
cultural r.
moral r.

relativistic

relativity
law of r.
r. of reality
special theory of r.

relaxant
depolarizing muscle r.
relaxation
applied r. (AR)
r. constant
differential r.
r. phase
progressive muscular r.
r. response
state of mindful r.
r. technique
r. technique training
therapeutic r.
r. therapy
r. time
r. training in adolescence
r. training in children
relaxation-induced anxiety (RIA)
relaxed
squarely face person, open posture, lean toward person, eye contact, r. (SOLER)
relearning method
release
dopamine r.
emotional r.
extended r. (ER)
r. of information
orgastic r.
r. phenomenon
pituitary prolactin r.
prolactin r.
r. therapy
releaser
relegate
relent
relentless
relevance
clinical r.
personal r.
r. of spirituality
relevant diagnostic criterion
reliability
r. coefficient
equivalent form r.
index of r.
interjudge r.
interobserver r.
interrater r.
r. of patient information
split-half r.
test-retest r.
reliable
r. diagnosis
r. history
reliance
hemispheric r.
reliant
relief
comic r.
Miles Nervine Nighttime Pain R.
pain r.
symptom r.
reliever
religion
Buddhist r.
Catholic r.
Christian r.
Eastern r.
Hindu r.
influence of r.
Mormon r.
Muslim r.
organized r.
Protestant Christian r.
salience of r.
Scientology r.
Sikh r.
religiosa
melancholia r.
religiosity
intrinsic r.
religio-terror
religious
r. activity
r. affiliation
r. approach
r. attitude
r. background
r. behavior
r. belief
r. commitment
r. community
r. conflict
r. conviction
r. cult
r. delusion
r. denomination
r. difference
r. dynamic
r. ecstasy
r. experience
explicitly r.
r. faith
r. fasting

NOTES

religious *(continued)*
r. healer
r. inclination
r. influence
r. insanity
r. institution
r. interest
r. intervention
r. language
r. life
r. mania
r. metaphor
r. milieu
r. nonbelief
r. object
r. obsession
r. organization
r. orientation
r. orthodoxy factor
r. person
r. perspective
r. practice
r. proscription
r. or spiritual problem
r. teaching
r. tenet
r. theme
r. tradition
r. upbringing
r. values
r. value system
religiously devout
relinquish
relinquishment
custody r.
relive
relocate
relocation
frequent r.
reluctance
reluctant
REM
rapid eye movement
REM behavior disorder (RBD)
REM period
REM sleep
REM sleep activity
REM sleep behavior
REM sleep behavior disorder
REM sleep efficiency
REM sleep rebound
REM sleep-related disorder
REM state
remand
remark
caustic r.
derogatory r.
disparaging r.
self-deprecatory r.
threatening r.
remarkable
remarriage
remarried
remarry
rematch
remedial
r. intervention
r. psychotherapy
r. teaching
remediation
cognitive r.
remedy
herbal r.
mystical r.
remilitarize
reminder
reminisce
reminiscence therapy
reminiscent
r. aura
r. neuralgia
reminiscing
remission (R)
early full r.
full r.
partial r.
period of r.
spontaneous r.
sustained full r.
sustained partial r.
transference r.
remitted substance abuser
remittent
remitting
r. dementia
r. schizophrenia
REM-onset sleep
remonstrate
remorse
feeling of r.
lack of r.
remorseful
remorseless
remote
r. attempter
r. episodic memory
r. recall
r. suicide attempt
remotivation
removed affect
remover
nail polish r.
remuneration
rename
render
rendezvous
renegade

renege
renegotiable
renewal
renifleur
renitent
Renpenning syndrome
renunciation
instinctual r.
REO
receptive-expressive observation
reorganization
plastic r.
recovery and r.
reorient
reorientation
reparation
reparative response
reparenting
repartee
repatriation
repay
repeat
r. abuser
r. sex offender
r. tendency
repeated
r. abuse
r. bullying
r. hand-washing
r. heavy drinker
r. infarct dementia
r. nighttime awakening
r. painful experiences
r. REM sleep interruptions
r. shifts in affective expression
r. substance self-administration
r. suicide attempts
repeatedly
repeater
accident r.
repeating
r. pattern
r. ritual
repent
repentance
repentant
repercussion
repersonalization
repertoire
r. of aggressive behavior
behavioral r.
repertory
repetition
r. compulsion
compulsive r.
r. by imitation
impaired r.
needless r.
r. reaction
senseless imitative word r.
sentence r.
r. of sound
stereotyped r.
trauma-related r.
repetition-compulsion principle
repetitious
r. activity
r. behavior
r. request
repetitive
r. checking behavior
r. complaints
r. convulsion
r. exploratory behavior
r. fire setting
r. hand washing
r. hitting
r. idea
r. imitative movement
r. impulse disorder
r. lying
r. motor activity
r. partial seizure
r. pattern
r. pattern of behavior
r. play
r. question
r. request
r. ritual
r. rumination
r. screaming
r. statement
r. transcranial magnetic stimulation (rTMS)
r. violence
r. vocalization
r. watching
replaceable
replacement
electrolyte r.
r. formation
hormone r.
r. memory
r. relationship

NOTES

replacement *(continued)*
r. technique
r. therapy
repletion
replication
reply
latency of r.
report
case r.
r. criminal
informant r.
mental status examination r. (MSER)
paucity of r.'s
phenomenal r.
retrospective r.
reportedly
reporting abuse
Reposans-10
repose
reprehend
reprehension
representation
coitus r.
collective r.
concrete r.
internal r.
preexisting r.
symbolic r.
representational system
representative
instinct r.
r. intelligence
r. sample
repress
repressed
r. emotion
r. feeling
r. impulse
r. instinctual drive
r. need
return of the r.
repressing emotional trauma
repression
cognitive approach to dreaming and r.
emotional r.
organic r.
primal r.
primary r.
proper r.
r. resistance
secondary r.
repressive
r. behavior
r. coping style
r. inspirational group psychotherapy
r. personality
repressor
reprieve
reprimand
reprisal
reproach
reprobate
reprocessing
eye movement r.
eye movement desensitization and r. (EMDR)
reproduce
reproduction
chain r.
visual r.
reproductive
r. assimilation
r. facilitation
r. failure
r. mortality
reprove
reptilian stare
repudiate
repugnance
repugnant
repulse
repulsion
repulsive
reputable
reputation
evil r.
repute
request
repetitious r.
repetitive r.
required
r. guardianship
r. relationship
r. task
requirement
performance r.
requisite
rescind
rescission
rescue
r. fantasy
r. mechanism
r. operation
rescuer
research
action r.
advocacy r.
Agency for Health Care Policy and R. (AHCPR)
applied r.
r. assistant
Australian Council for Educational R. (ACER)
behavioral r.
biologic r.
brain r.

r. clinic
comparative r.
consumer r.
cross-sectional r.
empirical r.
epidemiological r.
ethics of psychiatric r.
evaluation r.
field r.
genetic r.
infancy r.
r. initiative
Institute of Educational R. (IER)
Institute of Personality and R. (IPAR)
International Society for Sexually Transmitted Disease R.
intervention r.
r. interview
motivation r.
neurochemical r.
nonspecific r.
normatological r.
r. observation
operational r.
operations r. (OR)
personality r.
population r.
r. program
psychiatric r.
psychological r.
quasi-experimental r.
specificity of r.
taxonomic r.
twin r.

researcher
personality r.
psychiatric r.

resemblance
clinical r.

resemble

resent

resentful

resentment
covert r.

reservatus
coitus r.

reserve
cognitive r.
operant r.

reservist

reside

residence
intensive care community r.

residential
r. OCD program
r. placement
r. setting
r. treatment
r. treatment center (RTC)
r. treatment facility

resident physician

residual
r. amnesia
r. disability
r. impairment
r. negative symptom
r. pain
r. phase
r. positive symptom
r. psychotic symptom
r. schizophrenia
r. state

residual-type
r.-t. schizophrenia
r.-t. schizophrenic disorder

residue
archaic r.
day r.
night r.

resignation
neurotic r.

Resilience: Acceptance of Life and Self

resilient

resiniferatoxin receptor

resistance
analysis of r.
r. analysis
r. to bathing
r. to care
character r.
compliance masking covert r.
conscious r.
covert r.
ego r.
environmental r. (ER)
r. to extinction
galvanic skin r.
id r.
least r.
r. level
manifestation of r.
overt compliance masking covert r.
passive r.
patient r.

NOTES

resistance *(continued)*
psychogalvanic skin r. (PGSR)
repression r.
social r.
state of r.
superego r.
r. to thyroid hormone (RTH)
transference r.
treatment r.
unconscious r.
violent r.
resistant
r. attachment
r. depression
r. mood disorder
r. schizophrenia
seizure r.
treatment r.
resistentiae
locus minoris r.
resistiveness
resocialization
resolute
resolution
anxiety r.
conflict r.
crisis r.
peer-to-peer conflict r.
r. phase
r. phase of sexual response cycle
temporal r.
resolve conflict
resolving
r. conflict skills
r. emotional trauma
resonance
acoustic r.
r. disorder
resource
cluster of r.'s
community r.
r. for coping
deep inner r.
r. holding potential
human r.'s
intellectual r.
lacking social r.'s
mental health r.
neuropsychologic r.
psychological r.
r. state
resourceful
respect
boundary r.
mutual r.
respectable
respectful
respiration
Biot r.
bronchial r.
Cheyne-Stokes r.
diffusion r.
electrophrenic r.
internal r.
opposition r.
temperature, pulse, r. (TPR)
tissue r.
respiratory
r. anosmia
r. depression
r. impairment sleep disorder
r. pause
r. psychogenic disorder
respite
place of r.
r. time
resplendent
respondeat superior
respondent
r. behavior
r. condition
r. conditioning
respond to environment
responder
psychotherapy r. (PR)
response
abnormal r.
abnormal muscle r. (AMR)
achromatic color r.
r. acquiescence
acute stress r.
adaptive r.
adverse autonomic r.
adverse psychological r.
affect r.
aggressive r.
agitation r.
amygdala r.
anamnestic r.
anticipatory r.
antidepressant r.
antipsychotic r.
anxiety relief r.
anxiolytic r.
appropriate r.
appropriateness of emotional r.
auditory brainstem r. (ABR)
auditory evoked r.
autonomic r.
aversion r.
avoidance r.
barrier r.
blink r.
blunted r.
brain r.
brainstem auditory evoked r.
caffeine r.
catastrophic r.

cellular immunologic r.
center-surround r.
chaining r.
chromatic r.
chronic r.
cingulate r.
circular pattern r.
clasp-knife r.
clerical r.
clinical r.
cocaine-related r.
color r.
conditioned avoidance r.
conditioned drug r.
conditioned emotional r. (CER)
conditioned escape r.
confabulated detail r. (dD)
confabulated whole r. (DWR)
consistent r.
coping r.
cortical evoked r.
covert r.
criminal r.
culturally sanctioned r.
culturally unsanctioned r.
cumulative r.
r. curve
Cushing r.
delayed r.
r. deviation
differential r.
discrete emotional r.
r. dispersion
dissociative r.
dysphoric r.
dyspnea r.
dysregulated stress r.
electrodermal r. (EDR)
emotional r.
r. to environment
evoked r. (ER)
evoked potential r. (EPR)
evoked somatosensory r.
exaggerated startle r.
extensor plantar r.
eye blink r.
false-negative r.
false-positive r.
fastigial pressor r. (FPR)
fear r.
fight-or-flight r.
form r. (F)
free r.
frequency r.
frustration r.
galvanic skin r. (GSR)
generalization r.
genital r.
good form r. (F+)
heat defense r.
hedonic r.
r. hierarchy
hostile r.
human r. (h)
human figure parts r.
human movement r.
hyperactive sympathetic r.
hypnotic r.
immune r.
implicit r.
inadequate r.
inappropriate r.
incompatible r.
inconsistent r.
r. index
individual r.
inhibited sexual r.
instrumental r.
intense startle r.
intropunitive r.
involuntary r.
latency of r.
latent r.
level of r.
local r.
long latency r.
loss of r.
low-key r.
maladaptive r.
marriage r.
mediated r.
metabolic r.
morbid r.
motor r.
negative r.
negativistic r.
no r.
oculomotor r.
orienting r.
original r.
overt r.
r. to pain
paradigmatic r.
paradoxical r.
pathological r.
r. pattern

NOTES

response *(continued)*
penetration r.
perseverative r.
personal r.
physiologic r.
pilomotor r.
plantar r.
polarity r.
poor form r. (F-)
poor genital r.
popular r.
position r.
positive r.
postsaccadic neuronal r.
r. prevention
r. processing time
psychogalvanic r. (PGR)
psychological r.
psychologically mediated r.
psychophysiologic r.
rare detail r.
r. rate
reactive r.
recruiting r.
reinforcing drug r.
relaxation r.
reparative r.
reward-irrelevant r.
satiety r.
r. set
sexual r.
shading r. (ShR)
skin conductance orienting r. (SCOR)
small detail r.
somatosensory evoked r. (SER)
sonomotor r.
space r.
r. specificity
startle r.
stimulus r.
stress effect and immune r.
stress-related physiological r.
sympathetic r.
r. system
target r.
texture r.
thalamic r.
r. theory
therapeutic r.
thermoeffector r.
thermoregulatory r.
tissue-type metabolic r.
total r. (lz R)
treatment r.
unconditioned r. (UCR)
unexpected r.
unsanctioned r.
unusual detail r. (Dd)
unusual rare detail r. (dr)
vibrotactile r.
vista r.
visual evoked r. (VER)
whole r. (W, WR)

response-driven procedure

response-produced cue

response-specificity

responsibility
ascriptive r.
assigned r.
clinical r.
community r.
criminal r.
denial of r.
diminished r.
disavows r.
distribution of r.
excessive r.
feeling of r.
generational r.
homemaking r.
household r.
increased r.
individual r.
interpersonal r.
legal r.
limited r.
minimize r.
new r.
obsessive feelings of r.
patient r.
personal r.
position of r.
primary r.
sense of r.
serotonergic r.
sexual r.
social r.
test of criminal r.

responsible
r. eating habit
r. sexual behavior

responsive
treatment r.

responsiveness
abnormal r.
absence of emotional r.
affective r.
diminished r.
emotional r.
facial r.
mutual affective r.
OCD r.
reduced r.
threshold of r.

responsivity
emotional r.
mood r.

neuroleptic r.
treatment r.

REST
regressive electroshock treatment
restricted environment stimulation therapy

rest
r. home
metabolism at r.
r. pain
regional glucose metabolism at r.
r. tremor

restatement

rest-cure technique

restful

resting
r. anterior cingulate flow
r. energy expenditure
r. PET study
r. potential
r. state
r. tremor
r. wakefulness

restitution
cognitive r.
neurologic r.

restitutional symptoms of schizophrenia

restitutive therapy

restless
r. behavior
r. leg
r. leg syndrome
r. pacing

restlessness
motor r.
motoric r.
nocturnal r.
psychomotor r.

restrain

restraining
r. order
r. order violation
r. therapy

restraint
ankle r.
chemical r.
chest r.
compulsive r.
dietary r.
ethical r.
involuntary r.
lack of r.
r. law
leather r.
physical r.
4-point r.
Posey r.
seclusion and r. (S&R)
sign of r.
situational r.
soft r.
wrist r.

restricted
r. access to food
r. activity
r. behavior
r. diet
r. environment stimulation therapy (REST)
r. focus
r. interest
r. range of affect
r. range of emotional expression

restricting
r. behavior
r. type

restriction
activity r.
building r.
close watch r.
dietary r.
ego r.
r. endonuclease
r. fragment length polymorphism (RFLP)
open seclusion r.
shoe r.
sleep r.
unit r.

restrictive
r. attitude
r. behavior
r. criterion

restructuring
attitude r.
cognitive r.
perceptual r.
sexual attitude r. (SAR)
systematic rational r. (SRR)

restzustand schizophrenia

result
anomalous r.
biometric r.
concordant r.
positive r.

resumption

NOTES

R

resurgence
resuscitate
do not r. (DNR)
resuscitation
cardiopulmonary r. (CPR)
resuscitative snores
resymbolization
RET
rational emotive therapy
Ret, ret
retarded
retaliate
retaliation
retaliatory aggression
retardata
ejaculatio r.
retardation
American Association of Mental R. (AAMR)
arithmetical skills learning r.
borderline mental r.
cultural-familial mental r.
developmental r.
r. developmental delay disorder
frank mental r.
idiopathic language r.
incidental learning language r.
language skills learning r.
learning r.
mental r. (MR)
moderate mental r.
motor r.
perceptual r.
psychomotor r.
psychopathology of r.
r. psychopathology
psychosis with mental r.
psychosocial r.
reading skills learning r.
severe mental r.
simple r.
trichorrhexis nodosa with mental r.
unspecified mental r.
retarded (Ret, ret)
r. depression
r. development
educable mentally r. (EMR)
r. ejaculation
r. maturation
mentally r.
profoundly r.
r. schizophrenia
trainable mentally r. (TMR)
retch
retell
retention
r. control training
r. defect
fluid r.
informal r.
involuntary r.
memory r.
psychogenic r.
r. and recall
selective r.
r. in treatment
voluntary r.
retentive
anal r.
retest
RETHINK
recognize, empathize, think, hear, integrate, notice, keep
reticence
reticent
reticula (*pl. of* reticulum)
reticular
r. activating system (RAS)
r. thalamic nucleus
reticuloendothelial system
reticulum, pl. **reticula**
retifism
retinopathy
retirement
job r.
r. neurosis
r. planning
r. syndrome
retiring
retort
retrace
retract
retraction nystagmus
retrain
retraining
breathing r.
r. emotion
retreat
r. from reality
vegetative r.
York r.
retrenchment
ego r.
retribution
retributive rage
retrieval
information r.
limited-capacity r.
r. problem
r. task
word r.
retroactive
r. amnesia
r. displacement
r. inhibition (RI)
retroanterograde amnesia
retrocollic spasm
retrocollis

retrocursive absence
retroflexed rage
retroflexion
retrogasserian
retrogenesis
law of r.
retrograde
r. amnesia
r. degeneration
r. ejaculation
r. loss of memory
r. memory interference
retrography
retrogression
retropulsion of gait
retropulsive epilepsy
retrospect
retrospection
retrospective
r. experimental study design
r. falsification
r. gaps in memory
r. projection
r. report
r. ruminative jealousy
r. study
retrosplenial cingulate pathway
Rett
R. disorder
R. syndrome
return
law of diminishing r.
point of no r.
r. of the repressed
returning to home
reuniens
nucleus r.
reunion
reunite
reuptake
r. blockade
dopamine r.
r. inhibitor
reus
actus r.
revamp
revelation
revenant
revenge
desire for r.
r. murder
r. obsession
revengeful
reverberating circuit
revere
reverence
reverent
reverie
hypnagogic r.
reversal
r. of affect
behavior r.
deficit r.
r. formation
gender role r.
habit r.
r. learning
phase r.
role r.
sex r.
sleep r.
sudden financial r.
surgical sex r.
reverse
r. anorexia nervosa
r. causality
r. discrimination
r. diurnal variation
r. orientation
r. vegetative symptoms
reversed orientation
reversibility
reversible
r. affective disorder syndrome
r. amnesia
r. cause
r. cholinesterase inhibitor
r. cognitive impairment of depression
r. decortication
r. dementia
r. intoxication
r. memory impairment
r. schizophrenia
r. shock
reversion
revert
review
claim r.
clinical record r.
comprehensive r.
computer-assisted r.
concurrent r.
continued stay r. (CSR)
contract r.
critical r.

NOTES

review *(continued)*
drug use r. (DUR)
empirical r.
extended-care r.
extended-stay r.
medical r.
r. method
record r.
systematic r.
r. of systems (ROS)
treatment services r.
utilization r. (UR)
revile
revindication
revised
revision
Diagnostic and Statistical Manual of Mental Disorders, 4th Edition, Text R. (DSM-IV-TR)
r. process
secondary r.
revisionism
revitalize
revive
revivification
revocable
revocation of driver's license
revoke
revolution
sexual r.
revolutionary
revolutionist
revolutionize
revolver
revolving
r. door
r. door syndrome
revulsion
sexual stimuli r.
rewake
reward
r. circuitry
consummatory r.
delayed r.
r. dependence (RD)
external r.
extrinsic r.
feeling frightened; expecting bad things to happen; attitudes and actions that help; results and r. (FEAR)
intrinsic r.
potential external r.
psychic r.
r. by superego
r. system
token economy r.
reward-and-punishment program
reward-associated behavior
rewarding effect
reward-irrelevant response
RFLP
restriction fragment length polymorphism
rhathymia
rhembasmus
rheobase
rheoencephalogram
rheoencephalography
rheumatica
tetania r.
rheumatic psychogenic disorder
rheumatism
rheumatoid
rhigosis
rhigotic
rhinencephalon
rhinolalia clausa
rhinorrhea
rhinotillexomania
rho
Spearman r.
rhombencephalic sleep
rhomboidalis
rhomboidal sinus
rhotacism
rhyme
rhyming
r. delirium
r. slang
word r.
rhypophagy
rhythmic, rhythmical
r. chorea
r. contraction
r. mood
r. movement disorder
r. oscillation
r. sensory bombardment therapy (RSBT)
r. slow eye movement
r. tremor
r. twitch
rhythmopathy and depression
RI
retroactive inhibition
RIA
relaxation-induced anxiety
ribald
ribonucleic acid (RNA)
Ribot law of regression
Rican
Puerto R.
Richardson-Steele-Olszewski syndrome
Richards-Rundel syndrome
riche
nouveau r.
riddance phenomenon

ridden
instinct r.
riddling
rider
night r.
ridicule
fear of r.
ridiculous
Riese hearing
rifle
assault r.
rift
right
bill of r.'s
civil r.'s
fight for r.'s
gay r.'s
r. hemisphere
r. hemisphere cognitive skills
r. hemisphere dominance
human r.'s
r. to life
mentally retarded persons' r.'s
moral r.
parental r.'s
patient r.'s
Patient's Bill of R.'s
privacy r.
r. to refuse treatment
The Mental Health Bill of R.'s
visitation r.'s
r. wing authoritarianism (RWA)
r. to work
righteous
right-footed
right-hand dominant
right-handed
right-handedness
right-left
r.-l. confusion
r.-l. discrimination
r.-l. disorientation
right-minded
right-to-lifer
rigid
r. akinetic syndrome
r. attitude
r. body position
r. control
r. eating plan
r. family
r. posture
r. pupil
r. sleep practice
r. state
rigidity
affective r.
catatonic r.
cerebellar r.
clasp-knife r.
cogwheel r.
decerebrate r.
excessive r.
extensor r.
extrapyramidal r.
intellectual r.
lead-pipe r.
muscle r.
mydriatic r.
nuchal r.
ratchet r.
rigor
Riley-Day syndrome
Riluzole
ring
international child pornography r.
Japanese erection r. (JER)
Kayser-Fleischer r.
multistate drug distribution r.
ringleader
riot gun
riotous
risible
risk
accident r.
acute suicide r.
addictive r.
adolescent at r.
alcoholism r.
at r.
attributable r.
averse to r.
r. aversion
children at r.
depression r.
elevated r.
empiric r.
established r.
r. factor
r. factor for mortality
r. factor for violence
falling r.
health r.
high suicide r.
imminent r.
r. indicator

NOTES

risk *(continued)*
infant at r.
r. level
lifetime r.
long-term r.
minimal r.
morbid r.
mortality r.
r. paradigm
parent at r.
persistent r.
r. preference
r. profile
psychiatric r.
r. ratio (RR)
recurrence r.
r. reduction
relative r.
r. rescue rating (RRR)
schizophrenia r.
significant r.
suicide r.
r. of suicide attempt
r. taker
underestimating r.
violence r.
women at r.

risk-benefit
r.-b. assessment
r.-b. profile
r.-b. ratio

risk-reduction counseling

risk-taking
r.-t. behavior
sex-related r.-t.
sexual r.-t.

risky
r. sexual activity
r. sexual behavior

risque

risus
r. caninus
r. sardonicus

rite
r. of passage
puberty r.

Ritter
R. law
R. opening tetanus

Ritter-Rollet phenomenon

ritual
r. abuse
accepted r.
ADHD r.
r. behavior
body modification r.
checking and touching r.'s
cognitive r.
compulsive r.
degrading r.
hand-washing r.
healing r.
r. injury in OCD
r. ligature strangulation
marriage r.
masochistic r.
painful r.
presentational r.
r. prevention
r. reduction
repeating r.
repetitive r.
self-damage r.
sleep r.
touching r.

ritualism

ritualistic
r. behavior
r. fashion
r. thinking

ritualized makeup application

ritualizer

ritual-making

rival normative theory

rivalry
perceptual r.
sibling r.

rive

riverboat gambling

RLE
recent life event

RNA
ribonucleic acid
heterogeneous nuclear RNA
messenger RNA

RO
reality orientation
reality oriented

R/O
rule out

road
r. rage
yellow brick r. (YBR)

robber

robbery
drug-facilitated r.
fear of r.

Robertson pupil

robotic

robotism

robotize

robust

robustious

ROC
receiver operating characteristic

Rochester method

rock
acid r.

hard r.
r. and roll
soft r.

rocker

rocking
body r.

rodonalgia

rofecoxib

rogerian
r. group therapy
r. theory

rogue's gallery

roister

rolandic
r. epilepsy
r. fissure

Rolando
fissure of R.
R. zone

role
alternating r.
altruistic r.
r. ambiguity
anticipation of r.
attacker r.
behavior r.
r. boundary
caretaking r.
central r.
community r.
complementary r.
r. conflict
r. confusion
contributing r.
cross-sex r.
cultural r.
r. demand
dependent patient r.
r. deprivation
r. deviance
r. diffusion
discomfort with gender r.
etiologic r.
r. experimentation
explicit r.
feminine social r.
r. fixation
follower r.
r. function
gender r.
helper r.
implicit r.
r. insufficiency
integral r.
interpersonal r.
interpreter r.
leader r.
leadership r.
masculine social r.
maternal r.
r. model
noncomplementary r.
r. obligation
r. obsolescence
pathophysiologic r.
r. pattern
peacemaker r.
pivotal r.
r. playing
protector r.
regulatory r.
r. reversal
sex r.
r. shift
sick r.
social r.
r. specialization
spectator r.
stereotypical gender r.'s
r. strain
thematic r.
r. theory of personality
therapeutic r.
r. therapy
r. transition
r. transition in aging
victim r.
women's r.

role-enactment theory

role-play

role-playing

rolfing

roll
rock and r.
Spiegel eye r.

roller
r. coaster emotion
high r.

rollick

romance
family r.
r. fantasy
memory r.

Roman holiday

romantic
r. disappointment

NOTES

romantic *(continued)*
r. fantasy
r. intrigue
r. relationship
romanticism
romanticize
Romberg
R. sign
R. symptom
Romberg-Howship symptom
rombergism
rookie
room
behavior control r. (BCR)
r. and board
chill-out r.
consulting r.
dead r.
emergency r. (ER)
free field r.
Internet suicide chat r.
locked r.
padded r.
quiet r.
semiprivate r.
roomer
roommate conflict
rootedness
rooted obsession
roots of prejudice
Rorschach
R. card
R. projective technique
ROS
review of systems
rosa
mal de la r.
rose-colored glasses
Rosenbach law
Rosenthal syndrome
rosso
mal r.
rostral
r. medial prefrontal cortex
r. supplementary motor area
rostrum, pl. **rostra, rostrums**
rotary
r. nystagmus
r. vertigo
rotated factor
rotation
factor r.
varimax r.
rotatoria
chorea r.
rotatory
r. jaw movement
r. spasm
r. tic
rote
r. memory
r. recall
r. verbal learning
rotted obsession
rotunda
fenestra r.
Rouge
Khmer R.
rough-and-tumble play
roughness
roughshod
roulette
Russian r.
Rouse vs Cameron
route
cognitive r.
oral r.
routine
agreed-on r.
r. clinical care
complex finger r.
complex hand r.
constant r.
family r.
grimly adhered-to r.
motor r.
negligible r.
r. screening
r. skill
stereotyped r.
task-specific r.
r. use
roving
r. eye movement
r. ocular movement
row
death r.
skid r.
royal
R. College of Psychiatrists (RCP)
r. malady
RPM-R
Raven progressive matrices-R
RR
risk ratio
RRR
risk rescue rating
RRT
registered recreation therapist
RSBT
rhythmic sensory bombardment therapy
RT
rational therapy
reaction time
recreational therapy
RTC
residential treatment center

RTH
resistance to thyroid hormone
rTMS
repetitive transcranial magnetic stimulation
rub
r. out
r. up
rubber
burning r.
r. fetish
rubberist
rubbing
coin r.
rubella embryopathy
Rubinstein-Taybi syndrome
Rubin vase
rubric
ruckus
rudeness
rudimentary paranoia
rueful
rugged
ruination
ruinous
rule
r. of abstinence
American Law Institute r.
analytic r.
Anstie r.
assimilation r.
base r.
basic r.
r. bending
r. breaker
disregard for r.'s
dissimilation r.
Durham r.
r. of evidence
grandma r.
ground r.
group r.
Hebb r.
1-hour restraint r.
house r.
Jackson r.
mature minor r.
M'Naghten r.
morphological r.
neutralization r.
New Hampshire r.
OHIO r.
only-handle-it-once r.
r. out (R/O)
Pitres r.
r. preoccupation
redundancy r.
seclusion and restraint r.
sequencing r.
serious violations of r.'s
r. skills
syntactic r.
Tarasoff r.
r. of thumb
transformational r.
r. utilitarianism
violation of r.'s
ruler
ruling
r. of court
r. in tics
rumble
rumbling
ruminate
rumination
anxious r.
behavioral theory of r.
depressive r.
r. disorder
r. disorder of infancy
guilty r.
homicidal r.
manie de r.
morbid r.
neurotic r.
obsessional r.
obsessive r.
persistent r.
psychogenic r.
repetitive r.
suicidal r.
r. syndrome
ruminative
r. coping style
r. depression
r. idea
r. tension state
r. thought
r. worry
rumormonger
rumor spreading
run
r.'s in family
r. in
trial r.
runabout

NOTES

runaround
runaway
habitual r.
r. hotline
r. reaction
running
r. commentary
r. commentary hallucination
r. fit
runny nose
rural
r. psychiatry
r. society
ruralist
Russell
R. sign
R. syndrome
Russian roulette
russomania
ruthful
ruthless
RWA
right wing authoritarianism
Rx
prescription
therapy
RXR
9-*cis* retinoic acid receptor

7s
serial 7s
SA
Schizophrenics Anonymous
self-analysis
sensory awareness
Sexaholics Anonymous
social acquiescence
social age
suicide attempt
SAA
Sex Addicts Anonymous
sabotage
masochistic s.
s. of therapy
saboteur
sabulous
saccade
saccadic
s. eye movement
s. tracking
saccharate
sacerdotal
sacerdotalism
sacrament
sacramental
sacramentalist
sacrifice
sacrificial
sacrilege
sacrolisthesis
sacrosanct
SAD
seasonal affective disorder
separation anxiety disorder
social avoidance and distress
S-adenosylmethionine (SAMe)
sadism
anal s.
id s.
infantile s.
larval s.
manual s.
omnipotent infantile s.
oral s.
phallic s.
primal s.
sexual s.
superego s.
sadist
sexual s.
sadistic
s. act of rape
s. behavior
s. mutilation
s. patient
s. personality
s. personality disorder
s. rape act
s. sexual abuse
SADL, SADLs
simulated activities of daily living
sad mood
sadness
feeling of s.
frequent s.
induced s.
normal s.
s. period
profound s.
prolonged s.
recall-generated s.
sadomasochism (SM, S/M)
bondage and s. (BDSM)
sexual s.
sadomasochistic
s. personality disorder
s. relationship
s. sex
s. trend
SAD PERSONS
sex, age, depression, previous attempt, ethanol, rational thinking loss, separated, divorced, widowed, organized plan, no social support, stated future intent
SADR
suspected adverse drug reaction
Saenger sign
SAFE
support, autonomy, fusioning, empathy
safe
s. environment
s. place
s. sex
s. sex activity
safeguard
safekeeping
safety
community s.
contract for s.
s. device
s. of ego
factor of s. (FS)
s. motive
patient s.
sense of s.
therapeutic s.
s. valve
workplace s.

sagging posture
sagittal
s. orientation
s. plane
SAID
sexually acquired immunodeficiency
Saint (St.)
S. Dymphna disease
S. John's dance
S. Louis criteria for schizophrenia
S. Martin disease
S. Mathurin disease
saintly
salaam
s. convulsion
s. seizure
s. spasm
salacious
salad
word s.
sale
illegal drug s.
Saleto
salicylate
ammonium s.
amyl s.
salience
emotional s.
s. of religion
s. of spirituality
salient loading
saliva
s. screen for alcohol
s. smearing
salivation
sallow
salt
inorganic mercury s.
saltation
saltatoria
saltatory
s. chorea
s. conduction
s. evolution
s. spasm
salt-free diet
salubrious
salute
salvation
salvo
SAM
sex arousal mechanism
SAMe
S-adenosylmethionine
sameness
preoccupation with s.
same-sex
s.-s. disclosure
s.-s. group composition
s.-s. harassment
s.-s. marriage
s.-s. orientation
s.-s. peer
s.-s. sexual experience
s.-s. twins
Samoan
sample
cocaine-free urine s.
random s.
representative s.
s. standard deviation
sampling
area s.
behavior s.
block s.
controlled s.
samsara
SAN
slept all night
sanatorium, sanitarium
sanctification
sanctimonious
sanctimony
sanction
legal s.
social s.
sanctioned
culturally s.
sanctity
sanctuary
sanctum
sandbox marriage
Sander disease
Sandler
S. triad
S. view of depressive disorder
sandwich generation
sane
Sanfilippo
S. disease
S. syndrome
sangue dormido
sanguine constitutional type
sanguineous
sanitarium (*var. of* sanatorium)
sanity
SAPD
self-administration of psychoactive drug
sapience
sapphism
SAR
sexual attitude reassessment
sexual attitude restructuring
sarcasm
sarcastic
sardonic
s. grin
s. laugh

sardonicus
risus s.
sarmassation
SAT
systematized assertive therapy
satanic
s. cult
s. worship
satanism
satanist
Satan worship
satellite
s. clinic
s. housing
satellitosis
satiable
satiate
satiation
eating without s.
food s.
satiety
s. center
s. response
satisfaction
decreased job s.
impaired orgasm s.
job s.
life s.
marital s.
orgasm s.
patient s.
personal s.
relationship s.
sativa
Cannabis s.
Saturday night palsy
saturnine encephalopathy
satyriasis
satyrism
satyromania
Saunders-Sutton syndrome
savage attack
savagely
savagery
savant
idiot s.
linguistic s.
s. skill
save face
saver
face s.
savoir faire
savvy
sawtooth wave
saxonus
coitus s.
SBB
stimulation-bound behavior
SBD
supervisory behavior description
SBS
social breakdown syndrome
scabiomania
scaffolding
scale
absolute rating s.
Brief Psychiatric Rating S. (BPRS)
Brief Psychiatric Rating S.-Expanded (BPRS-E)
fish s.
modified overt aggression s. (MOAS)
scaling
age-grade s.
item s.
scalp
s. contusion
s. lock
scam
SCAN
suspected child abuse/neglect
scan
baseline s.
brain SPECT s.
CAT s.
computerized tomography s.
emission tomography s.
eye s.
genome s.
longitudinal s.
single-photon emission CT s.
scandal
sex s.
scandale
succès de s.
scandalize
scandalmonger
scandalous
scanner
neuro-optimized IGE LX System s.
scanning
s. communication board
comparative s.
eye s.
radioisotope brain s.

NOTES

scanning *(continued)*
s. speech
s. visage
scapegoat
scapegoating communication pattern
scaphocephalic idiocy
scar
emotional s.
multiple surgical s.'s
psychic s.
psychological s.
scared
scaremonger
scarfing
scarify
scarlet letter
Scarpa method
scary
scathe
scathing
scatologia
telephone s.
scatological, scatologic
s. language
scatology
scatophagy
scatter
s. child
s. diagram
scatteration
scatterbrained
scattering
scavenger
free radical s.
SCD
service-connected disability
scelalgia
scelotyrbe
scenario
physician-patient s.
scene
high-emotion s.
primal s.
traumatic s.
scent
psychology of s.
schadenfreude
schedule
S. I–IV
abnormal sleep-wake s.
altered sleep s.
child assessment s. (CAS)
s. for clinical assessment in neuropsychiatry
continuous reinforcement s.
coping with bipolar prodromes s.
developmental s.
s. drug
fixed-interval reinforcement s.
fixed-ratio reinforcement s.
s. II substance
interest s.
intermittent reinforcement s.
medication taper s.
mental health diagnostic interview s.
mental status s. (MSS)
National Institute of Mental Health-Diagnostic Interval S. (NIMH-DIS)
positive and negative affect s.
s. preoccupation
regular eating s.
regular sleeping s.
regular waking s.
s. of reinforcement
reinforcement s.
shifting sleep-work s.
sleep-wake s.
social functioning s.
status s.
s. for Tourette syndrome and other behavioral syndromes
variable-interval reinforcement s.
vocational interest s. (VIS)
work s.
Scheid
cyanotic syndrome of S.
S. cyanotic syndrome
schema, pl. **schemata**
body s.
cognitive s.
Kraepelin s.
perceptual s.
schematic mental model
scheme
Schicksal analysis
Schirmer syndrome
schism
marital s.
schismatic
schismatize
schizencephalic microcephaly
schizencephaly
schizoaffective
s. disorder
s. disorder, bipolar type
s. disorder, depressed
s. disorder, manic
s. episode
s. psychosis
s. schizophrenia
s. syndrome
schizobipolar
schizocaria
schizogen
schizogyria

schizoid
- s. composite description
- s. diagnostic prototype
- s. disorder of childhood
- s. fantasy
- s. feature
- s. neurotic personality disorder
- s. personality
- s. position
- s. Q factor
- s. trait

schizoidia

schizoidism

schizoid-schizotypal personality disorder (SSPD)

schizomania

schizomanic

schizomimetic

schizophasia

schizophrasia

schizophrene

schizophrenese

schizophrenia (SZ)
- active-phase symptom of s.
- acute simple-type s.
- acute undifferentiated s.
- adult s.
- alternative dimensional descriptor for s.
- ambulatory s.
- Andreasen positive and negative symptoms of s.
- arrest of s.
- atypical s.
- behavioral disorganization in s.
- borderline s. (BS)
- burned-out anergic s.
- catastrophic s.
- catatonic s.
- catatonic-type s.
- cenesthopathic s.
- childhood s.
- childhood-onset s.
- chronic s.
- chronic undifferentiated s.
- clearcut s.
- coenesthetic s.
- compensation s.
- cyclic s.
- 3-day s.
- deficit s.
- s. deliriosa
- delusion in s.
- depressed schizoaffective s.
- derailment in s.
- diathesis-stress theory of s.
- disorganized s.
- disorganized factor in s.
- disorganized speech in s.
- disorganized-type s.
- distorted communication in s.
- distorted language in s.
- double bind theory of s.
- early-onset s.
- engrafted s.
- exaggerated communication in s.
- exaggerated inferential thinking in s.
- excited schizoaffective s.
- 3-factor dimensional model of s.
- familial transmission of s.
- Finnish adoptive family study of s.
- first-episode s.
- flexibilitas cerea s.
- fragmentary hallucination in s.
- grandiose-type s.
- hebephrenic s.
- hypofrontality hypothesis in s.
- iatrogenic s.
- incipient s.
- s. index
- individual with s.
- induced s.
- jealous-type s.
- larval s.
- late-life s.
- latent s.
- late-onset s.
- medication-resistant s.
- mixed s.
- mixed-type s.
- negative-symptom s.
- nondeficit s.
- nonkraepelinian chronic s.
- nonregressive s.
- nonsystematic s.
- nuclear s.
- oneiroid s.
- paranoid s.
- paranoid-type s.
- paraphrenic s.
- Pavlov theory of s.
- persecutory-type s.
- s. phase
- positive s.
- prepsychotic s.

NOTES

schizophrenia *(continued)*
primary s.
process s.
prodromal phase of s.
prolonged prodrome of s.
prototypical s.
pseudoautosomal locus for s.
pseudoneurotic s.
pseudopsychopathic s.
s. psychosis
psychotic dimension of s.
psychotic disorganization in s.
reactive s.
recent-onset s.
recidivism in s.
refractory s.
regressive symptoms of s.
remitting s.
residual s.
residual-type s.
resistant s.
restitutional symptoms of s.
restzustand s.
retarded s.
reversible s.
s. risk
Saint Louis criteria for s.
schizoaffective s.
schizophreniform s.
schizophreniform-type s.
Schneider diagnostic system for s.
Selvini-Palazzoli model of s.
simple s.
simple-type s.
s. simplex
somatic s.
s. spectrum
s. spectrum disorder
subchronic s.
s. symptom
s. syndrome
systematic s.
toxic s.
treatment-refractory s.
treatment-resistant s.
undifferentiated s.
undifferentiated-type s.
unspecified s.
water balance in s.
s. with childhood onset
withdrawn catatonic s.
s. with premorbid asociality (SPA)
s. with premorbid association (SPA)

schizophrenia-prone individual

schizophrenic
s. affect
anergic s.
S.'s Anonymous (SA)
s. attack
burned-out s.
s. catalepsy
s. catatonia
s. defect state
s. dementia
s. diagnosis
s. disorder
s. episode
s. exacerbation
s. excitement
s. factor
s. genotype
s. illness
s. inpatient
International Society for the Psychologic Treatment of S.'s
neuroleptic-resistant s.
s. paranoid psychosis
s. patient
s. personality
s. process
s. reaction
s. reaction, acute paranoid (SR/AP)
s. reaction, acute undifferentiated (SR/AU)
s. reaction, chronic paranoid (SR/CP)
s. reaction, chronic undifferentiated (SR/CU)
s. residual state (SRS)
s. spectrum (SS)
subchronic s.
s. surrender
s. symptom
s. syndrome
s. syndrome of childhood
treatment-resistant s.

schizophrenic-affective psychosis

schizophreniform
s. attack
s. diagnosis
s. disorder
s. patient
s. psychosis
s. schizophrenia

schizophreniform-type schizophrenia

schizophrenosis

schizotaxia

schizothemia

schizothyme

schizothymia
introverted s.
schizotypal s.

schizothymic personality

schizotonia

schizotypal
s. category
s. patient

s. personality disorder
s. schizoid personality
s. schizothymia
schizotypy
schmaltz
schnauzkrampf
Schneider
S. definition of personality
S. diagnostic system for schizophrenia
S. first-rank symptom
schneiderian
s. criteria for depressive personality
s. delusion
s. first-rank symptom
schneiderian-type papilloma
scholarly
scholastic attainment
school
s. achievement
s. adjustment
s. advisor
s. age
alternative s.
s. aversion
s. counselor
s. culture
day s.
s. difficulty
s. discipline problem
s. dropout
s. dysfunction
s. entering problem
existential s.
s. functioning
s. functioning impairment
s. handicap condition
s. history
humanistic s.
s. language
middle s.
missed s.
s. nurse
s. performance
s. phobia
problem in s.
s. refusal
s. refusal syndrome
senior high s.
s. sickness
s. support system
s. of thought
s. truancy
school-age
s.-a. child
s.-a. testing
school-based
s.-b. child-and-parent-focused psychosocial treatment
s.-b. intervention
Schooler-Kane criteria
schooling
home s.
poor s.
schoolmaster
Schreber case
Schuele sign
Schüller phenomenon
Schutz measure
schwannoma
sciatica
science
applied s.
Bachelor of Medical S.
behavioral s.
cognitive s.
exact s.
S. Research Associates (SRA)
social s.
scientific
s. credibility
s. empiricism
s. method
s. proof
s. psychopathology
scientism
scientist
Scientology religion
scierneuropsia
scieropia
sciolism
sciosophy
scissor gait
sclera, pl. **sclerae**
injected s.
scleresis
pavor s.
sclerneuropsia
scleropia
sclerosis, pl. **scleroses**
Canavan s.
combined s.
diffuse s.
focal s.
hippocampal s.
insular s.

NOTES

sclerosis *(continued)*
lobar s.
mantle s.
s. of white matter
sclerotica
eutonia s.
scleroticans
sclerotic area
sclerotome area
scoliosis
scoop
SCOPE
systematic, complete, objective, practical, empirical
scope of treatment
scopolagnia
scopomorphinism
scopophilia
scoptophilia
SCOR
skin conductance orienting response
scoracratia
score
age s.
avoidance s.
Barnes global s.
BPRS anxiety-depression s.
BPRS total s.
BPRS withdrawal/retardation s.
Charlson comorbidity s.
chronic disease s.
clinical global impressions severity and improvement s.
clinical performance s. (CPS)
cognitive s.
composite s.
compulsion s.
conservative cutoff s.
critical s.
cutoff s.
depression s.
descriptor s.
dichotomization of s.
s. discrimination
elevated s.
emotional memory s.
endpoint CGI s.
event recall s.
factor s.
finger-tapping s.
general knowledge s.
global aggression s.
global clinical impression s.
Hachinski ischemic s.
intelligence s.
intrusion s.
IS total s.
liberal cutoff s.
logarithm of odds s.
logical memory subtest s.
mania rating s.
mean total weighted sum s.
memory s.
mood cluster s.
narcissistic Q s.
negative s.
numerical s.
overall defensive functioning s.
overprotection s.
pain and distress s.
peak s.
percentile s.
performance s.
personality disorder s.
personal memory s.
positive s.
practical social judgment s.
Q s.
quantitative s.
raw s.
SANS total s.
Simpson-Angus total s.
social judgment s.
speech discrimination s. (SDS)
standard s.
subclinical s.
subtest scale s.
sum s.
summary s.
T s.
total AIMS s.
total emotional memory s.
total symptom s.
total weighted sum s.
verbal weighted sum s.
weighted sum s.
word discrimination s.
Z s.
scorecard
scoring
s. coefficient
objective s.
scorn
scornful
Scorpio
scotoma, pl. **scotomata**
absolute s.
cecocentral s.
central s.
dense s.
flittering s.
fortification s.
homogenous scintillating s.
mental s.
negative s.
paracentral s.
relative s.
scotomization

scotophilia
scourge
scowl
scrappy
scratch fear
scratching
excessive skin s.
scrawny
scream
primal s.
screamer
screaming
repetitive s.
screech
screen
age-adjusted genome s.
blank s.
blood drug s.
s. for caregiver burden
cocaine-free urine s.
s. defense
dream s.
drug s.
s. fantasy
gambling s.
genome s.
heavy metal s.
memory s.
7-minute s.
opiate-free urine s.
s. out irrelevant stimulus
sex-adjusted genome s.
simple drug s.
smoke s.
syphilis s.
tox s.
toxicology s.
urine drug s.
Urine Luck adulterant for urine drug s.
urine toxicology s.
screener
screening
s. for alcohol
developmental s.
s. examination
fetal s.
genetic s.
illiteracy s.
language s.
organicity s.
periodic s.
polymorphism s.
preemployment drug s.
s. question
routine s.
S. for Somatoform Symptoms
toxicology s.
scribble
scribomania
script
s. analysis
life s.
sexual s.
scriptorius
calamus s.
scrotal pain
scrub
scruffy
scruple
decoration s.
defloration s.
virginity s.
scrupulosity
scrupulous
scrupulously observant
scrutinize
scrutiny
SCS
subacute confusional state
sculpting
family s.
scum
scurrile
scurrility
scurrilous
scurry
Scutellaria lateriflora
S-D
suicide-depression
SD
standard deviation
Sd
stimulus drive
SDAT
senile dementia of Alzheimer type
SDB
sleep-disordered breathing
SDD
specific developmental disorder
sporadic depressive disease
SDL
self-directed learning
SDR
sequential diagrammatic reformulation

NOTES

S

SDS
sensory deprivation syndrome
speech discrimination score
seaman mania
seamstress' cramp
seamy
sear
search
s. for parent
strip s.
transderivational s.
s. warrant
word s.
searching
symptom s.
searchingly
searing pain
seasonal
s. affective disorder (SAD)
s. affective disorder syndrome
s. energy syndrome
s. factor
s. migraine
s. migraine headache
s. mood disorder
s. mood swing
s. pattern
seasonal-related psychosocial stressor
season of birth
seasoned
seat
driver's s.
Seattle Longitudinal Study
secandi
mania s.
secern
secession
Seckel syndrome
seclude
secluded environment
seclusion
involuntary s.
s. law
locked door s.
s. need
office s.
s. and restraint (S&R)
s. and restraint rule
unlocked s.
voluntary s.
seclusive personality
second
s. childhood
s. fiddle
s. generation
s. guess
s. impact syndrome
s. messenger
s. negative phase
s. opinion
s. signaling system
s. thought
secondary
s. amenorrhea
s. anorgasmy
s. autism
s. autoerotism
s. care
s. defense symptom
s. degeneration
s. delirium
s. dementia
s. depression
s. deviance
s. diagnosis
s. drive
s. effect
s. elaboration
s. elaboration of dream
s. emotional problem
s. environment
s. erectile dysfunction
s. fantasy
s. gain
s. generalized epilepsy
s. identification
s. impotence
s. integration
s. mania
s. mental deficiency
s. mood disorder
s. morbidity
s. motivation
s. narcissism
s. orgasmic dysfunction
s. pain
s. personality
s. personality trait
s. prevention
s. process
s. process thinking
s. psychic process
s. reinforcement
s. reinforcer
s. repression
s. retarded ejaculation
s. revision
s. reward conditioning
s. self
s. sensation
s. sex characteristic
s. sleep disorder
s. stress
s. syphilis
s. transitional object
s. verbal memory
second-class
second-generation antipsychotic drug

second-line
s.-l. agent
s.-l. medication
s.-l. therapy
second-messenger system
second-order conditioning
second-rate
secrecy
secret
s. ceremony
s. control
s. society
secretase inhibitor
secretin
secretion
cortisol s.
leptin s.
secretive manner
sect
sectarian
section
axial s.
coronal s.
S. Eight
pituitary stalk s.
psychiatric services s. (PSS)
sectionalism
sector
secularism
secularist
secular trend
secure
s. attachment
s. attachment style
s. base effect
s. communication
s. correspondence
s. environment
security
s. blanket
s. breach
breach of s.
computer s.
emotional s.
false sense of s.
maximum s.
s. operation
Sedapap
sedate
sedation
acute s.
daytime s.
prolonged s.
s. threshold
unnecessary s.
sedative
s. abuse
s. abuser
s. addiction
s. antihistamine
Battley s.
s. delirium
s. dependence
s. drug
s. effect
s. hallucinogen
s.-, hypnotic-, or anxiolytic-induced anxiety disorder
s.-, hypnotic-, or anxiolytic-induced persisting dementia
s. intoxication
s. occupation
s. overdose
s. property
short-acting s.
s. use disorder
s. withdrawal
sedative-hypnotic
s.-h. agent
s.-h. drug
s.-h. withdrawal symptom
sedative-induced
s.-i. anxiety
s.-i. disorder
s.-i. persisting dementia
s.-i. psychotic disorder with delusions
s.-i. psychotic disorder with hallucinations
sedativism
sedentary lifestyle
sedimentation
sedition
seditious
seduce
seducement
seducer
seduction
infantile s.
seductive
s. behavior
s. personality
s. personality disorder
s. tendency
seductress
sedulous

NOTES

seed psychosurgery
seedy
seeker
- care s.
- fact s.
- minor asylum s.
- spiritual s.
- unaccompanied adolescent asylum s.

seeking
- help s.
- novelty s.
- outpatient psychiatric help s.
- pleasure s.
- reassurance s.
- sensation s.
- sympathy s.

seeming
seemingly
seer
seeress
seethe
seething
Seglas-type paranoia
segment
- adrenal s.

segmental
- s. analysis
- s. anesthesia
- s. neuritis
- s. neuropathy

segmentation
- atlas-based s. (ABSEG)

segregate
segregated community
segregation
- administrative s.
- s. analysis study
- disciplinary s.
- s. hypothesis
- perceptual s.

segregationist
SEH
severe emotional handicap
Seitelberger disease
seizure
- absence s.
- s. activity
- acute s.
- akinetic s.
- alcohol as cause of s.
- alcohol-related s.
- alcohol withdrawal s.
- aphasic s.
- apneic s.
- apoplectiform s.
- asteric s.
- asymptomatic s.
- atonic absence s.
- atypical absence s.
- audiogenic s. (AGS)
- auditory s.
- automatic s.
- autonomic s.
- bilateral myoclonic s.
- brain s.
- cardiovascular s.
- central s.
- centrencephalic s.
- cephalic s.
- cerebellar s.
- cerebral s.
- cerebrospinal s.
- clonic s.
- clonic-tonic-clonic s.
- complex partial s. (CPS)
- continuing petit mal s.'s
- conversion s.
- convulsive s.
- coordinate s.
- cryptogenic s.
- diencephalic s.
- dose-dependent s.
- drug-induced s.
- drug withdrawal s.
- s. dyscontrol
- elementary partial s.
- emotional cause of s.
- epilepsia partialis continua s.
- s. epilepsy
- epileptic s.
- epileptiform s.
- erotic s.
- essential s.
- febrile s.
- fluent aphasic s.
- focal s.
- fragmentary s.
- s. frequency (SF)
- generalized tonic-clonic s.
- grand mal s.
- gustatory s.
- s. history
- hysterical s.
- iatrogenic s.
- ictal confusional s.
- ictal depression phase of s.
- infantile s.
- jackknife s.
- jacksonian s.
- major motor s.
- s. management
- massive s.
- maximal electroshock s. (MES)
- mimetic s.
- mimic s.
- s. monitoring
- myoclonic s.
- new-onset s.

nocturnal s.
nonfluent aphasic s.
olfactory psychomotor s.
paroxysmal s.
partial complex s.
partial sensory s.
partial tonic s.
petit mal variant s.
phase of s.
photogenic s.
post-ECT s.
postictal depression phase of s.
posttraumatic s.
postural s.
precentral s.
premonition of s.
primary s.
psychic s.
psychogenic s.
psychomotor s.
puerperal s.
recurrent s.
reflex s.
repetitive partial s.
s. resistant
salaam s.
s. sensitive (SS)
sensory-evoked s.
simple partial s. (SPS)
situation-related s.
sleep-related epileptic s.
somatosensory s.
spasmodic s.
spontaneous s.
subclinical s.
subjective s.
symptomatic s.
temporal lobe s.
tetanic s.
s. threshold
tonic s.
tonic-clonic s.
traumatic s.
typical absence s.
uncinate s.
unilateral s.
uremic s.
vertiginous s.
visual s.
withdrawal s.

sejunction

sejunctiva
dementia s.

selection
adverse s.
s. bias
internal s.
item s.
ligand s.
natural s.
personnel s.

selective
s. abstraction
s. amnesia
s. attachment
s. attention
s. auditory agnosia
s. deafness
s. inattention
s. memory
s. mutism
s. norepinephrine reuptake inhibitor
s. preventive intervention
s. retention
s. serotonin reuptake inhibitor (SSRI)
s. service
s. silence
s. speech perception alteration

selectivity
s. of attention
mesolimbic s.
motivational s.

self, pl. **selves**
acceptance of s.
actual s.
aggression against s.
bad s.
bipolar s.
creative s.
danger to s.
death of s.
deformation of s.
disturbed sense of s.
empirical s.
ethical s.
exaggerated sense of s.
faith in s.
fragile sense of s.
fragmented sense of s.
glorified s.
grandiose s.
harming s.
hidden s.
idealized s.
looking-glass s.

S

NOTES

self *(continued)*
multiple domains of s.
nonturning against s. (NTS)
not turning against s.
personified s.
phenomenal s.
physical aggression against s.
pride in s.
real s.
reckless disregard for safety of s.
Resilience: Acceptance of Life and S.
secondary s.
sense of s.
subconscious s.
subliminal s.
true s.
turning against s. (TAS)
turning aggression against s.
self-abandoned
self-abasement
self-abnegation
self-absorbed
s.-a. mania
s.-a. tendency
self-absorption
intimacy vs s.-a.
self-abuse
self-acceptance
self-accusation
delusion of s.-a.
self-actualization
self-administer
self-administration
s.-a. of psychoactive drug (SAPD)
repeated substance s.-a.
self-aggrandizement
self-aggrandizing
self-alienation
self-analysis (SA)
self-anger
self-annoyance
self-appointed
self-appraisal
self-asphyxiation
self-assertion
self-assurance
self-assured
self-assuring thought
self-attribution of guilt
self-aware
self-awareness
objective s.-a.
self-belief
self-blame
self-blaming depression
self-bondage
self-burning
self-care
s.-c. activity
s.-c. deficit
diabetes s.-c.
s.-c. dysfunction
impaired s.-c.
poor s.-c.
s.-c. skill
self-censure
self-centered attitude
self-centeredness
self-chosen ethical principle
self-commitment
self-comparison
negative s.-c.
self-concealment
self-concept
fractured s.-c.
narcissistic s.-c.
negative s.-c.
self-condemnation
self-condemning
self-confidence
lack of s.-c.
low s.-c.
poor s.-c.
self-conflict
undisciplined s.-c.
self-consciousness
interpersonal s.-c.
self-construal
self-contained
self-content
self-control
s.-c. pain control
s.-c. technique
s.-c. therapy
self-correlation
self-critical attitude
self-criticism
pervasive s.-c.
self-cutting
delicate s.-c.
self-damage ritual
self-damaging
s.-d. behavior
s.-d. impulsivity
self-debasement
self-deceiving
self-deception
self-defeat
self-defeating
s.-d. behavior
s.-d. personality
s.-d. personality disorder
s.-d. thinking
s.-d. trait

self-defense
fighting, injuries, sex, threats, s.-d. (FISTS)
self-deluding
self-denial
self-deprecating thought
self-deprecation
self-deprecatory remark
self-deprivation
self-derogation
self-derogatory
s.-d. concept
s.-d. content
s.-d. theme
self-described
s.-d. agnostic
s.-d. smoker
self-desensitization
self-destruction
self-destructive
s.-d. adolescent
s.-d. behavior
s.-d. hallucination
s.-d. impulse
s.-d. patient
s.-d. pattern
s.-d. urge
self-destructiveness
self-determination
self-development
self-devoted
self-differentiation
self-directed
s.-d. aggression
s.-d. exposure
s.-d. learning (SDL)
s.-d. writing
self-direction
self-disapproval
self-discipline
lack of s.-d.
self-disciplined
self-disclosure
s.-d. anxiety
emotional s.-d.
guarded s.-d.
s.-d. pattern
self-discovery
self-disgust
self-distrust
self-doubt
self-dramatization
self-dramatizing behavior
self-dynamism
self-effacement
self-efficacy and outcome expectation approach
self-emancipation
self-energizing
self-enrichment
self-esteem
adolescent s.-e.
covert s.-e.
denigrated s.-e.
inflated s.-e.
overt s.-e.
s.-e. regulation
self-estrangement
self-evident
self-examination
self-excoriation
self-exiled
self-experience
self-exposure therapy
self-expression
self-extension
self-extinction
self-feeding
self-fellator
self-fulfilling prophecy
self-fulfillment
self-given
self-guided
self-handicapping strategy
self-harm
s.-h. behavior
contract against s.-h.
deliberate s.-h. (DSH)
self-harming
s.-h. act
s.-h. behavior
self-hate
self-hatred
self-healing
self-help
belief system of s.-h.
s.-h. clearinghouse
s.-h. group
s.-h. manual
s.-h. participant
s.-h. question
s.-h. skill
self-helper
inner s.-h.
self-hypnorelaxation
self-hypnosis

NOTES

self-identification
self-identity
self-image
impaired s.-i.
negative s.-i.
unstable s.-i.
self-importance
self-imposed fasting
self-impression
self-incriminating
self-incrimination
self-induced
s.-i. alopecia
s.-i. anxiety
s.-i. dermatitis artefacta
s.-i. disease
s.-i. factitial dermatitis
s.-i. hair loss
s.-i. injury
s.-i. vomiting
self-indulgence
self-inflicted (SI)
s.-i. bodily injury
s.-i. chemical injury
s.-i. dermatitis neglecta
s.-i. gunshot wound
s.-i. hair cutting
s.-i. head shaving
s.-i. lesion
s.-i. physical injury
s.-i. skin cutting
s.-i. stab wound
s.-i. thermal injury
s.-i. trauma
s.-i. wound (SIW)
self-injurious behavior (SIB)
self-injury
adult s.-i.
method of s.-i.
motivation for s.-i.
pattern of s.-i.
self-interest
self-inventory
selfish
self-knowledge
selfless
self-limited process
self-limiting
self-loathing
self-love
self-made
self-managed reinforcement
self-management
diabetes s.-m.
self-manipulation
self-maximization
self-medicate
self-medicating attitude
self-medication hypothesis
self-mutilation
history of s.-m.
self-mutilative behavior
self-mutilator
self-neglect
self-object transference
self-observation
self-opinion
exaggerated s.-o.
self-opinionated
self-organization
primitive aggressive s.-o. (PASO)
self-painting
self-peeping
narcissistic s.-p.
self-perceived cognitive disorder
self-perception
self-perpetuated disease
self-pity
self-pitying constellation
self-portrait
self-possessed
self-preservation
self-pressuring
self-pride
self-produced
self-protective
self-psychology
self-punish
self-punishing behavior
self-punishment
expiatory s.-p.
illness as s.-p.
self-rated
s.-r. functioning
s.-r. impact of disease
s.-r. improvement
self-rating
self-realization
self-recognition
self-reference value
self-referential
self-reflection
self-regard
self-regulation
self-regulatory
s.-r. ability
s.-r. capacity
s.-r. strategy
self-reinforcement
cognitive s.-r.
self-related thought
self-reliance training
self-reliant
self-renewal
self-report
s.-r. assessment
childhood maltreatment history s.-r.
s.-r. data

s.-r. format
s.-r. measure
s.-r. study
young adult s.-r.
youth s.-r.

self-reported
s.-r. aggression
s.-r. anxiety
s.-r. case
s.-r. depression
s.-r. guilt
s.-r. helplessness
s.-r. mood
s.-r. pessimism
s.-r. sinfulness
s.-r. symptom
s.-r. worthlessness

self-reporting
self-reproach
self-restraint
self-revealing
self-ridicule
self-righteous
self-role concept
self-sacrifice
self-satisfaction
self-searching
self-seeking
self-sentience
self-serving
self-soothing
s.-s. act
s.-s. capacity
s.-s. coping skill
impaired s.-s.
s.-s. technique

self-starter
self-starvation
self-stimulating
self-stimulation
intracranial s.-s.

self-stimulatory behavior
self-strangulation
self-study
self-styled
self-sufficient
self-support
youth s.-s.

self-supporting
self-supportive
self-suppression
self-suspicion
self-sustaining
self-system
self-talk
self-taught
self-titrate
self-tolerance
self-torture
self-treatment
self-trust
self-understanding
self-will
self-willed
self-worship
self-worth
inflated s.-w.

Seligman
S. theory of depression
S. view of depressive disorders

sella, pl. **sellae**
sell short
Selter disease
selves (*pl. of* self)
Selvini-Palazzoli model of schizophrenia
Selye
adaptation syndrome of S.

SEM
standard error of mean

semantic
s. aberration
s. activation
s. aphasia
s. argument
s. argument communication pattern
s.'s of autism
behavioral s.'s
s. category
s. clustering
s. cue
s. dementia
s. differential
s. dissociation
extension s.'s
general s.'s
generative s.'s
s. jargon
s. memory
s. memory function
s. pragmatic disorder
s. process
s. processing
s. psychosis
quantitative s.'s
referential s.'s
s. relatedness

NOTES

semantic *(continued)*
s. relationship
s. therapy
semantogenic disorder
semblance
semeiopathic (*var. of* semiopathic)
semeiosis (*var. of* semiosis)
semeiotic (*var. of* semiotic)
semen
s. fear
s. loss
loss of s.
semiautomatic
s. action
s. quality
semicomatose
semiconscious
semicretinism
semidarkness
semideify
semidominant
semierect
semi-independent
semilethal
semiliterate
semimystical
seminarcosis
seminomad
seminude
semiopathic, semeiopathic
semiosis, semeiosis
semiotic, semeiotic
s. function
semipermeable
semiprivate room
semiquantitative
semireligious
semiretirement
semisacred
semisecret
semiskilled employee
semisleep
state of s.
semistructured diagnostic interview
semitendinous
Semon-Hering theory
Semon law
Semon-Rosenbach law
send up
senectitude
senescence
senescent pedophilia
senile
s. brain syndrome
s. chorea
s. degeneration
s. delirium
s. dementia
s. dementia of Alzheimer type (SDAT)
s. dementia confusional state
s. depression
s. deterioration
s. epilepsy
s. imbecility
s. insanity
s. involution
s. mania
s. melancholia
s. memory
s. neurosis
s. organic psychotic state
s. osteoporosis
s. paranoia
s. paranoid psychosis
s. paranoid reaction
s. paranoid state
s. paraplegia
s. paroxysmal psychosis
s. plaque
s. psychoneurosis
s. psychotic mental disorder
s. tremor
senilis
alopecia s.
paranoia s.
sexualitas s.
senility
senior
s. citizen
s. citizen community
s. high school
seniority
senium praecox
sensate
s. focus
s. focus approach
s. focus exercise
s. focus learning
s. focus-oriented therapy
sensation
abnormal tactile s.
abnormal taste s.
altered s.
anxiety-related s.
autonomic s.
bodily s.
buzzing s.
creeping-crawling s.
delayed s.
diminished s.
drug-induced floating s.
s. of ejaculatory inevitability
epicritic s.
facial s.
feeling s.
fine tactile s.

floating-like s.
genital s.
girdle s.
s. increment
kinesthetic s.
light touch s.
loss of s.
mental s.
numbing s.
objective s.
out-of-body s.
out-of-mind s.
peripheral s.
phantom s.
physical s.
pins-and-needles s.
pin-sticking s.
preputial s.
primary s.
proprioceptive s.
referred s.
reflex s.
secondary s.
s. seeking
sexual s.
s. of slowed time
smothering s.
special s.
sticking s.
subjective s.
superficial s.
tactile s.
taste s.
temperature s.
tingling s.
touch s.
transferred s.
visual s.

sensational
sensationalism
sensationalize
sensation-focused apprehension
sensation-seeking trait
sense

s. of alienation
s. of apprehension
s. of arousal
s. of attachment
s. of belonging
s. of betrayal
s. of bodily change
chemical s.
s. of commitment
common s.
s. of community
s. of concern
s. of continuity
s. of control
s. of detachment
s. of empowerment
s. of entitlement
equilibratory s.
s. of equilibrium
s. of estrangement
external s.
s. of failure
s. of fatigue
s. of foreshortened future
s. of humor
s. of identity
s. of impending doom
s. of ineffectiveness
internalized s.
s. of intimacy
joint s.
kinesthetic s.
labyrinthine s.
make s.
s. of mastery
muscular s.
no s.
s. of numbing
obstacle s.
s. of ownership
s. of place
position s.
posture s.
pressure s.
s. of reality
s. of responsibility
s. of righteous indignation
s. of safety
s. of self
seventh s.
s. of shame
sixth s.
space s.
special s.
static s.
stimulation of s. (SOS)
street s.
s. of superiority
tactile s.
temperature s.
thermal s.
thermic s.

NOTES

sense *(continued)*
time s.
touch s.
s. of trust
s. of uniqueness
visceral s.
s. of well-being
s. of wellness
s. of wholeness
senseless imitative word repetition
sensibility
aesthetic s.
articular s.
bone s.
cortical s.
deep s.
dissociation s.
epicritic s.
mesoblastic s.
proprioceptive s.
protopathic s.
splanchnesthetic s.
vibratory s.
sensible
sensiferous
sensigenous
sensimeter
sensing
sensitive
emotionally s.
s. measure
seizure s. (SS)
sensitivity
absolute s.
alcohol s.
anxiety s. (AS)
baroreflex s.
chemical s.
cold s.
contrast s.
cosmic s.
cultural s.
deep-pressure s.
s. to diversity
dopamine receptor s.
enhanced s.
feedback s.
general stress s.
high s.
interpersonal s.
loss of s.
pharmacologic s.
s. reaction of adolescence
s. reaction of childhood
reassurance s.
rejection s.
separation s.
substance s.
s. training
s. training group
warm s.
sensitization
behavioral s.
covert s.
overt s.
perceptual s.
sensomobility
sensomotor
sensoria (*pl. of* sensorium)
sensorial
s. epilepsy
s. hyperarousal
s. hypersensitivity
s. idiocy
sensorimotor
s. act
s. arc
s. behavior
s. development
s. gating
s. intelligence period
s. phase
s. skill
s. stage
s. system
s. theory
sensorium, pl. **sensoria, sensoriums**
clear s.
clouded s.
s. cloudiness
cloudy s.
s. distortion
sensorivasomotor
sensor operation
sensory
s. acuity
s. alexia
s. amusia
s. anesthesia
s. aphasia
s. apraxia
s. association area
s. ataxia
s. aura
s. awareness (SA)
s. bondage
s. charge
s. conversion symptom
s. cortex
s. cue
s. defect
s. deficit
s. deprivation
s. deprivation syndrome (SDS)
s. difficulty
s. dimension
s. discrimination
s. dissociation

s. dissociation syndrome
s. disturbance
s. environment
s. evoked potential (SEP)
s. experience
s. extinction
s. function
s. functioning
s. image
s. impairment
s. impression
s. inattention
s. information
s. integration
s. integration dysfunction (SID)
s. interface
s. level
s. load
s. modality
s. neglect
s. nerve
s. neuron
s. neuronopathy
s. overload
s. paralysis
s. perception
s. phantom
s. phenomenon
s. process
s. processing area
s. psychosis
s. receptor
s. shock
s. stimulation
s. stimulus
s. threshold

sensory-evoked seizure
sensory-induced epilepsy
sensory-precipitated epilepsy
sensualism
sensuality
sensualize
sensual pleasure
sensum
sensuosity
sensuous
sentence
s. completion
complex s.
death s.
jail s.
life s.
prison s.
s. repetition

sentencing
sentential language level
senticosus
Eleutherococcus s.

sentience
sentient
sentiment
anti-Muslim s.
public s.

sentimentality
sentimental value
sentinel activity
SEP
sensory evoked potential
somatosensory evoked potential

separable
separate
separated
s. from spouse
legally s. (LS)
s. status

separation
affective s.
s. agreement
s. anxiety
s. anxiety disorder (SAD)
s. anxiety disorder of childhood
s. distress
early s.
family s.
s. from parent
legal s.
parental s.
prolonged s.
s. sensitivity
sibling s.
traumatic s.
trial s.
twin s.

separation-individuation
s.-i. phase
s.-i. process

separative
septal
s. area
s. region

September 11, 2001
septicemia psychosis
septooptic dysplasia
septuagenarian
septum pellucidum

NOTES

septuplet
sepulture
sequela, pl. **sequelae**
caffeine s.
caffeine-related s.
clinical s.
clinically adverse s.
underdiagnosed s.
untreated s.
sequence
elaborate dream s.
s. of events
genetic s.
Luria hand s.
meaningless syllable s.
s. memory
phase s.
storylike dream s.
sequencing
s. ability
auditory s.
s. disability
letter-number s.
s. rule
sequential
s. diagrammatic reformulation (SDR)
s. dose
s. memory
s. multiple analyses (SMA)
sequester
sequestrate
sequestration
sequitur
non s.
SER
somatosensory evoked response
sera (*pl. of* serum)
serendipity
serene
serenity
serge
sergeant
gunnery s.
serial
s. assaulter
s. child molester
s. epilepsy
s. killer
s. linguistic expectation
s. list learning
s. mental status exams
s. murderer
s. observation
s. problem-solving approach
s. processing
s. 7s
seriatim function
series
experimental s.
s. of numbers
serious
s. assaultive act
s. consequence
s. desire for death
s. impairment
s. traumatic stress
s. violations of rules
seriously wounded in action (SWA)
serious-minded
sermon fear
sermonize
serology
serostatus
serotonergic
s. activity
s. agent
s. antidepressant
s. anxiolytic
s. deficiency hypothesis
s. deficit
s. neuron
s. neurotransmission
s. pathway
s. pharmacology
s. raphe nucleus
s. receptor
s. responsibility
s. side effect
s. synapse
s. system
s. tract
serotonin-dopamine
serotonin-norepinephrine reuptake inhibitor
Seroxat
serpent
serpentina
Rauwolfia s.
SERT
serotonin transporter
serum, pl. **sera**
s. diagnosis
s. level
s. sickness
s. testosterone
truth s.
s. vitamin A
service
access to healthcare s.'s
adjunctive mental health s.
Adult Protective S.'s (APS)
ambulatory mental health s.
American Psychiatry Association-Center for Mental Health S.'s
basic methadone s.

Center for Mental Health S.'s (CMHS)
child inpatient s.
child mental health s.
child outpatient s.
Children's Protective S.'s (CPS)
Civilian Health and Medical Program of the Uniformed S. (CHAMPUS)
community s.
comprehensive s.
consultation-liaison s.
Council on Psychiatric S.'s
counseling s.
Department of Health and Human S.'s (DHHS)
disability determination s. (DDS)
emergency s. (ES)
enhanced standard methadone s.
environment-centered s.
geriatric psychiatry inpatient s.
Health and Human S.'s (HHS)
Indian Health S. (IHS)
inpatient s.
Memphis Educational Model Providing Handicapped Infant S.'s (MEMPHIS)
mental health s.
mutual help s.'s
outreach s.'s
patient-centered s.'s
patient and family s.'s (PFS)
peer-helping s.
psychiatric emergency s. (PES)
psychiatry inpatient s.
psychosocial s.
recreational s.
selective s.
sleep disorder s.
social s. (SS)
social and rehabilitation s. (SRS)
special educational s.
system to plan early childhood s.'s (SPECS)
The Center for Mental Health S.'s
United States Public Health S. (USPHS)
vocational s.

service-connected disability (SCD)
servile
servitude
Serzone
SES
socioeconomic status
session
adjunctive individual s.
buzz s.
dyadic s.
education-focused s.
fixed-ended s.
group psychotherapy s.
individual psychotherapy s.
learning s.
marathon s.
open-ended s.
orientation s.
play s.
psychotherapy s.
rap s.
skull s.
therapy s.
4-way s.

SET
support, empathy and truth
set
s. about
acquiescent response s.
s. aside
data s.
difficulty in changing response s.
empty s.
s. eyes on
s. foot on
Health Plan Employer Data and Information S.
jet s.
learning s.
s. limits
mental s.
mind s.
s. in motion
s. one straight
s. in one's ways
perceptual s.
perseveration s.
polyethic criteria s.
postural s.
response s.
single criterion s.
s. the stage
substance-specific intoxication criteria s.'s
substance-specific withdrawal criteria s.'s
SWAP-200 item s.

NOTES

setback
set-by-age dosing
setter
fire s. (FS)
setting
behavior s.
clinical practice s.
community s.
deliberate fire s.
dimensional s.
educational s.
emergency psychiatric s.
experimental psychometric s.
fire s.
forensic s.
geriatric healthcare s.
goal s.
group s.
home s.
hospital s.
inpatient psychiatric s.
institutional s.
intentional fire s.
limit s.
outpatient mental health clinic s.
partial hospital s.
population s.
primary care s.
psychiatric s.
psychometric s.
psychosocial s.
real-world s.
repetitive fire s.
residential s.
social s.
vocational goal s.
settle
seventh sense
sever
severable
severalty
severance
severe
s. anxiety
s. ataxia
s. decompensation
s. dementia
s. depression
s. diffuse brain dysfunction
s. disability
s. dissociative symptom
s. emotional handicap (SEH)
s. environmental deprivation
s. guilt
s. impairment
s. intoxication
s. life stress
s. mental retardation
s. mental subnormality
s. stressor
s. trauma
severely
s. compromised
s. mentally impaired (SMI)
severity
addiction s.
baseline s.
compulsive s.
dementia s.
depression s.
disease s.
hyperintensity s.
s. of intent
s. of lethality
MOAS s.
objective s.
psychiatric s.
s. specifier
s. of worry
sewing spasm
sex
s. addict
S. Addicts Anonymous (SAA)
adult-child s.
s., age, depression, previous attempt, ethanol, rational thinking loss, separated, divorced, widowed, organized plan, no social support, stated future intent (SAD PERSONS)
anal s.
s. appeal
s. arousal mechanism (SAM)
assigned s.
s. assignment
biologic s.
casual s.
s. change
s. characteristic
s. chromatin
s. chromosome
s. clinic
compulsive s.
consensual s.
s. counseling
s. crime
s. determination
s. differentiation
s. drive
s. education
extramarital s.
fair s.
s. fear
forced s.
s. hormone
indeterminate s.
s. infantilism

S. Information and Education Council of the US (SIECUS)
s. interest
intermediate s.
Internet s.
s. inventory (SI)
s. kitten
s. limitation
s. linkage
s. market
900-number s.
s. object
s. offender (SO)
s. offense
opposite biological s.
oral s.
orogenital s.
parental attitude toward s.
s. partner
s. perversion
s. play
s. play with peers
s. play with sibling
premarital s.
s. preselection
promiscuous s.
s. ratio
s. reassignment
s. reassignment surgery (SRS)
s. reversal
s. role
s. role inversion
sadomasochistic s.
safe s.
s. scandal
s. specific
s. steroid
s. symbol
telephone s.
s. therapy
third s.
s. toy
s. trading
trading s.
s. typing
unprotected s.
unwanted anal s.
unwanted oral s.
unwanted vaginal s.

sex-adjusted genome screen
Sexaholics Anonymous (SA)
sex-conditioned character
sex-hormone binding globulin (SHBG)
sexism
sexist
sexless
sex-limited character
sex-linked character
sexological examination
sexology
sexopathy
sexploitation
sex-related

s.-r. HIV risk behavior
s.-r. risk-taking

sex-role behavior
sex-specific rate
sexual

s. aberration
s. abstinence
s. abuse
s. abuse of adult
s. abuse of child
s. abuse history
s. abuse status
s. acting out
s. activity
s. adaptation
s. addiction
s. adjustment
s. advance
s. adventurousness
s. aggression
s. anesthesia
s. anomaly
s. anxiety
s. arousal
s. arousal disorder
s. assault
s. assault by acquaintance
s. assault by stranger
s. attitude
s. attitude reassessment (SAR)
s. attitude restructuring (SAR)
s. attraction
s. aversion
s. aversion disorder
s. boundary violation
s. climax
s. coercion
s. commentary
s. compulsion
s. concern
s. contact
s. culture
s. curiosity

NOTES

sexual *(continued)*
s. delusion
s. demand
s. desire
s. desire disorder
s. development
s. deviance
s. deviance disorder
s. deviant
s. deviation
s. deviation neurotic disorder
s. differentiation
s. dimorphism
s. discrimination
s. domination
s. dysfunction
s. dysfunction due to general medical condition
s. encounter
s. energy
s. erethism
s. escapade
s. excitement
s. exhibition
s. experience
s. experimentation
s. exposure trauma
s. expression
s. fantasy
s. fantasy aid
s. favor
s. favor for crack
s. fear
s. feeling
s. fetish
s. frequency
s. frigidity
s. function
s. functioning
s. and gender identity disorder
s. gratification
s. harassment (SH)
s. identity
s. impairment
s. impotence
s. impulse
s. inappropriateness
s. incident
s. indifference
s. indiscretion
s. infantilism
s. inhibition
s. instinct
s. interaction
s. intercourse
s. interest
s. intimacy
s. intrigue
s. inversion
s. jealousy
s. learning
s. liaison
s. libido
s. life
s. love
s. maladjustment
s. marketplace
s. masochism
s. matching
s. maturity rating
s. melancholia
s. misbehavior
s. misconduct
s. mores
s. motivation
s. motive state
s. myth
s. nature
s. negativism
s. neurasthenia
s. neurosis
s. obsession
s. offense
s. opportunity
s. orientation
s. orientation distress
s. orientation disturbance
overtly s.
s. pain
s. pain disorder
s. partner
s. performance
s. perversion
s. pervert
s. physiology
s. pleasure
s. polarization
s. position
s. posturing
s. potency
s. predation behavior
s. predator
s. preference
s. preoccupation
s. promiscuity
s. provocation
s. prowess
s. psychogenic disorder
s. psychopath
s. psychopathy
s. reassignment
s. regulation
s. rehabilitation
s. relation
s. relationship
s. response
s. response cycle
s. responsibility

s. revolution
s. risk-taking
s. sadism
s. sadist
s. sadomasochism
s. script
s. sensation
s. side effect
s. soliloquy
s. stimulation
s. stimuli revulsion
s. stimulus
s. surrogate
s. symptom
s. symptom grouping
s. synergism
s. tension
s. thought
s. touching
s. trauma
s. urge
s. vandalism
s. violence

sexualis
psychopathia s.

sexualism

sexualitas senilis

sexuality
s. conversion therapy
extramarital s.
human s.
inappropriate s.
infantile s.
pathologic s.
perverted s.
polymorphous perverse s.
s. theory

sexualization

sexualize

sexually
s. abused child
s. acquired immunodeficiency (SAID)
s. active
s. arousing behavior
s. arousing fantasy
s. charged magazine
s. charged movie
s. charged television
s. dangerous
S. Dangerous Persons Act
s. dimorphic
s. gratified
s. inappropriate behavior
s. intimate
s. involved
s. maladjusted
s. motivated
s. seductive behavior
s. stimulated
s. suggestive
s. transmitted condition (STC)
s. transmitted disease (STD)
s. violated
s. violent
s. violent nature
s. violent offense
S. Violent Persons Commitment Act
s. violent predator

SF
seizure frequency

SF-1
steroidogenic factor-1

S factor

SFLE
stress from life experience

SH
sexual harassment
social history
state hospital

S&H
speech and hearing

sha
Gwa S.

shabby

shabu

shackle

shading
emotional s.
s. response (ShR)
s. response to black areas (Fc)
s. response to gray areas (Fc)

shadow
s. dance
object s.
s. mask technique
s. play

shakily

shakiness

shaking
fist s.
hand s.
s. palsy
s. tremor
s. voice

NOTES

shaky
shallow
s. affect
s. expression
sham
s. disorder
s. feeding
s. movement vertigo
s. rage
shaman
shamanism
shamanistic thought disorder
shambles
shame
feeling of s.
overt sign of s.
profound s.
sense of s.
shame-aversion therapy
shamefaced
shameful
shamus
shape
s. analysis
body s.
s. concern
good s.
overvaluation of s.
shaping
behavior s.
shared
s. delusional belief
s. grammar
s. language
s. mechanism
s. paranoid disorder
s. phenomenological feature
s. psychotic disorder
s. relationship
s. thought pattern
s. understanding
sharing
expression of s.
needle s.
s. of values
sharp
intellectually s.
s. object
sharpen
sharp-eyed
sharp-sighted
sharp-tongued
sharp-witted
shaving
s. cramp
self-inflicted head s.
SHBG
sex-hormone binding globulin
SHCU
state hospital children's unit
Shedler-Western Assessment Procedure-200 (SWAP-200)
sheepish
sheet
personal data s.
s. sign
timed behavioral rating s. (TBRS)
shell shock
shell-shocked
shelter
battered women's s.
s. facility
homeless s.
sheltered
s. home
s. life
s. workshop
s. workshop placement
shenjing shuairuo
shen-k'uei, shenkui
Sherman paradox
shield
ideational s.
shift
s. ability
abrupt topic s.
attention s.
s. in attitude
binaural s.
biobehavioral s.
Doppler s.
functional s.
gradual topic s.
s. masking technique
s. in mood
mood s.
paradigm s.
paradigmatic s.
phase s.
precipitous mood s.
s. referential index
role s.
temporary threshold s. (TTS)
s. work-related sleep disorder
s. work-type dyssomnia
shifting
associative s.
idiosyncratic topic s.
s. sleep-work schedule
topic s.
shiftless
shin-byung
shinkeishitsu
shivering thermogenesis
shock
break s.
cultural s.

culture s.
deferred s.
delayed s.
delirious s.
electrical s.
electric skin s.
electroconvulsive s. (ECS)
erethismic s.
s. exhibitionism
s. fear
future s.
insulin s.
irreversible s.
mental s.
neurogenic s.
primary s.
psychic s.
psychodramatic s.
s. psychosis
s. reaction
reversible s.
sensory s.
shell s.
spinal s.
s. stage
s. syndrome
s. therapy (ST)
transplantation s.
s. treatment
s. troops
vasogenic s.

shocky
shoddy
shoe
s. fetish
s. restriction

shook jong
shook-up
shooting
accidental s.
Columbine High School s.
drive-by s.
s. gallery
s. pain
s. rampage
s. spree

shoot-up
shopaholic
shoplift
shoplifting
shopping
s. addict
s. addiction
binge s.
doctor s.
s. spree

short
s. cycle
fall s.
s. fuse
s. half-life
s. REM latency
sell s.
s. shrift
s. sleep duration
s. sleeper
s. sleep latency
s. stare epilepsy
s. stature
stop s.
s. temper
s. test of mental status

short-acting
s.-a. benzodiazepine
s.-a. hypnotic agent
s.-a. sedative

shortcoming
short-contact psychotherapy
shortening reaction
shortfall
short-lasting drug effect
short-lived schizophrenic affect
shortness of breath (SOB)
short-sighted
short-spoken
short-tempered
short-term
s.-t. anxiety-provoking psychotherapy (STAPP)
s.-t. care facility
s.-t. commitment
s.-t. consequence
s.-t. declarative memory
s.-t. dynamic psychotherapy
s.-t. goal (STG)
s.-t. hospitalization
s.-t. hypoxia
s.-t. insomnia
s.-t. insurance
s.-t. maintenance
s.-t. memory (STM)
s.-t. psychotherapy technique
s.-t. recall
s.-t. therapy
s.-t. treatment

short-timer

NOTES

S

shotgun
.410-gauge s.
s. marriage
s. wedding
shoulder
cold s.
stooped s.'s
shouldered
showdown
shower
showman
showy
ShR
shading response
shrapnel
grenade s.
shrewd
shrewish
shriek
shrift
short s.
shrill
shrink
shrinking retrograde amnesia
shroud
shrug off
shuairuo
shenjing s.
shuffling
s. gait
s. steps
shuk yang
shun
shunt
shut
s. in
s. out
s. up
shut-eye
shut-in personality
shyness
s. disorder
s. disorder of childhood
SI
self-inflicted
sex inventory
social introversion
stimulation index
structure of intellect
systematic inquiry
sialidosis
sialoaerophagy
sialorrhea
Siamese twins
SIB
self-injurious behavior
sibling
abusive s.
biologic s.
s. bond
childhood loss of s.
s. jealousy
s. profile
s. relation
s. relational problem
s. rivalry
s. separation
sex play with s.
s. subsystem
sibship method
sicchasia
sick
s. headache
s. leave
s. role
s. thought
sicken
sickening
sickle flap
sickness
altitude s.
s. behavior
chronic African sleeping s.
decompression s.
falling s.
ghost s.
laughing s.
motion s.
school s.
serum s.
sleeping s.
sick-out
SID
sensory integration dysfunction
side
deep s.
s. effect
s. effect drug profile
2-sided message
side-glance
sideline
sideration
siderodromomania
sidetrack
SIDS
sudden infant death syndrome
SIECUS
Sex Information and Education Council of the US
sigh
premonitory s.
sighing
sighted
sightedness
sightless
sigil
sigma receptor
sigmatism

sign
accessory s.
s. of alcohol intoxication
arithmetic s.
Babinski s.
Battle s.
s. blindness
brainstem s.
Cantelli s.
cardinal s.
cerebellar s.
cerebral s.
characteristic s.
Claude hyperkinesis s.
clinical s.
contralateral s.
conventional s.
s. depression
doll's eye s.
early warning s.
echo s.
Escherich s.
extrapyramidal s.
eyelash s.
eye roll s.
fan s.
frontal release s.
Fukuda s.
Gordon s.
Gorlin s.
Hoffmann s.
iconic s.
s. of impending violence
indexical s.
Jackson s.
Joffroy s.
Kernig s.
s. language
Legendre s.
Leichtenstern s.
Leri s.
Lichtheim s.
local s.
Macewen s.
Magnan s.
Mannkopf s.
Masini s.
matchbox s.
melancholic s.
mirror s.
motor s.
neurovegetative s.
nonextrapyramidal neurologic s.
objective s.
omega s.
operational s.
s. of orbicularis
s. out
pathognomonic s.
physical s.
Pitres s.
positive frontal release s.
premonitory s.
prodromal s.
pseudo-Graefe s.
psychotic s.
s. of restraint
Romberg s.
root s.
Russell s.
Saenger s.
Schuele s.
sheet s.
Signorelli s.
Simon s.
spine s.
telltale s.
Uhthoff s.
vegetative s.
vital s. (VS)
von Graefe s.
Westphal s.
withdrawal s.
Woltman s.

signal
acoustic s.
bilateral contralateral routing of s.'s (BICROS)
s. detection
focal contralateral routing of s.'s (FOCALCROS)
gamma band s.
s. hyperintensity
ideomotor s.
increased s.
ipsilateral frontal routing of s.'s (IFROS)
leptin s.
s. theory of anxiety
s. transduction alteration

signaling
calcium s.
chemical s.

signalize

signalment

signal-noise characteristic

NOTES

signal-transducing
s.-t. guanine-nucleotide binding protein
signed
s. communication
s. consent form
s. out against medical advice (SOAMA)
signer
deaf s.
significance
affective s.
emotional s.
s. level
nonparametric test of s.
parametric test of s.
statistical s.
test of s.
significant
clinically s.
s. conflict
s. deterioration
s. difference
s. impairment
s. life event
s. loss
s. medical illness
not s. (NS)
s. other
s. range
s. risk
s. risk factor
s. sleep disturbance
statistically s.
s. supporting person
s. trend
s. weight loss
signify
Signorelli sign
Sikh religion
siknis
grisi s.
sildenafil citrate
silence
code of s.
s. communication pattern
electrocerebral s. (ECS)
selective s.
teen s.
tyranny of s.
silencer
silent
s. area
s. blocking in speech
s. cerebral infarction
s. generation
s. period
s. speech blockade
s. treatment
silicone implant
silliness
childlike s.
silly affect
silver
s. bullet
s. cord syndrome
s. lining
silver-tongued
similarity, pl. **similarities**
assumed s.
s. disorder of aphasia
vocabulary, information, block design, s. (VIBS, vibs)
simmer down
Simon sign
simple
s. absence
s. affective depression
s. alcoholic drunkenness
s. aphasia
s. aspect of fear conditioning
s. confrontation
s. delusion
s. depressive dementia
s. deterioration
s. deterioration senile psychosis
s. deteriorative disorder
s. drug screen
s. figure
s. hallucination
s. motor tic
s. obesity
s. paranoid reaction
s. paranoid state
s. partial seizure (SPS)
s. phobia
s. retardation
s. schizophrenia
s. senile dementia
s. task
s. vocal tic
simpleminded
simpleness
simple-type
s.-t. arteriosclerotic psychosis
s.-t. schizophrenia
simplex
melancholia s.
paranoia s.
purpura s.
schizophrenia s.
Simpson-Angus total score
simulant
simulate
simulated
s. activities of daily living (SADL, SADLs)

s. intercourse
s. presence therapy
simulation
conscious s.
simulee
folie s.
simulis
simultanagnosia, simultagnosia
simultanée
folie s.
simultaneous insanity
sin
capital s.
cardinal s.
deadly s.
delusion of s.
mortal s.
perceived s.
venial s.
sine
s. delirio
s. qua non
s. wave
s. wave unilateral ECT
sinful feeling
sinfulness
delusion of s.
self-reported s.
single
s. combat
s. criterion set
s. custody
s. diagnosis
s. episode
s. major locus (SML)
s. major locus model
s. nucleotide polymorphism
s. psychotic reaction
single-agent oral strategy
single-episode
s.-e. chronic mania
s.-e. depressive psychosis
s.-e. psychotic depression
single-handed
single-item indicator
single-minded
singleness
single-parent
s.-p. family
s.-p. home
single-photon emission CT scan
singles community
single-track
single-valued
single-word stage
singly
singsong fashion
singularity
singultus
sinica
Ephedra s.
sinister
sinistrad
sinistral
sinistrality
sinistromanual
sinistropedal
sinkable
sinkage
sinking feeling
sinner
sinning
sinography
sinus, pl. **sinus, sinuses**
rhomboidal s.
siren song
sissified
sissy behavior
sisterhood
sister-in-law
sisterly
sister-sister dyad
Sisyphus dream
SIT
stress inoculation training
sit
s. in
s. out
site
binding s.
dopamine uptake s.
recognition s.
uptake s.
sitieirgia
sitomania
sitting
s. balance
s. fear
situation
acute maladjustment s.
s. anxiety
anxiety-producing s.
anxiety-provoking s.
Asch s.
clinical s.
cluster of s.'s

NOTES

situation *(continued)*
s. cluster
conflictual s.
crisis s.
danger s.
dangerous s.
direful s.
disaster s.
dreaded s.
educational s.
either-or s.
emergency s.
emotion-laden s.
s. ethics
exile s.
family s.
feared single performance s.
high-risk gambling s.
histrionic s.
living s.
low-activity s.
low-stimulation s.
s. neurosis
oedipal s.
one-to-one s.
open-cue s.
peer interactional s.
performance s.
phobic s.
previously stabilizing social s.
psychoanalytic s.
real-world s.
social s.
stabilizing social s.
taxonomy of problematic social s. (TOPS)
triage s.
triggering s.
volatile s.

situational
s. anger disorder with aggression
s. anger disorder without aggression
s. anxiety
s. attribution
s. crisis
s. depression
s. disturbance
s. ethics
s. homosexuality
s. hypoactive sexual desire
s. insomnia
s. orgasmic dysfunction
s. panic
s. perception
s. posttraumatic neurosis
s. psychosis
s. restraint
s. sexual dysfunction
s. stressor
s. stress reaction
s. therapy
s. tic variation
s. trigger
s. variable

situationally
s. appropriate atmosphere
s. bound
s. bound panic attack
s. optimistic atmosphere
s. predisposed
s. predisposed panic attack

situational-type
s.-t. dyspareunia
s.-t. female orgasmic disorder
s.-t. female sexual arousal disorder

situation-related
s.-r. epilepsy
s.-r. seizure

situs analysis

sitzkrieg

SIW
self-inflicted wound

sixth sense

size
body s.
class s.
effect s.
internal architecture neuronal s.
neuronal s.
optimal group s.
s. perception
ventricle s.

skeptic

skeptical

skepticism
adolescent s.

sketchy

skew
s. deviation
s. distribution
marital s.

SKI
skill indicator

skid-row
s.-r. bum
s.-r. derelict

skid row

skill
abstraction s.
academic organizational s.
activities of daily living s.'s (ADLS)
adaptation s.
adaptive s.
s. area
assertiveness s.
attentional s.

auditory s.
basic s.
calculation s.
communication s.
communicative s.
conceptual s.
conflict resolution s.
conversational s.
coping s.
core mindfulness s.
daily living s.
decision-making s.
decoding s.
developmental s.
distress tolerance s.
ego coping s.
encoding s.
expressive language s.
fine motor s.
functional s.
generic s.
graphomotor s.
gross motor s.
health literacy s.
higher level s.
improved communication s.'s
s. indicator (SKI)
intellectual s.
interpersonal effectiveness s.
leisure s.
mathematical s.
memory s.
mental s.
mindfulness s.
motor s.
negotiating goals s.
negotiating routine s.
negotiating rules s.
nonconfrontational communication s.
numerical reasoning s.'s
oral language s.
organizational s.'s
parenting s.
people s.'s
perceptual s.
perceptus motor s.
perspective-taking s.'s
physical s.
poor language s.'s
positive communication s.'s
problem-solving s.'s
reasoning and memory s.'s
resolving conflict s.'s
right hemisphere cognitive s.'s
routine s.
rule s.'s
savant s.
self-care s.
self-help s.
self-soothing coping s.
sensorimotor s.
social s.
socialization s.
stress adaptability s.
s. training
uncoordinated motor s.
unrefined motor s.
visual perceptual s.
visuomotor problem-solving s.
vocabulary s.
word-attack s.
word-finding s.
word-recognition s.

skilled
s. nursing care (SNC)
s. nursing facility placement
s. worker

skillful

skill-less

skimming

skimpy

skin
s. of animals
clammy s.
s. conductance orienting response (SCOR)
s. disease
s. disease fear
s. eroticism
s. eruption
s. friability
glossy s.
s. injury fear
on the s.
s. picking
s. psychogenic disorder
s. pulling
taut facial s.
under the s.

skinhead gang member

Skinner box

skinnerian conditioning

skinny

skip
s. bail
s. class

NOTES

skip *(continued)*
s. meals
s. out
s. town
skipping
grade s.
skirmish
skirt the issue
skittish
skulk
skull
s. asymmetry
s. and crossbones
maplike s.
s. session
steeple s.
skullcap
sky marshal
skyscraper fear
slacken
slain
slamming
door s.
slander
slanderous
slang
rhyming s.
slap down
slasher
slashing
throat s.
slattern
slatternly
slaughter
slaughterous
slave
s. driver
s. system component
slavery
slavish
slay
slayer
SLC
sociopolitical locus of control
sleaze
sleazy
sledgehammer
sleep
abnormal behavior during s.
s. abnormality
abnormal physiological event during s.
activated s.
active s.
s. activity
aging effect on s.
alcohol-induced nighttime s.
s. architecture
s. arousal
arousal from s.
s. attack
s. behavior disorder
s. bruxism
s. change
s. change in aging
circadian phase of s.
s. complaint
confusional arousal from s.
consolidated s.
s. continuity
s. continuity disturbance
s. continuity variable
continuous s.
crescendo s.
curtailed s.
s. cycle
decreased need for s.
deep s.
s. deficit
delta-wave s.
s. and depression
s. deprivation
depth of s.
s. diary
s. disorder due to general medical condition
s. disorder insomnia
s. disorder service
disorders of initiating and maintaining s. (DIMS)
s. disruption
s. dissociation
disturbed s.
dreamless s.
s. drunkenness
s. duration
s. dysfunction
easily disturbed s.
s. efficiency
electric s.
electrotherapeutic s.
s. elevation
environmental disturbance of s.
s. epilepsy
s. erection
erratic s.
excessive s.
s. fear
fitful s.
forced s.
s. fragmentation
fragmented nighttime s.
s. hygiene
hypnotic s.
impaired s.
indeterminate s.
s. influence
s. initiation

insufficient nocturnal s.
s. interference
s. interruption
s. inversion
irresistible s.
s. latency
light s. (LS)
s. loss
s. mechanism
s. medicine
s. movement
need for s.
nonrestorative s.
NREM s.
s. numbness
s. onset
onset of s.
s. organization
panic attack during s.
paradoxic s.
paradoxical s.
s. paralysis
paroxysmal s.
s. pattern
s. phase
s. phase dyssomnia
s. phase syndrome
pontine s.
s. posture
primary disorder of s.
s. problem
problem initiating s.
problem maintaining s.
prolonged nocturnal s.
s. psychogenic disorder
quality of s.
quiet s.
rapid eye movement s.
REM s.
REM-onset s.
S. Research Society
s. restriction
s. reversal
rhombencephalic s.
s. ritual
slow-wave s. (SWS)
s. spindle
s. spindle on EEG
s. stage
s. starts disorder
s. state
s. state misperception
telencephalic s.
s. tendency
s. terror
s. terror disorder
s. terror episode
s. terror event
s. therapy
s. time
transitional s. (TS)
s. treatment
twilight s.
undisturbed nocturnal s.
unintended s.
yen s.

sleep-associated movement disorder

sleep-awake experience list (SWEL)

sleep-deprived EEG

sleep-disordered breathing (SDB)

sleep-electroshock therapy

sleeper

s. hold
short s.

sleep-induced respiratory impairment

sleep-inducing peptide

sleepiness

disorder of excessive s.
excessive daytime s. (EDS)
pathologic s.
physiologic s.

sleeping

s. drunkenness
s. partner
s. pill
s. sickness

sleepless

sleeplessness

s. associated with acute emotional conflicts or reaction
s. associated with anxiety
s. associated with conditional arousal
s. associated with depression
s. associated with intermittent emotional conflicts or reaction
s. associated with psychosis

sleep-onset

s.-o. episode
s.-o. insomnia
s.-o. REM period

sleep-related

s.-r. abnormal swallowing syndrome
s.-r. asthma
s.-r. bruxism
s.-r. cluster headache

NOTES

S

sleep-related *(continued)*
s.-r. epilepsy
s.-r. epileptic seizure
s.-r. groaning
s.-r. hallucination
s.-r. head banging
s.-r. myoclonus syndrome
sleeptalking disorder
sleep-wake
s.-w. abnormality
s.-w. cycle
s.-w. rhythm
s.-w. schedule
s.-w. schedule disorder
s.-w. system
s.-w. transition
s.-w. transition disorder
sleepwalker
sleepwalking
s. behavior
s. disorder
sleeve graft
sleight
slept all night (SAN)
SLI
speech and language impaired
sliding of meaning
slight
s. defect
inner s.
slink
slip
freudian s.
s. knot
slippage
cognitive s.
slipshod
slope
gradient s.
sloppy appearance
slothful
slot machine gambling
slough
s. off
s. over
slovenly
slow
s. double taper
s. euthanasia
s. learner
s. metabolizer patient
s. rate of language development
s. speech
start low and go s.
s. virus
slowed
s. gait
s. thinking
slow-frequency EEG activity
slowing
motor s.
psychomotor s.
slowness
obsessional s.
s. of thought
slow-tempered
slow-wave
s.-w. sleep (SWS)
s.-w. sleep stability
slow-witted
sluggard
sluggish
sluggishness
slum
slumber
affective s.
slumlord
slumming
slump
slumped posture
slur
racial s.
verbal s.
slurred speech
slut
sly
SM, S/M
sadomasochism
SMA
sequential multiple analyses
supplementary motor area
smacking
lip s.
small
s. detail response
s. penis complex
s. talk
small-amplitude rapid tremor
small-minded
small-mindedness
small-time
smashing
SMD
stereotypic movement disorder
smear
blood s.
smearing
saliva s.
smell
s. blindness
s. imagery
SMH
state mental hospital
SMI
severely mentally impaired
smile
endogenous s.
exogenous s.

forced s.
social s.
smirk
smite
Smith-Lemli-Opitz syndrome
SML
single major locus
SML model
smoke
drug s.
s. screen
smoked
never s.
smoker
abstinent tobacco s.
acutely abstinent tobacco s.
alcoholic s.
chain s.
heavy s.
pack-per-day s.
pregnant s.
self-described s.
tobacco s.
smoker's syndrome
smoking
s. abstinence
s. behavior
s. cessation
s. exposure
guided s.
s. history
household s.
peer s.
prenatal s.
rapid s.
s. relapse
stopped s.
smoking-related reduction
smooth pursuit eye movement (SPEM)
smooth-tongued
smothering sensation
smother love
smug
smuggle
smuggler
smut
smutty
snake symbol
snap
s. back
s. finger
snapping
finger s.
s. off
snappish
snappy
snapshot
cross-sectional s.
snare
snarl
snatcher
child s.
purse s.
snatching
body s.
SNC
skilled nursing care
sneaky
snide
sniffing
s. death
glue s.
inhalant s.
snipe
snippy
snit
snitch
snivel
snob appeal
snobbery
snobbish
snooping
data s.
snoopy
snore
resuscitative s.
snorting
drug s.
snout reflex
snow
s. fear
s. job
s. under
SNR
specific neurotic syndrome
SNS
sympathetic nervous system
snub-nose pistol
snuff
cohoba s.
SO
sex offender
SOAMA
signed out against medical advice

NOTES

soapbox
soaring
SOB
shortness of breath
sobbing
sober
soberness
sobersided
sobriety
white knuckling s.
Youth Enjoying S. (YES)
sob story
SOC
state of consciousness
so-called
sociability
change in s.
heightened s.
sociable
social
s. abulia
s. acceptance
s. acquiescence (SA)
s. acting out
s. activity
s. adaptation
s. adjustment
s. adjustment measure
s. age (SA)
s. alienation
s. anhedonia
s. anorexia
s. anthropology
s. anxiety
s. anxiety disorder
s. apprehensiveness
s. approval
s. assistance
s. atom
s. attachment
s. attraction
s. attribution
s. avoidance and distortion
s. avoidance and distress (SAD)
s. awkwardness
s. babbling
s. barrier
s. beverage
s. breakdown syndrome (SBS)
s. casework
s. causation theory
s. class
s. class and mental illness
s. climber
s. club
s. cognition
s. communication
s. competence
s. compliance
s. concern
s. conformity
s. connectedness
s. connection
s. consciousness
s. consequence
s. construction
s. contact
s. context
s. control
s. cripple
s. cue
s. darwinism
s. dependence
s. deprivation
s. deprivation syndrome
s. desirability
s. detachment
s. detoxification
s. development
s. deviance
s. diagnosis
s. disability syndrome
s. disapproval
s. disconnection
s. disease
s. distance
s. dominance
s. dominance theory
s. drinker
s. drinking
s. dyad
s. dysfunction
s. dysmaturation
s. eating
s. ecology
s. engineering
s. environment
s. etiology
s. evaluation
s. facilitation
s. fear
s. function
s. functioning
s. functioning impairment
s. functioning level
s. functioning schedule
s. gambling
s. gesture speech
s. goal
s. harmony
s. and health assessment
s. hierarchy
s. history (SH)
s. hunger
s. identification
s. identity
s. ignorance
s. immaturity

s. impairment rating
s. implication
s. inadequacy
s. inappropriateness
s. inattentiveness
s. ineptness
s. inhibition
s. insecurity
s. instinct
s. integration
s. integration-disintegration model
s. intelligence
s. interaction
s. interaction therapy
s. interest
s. introversion (SI)
s. island
s. isolate
s. isolation
s. isolation syndrome
s. judgment
s. judgment score
s. justice
s. label
s. learning experience
s. learning group therapy
s. learning theory
s. loss
s. maladaptation
s. maladjustment
s. masochism
s. maturation
s. medicine
s. mores
s. network
s. network therapy
s. niche
s. norm
s. objective
s. opportunity
s. outcast
s. overdependence
s. perception
s. performance
s. persecution
s. phobia
s. phobic-like behavior
s. poison
s. policy
s. policy planning
s. pressure
s. problem
s. process
s. property
s. psychiatry
s. psychologist
s. psychology
s. quotient (SQ)
s. readjustment
s. recovery
s. reference group
s. rehabilitation
s. and rehabilitation service (SRS)
s. reinforcement
s. relatedness
s. relatedness disturbance
s. relations deficit
s. relationship
s. resistance
s. responsibility
s. risk factor
s. role
s. role disability
s. sanction
s. science
S. Security Administration (SSA)
s. selection theory
s. service (SS)
s. service agency
s. service consultation
s. setting
s. situation
s. situation avoidance
s. skill
s. skills deficit
s. skills deterioration
s. skills training (SST)
s. smile
s. standard
s. status
s. stereotypical behavior
s. stimulation
s. strata
s. stress
s. stressor
s. structure
s. support
s. support after treatment
s. support during treatment
s. taboo
s. tension
s. tolerance
s. toxicity
s. trap
s. type
s. undesirable

NOTES

social *(continued)*
s. value
s. viscosity
s. welfare
s. welfare organization
s. withdrawal
s. withdrawal of childhood
s. work
s. worker
s. zeitgeber
s. zone
social-emotional functioning
socialist
socialistic
socialite
sociality
socialization
adolescent s.
adult s.
s. skill
socialize
socialized
s. childhood truancy
s. conduct disorder
s. delinquency
s. dementia
s. disturbance
s. medicine
s. runaway reaction
socially
s. acceptable behavior
s. adhesive
s. alienated
s. amiable
s. beneficial
s. disabling
s. disruptive environment
s. dysfunctional
s. dysfunctional adolescent
s. effective
s. functional
s. harmful
s. intimate model
s. neutral
s. unacceptable behavior
s. undesirable behavior
s. withdrawn
social-minded
social-minded
societal
s. bias
s. force
s. implication
s. norm
s. reaction theory
s. structure
society
American Pain S. (APS)
American Psychological S. (APS)
American Psychosomatic S.
Behavior Therapy and Research S. (BTRS)
S. of Biological Psychiatry
demand of s.
S. for Developmental and Behavioral Pediatrics
Hemlock S.
S. for Industrial and Organizational Psychology
s. level
majority s.
Northern California Psychiatric S.
Orange County Psychiatric S.
Orphan Train Heritage S.
postconflict s.
rural s.
secret s.
Sleep Research S.
Southern California Psychiatric S.
traditional s.
Vienna Psychoanalytic S.
Wednesday Evening S.
sociobiology
sociocenter
sociocentric
sociocentrism
sociocosm
sociocultural
s. ambiance
s. background
s. foundation
s. milieu
s. trend
sociodemographic
s. background
s. composition
s. feature
s. measure
s. variable
socioeconomic
s. background
s. class
s. group
s. life change
s. status (SES)
socioenvironmental therapy
sociofugal space
sociogenesis
sociogenic
sociogram
objective s.
perceptual s.
sociolinguistic
sociologese
sociologic
sociological
sociology
clinical s.

industrial s.
medical s.
sociomedical
sociometric distance
sociometrist
sociometry
sociopath
sociopathic
s. behavior
s. personality
s. personality disorder (SPD)
s. personality disturbance (SPD)
sociopathology
sociopathy
sociopolitical
s. agenda
s. locus of control (SLC)
s. position
s. reality
sociopsychological
socioreligious
sociosexual
sociotaxis
sociotherapy
socratic questioning
sodium
s. barbital
s. lactate
s. valproate
sodium-responsive periodic paralysis
sodomist
sodomize
sodomy
soft
s. chancre
s. diet
s. line
s. psychotic-like phenomenon
s. psychotic symptom
s. restraint
s. rock
s. speech
s. spot
s. touch
softheaded
softhearted
softliner
soft-pedal
soft-spoken
soiled
soiling
solace
soldier
s. in armed conflict
s. of fortune
s.'s heart
soldiering
solely
solemn
s. affect
s. vow
solemnity
solemnize
SOLER
squarely face person, open posture, lean toward person, eye contact, relaxed
Solian
solicit
solicitation
solicitous spouse behavior
solicitude
solidarity
solidify
soliloquize
soliloquy
sexual s.
solipsism
solitariness
solitary
s. activity
s. aggressive-type conduct
s. aggressive-type conduct disorder
s. confinement
s. hunter syndrome
s. stealing
solitude
solitudinarian
solo sexual activity
solution
s. analysis
auxiliary s.
comprehensive s.
expansive s.
major s.
masochistic s.
Methylin oral s.
The Centre for Mental Health S.'s
solution-focused therapy
solvable
solvent
s. abuse
s. dementia
s. dependence
volatile s.
Soma

NOTES

somata
neuronal s.
somatagnosia
somatalgia
somatesthesia
somatesthetic area
somatic
s. antidepressant
s. antidepressant treatment
s. category
s. cell
s. complaint
s. delusion
s. focus
s. hallucination
s. marker
s. memory
s. obsession
s. paranoid disorder
s. problem
s. psychosis
s. schizophrenia
s. subtype
s. symptom
s. therapy
s. treatment for depression
s. type
somatist
somatization
s. neurotic disorder
s. pain symptom
s. pseudoneurological symptom
s. reaction
s. sexual symptom
s. tendency
somatized
s. depression
s. plea for treatment
somatizing
s. clinical depression
s. disorder
somatoform
s. dissociation
s. interface disorder
s. pain
s. pain disorder (SPD)
somatognosia
somatology
somatometry
somatomotor epilepsy
somatopathic drinking
somatophrenia
somatopsychiatric comorbidity
somatopsychic disorder
somatopsychosis
somatosensory
s. cortex of right hemisphere of brain
s. epilepsy
s. evoked potential (SEP)
s. evoked response (SER)
s. seizure
s. system
somatosexual
somatosexuality
somatotherapy
somatotonia
somatotopagnosis, somatotopagnosia
somatotopic
somatotype
somatotypology
somatron table
somber mood
some degree of range
somesthesia
somesthetic
s. area
s. system
sommeil
tic de s.
somnambulance
somnambulant
somnambulate
somnambulic epilepsy
somnambulism
cataleptic s.
monoideic s.
polyideic s.
somnambulist
somnambulistic trance
somnial
somnifacient
somniferous
somniferum
Papaver s.
somnific
somnifugous
somniloquence, somniloquism
somniloquist
somniloquy
somnipathist
somnipathy
somnocinematograph
somnolence, somnolency
daytime s.
disorder of excessive s. (DOES)
excessive daytime s.
treatment-emergent s.
somnolent detachment
somnolentia
somnolescent
somnolism
somopsychosis
son
favorite s.
Sonata

song
rap s.
siren s.
son-in-law
sonogram
sonomotor response
sonorous
soothe
soothing
soothsayer
sophism
sophist
sophistic
sophisticate
sophistication
sophistry
sophomania
sophomoric
sopiet
sopor
soporiferous
soporifical
soporific drug dependence
soporose, soporous
sorbitol
sorcerer
sorceress
sorcerous
sorcery
sordid
sore
venereal s.
sororate
sorority
sorrow
overt sign of s.
sorrowful
sorrow-provoking stimuli
sort
out of s.'s
sortie
sortilege
sorting polarities
SOS
stimulation of sense
sosies
illusion des s.
SOT
stream of thought
sot
soteira
Sotos syndrome
soul
s. blindness
folk s.
s. loss
s. mate
negative ruler of s.
s. pain
world s.
soulful
soulless
soul-searching
sound
abnormal stoppage of s.
air-blade s.
s. analysis
attention to s.
s. blending
clucking s.
coconut s.
s. fear
s. inside head
opening s.
s. outside head
perception of s.
repetition of s.
s. symbolism
s. therapy
sounding board
soundless voice
soundly
soundness
sound-symbol association
soup kitchen
source
anxiety s.
collateral s.
external s.
nonself s.
potent pleasure s.
s. of sexual knowledge
sour grapes mechanism
sourness fear
South Beach diet
Southeast Asian refugee
Southern California Psychiatric Society
SP
scale of psychosis
systolic pressure
SPA
schizophrenia with premorbid asociality
schizophrenia with premorbid association
space
brain s.

NOTES

S

space *(continued)*
- s. context
- defensible s.
- detail response to small white s. (Dds)
- enclosed s.
- ethological model of personal s.
- inner s.
- life s.
- open s.
- s. perception
- personal s.
- s. response
- s. sense
- sociofugal s.

spacer

spacing

span
- apprehension s.
- attention s.
- s. of attention
- auditory s.
- auditory memory s. (AMS)
- comprehension s.
- digit s. (DS)
- eye-voice s.
- life s.
- limited attention s.
- liver s.
- memory s.
- narrowed attention s.

spanking

spar

sparing
- extrapyramidal symptom s.

Spartan diet

spasm
- affect s.
- anorectal s.
- canine s.
- carpopedal s.
- clonic s.
- cynic s.
- dancing s.
- functional s.
- habit s.
- hemifacial s.
- histrionic s.
- infantile s.
- intention s.
- masticatory s.
- mimic s.
- mobile s.
- muscle s.
- nictitating s.
- nodding s.
- occupational s.
- phonic s.
- progressive torsion s.
- retrocollic s.
- rotatory s.
- salaam s.
- saltatory s.
- sewing s.
- synclonic s.
- tailor's s.
- s. and tic
- tonic s.
- tonoclonic s.
- tooth s.
- vasomotor s.
- winking s.

spasmodic
- s. convulsion
- s. diathesis
- s. dysphonia
- s. laughter
- s. laughter syndrome
- s. mydriasis
- s. seizure
- s. tic
- s. winking syndrome

spasmodica
- tabes s.

spasmodicus

spasmology

spasmolygmus

spasmolysis

spasmolytic

spasmophemia

spasmophilia

spasmus
- s. caninus
- s. coordinatus
- s. nictitans
- s. nutans

spastic
- s. abasia
- s. amaurotic axonal idiocy
- s. aphonia
- s. diplegia
- s. dysphonia
- s. gait
- s. hemiplegia
- s. micosis
- s. miosis
- s. mydriasis
- s. state
- s. torticollis

spastica
- dysphonia s.

spasticity
- clasp-knife s.
- s. of conjugate gaze
- flexor s.

spat

spate

spatial
s. ability
s. agnosia
s. agraphia
s. aptitude
s. balance
s. behavior
s. contiguity
s. disorganization
s. disorientation
s. distortion
s. localization
s. music
s. neglect
s. nonrecognition
s. organization
s. orientation
s. summation
s. task
spatially
spatial-temporal context
SPD
sociopathic personality disorder
sociopathic personality disturbance
somatoform pain disorder
speak
s. out
s. up
speaking
avoidance s.
s. capacity
spearhead
Spearman
S. 2-factor theory
S. rho
special
s. education
s. educational service
s. education need
s. jury
s. needs probation
s. power
s. relationship to deity theme
s. relationship to famous person theme
s. sensation
s. sense
s. sex offender
s. talent
s. theory of relativity
specialist
addiction s.
certified addiction disease s.
child development s.
learning disabilities s.
mental health s.
specialization
role s.
specialized
s. foster care
s. language assessment
specialty
American Board of Medical S.'s (ABMS)
s. mental health treatment
species
allopatric s.
specific
s. academic or work inhibition
s. action potential
s. culture, age, and gender features
s. delay
s. developmental disorder (SDD)
s. dynamic pattern
s. effect
s. gender feature
s. learning disability
s. neurotic syndrome (SNR)
s. neurotransmitter
s. pathophysiological mechanism
s. phobia
s. psychotherapy
s. reading difficulty (SRD)
s. reading disability
s. sensory cue
sex s.
s. situational stressor
s. symptom
s. system
specification
job s.
specificity
criterion of s.
s. hypothesis
individual response s.
IR s.
physiologic response s.
s. of research
response s.
stimulus s.
symptom s.
treatment s.
specified
not otherwise s. (NOS)
specifier
course s.

NOTES

specifier *(continued)*
longitudinal course s.
severity s.
subtype and/or s.
type s.
speciosity
specious
SPECS
system to plan early childhood services
spectacle
spectacular
spectator
s. role
s. therapy
spectra (*pl. of* spectrum)
spectral
s. relationship
s. relationship to deity
s. relationship to famous person
spectrin
brain s.
spectrometry
spectroscopy
magnetic resonance s. (MRS)
point-resolved s. (PRESS)
spectrum, pl. **spectra, spectrums**
acoustic s.
band s.
bipolar s.
bulimic-anorexic s.
s. disorder
fortification s.
impulsive s.
panic-agoraphobic s.
psychotherapeutic s.
schizophrenia s.
schizophrenic s. (SS)
speculate
speculation
speculative
speech
absent s.
accelerated s.
s. act
agrammatic s.
alaryngeal s.
alteration in rate of s.
antiexpectancy s.
s. apraxia
aprosodic s.
s. aprosody
arrest of s.
articulation of s.
s. aspect
ataxic s.
audible blocking in s.
automatic s.
bilateral s.
bizarre s.
blocked s.
buccal s.
cerebellar s.
circumstantial s.
cleft palate s.
clipped s.
condescending s.
confused s.
s. content
cued s.
delayed s.
s. derailment
s. developmental delay disorder
s. difficulty
digressed s.
s. disability
disconnect s.
s. discrimination score (SDS)
s. disfluency
disorganized s.
s. disorientation
distractible s.
s. disturbance
dramatic s.
s. in dream
droning s.
dysarthric s.
s. dysfunction
s. dyspraxia
dysrhythmic s.
echo s.
egocentric s.
emotional s.
emotive s.
emphatic s.
euphoric s.
excessively impressionistic s.
excessively loud s.
excessively soft s.
executive s.
explosive s.
external s.
fast s.
figure of s.
flaccid s.
s. fluency
fluent aphasic s.
fluent paraphasic s.
s. hallucination
halting s.
s. and hearing (S&H)
hesitant s.
hyperkinetic s.
hypokinetic s.
imitative s.
impoverished s.
incessant s.
incoherent s.
incomprehensible s.

increased s.
infantile s.
s. inflection
s. intention center
internalized s.
involuntary pause in s.
labyrinthine s.
lack of s.
laconic s.
s. and language behavior
s. and language disorder
s. and language impaired (SLI)
loud s.
manic s.
s. mannerism
mimic s.
minimal spontaneous s.
mirror s.
s. monitoring center
monosyllabic s.
monotone s.
monotonous s.
s. and motor mapping
narrative s.
nonfluent aphasic s.
nonsensical s.
odd s.
organ s.
organic s.
overconcrete s.
over-elaborate s.
parasocial s.
s. pattern
paucity of s.
pause in s.
s. perception
s. perception region
s. perception system
performative s.
perseverative s.
phantom s.
plateau s.
s. poverty
poverty of content of s.
pressure of s.
pressured s.
s. processing
s. processing alteration
s. processing impairment
psychotic s.
quality of s.
quantity of s.
rambling flow of s.
rapid s.
rate of production of s.
s. reception threshold (SRT)
scanning s.
silent blocking in s.
slow s.
slurred s.
social gesture s.
soft s.
spoken s.
spontaneous s.
staccato s.
stilted s.
s. structure
subvocal s.
syllabic s.
tangential s.
s. therapy
threatening s.
s. tracking
s. tracking alteration
tremulous s.
underproductive s.
unintelligible s.
unstoppable flow of s.
vague s.
well-articulated s.
whispered s.

speechless

speech-motor deficit

speech-reading aphasia

speed

s. of information processing disturbance
mental s.
motor s.
perceptual s.
s. of processing
psychomotor s.
s. quotient
s. of thought
verbal perceptual s.
visual perceptual s.

spell

breathholding s.
crying s.
dizzy s.
doubting s.
s.'s of doubting and brooding
s. out
staring s.
vacant s.

spellbind

NOTES

spellbound
spelling
s. difficulty
s. dyspraxia
finger s.
s. grade equivalent
SPEM
smooth pursuit eye movement
spender
binge s.
spending
excessive s.
s. spree
spes phthisica
sphere
conflict-free s.
oriented in all s.'s
personality s.
psychosexual s.
spheresthesia
sphincter
s. control
s. morality
spider fantasy
Spiegel eye roll
Spielmeyer acute swelling
spike
peak absorption s.
spike-and-wave complex
spiked
s. hair
s. profile
spinal
s. anesthesia
s. ataxia
s. paralysis
s. pyramidotomy
s. shock
s. stroke
s. tap
s. trigeminal nucleus
spinalis
commotio s.
tabes s.
spindle
sleep s.
spine
poker s.
s. sign
spineless
spinifugal
spinipetal
spinning
spinogalvanization
spinoreticulothalamic pathway
spinothalamic
spinster
spiral
spirit
acquisitive s.
ancestral s.
community s.
controlling external s.
evil s.
external s.
neutral s.
possessed by s.
s. possession
s. writing
spirited
spiritism
spiritless
spiritual
s. activity
s. advice
s. advisor
s. approach
s. assessment
s. attitude
s. awareness
s. behavior
s. concern
s. counselor
devoutly s.
s. dimension
s. dimension in psychiatry
s. direction
s. distress
s. domain
s. emergence syndrome
s. emergency
s. emptiness
s. exercise
s. factor
s. focus group
s. function
s. guidance
s. guide
s. healing
s. impairment
s. inclination
s. intervention
s. issue
s. leadership
s. medium
s. orientation
s. pain
s. person
s. pilgrimage
s. possession
s. possession experience
s. practice
s. seeker
s. strength
s. value
spiritualism

spirituality
awareness of s.
personal s.
relevance of s.
salience of s.
spiritually homeless
spiteful
spite reaction
spitting
chewing and s.
splanchnesthesia
splanchnesthetic sensibility
splanchnic anesthesia
splenetic
splenium, pl. **splenia**
s. tissue
splinter
s. function
s. group
split
s. brain
s. custody
s. in ego
s. personality
split-brain preparation
split-half
s.-h. reliability
s.-h. reliability coefficient
split-off and denied experience
split-screen phenomenon
splitting
s. behavior
brain s.
ego s.
time s.
splurge
stealing s.
spoiled child reaction
spoken
s. language
s. language disorder
s. language impairment
s. language quotient
s. speech
spontaneity
parental s.
s. state
Theater of S.
s. training
spontaneous
s. abortion
s. convulsion
s. drawing
s. dyskinesia
s. imitation
s. improvement
s. laughter
s. movement
s. narrative discourse
s. panic attack
s. recovery
s. remission
s. seizure
s. speech
sporadic
s. depression
s. depressive disease (SDD)
sporotrichositic chancre
sport
s.'s betting
s.'s betting gambling
wheelchair s.'s
spot
blind s.
cold s.
figurative blind s.
hypnogenic s.
mental blind s.
pink s.
soft s.
temperature s.
touch s.
Trousseau s.
spousal
s. abuse
s. loss
s. loss through death
s. rape
spouse
s. abandonment
s. abuse
s. abuse index
s. abuser
battered s.
death of s.
distraught s.
dominant s.
s. rape
separated from s.
s. subsystem
spreading
s. depression
rumor s.
spree
buying s.
shooting s.

NOTES

spree *(continued)*
shopping s.
spending s.
spring finger
springing mydriasis
sprouting
hippocampal s.
spurious finding
spurt
end s.
initial s.
SQ
social quotient
status quo
squander mania
squarely face person, open posture, lean toward person, eye contact, relaxed (SOLER)
squeeze technique
SR
Ritalin SR
S&R
seclusion and restraint
SRA
Science Research Associates
SR/AP
schizophrenic reaction, acute paranoid
SR/AU
schizophrenic reaction, acute undifferentiated
SR/CP
schizophrenic reaction, chronic paranoid
SR/CU
schizophrenic reaction, chronic undifferentiated
SRD
specific reading difficulty
SRI
serotonin reuptake inhibitor
SRR
systematic rational restructuring
SRS
schizophrenic residual state
sex reassignment surgery
social and rehabilitation service
SRT
speech reception threshold
SS
schizophrenic spectrum
seizure sensitive
social service
SSA
Social Security Administration
SSN
superior salivary nucleus
SSOP
Standard System of Psychiatry
SSPD
schizoid-schizotypal personality disorder
SSRI
selective serotonin reuptake inhibitor
SSRI discontinuation
SSRI-induced
SSRI-i. anorgasmy
SSRI-i. bruxism
SSRI-i. erectile dysfunction
SSRI-i. sexual disturbance
SSRI-i. sexual side effect
SST
social skills training
ST
shock therapy
St.
Saint
St. John's wort
St. Louis hysteria
St. Vitus dance
stabbing pain
stability
behavioral s.
biopsychosocial s.
clinical s.
s. of ego
emotional s.
family s.
job s.
marital s.
s. of marriage
mental s.
occupational s.
personality trait s.
relative slow-wave sleep s.
slow-wave sleep s.
stabilization
acute s.
crisis s.
in-home crisis s.
mood s.
stabilize
stabilizer
mood s.
stabilizing social situation
stable
s. ego structure
emotionally s.
s. personality
relatively s.
s. sleep difficulty
s. sleep-wake pattern
s. therapeutic relationship
stably unstable
staccato speech
stacking
s. anchor
card s.
staff
consulting s.

medical s.
s. member
stage
adolescent developmental s.
adulthood developmental s.
alarm reaction s.
anal s.
anal-expulsive s.
attending to language s.
autonomous s.
biting s.
childhood developmental s.
cognitive development s.
concrete operation s.
concrete operational s.
confrontation s.
s.'s of death and dying
dementia s.
developmental s.
equality s.
equity s.
s. of exhaustion
exhaustion s.
formal operation s.
s. fright
functional assessment s.
genital s.
grammar development s.
grammar formation s.
group s.
heteronomous s.
HIV illness s.
individuation s.
infancy developmental s.
initial s.
intuitive s.
late-life developmental s.
latency s.
life s.
locomotor-genital s.
s. 3 mania
manipulation s.
muscular-anal s.
oedipal s.
oral s.
oral-sensory s.
2o-word messages s.
phallic s.
physioplastic s.
Piaget cognitive development s.
postambivalent phase s.
preattachment s.
preclinical s.
preconceptual s.
pregenital s.
preoedipal s.
preoperational thought s.
psychosexual s.
pubertal s.
question s.
recovery s.
rehabilitation s.
sensorimotor s.
set the s.
shock s.
single-word s.
sleep s.
symbiotic s.
symptom experience s.
toddler s.
true communication s.
urethral s.
staggering gait
staging
functional assessment s.
stagnation
generativity vs s.
stain
toluidine blue s.
stake
stalemate
analytic s.
stalker
nonviolent s.
s. preoccupation
violent s.
stalking
s. behavior
s. law
s. victim
violence in s.
stammer
stammering of bladder
stamp
date s.
digit s.
stance
approach-avoidance s.
combative s.
defensive adultomorphic s.
masochistic s.
norm-assertive s.
stand
s. out
standard
s. antipsychotic therapy

NOTES

standard *(continued)*
s. behavior
best interest s.
s. of care
competency s.
s.'s development
s. deviation (SD)
s. dose
s. dose administration
double s.
s. error
s. error of difference
s. error of mean (SEM)
foreign s.
s.'s implementation
judgment s.
s. kinetic model
legal s.
s. of living
s. methadone maintenance treatment program
normative s.
s. of performance
s. practice
s. probation
s. psychiatric nomenclature
psychometric s.
s. rating procedure
s. reference
s. score
social s.
S. System of Psychiatry (SSOP)
standardization
standardize
standardized
s. assessment
s. cognitive assessment technique
standing balance
standoff
Stanford-Binet
Stanley Foundation bipolar network
STAPP
short-term anxiety-provoking psychotherapy
starch
s. eater
s. eating
stare
blank s.
s. down
empty s.
manic s.
postbasic s.
reptilian s.
unblinking s.
vacant s.
star fear
staring
s. face
s. facial expression
s. spell
starter marriage
startle
s. abnormality
acoustic s.
affective modulation of s.
s. epilepsy
s. reaction
s. reflex
s. response
s. syndrome
s. technique
startling stimulus
start low and go slow
starvation fasting
starve
stash
stasis
libido s.
state
absent s.
across identity s.
activated s.
active s.
acute s.
acute confusional s. (ACS)
adrenergic response s.
adult ego s.
affect s.
affective and paranoid s.
agitated s.
alcoholic confusional s.
alcoholic paranoid s.
alcoholic twilight s.
alcohol-induced paranoid s.
alcohol paranoid s.
alert awake s.
s. of alertness
alpha s.
altered s.
amnesic s.
amnestic s.
anxiety s. (AS)
anxiety tension s. (ATS)
apallic s.
appetitive s.
apprehension s.
arousal s.
arteriosclerotic dementia confusional s.
arteriosclerotic paranoid s.
arteriosclerotic psychosis confusional s.
atypical neurotic anxiety s.
awake s.
borderline s.
break s.
calm wakefulness s.

catatonic s.
central excitatory s.
central motive s.
chronic deficit s.
chronic delusional s.
clear twilight s.
climacteric paranoid s.
clouded s.
cognitive s.
S. Comprehensive Mental Health Plan Act of 1986
confusional twilight s.
conscious s.
s. of consciousness (SOC)
constitutional psychopathic s. (CPS)
convulsive s.
delirium-like s.
s. dependence
depressed manic s.
depressive mixed s.
desire s.
dietary s.
diffusional s.
discrete behavioral s.
disorganized s.
dissociated s.
dissociative s.
dream s.
dreamlike s.
dreamy s.
drug-induced confusional s.
drug-induced hallucinatory s.
drug-induced paranoid s.
drug-induced semihypnotic s.
drug-like desire s.
drug psychosis hallucinatory s.
dysequilibrium s.
dysphoric manic s.
ego s.
elusive illness s.
emotional s.
end s.
epileptic clouded s.
epileptic confusional s. (ECS)
epileptic twilight s.
erotomanic delusional s.
euthymic s.
excited s.
exhaustion s.
explosive psychotic s.
s. factor
fatigue s.
fluctuating ego s.
fugue s.
fusion s.
generalized neurotic anxiety s.
general mood s.
global attractor s.
hallucinatory s.
s. of heightened attention
heightened attention s.
heightened awareness s.
s. of heightened awareness
homicidal s.
s. hospital (SH)
s. hospital children's unit (SHCU)
hyperadrenergic s.
hypereridic s.
hyperpathic s.
hypnagogic s.
hypnoid s.
hypnopompic s.
hypnotic s.
hypodopaminergic s.
hysterical coma-like s.
hysterical fugue s.
identity s.
immobile s.
internal s.
involutional paranoid s.
lacunar s.
litigious delusional s.
local excitatory s.
locked in s.
manic s.
marasmic s.
s. marker of heavy drinking
menopausal paranoid s.
mental s.
s. mental hospital (SMH)
merger s.
s. of mind
s. of mindful relaxation
mixed bipolar s.
mixed mood s.
mood s.
moribund s.
multiple ego s.'s
mute s.
negative mood s.
neurotic anxiety s.
neurotic depressive s.
nonresponsive s.
obsessional s.
obsessive-ruminative tension s.
oneiroid s.

NOTES

state *(continued)*
opposite affect s.
oral s.
organic psychotic s.
pain s.
panic attack neurotic anxiety s.
panic-free s.
paranoia querulans paranoid s.
paranoid litigious s.
paraphonic s.
paraphrenia paranoid s.
parasomniac conscious s.
parent ego s.
pathological mood s.
perfection s.
perplexity s.
persistent vegetative s. (PVS)
phobic s.
possession trance s.
postanoxic s.
postepileptic twilight s.
postictal s.
postoperative confusional s.
premenstrual tension s.
premorbid s.
presenile dementia confusional s.
presenile organic psychotic s.
profile of mood s.'s (POMS)
prolonged transition to fully awake s.
s. psychiatric institution
psychogenic twilight s.
psychological s.
psychopathic s.
psychotic s.
rapid eye movement s.
reactive confusional s.
refractory s.
REM s.
residual s.
s. of resistance
resource s.
resting s.
rigid s.
ruminative tension s.
schizophrenic defect s.
schizophrenic residual s. (SRS)
s. of semisleep
senile dementia confusional s.
senile organic psychotic s.
senile paranoid s.
sexual motive s.
simple paranoid s.
sleep s.
spastic s.
spontaneity s.
s. statute
steady s.
subacute confusional s. (SCS)
subacute delirious s.
subacute irritable depressive s.
subdelirious s.
subdued s.
substance-induced s.
subsyndromal s.
tension s.
toxic confusional s.
toxic drug s.
trance s.
trancelike s.
transcendental s.
transient postictal confusional s.
traumatic defect s.
twilight confusional s.
unresponsive s.
vegetative s.
visceral emotional s.
wakeful s.
withdrawal s.

stated
s. age
s. desire

state-dependent
s.-d. learning
s.-d. measure
s.-d. memory

statement
fashion s.
nonsensical s.
opening s.
personality-descriptive s.
repetitive s.
suicidal s.
SWAP-200 s.

state-of-the-art
s.-o.-t.-a. analysis
s.-o.-t.-a. analysis technique

state-trait interaction

static
s. ataxia
s. convulsion
s. dementia
s. demography
s. encephalopathy
s. infantilism
s. sense
s. steadiness
s. tremor

station
obligatory relay s.

statistic
s.'s collection
descriptive s.
inferential s.
National Center for Health S.'s
psychiatric s.
vital s.'s

statistical
s. artifact
s. deviation
s. inference
s. mean
s. median
s. significance
s. trend
statistically
s. significant
s. significant improvement
stature
psychosocially determined short s.
short s.
status
absence s.
acute change in mental s.
altered mental s.
ambulatory s.
s. aura
baseline mental s.
biologic s.
s. choreicus
clinical s.
cognitive s.
confident s.
s. cribrosus
s. criticus
current cognitive s.
degenerative s.
s. degenerativus
s. deterioration
disordered mental s.
divorce s.
s. dysgraphicus
s. dysraphicus
elopement s. (ES)
s. epilepsy
s. epilepticus
s. epilepticus organic psychosis
ethnic s.
s. examination
female biological s.
functional s.
general cognitive s.
grand mal s.
health s.
higher s.
s. hypnoticus
s. hypoplasticus
immigrant s.
s. index
s. indicator
s. lacunaris
latchkey s.
male biological s.
marital s.
menopausal s.
mental s.
s. nervosus
nutritional s.
s. offender
open-ward s.
parent's marital s.
parole s.
partner s.
petit mal s.
postoperative s.
preepisode s.
proband s.
probation s.
prognostic s.
s. quo (SQ)
s. raptus
s. schedule
separated s.
sexual abuse s.
short test of mental s.
social s.
socioeconomic s. (SES)
suicide s.
symptomatic s.
temporal lobe s.
uncertain biological s.
s. value
s. vertiginosus
widowed s.
statute
federal s.
state s.
statutory
s. criteria
s. offense
s. rape
statuvolence
statuvolent
Stauder lethal catatonia
staunch
stauroplegia
stay
estimated length of s.
inpatient s.
length of s. (LOS)
length of patient s. (LOPS)
s. on task

NOTES

STC
sexually transmitted condition
STD
sexually transmitted disease
steadiness
static s.
steady
s. gait
s. state
steady-state
s.-s. dose
s.-s. equilibrium
s.-s. method
s.-s. regimen
stealing
s. an anchor
compulsive s.
s. impulse
solitary s.
s. splurge
stealth
steamy
Stearns alcoholic amentia
steatosis
hepatic s.
Steele-Richardson-Olszewski disease
steeple skull
stem completion
stenosis, pl. **stenoses**
artery s.
stenostenosis
step
shuffling s.'s
12-step
12-s. meeting
12-s. program
12-s. program for substance abuse
stepbrother
stepchild
2-step command
stepdaughter
stepfather
stepmother
steppage gait
stepparent
steppingstone theory
steprelation
stepsister
stepson
3-step task
stepwise deterioration
stereoagnosis
stereoanesthesia
stereoelectroencephalography
stereoencephalometry
stereognosis
stereognostic perception
stereopathy
stereopsyche
stereoscopic vision
stereotaxic coordinate system
stereotaxis, stereotaxy
stereotype
cultural s.
stereotyped
s. activity
s. attitude
s. behavior
s. body movement
s. emotion
s. interest
s. motor movement
s. movement disorder
s. repetition
s. routine
s. stress
s. vocalization
stereotypic
s. motor movement
s. movement disorder (SMD)
stereotypical
s. behavior
s. gender roles
stereotyping
stereotypy, pl. **stereotypies**
s. and habit disorder
oral s.
sterile
sterility
elective s.
sterilization
mental patient s.
sterilize
stern
Sternberg paradigm
steroid
anabolic s.
anabolic-androgenic s. (AAS)
s. psychosis
sex s.
s. withdrawal syndrome
steroid-induced
s.-i. delirium
s.-i. mania
s.-i. mood disorder
steroidogenic factor-1 (SF-1)
stethoparalysis
stethospasm
Stewart-Morel syndrome
STG
short-term goal
sticking sensation
stiff neck
stiffness
tongue s.
stifle
stigma, pl. **stigmas, stigmata**
s. change

external s.
medication s.
s. of psychosis
psychosocial s.
s. of venipuncture

stigmatic
stigmatism
stigmatization
stigmatized
stiletto
stillbirth
stilted
s. attitude
s. speech
s. view

stimulant
s. abuse
amphetamine-type s. (ATS)
beta s.
chimeric s.
s. choice
CNS s.
dopaminergic s.
s. effect
s. overdose
psychomotor s.
s. therapy
s. tolerance
s. treatment

stimulant-dependent sleep disorder
stimulant-induced
s.-i. insomnia
s.-i. postural tremor

stimulate
stimulated
sexually s.

stimulating
s. environment
s. experience
s. occupation

stimulation
s. adjustment
amygdaloid s.
audiovisual brain s.
autogenital s.
brain s.
chemical s.
chimeric s.
clitoral s.
cocaine-induced dopamine s.
cognitive s.
s. condition
conditioned s.
direct genital s.
dopamine s.
dorsal column s.
double simultaneous s. (DSS)
electrical intracranial s.
electrical transcranial s. (ETS)
emotional s.
endogenous s.
environmental s. (ES)
epileptogenic s.
exogenous s.
external s.
s. fatigue
fixed-dose s.
functional electrical s. (FES)
genital s.
s. index (SI)
insufficient s.
intracranial s. (ICS)
manual s.
minimizing s.
noncoital s.
olfactory s.
oral s.
pathway s.
percutaneous s.
s. PET study
photic s.
postsynaptic s.
s. ratio
repetitive transcranial magnetic s. (rTMS)
s. of sense (SOS)
sensory s.
serotonin s.
sexual s.
social s.
subliminal s.
supranormal s.
sympathetic s.
synesthetic s.
tactile genital s.
tetanic s.
therapeutic electric s.
thyrotropin-releasing hormone s.
transcranial magnetic s. (TMS)
vagus nerve s. (VNS)
visual s.

stimulation-bound behavior (SBB)
stimulation-related adverse effect
stimulator
Caldwell high speed magnetic s.

stimulus, pl. **stimuli**

NOTES

stimulus *(continued)*
accidental s.
adequate s.
alerting s.
ambiguous external s.
angry reaction to minor s.
anxiolytic s.
auditory s.
aversive s.
s. avoidance
chemical s.
conditioned s. (CS)
s. control
discriminant s.
discriminative s.
distracting stimuli
dream s.
s. drive (Sd)
effective s.
emotional s.
emotionally provoking s.
emotion-related feedback s.
emotive s.
environmental s.
epileptogenic s.
erotic s.
excitatory s.
external speech s.
s. fading
fatness s.
frightening s.
s. generalization
heterologous s.
homologous s.
inadequate s.
incidental s.
ineffective s.
internal s.
irrelevant external s.
liminal s.
masking s.
maximal s.
method of constant stimuli
minor s.
musical s.
neutral s.
novel s.
noxious s.
outside s.
s. overload
painful s.
paraphiliac s.
pedophilic s.
perceptual emotive s.
pharmacological s.
phobic s.
pleasant s.
pleasurable stimuli
provocative s.
provoking s.
psychosensory s.
reaction to minor s.
real external s.
real-life s.
reinforcing s.
s. response
screen out irrelevant s.
sensory s.
sexual s.
sorrow-provoking stimuli
s. specificity
startling s.
subliminal s.
s. substitution
subthreshold s.
summation of stimuli
supramaximal s.
tactile s.
target s.
s. tension
terrifying s.
s. therapy
thermal s.
s. threshold
threshold s.
train-of-four s.
triggering s.
unconditioned s. (UCS)
visual s.
visuospatial s.
s. word

stimulus-bound
stimulus-independent thought
stimulus-response theory
stimulus-sensitive myoclonus
stinginess
stinging pain
stingy
stir fever
Stirling County study
stirred-up emotion
STM
short-term memory
Stockholm syndrome
stocking-and-glove
s.-a.-g. anesthesia
s.-a.-g. sensory loss
stocking anesthesia
stocking-glove
stoic
stoichiometric change
stoker's cramp
stolen
stomach
nervous s.
stonewall
Stony Brook High Risk Project
stooped shoulders

stop
s., look and listen intervention
s. short
s. signal task
stop-and-think technique
stopped smoking
stopping
s. task
thought s.
stop-start technique
storage
iconic s.
long-term s.
memory s.
store
cellular s.
high-energy cellular s.
storm
emotional s.
Operation Desert S. (ODS)
storm-and-stress period
stormed defense
storminess
stormy personality
story
s. fear
horror s.
s. memory
sob s.
storylike dream sequence
storyteller
storytelling
unbelievable s.
strabismus
straight
s. and narrow
set one s.
strain
financial s.
interpersonal s.
job s.
physical s.
psychological s.
role s.
vocational s.
straitjacket
chemical s.
straits
dire s.
strangalesthesia
strange behavior pattern
strangeness fear
stranger
s. anxiety
s. fear
sexual assault by s.
strangle
stranglehold
strangulated affect
strangulation
s. ligature
ritual ligature s.
strata (*pl. of* stratum)
strategic
s. compliance
s. family therapy
s. intervention
s. planning
strategically
strategist
strategy
acceptance s.
adjunctive s.
age-appropriate s.
alternative s.
augmentation s.
bibliotherapeutic s.
candidate gene s.
challenge s.
coactive s.
cognitive s.
combination s.
conflict resolution s.
coping s.
crisis management s.
dangerous coping s.
data reanalysis s.
defense s.
dose-reduction s.
empirical-rational s.
family-centered s.
gambling s.
genetic s.
hockey stick s.
inference s.
learning s.
loading s.
low-dose s.
maladaptive coping s.
maladaptive problem-solving s.
maternal problem-solving s.
memory retrieval s.
mnemonic s.
optimal treatment s.
polygamous s.

NOTES

strategy *(continued)*
precursor load s.
problem-solving s.
protective survival s.
reality-oriented supportive s.
reanalysis s.
self-handicapping s.
self-regulatory s.
single-agent oral s.
survival s.
therapeutic s.
treatment evaluation s.
treatment package s.
validation s.
visual representation s.
stratification
population s.
post hoc s.
stratum, pl. **strata**
social strata
stream
breath s.
s. of consciousness
s. of mental activity
s. of thought (SOT)
street
s. addict
s. drug
s. fear
s. gang
s. people
s. person
s. sense
s. talk
streetperson
streetwalker
strength
antagonistic muscle s.
associative s.
effective habit s.
ego s. (ES)
fatigue s.
habit s.
human s.
muscle s.
personal s.
psychological s.
spiritual s.
s.'s and weaknesses
strenuous
stress
acute foot-shock s.
adaptability to s.
s. adaptability skill
s. audit
biologic s.
caregiver s.
catastrophic s.
causative s.
chronic s.
combat s.
contrastive s.
day-to-day s.
disabling s.
s. disorder
disorders of extreme s., not otherwise specified (DESNOS)
effect of s.
s. effect and immune response
s. effect in old age
s. effect on adult
s. effect on adult thinking
s. effect on learning
s. effect on memory
ego s.
emotional s.
environmental s.
exceptional s.
excessive s.
executive s.
exogenous s.
family s.
fatigue s.
fight-or-flight s.
s. from life experience (SFLE)
iambic s.
identifiable s.
s. immunity
s. inoculation
s. inoculation training (SIT)
s. interview
intolerance of s.
job s.
job-related s.
s. level
level of psychosocial s.
life s.
major life s.
s. management
s. management style
marital s.
maternal s.
medical s.
mental s.
nonspecific s.
occupational s.
overwhelming s.
perceived s.
physical s.
postdisaster s.
precipitating s.
s. prevention
primary s.
psychological s.
s. psychosis
psychosocial s.
s. reaction
reaction to life s.

s. reduction
s. response pattern
s. response syndrome
secondary s.
serious traumatic s.
severe life s.
s. situational reaction
social s.
stereotyped s.
subjective s.
temporary s.
tertiary s.
s. theory
transient emotional s.
trauma-related s.
traumatic s.
trochaic s.
war-related s.
weak s.
stress-altered startle reflex
stress-diathesis model
stress-driven diathesis
stressful
s. divorce
s. encounter
s. environment
s. life event
s. life experience
s. mate
s. precipitating event
psychologically s.
stress-illness process
stress-induced
s.-i. alopecia
s.-i. cognitive impairment
s.-i. immune system alteration
s.-i. personality disorder
s.-i. reactive bowel
stressor
brief reactive psychosis with marked s.'s
childhood s.
chronic s.
cumulative s.'s
disaster s.
early life s.
educational s.
environmental s.
external s.
extreme s.
identifiable s.
internal s.
life s.
maladaptive reaction to s.
naturalistic s.
postmigration s.
premigration s.
psychosocial s.
race-related s.
seasonal-related psychosocial s.
severe s.
situational s.
social s.
specific situational s.
traumatic s.
s. uncontrollability
stress-precipitating tremor
stress-related
s.-r. amenorrhea
s.-r. disorder
s.-r. disturbance
s.-r. illness
s.-r. paranoid ideation
s.-r. physiological response
s.-r. psychopathology
s.-r. psychophysiological problem
s.-r. syndrome
stress-strain relationship
stria, pl. **striae**
acoustic s.
s. terminalis
striatal
s. hypometabolism
s. metabolism
striatocerebral tremor
striatofrontal
s. circuitry
s. dysfunction
striatum
corpus s.
striatus-orbitofrontal metabolism
stricken
pain s.
strict parent
strident
stridor
strife
family s.
strike
hunger s.
3-strikes law
stringent
stripper
strip search
striptease

NOTES

striving
emancipatory s.
maintenance s.
s. for superiority
stroke
cocaine-related s.
emotional s.
hallucinogen-related s.
lacunar s.
National Institute of Neurological and Communicative Disorders and S.
spinal s.
stroking
strong
s. craving
s. impulse
strongly held idea
strong-minded
strong-willed
Stroop effect
structural
s. ambiguity
s. analysis of social behavior
s. atrophy
s. balance
s. brain abnormality
s. brain imaging
s. change
s. clinical interview
s. diagnosis
s. embeddedness
s. family therapy
s. gene
s. injury
s. integration
s. magnetic resonance imaging
s. MRI
s. neuroimaging
s. pathology
s. profile
s. strategic therapy
s. theory
structuralism
structure
abnormal brain s.
alteration of memory s.
base s.
brain s.
character s.
cognitive s.
cooperative reward s.
cortical s.
deep s.
depressive character s.
dysphoric character s.
ego s.
external s.
field s.
functional superego s.
group s.
hierarchical s.
hypoactive limbic s.
individualistic reward s.
initiating s.
s. of intellect (SI)
intermediate s.
knowledge s.
lack of s.
limbic s.
medial temporal s.
mental s.
narcissistic character s.
neural s.
organizational s.
pedigree s.
perceptual s.
personality s.
pragmatic s.
social s.
societal s.
speech s.
stable ego s.
superego s.
surface s.
syntactic language s.
underlying s.
unique pedigree s.
white matter s.
structured
s. clinical interview
s. environment
s. hallucination
s. interactional group
s. interactional group psychotherapy
s. interview for assessing perceptual anomalies
s. milieu
s. task
s. verbal information
structured-based ethics
struggle
s. behavior
leadership power s.
power s.
strychnine
aloin, belladonna, s. (ABS)
belladonna alkaloid
strychninism
strychnomania
stubborn
stubbornly defiant
student
above-average s.
at-risk high school s.
at-risk middle school s.
average s.

below-average s.
college s.

study

adoption s.
Allport A-S reaction s.
analog s.
autopsy s.
bidirectional selection s.
biochemical s.
biophysical s.
blind s.
Bonn early recognition s.
brain imaging s.
brain potential s.
brain structure s.
case control s.
case history s.
Child Health and Development S.
Children's Health S. (CHS)
clinical comparison s.
cohort s.
community s.
Conflict and Management Of Relationships s. (CONAMORE)
correlation s.
crossover s.
cross-sectional s.
s. design
diachronic s.
double-blind s.
double-blind drug s.
Dunedin Multidisciplinary Health and Development S.
Early Developmental Stages of Psychopathology S.'s
ECA s.
ecological s.
electrodiagnostic s.
emotional fatigue s.
empirical s.
epidemiological s.
ethological s.
event-related brain potentials s.
experimental s. (ES)
family risk s.
followup s.
functional brain imaging s.
gambling impact and behavior s.
genetic linkage s.
s. group
high-risk s.
hysteria s.
imaging s.
International Society for Traumatic Stress S.'s
Isle of Wight s.
laboratory s.
longitudinal s.
long-term naturalistic s.
MacArthur violence risk assessment s.
Marcé s.
Masters and Johnson s.
Medical Outcomes S. (MOS)
Midtown Manhattan s.
moon-phase s.
multivariate s.
National Comorbidity S. (NCS)
National Vietnam Veterans Readjustment S. (NVVRS)
naturalistic followup s.
nerve conduction s.
neurophysiological s.
New Haven s.
New York longitudinal s. (NYLS)
nocturnal penile tumescence s.
noninvasive brain imaging s.
outcome s.
parametric s.
pathological s.
pedigree s.
phenotypic s.
picture frustration s. (PFS)
pilot s.
placebo-controlled drug s.
postmortem s.
prediction s.
Prenatal Determinants of Schizophrenia S.
Prevention of Suicide in Primary Care Elderly: Collaborative S. (PROSPECT)
prospective s.
psychological autopsy s.
Quality of Life, Effectiveness, Safety, and Tolerability S. (Q.U.E.S.T.)
resting PET s.
retrospective s.
Seattle Longitudinal S.
segregation analysis s.
self-report s.
stimulation PET s.
Stirling County s.
synchronic s.
systematic s.

NOTES

study *(continued)*
time and motion s.'s
time-motion s.
Treatment for Adolescents with Depression S.
twin s.'s
ultrastructural s.
United States-United Kingdom S.
S. of Values (SV)
Vantaa depression s. (VDS)
stumbling
syllable s.
stump
s. hallucination
s. neuralgia
stun gun
stunt
dangerous s.
stupefacient, stupefactive
stupefaction
stupefy
stupemania
stupidity
stupor
affective s.
akinetic s.
alcoholic s.
anergic s.
benign s.
Cairns s.
catatonic s.
delusion s.
s. and depression
depressive s.
diencephalic s.
emotional s.
epileptic s.
examination s.
exhaustive s.
frank catatonic s.
lethargic s.
malignant s.
s. mania
manic s.
postconvulsive s.
psychogenic s.
psychomotor s.
stuporosa
melancholia s.
stuporous
s. catatonia
s. depression
s. exhaustion
s. manic-depressive psychosis
s. melancholia
s. patient
stuporous-type manic-depressive psychosis
stutter
stutterer
stuttering
s. block theory
s. gait
hysterical s.
labiochoreic s.
style
adaptive s.
aggressive attributional s.
ambivalent attachment s.
analysis of coping s.
arrogant s.
attachment s.
attributional s.
avoidance s.
avoidant s.
borderline personality s.
cognitive s.
coping s.
deceitful s.
deception s.
dispositional coping s.
dramatic interpersonal s.
dysfunctional family s.
dysfunctional personality s.
interpersonal s.
intrapsychic s.
introtensive personality s.
introtensive problem-solving s.
introversive problem-solving s.
s. of leadership and management
linguistic s.
neurotic s.
obsessive neurotic s.
parenting s.
perceptual s.
problem-solving s.
repressive coping s.
ruminative coping s.
secure attachment s.
stress management s.
stymie
subacute
s. confusional insanity
s. confusional state (SCS)
s. delirious state
s. delirium
s. irritable depressive state
s. organic reaction
s. posttraumatic organic psychosis
s. psychoorganic syndrome
s. spongiform encephalopathy
subaffective
s. disorder
s. dysthymia
subantigen
subaverage
s. academic functioning

s. intellectual functioning
s. motor coordination
subcategory
subception
subchronic
s. schizophrenia
s. schizophrenic
subclass
subclassification
subclavian steal syndrome
subclinical
s. absence
s. depressive symptom
s. range
s. score
s. seizure
s. syndrome
subcoma therapy
subconscious
s. awareness
s. memory
s. mind
s. perception
s. self
subconsciousness
subcortical
s. alexia
s. arteriosclerotic encephalopathy
s. brain involvement
s. condition
s. dementia
s. dysfunction model
s. gray matter
s. gray matter area
s. gray matter hyperintensity
s. gray region
s. motor aphasia
s. neglect
s. pathology
s. white matter
subcortical-frontal lobe abnormality
subcultural language
subculture norm
subcutaneous injection
subdelirious state
subdelirium
subdivision
hippocampal formation s.
subdue
difficult to s.
subdued state
subdural
subfactor
borderline s.
dysphoric s.
subgenual cingulate region
subgroup
cultural s.
diagnostic s.
ethnic s.
phenomenological s.
subgrundation
subiculum, pl. **subicula**
subject
caffeine-abstinent s.
ego s.
normal s.
subjective
s. criticism
s. depression
s. distortion
s. distress
s. doubles
s. drive
s. effect
s. emotional feeling
s. equality
s. error
s. experience
s. fear
s. incompetence
s. insomnia complaint
s. manifestation
s. mentation
s. mood change
s., objective, assessment, plan
s. orientation
s. pain
s. plane
s. psychology
s. psychostimulation
s. seizure
s. sensation
s. sleep characteristic
s. stress
s. symptom
s. unit of distress rating
s. vertigo
s. vision
s. well-being
subjectively unpleasant feeling
subjectivism factor
subjectivity
overwhelmed s.
subjugate

NOTES

subjunctive mood
sublimate
sublimation
s. defense mechanism
s. difficulty
sublime
subliminal
s. behavior
s. consciousness
s. excitation
s. fringe
s. learning
s. message
s. perception
s. self
s. stimulation
s. stimulus
s. suggestion
s. thirst
sublimity
sublingual
s. gland
s. medication
submachine gun
submania
submerge
submerged individual need
submission
authoritarian s.
domination and s.
submissive behavior
submissiveness
submodality
critical s.
subnormal
educationally s. (ESN)
s. intelligence
subnormality
mental s.
moderate mental s.
profound mental s.
severe mental s.
subnucleus
amygdala s.
suboccipital
s. decompression
s. headache
s. neuralgia
s. neuritis
s. puncture
suboptimal
s. treatment
s. treatment modality
subordinate
s. association
s. position
subordination
subphase
rapprochement s.
subplate zone
subpoena duces tecum
subpoenaed
subpotent
subpsyche
subscribe
subsequent
s. amnesia
s. development
s. trauma
subservient
subshock therapy
subsidiation
subsidize
subsidy
subsist
subsistence diet
subsocial
subsonic
subspecialty
substance
s. abuse
s. abuse counselor
s. abuse and dependence
s. abuse disorder
S. Abuse Mental Health Services Administration
s. abuser
s. abuse treatment
s. abuse treatment facility
s. addiction
amphetamine-like s.
anxiolytic s.
behavior-altering s.
caffeinated s.
controlled s.
s. dependence disorder
ego s.
endogenously produced s.
s. group
illicit psychoactive s.
s. intoxication
s. K
long-half-life anxiolytic s.
mind-altering s.
mood-altering s.
nontoxic s.
pineal s.
psychoactive s.
schedule II s.
s. sensitivity
s. tolerance
toxic s.
s. use
s. use disorder (SUD)
s. withdrawal delirium
s. withdrawal tremor
substance-abuse persisting dementia
substance-abusing parent

substance-bound behavior
substance-induced
s.-i. anxiety
s.-i. chronic psychosis
s.-i. delirium
s.-i. dystonia
s.-i. etiology
s.-i. excitement
s.-i. intoxication
s.-i. manic episode
s.-i. organic mental disorder
s.-i. perception
s.-i. persisting dementia
s.-i. presentation
s.-i. psychotic disorder
s.-i. psychotic disorder with delusions
s.-i. sexual dysfunction
s.-i. state
s.-i. symptomatology
s.-i. syndrome
substance-related
s.-r. cause
s.-r. disorder
s.-r. legal problem
s.-r. syndrome
substance-seeking behavior
substance-specific
s.-s. intoxication criteria sets
s.-s. withdrawal
s.-s. withdrawal criteria sets
substandard
substantia
s. innominata
s. nigra
substantial comorbidity
substantive universals
substitute
displacement s.
father s.
s. formation
mother s.
s. object
opioid s.
regressive s.
substituted amphetamine
substituting
s. behavior
s. feeling
s. thought
substitution
s. accuracy code
s. analysis
s. defense mechanism
digit symbol s.
s. disorder
s. efficiency code
stimulus s.
symptom s.
substitutive
s. agent therapy
s. medication
s. reaction type
substrate
biologic s.
brain s.
complete s.
neural s.
partial s.
subsultus
s. clonus
s. tendinum
subsume
subsyndromal
s. bipolar mood fluctuation
s. depression
s. depressive symptom
s. mood symptom
s. state
s. thought disorder
subsystem
s. boundary
cognitive s.
depreciated s.
executive s.
individual s.
interacting cognitive s.
parallel s.
parent s.
sibling s.
spouse s.
subteen
subtemporal decompression
subtetanic
subthalamic nucleus
subtherapeutic dose
subthreshold
s. presentation
s. stimulus
subtle
s. gesture
s. meaning
s. memory problem
s. symptom
subtype
s. and/or specifier

NOTES

subtype *(continued)*
Central European s.
clinical s.
delusional s.
depression s.
diagnostic s.
disorganized s.
Eastern s.
erotomanic s.
grandiose s.
jealous s.
kraepelinian s.
male alcoholism s.
persecutory s.
psychotic depressive s.
somatic s.
Western s.
subunit
beta s.
suburban community
subversion
subversive
subvocal speech
subwaking
succedaneum
caput s.
succeed
succès de scandale
success
cumulative probability of s. (CPS)
s. experience
failure through s.
lack of academic s.
lack of vocational s.
s. neurosis
outlet for s.
therapeutic s.
successful suicide
successive approximation
succinct
succinimide
succinylcholine
succorance need
succubus
succumb
sucking
s. behavior
finger s.
s. reflex
s. technique
thumb s.
suckling
eternal s.
SUD
substance use disorder
sudden
s. ambush
s. cheerfulness
s. death
s. fear
s. financial reversal
s. infant death syndrome (SIDS)
s. insight
s. motor movement
s. onset
s. onset of symptoms
s. vocalization
sudden-onset headache
Sudeck syndrome
sudomotor component
suffer
suffering
anticipated emotional s.
s. death
ego s.
emotional s.
s. hero daydream
mental s.
sufficient quantity
suffocate
suffocating attachment
suffocation
s. fear
s. hysterics
s. panicker
traumatic s.
suffrage
female s.
sugar
blood s.
suggestibility
disturbance in s.
s. effect
suggestible
suggestion
affective s.
hypnotic s.
posthypnotic s.
prestige s.
subliminal s.
s. therapy
s. under hypnosis
verbal s.
suggestive
s. medicine
s. psychotherapy
sexually s.
s. therapeutics
suicidal
s. act
actively s.
s. behavior
s. crisis
s. depressed patient
s. emergency
s. feature
s. gesture
s. ideation

s. intent
s. intention
s. melancholia
s. obsession
s. plan
s. potential
s. preoccupation
s. rumination
s. statement
s. thinking
s. thought
suicidality
suicide
s. acceptability
accidental s.
accomplished s.
s. act
adolescent s.
alcohol-related risk for s.
altruistic s.
anomic s.
assisted s.
s. attempt (SA)
s. attempter
s. attempt history
s. attempt rate
s. behavior
s. in children
cluster s.
s. cluster
collective s.
completed s.
s. completion
compulsive s.
contract against s.
copycat s.
deterrent to s.
Durkheim theory of s.
egotistic s.
elderly s.
focal s.
s. gesture
half-hearted attempt at s.
s. by hanging
s. hotline
impulsive s.
s. incidence
s. intent
s. inventory
s. lethality
s. letter
s. means
s. method
s. motivation
s. note
s. pact
physician-assisted s.
s. plan
s. potential
s. precaution
s. predictor
s. predisposition
s. prevalence
s. prevention
s. prevention center
psychic s.
psychological s.
rational s.
s. risk
s. risk assessment
s. risk factor
s. status
successful s.
s. survivor syndrome
s. talk
teenage s.
s. tendency
thought of s.
s. threat
threat of imminent s.
s. victim
s. vulnerability
suicide-depression (S-D)
suicidology
American Association of S. (AAS)
suigenderism
suit
paternity s.
sukra prameha
sulcal prefrontal cortex
sulcus, pl. **sulci**
calcarine s.
callosal s.
central s.
cingulate s.
flattened s.
frontal s.
inferior frontal s.
inferior temporal s.
middle frontal s.
occipital s.
postcentral s.
precentral s.
superior frontal s.
superior temporal s.

NOTES

sulcus *(continued)*
temporal s.
terminal s.
Sulpiride
sultry
sumatriptan
summary score
summation
spatial s.
s. of stimuli
sum score
Sunday neurosis
sundowner
s. effect
s. syndrome
sundowning behavior
sundown syndrome
sunlight fear
sunrise
s. fear
s. syndrome
suo yang
superachiever
superambitious
supercautious
supercilious
superconfident
supercriminal
superego
s. anxiety
autonomous s.
s. control
s. disturbance
double s.
s. functioning
group s.
heteronomous s.
s. lacuna
parasite of s.
parasitic s.
primitive s.
s. resistance
reward by s.
s. sadism
s. structure
superexcitation
superficial
s. affect
s. charm
s. idiot
s. pain
s. psychotherapy
s. sensation
superfluous
superhit
superhuman
superimposed
s. delirium
s. dementia
superintelligent
superior
s. frontal sulcus
s. functioning
s. intelligence
s. manner
s. paraplegia
respondeat s.
s. salivary nucleus (SSN)
s. temporal auditory cortical area
s. temporal sulcus
superiority
s. complex
s. feeling
intellectual s.
sense of s.
striving for s.
superlative
superman
supermoron
supermotility
supernatural
supernaturalism
supernormal
supernumerary
superordinate
superpersonal unconscious
superpower
supersensible
supersensory
supersexuality
superstar
superstition
superstitious
s. behavior
s. control
supervalent thought
supervised
s. after-school activity
s. probation
supervision
boundaries in postanalytic s.
one-on-one s.
person in need of s.
postanalytic s.
supervisor
supervisory
s. behavior description (SBD)
s. relationship
superwoman
supinator jerk
supplement
dietary s.
herbal s.
Medicare s.
supplementary motor area (SMA)
supplementation
oral s.
supplicate

supplicatory
supply
drug s.
emotional s.
support
artificial life s.
s., autonomy, fusioning, empathy (SAFE)
behavioral s.
child s.
community s.
considerable external s.
constructive s.
decision s.
emotional s.
s., empathy and truth (SET)
empirical s.
environmental s.
external s.
family s.
financial s.
s. group
informational s.
instrumental s.
lack of family s.
limited social s.
mediators of social s. (MOSS)
number of s.'s
peer s.
physical s.
social s.
s. system
s. team
supported employment program
supporter
supporting
s. data
s. evidence
supportive
s. confrontation
s. ego
s. group therapy
s. housing
s. medication
s. medication clinic
not s.
s. psychotherapy
reality-adaptive s.
s. relationship
s. talk-down
s. validation
supportive-expressive psychotherapy
suppressant
appetite s.
suppressed anger
suppression
conditioned s.
s. of feelings
s. neurosis
rebound s.
thought s.
suppressive therapy
suppurative
suprachiasmatic nucleus
supraclinoid
supraindividual
supraliminal
supramarginal/angular cortex
supramaximal stimulus
supranormal stimulation
supranuclear
s. gaze palsy
s. paralysis
supraoptic nucleus
supraorbital neuralgia
suprarational
suprasegmental analysis
suprasellar
supratentorial overlay
suprathreshold ECT
supremacist
white s.
supremacy
supreme
s. being
s. court
supremo
surcease
surdimutism
surdity
surety
surface
s. affability
s. ego
s. structure
surfeit
surge
surgency
surgent growth
surgery
multiple s.'s
plastic s.
sex reassignment s. (SRS)
surgical
s. addiction

NOTES

surgical *(continued)*
s. brain trauma organic psychosis
s. procedure
s. sex reassignment
s. sex reversal
surly
surmise
surmount
surreal
surrealism
surrealistic
surrender
schizophrenic s.
will to s.
surreptitious bloodletting
surrogate
s. decision maker
s. father
s. mother
mother s.
s. parent
sexual s.
s. sexual partner
surroundings
familiar s.
indifferent to s.
oblivious to s.
reduced awareness of s.
surveillance protocol
survey data
surveyor
survival
s. belief
s. of fittest
nerve cell s.
s. skills workshop
s. strategy
s. time
survivalist
surviving
s. family member
s. parent
survivor
s. of abuse
s. of death
s. guilt
Holocaust s.
s. of neglect
s. syndrome
torture s.
trauma s.
susceptibility
environmental s.
s. factor
genetic s.
s. locus
s. locus for autism
susceptible individual
suspect
murder s.
suspected
s. adverse drug reaction (SADR)
s. awareness
s. child abuse/neglect (SCAN)
s. disease
suspended animation
suspension
suspicion
suspicious
s. behavior
s. ideation
suspiciousness
chronic s.
sustain
sustainability of change
sustained
s. attention
s. belief
s. compliance
s. emotion
s. fatigue
s. full remission
s. manner
s. partial remission
s. position
sustenance of life
sustentation
susto
SV
Study of Values
SWA
seriously wounded in action
swagger
swallow-belch method
swallowing
air s.
s. automatism
difficulty s.
SWAP-200
Shedler-Western Assessment Procedure-200
SWAP-200 assessment procedure
SWAP-200 description
SWAP-200 item
SWAP-200 item set
SWAP-200 statement
swapping
partner s.
swastika
swat
swaying
body s.
s. gait
swear
swearing
compulsive s.
sweetheart contract

sweet-lemon mechanism
SWEL
sleep-awake experience list
swelled head
swelling
brain s.
Spielmeyer acute s.
swill
swimming in head
swindle
swindler
epileptic s.
pathologic s.
pathological s.
swing
compensatory mood s.
cyclic mood s.
decreased arm s.
dramatic behavioral s.
energy s.
mood s.
s. phase control
rebound mood s.
seasonal mood s.
swinging
major mood s.
switch
s. process
s. referential index
swollen
s. extremity
s. eye
s. neuron
SWS
slow-wave sleep
Sx
symptom
sycophant
syllabic speech
syllable stumbling
syllogistic reasoning
symbion
symbiosis
dyadic s.
triadic s.
symbiotic
s. attachment
s. infantile psychosis
s. marriage
s. phase
s. psychosis of childhood
s. relatedness
s. stage
symbol
association of sounds and s.'s
digit s. (DS)
mathematical s.
memory s.
phallic s.
picture s.'s (PICSYMS)
sex s.
snake s.
universal s.
Wing s.
symbolia
symbolic
s. anxiety
s. categorization
s. computation
s. displacement
s. elaboration
s. function
s. loss
s. mastery
s. masturbation
s. meaning
s. persona
s. play
s. realization
s. representation
s. thinking
s. thought
s. value
s. wounding
symbolically
performing s.
symbolism
anagogic s.
cryptogenic s.
dream s.
functional s.
material s.
metaphoric s.
sound s.
threshold s.
true s.
symbolization defense mechanism
symmetric distal neuropathy
symmetromania
symmetry obsession
sympathectomy
chemical s.
periarterial s.
sympathetic
s. discharge
s. dysfunction

S

NOTES

sympathetic *(continued)*
s. epilepsy
s. hypertonia
s. imbalance
s. nerve ending
s. nervous system (SNS)
s. nervous system-medicated vasoconstriction
s. output
s. response
s. stimulation
s. stress reaction
sympathetica
ptosis s.
sympathic
sympathiconeuritis
sympathicopathy
sympathicotonia
sympathicotonic
sympathicotripsy
sympathism
sympathist
sympathizer
sympathoadrenal hyperactivity
sympathomimetic
s. abuse
s. addiction
s. agent
s. delirium
s. delusional disorder
s. drug
s. effect
s. intoxication
s. withdrawal
sympathomimetic-induced thermogenesis
sympathy seeking
symptom (Sx)
abstinence s.
accessory s.
active-phase s.
active psychotic s.
acute s.
adjustment reaction physical s.
adolescent depression s.
adolescent depressive s.
affective s.
alcoholic s.
s. amplification
anchor s.
anxiety s.
arousal s.
array of s.'s
s. assessment
attention deficit s.
atypical factitious disorder with physical s.'s
auditory s.
autoplastic s.
avoidance s.
avoidant s.
baseline s.
behavioral dysfunction s.
benzodiazepine withdrawal s.
s. of bereavement
biologic dysfunction s.
biphasic s.
bodily s.
body-related obsessive-like s.
cardiac s.
cardinal s.
catatonic s.
s. categorization
chronicity of s.'s
chronology of s.'s
clinical s.
clinician-rated cognitive s.
cluster of s.'s
cluster C, D s.'s
cocaine withdrawal s.
cognitive s.
s. complex
compulsive s.
constellation of signs and s.'s
conversion s.
s. criteria
s. crystallization
culturally sanctioned s.
cyclical pattern of s.'s
debilitating dysphoric s.
deficit s.
delusion s.
depression s.
depressive s.
s. diary
s. dimension
disabling psychiatric s.
disaster-related avoidant s.
disaster-related intrusive s.
discrete s.
dishonest simulation of s.'s
disorganization dimension of positive schizophrenic s.'s
dissociative s.
drug-induced negative s.
eating s.
eclamptic s.
emotional s.
equivalent s.
s. evaluation
exacerbated s.
s. exacerbation
s. experience stage
extrapyramidal s. (EPS)
extrapyramidal syndrome s.
fatigue s.
feigned s.
first-rank s. (FRS)
first-rank psychotic s.

florid s.
fluctuating cognitive s.'s
food-related obsessive-like s.
s. formation
frank psychotic s.
s. free
Frenkel s.
fundamental s.
general s.
generic negative s.
Gordon s.
gramophone s.
s. group
s. grouping
heritable s.
hiding s.'s
hyperarousal s.
hypnotic withdrawal s.
hypochondriacal s.
impairment s.
individual depressive s.
induced factitious s.
insomnia s.
intentionally produced s.
intrusive s.
key s.
s. level
localization of s.'s
Macewen s.
manic s.
manifest s.
manifestly observable s.
s. measure
medical s.
mental s.
minimal residual s.
mood s.
motor conversion s.
movement s.
multiple medically unexplained s.'s (MMUS)
negative s.
neurobehavioral s.
neuroethological s.
s. neurosis
neurovegetative s.
nicotine withdrawal s.
nonbizarre s.
nonpsychotic onset of s.'s
nonpsychotic signs and s.'s
numbing s.
objective s.
obsessive-compulsive s.
onset of s.'s
organ-specific s.
overall depressive s.
s. overlap
pain s.
painful s.
panic s.
panic-like s.
panic-related s.
perceptual s.
persisting mental s.
phylogenetic s.
physical signs and s.'s
positive schizophrenic s.'s
possession trance s.
posttraumatic stress s.
preexisting s.
preexisting mental disorder s.
premonitory s.
s. presentation
presenting s.
primary defense s.
primary enduring negative s.
primary nonenduring negative s.
principal s.
prodromal psychotic s.
productive s.'s
s. profile
s. progression
prominent mood s.
proxy s.
psychiatric s.
psychogenic physical s.
psychological dysfunction s.
psychological-related s.'s
psychological signs and s.'s
psychomotor s.
psychopathology s.
psychosensory s.
psychosexual s.
psychosomatic s.
psychotic signs and s.'s
s. rating
recurring s.
s. reduction
reexperiencing perceptual s.
s. relief
s. relief through hypnosis
residual negative s.
residual positive s.
residual psychotic s.
s. response pattern
reverse vegetative s.'s

NOTES

symptom *(continued)*
Romberg s.
Romberg-Howship s.
scale for assessment of negative s.'s
schizophrenia s.
schizophrenic s.
Schneider first-rank s.
schneiderian first-rank s.
Screening for Somatoform S.'s
s. searching
secondary defense s.
sedative-hypnotic withdrawal s.
self-reported s.
sensory conversion s.
severe dissociative s.
sexual s.
soft psychotic s.
somatic s.
somatization pain s.
somatization pseudoneurological s.
somatization sexual s.
specific s.
s. specificity
subclinical depressive s.
subjective s.
s. substitution
subsyndromal depressive s.
subsyndromal mood s.
subtle s.
sudden onset of s.'s
target s.
tic s.
total s.
trauma-type s.
treatment-resistant s.
troublesome s.
unintentionally produced s.
unpleasant withdrawal s.
vegetative s.
visual s.
withdrawal s.
worrying s.
s. worsening

symptomatic
s. act
acutely s.
s. depression
s. disadvantage
s. epilepsy
s. headache
s. impotence
s. indication
s. management
s. neuralgia
s. paramyotonia
s. patient
s. perspective
s. presentation
s. progression
s. psychosis
s. reaction
s. seizure
s. status
s. therapy
s. treatment

symptomatica
alopecia s.
indicatio s.

symptomatically reactive

symptomatize

symptomatology
acute psychiatric s.
depressive s.
mood s.
negative s.
panic s.
psychotic s.
substance-induced s.

symptom-based drug choice

symptom-free

symptom-related predictor

synagogue

synaphoceptor

synapse, pl. **synapses**
chemical s.
cholinergic s.
conjoint synapses
dopaminergic s.
electrical s.
excitatory s.
s. formation
noradrenergic s.
serotonergic s.
viable s.

synapsin I, II, III

synaptic
s. activity
s. compartment
s. compensation
s. plasticity
s. transmission
s. vesicle
s. vesicle recycling

synaptobrevin

synaptogenesis

synaptotagmin

synchronic study

synchronization
event-related s.

synchronous

synchrony
bilateral s.
gamma s.

synclonic spasm

synclonus

syncopal

syncope
hysterical s.
laryngeal s.
local s.
micturition s.
postural s.
vasomotor s.
vasopressor s.
vasovagal s.
syncopic
syncretic
s. thinking
s. thought
syncretism
syndrome
aberrant motivational s.
absence s.
abstinence s.
abused child s.
Acosta s.
acquired immunodeficiency s. (AIDS)
acroparesthesia s.
acute brain s. (ABS)
acute organic brain s.
acute posttraumatic stress s.
acute psychoorganic s.
Adams-Stokes s.
adaptation s.
addiction s.
addictive s.
adiposogenital s.
adjustment reaction physical s.
adrenogenital s. (AGS)
advanced sleep-phase s. (ASPS)
affective disorder s.
Aicardi s.
air pollution s. (APS)
akinetic-abulic s.
alcohol abstinence s.
alcohol amnestic s.
alcohol dependence s.
alcoholic brain s.
alcoholic malabsorption s.
alcohol-induced organic mental s.
alcohol withdrawal s.
Alice in Wonderland s.
alveolar hypoventilation s.
Alzheimer s.
amnesic s.
amnestic confabulatory s.
amotivational s.
androgen insensitivity s.
Angelucci s.
anger and violence psychiatric s.
angry woman s.
anticholinergic s.
antimotivational s.
Anton s.
anxiety s.
anxiety-related psychiatric s.
apallic s.
apathy s.
s. aphasia
approximate answer s.
s. of approximate relevant answers
asphyctic s.
atypical or mixed organic brain s.
autoscopic s.
aviator's effort s.
avoidance s.
Balint s.
Bardet-Biedl s.
battered child s. (BCS)
battered spouse s.
battered woman s. (BWS)
behavioral assessment of dysexecutive s. (BADS)
behavioral reaction brain s.
behavior, speech, and other s.'s
Behr s.
benzodiazepine discontinuation s.
Bianchi s.
black patch s.
blue velvet s.
Bonnet s.
Bonnevie-Ullrich s.
Bonnier s.
Borjeson-Forssman-Lehmann s.
bradykinetic s.
brain psychoorganic s.
Briquet s.
Brissaud s.
Brissaud-Marie s.
Brissaud-Sicard s.
Bristowe s.
Brown-Sequard s.
buffoonery s.
burnout s.
callosal disconnection s.
Capgras s.
capsulothalamic s.
cardiopulmonary-obesity s.
carinatum s.
catastrophic ancataplexy s.
catatonic s.

NOTES

syndrome *(continued)*
cat-cry s.
cat's eye s. (CES)
characteristic withdrawal s.
Charles Bonnet s.
child abuse s.
childhood-onset Tourette s.
childhood Tourette s.
China s.
choreiform s.
chromosome 21-trisomy s.
chronic alcoholic brain s. (CABS)
chronic brain s. (CBS)
chronic fatigue s. (CFS)
chronic hyperventilation s.
Cinderella s.
Citelli s.
Claude s.
Clerambault erotomania s.
clinical poverty s.
cloverleaf skull s.
clumsiness s.
clumsy child s.
Cohen s.
Collet-Sicard s.
compulsive swearing s.
concentration camp s. (CCS)
concussion s.
confused language s. (CLS)
contralateral neglect s.
Cornelia de Lange s.
corpus callosum s.
Cotard s.
Creutzfeldt-Jakob s.
cri du chat s.
Crigler-Najjar s., type 1 and 2
Crouzon s.
crush s.
crying cat s.
cryptogenic epileptic s.
cult indoctrination s.
culture-bound s.
culture-specific s.
cyclic vomiting s.
DaCosta s.
de Clerambault s.
de Lange s.
delayed sleep-phase s.
Delilah s.
delusional misidentification s.
delusional transient organic s.
dementia s.
dementia-aphonia s.
dementia-related psychiatric s.
dependence s.
depersonalization s.
depression-related psychiatric s.
depressive s.
depressive-type psychoorganic s.
deprivation s.
De Sanctis-Cacchione s.
s. of deviously relevant answers
dialysis encephalopathy s.
dietary chaos s.
disconnection s.
discontinuation s.
disorganization s.
displaced child s.
dissociation s.
Don Juan s.
drug-induced s.
drug withdrawal s.
Dubowitz s.
dysexecutive s.
dysmnesic s.
dyspraxia s.
ectopic ACTH s.
Edwards s.
effort s.
Ehret s.
Eisenlohr s.
Ekbom s.
electroshock-induced psychotic s.
Elpenor s.
elusive s.
empty nest s.
environmental dependency s.
epileptic s. (ES)
episodic dyscontrol s.
Epstein-Barr s.
exhaustion s.
exploding head s.
extrapyramidal s. (EPS)
failure-to-grow s.
failure-to-thrive s.
false memory s.
fatigue s.
feminizing testes s.
fetal alcohol s. (FAS)
fetal hydantoin s.
Figueira s.
flashing pain s.
fluid retention s. (FRS)
Flynn-Aird s.
focal brain s.
fragile X s. (FMR1)
fragmented s.
Fregoli s.
Freud s.
Fröhlich s.
frontal lobe s.
full s.
full-blown s.
functional psychiatric s.
Ganser s.
Gelineau s.
gender difference psychiatric s.
gender dysphoria s.

general adaptation s. (GAS)
Gilles de la Tourette s.
Gjessing s.
Goldenhar s.
Goliath s.
Gowers s.
gray-out s.
Guillain-Barré s.
Gulf War s.
hallucinatory transient organic s.
hallucinatory-type psychoorganic s.
happy puppet s.
headache s.
head-bobbing doll s.
Heller s.
hepatorenal s.
Herrmann s.
Hinman s.
holiday s.
hospital addiction s.
housewife s.
hyperactive child s. (HACS)
hyperkinetic behavior s. (HBS)
hypernyctohemeral s.
hypersensitivity s.
hyperventilation s. (HVS)
hypokinetic s.
immune deficiency s.
impostor s.
indifference to pain s.
infectious-exhaustive s.
intensive care s.
interictal behavior s.
intermediate brain s.
intoxication s.
irritable bowel s. (IBS)
isolation s.
Joubert s.
jumping Frenchmen of Maine s.
Kallmann s.
Kanner s.
Kleine-Levin s.
Klinefelter s.
Klippel-Feil s.
Klüver-Bucy s.
koro s.
Korsakoff s.
Krabbe s.
lacunar s.
Landau-Kleffner s.
Landry-Guillain-Barré s.
Lasègue s.
latah s.
Laurence-Biedl s.
Laurence-Moon s.
Laurence-Moon-Bardet-Biedl s.
Laurence-Moon-Biedl s.
laxative abuse s. (LAS)
Lesch-Nyhan s.
lobotomy s.
Louis-Bar s.
Madame Butterfly s.
Mad Hatter s.
Magenblase s.
Main s.
major psychiatric s.
male climacteric s.
malpractice stress s.
manic s.
manic-depressive s.
Marie-Robinson s.
marker X s.
Martin-Bell s.
Mast s.
maternal deprivation s.
medial frontal lobe s.
medical s.
medullary s.
menstrual-associated s.
metabolic s.
metabolic s. X
Millard-Gubler s.
Milles s.
mood swing s.
Moore s.
Morgagni s.
Moynahan s.
Muenzer-Rosenthal s.
multiimpulsivity s.
Munchausen by proxy s.
myasthenic s.
narcolepsy-cataplexy s.
neglect s.
neonatal abstinence s.
nest s.
Neumann s.
neurobehavioral s.
neurocutaneous s.
neurogenic shock s.
neuroleptic malignant s. (NMS)
neurotic reaction brain s.
Nielsen s.
night eating s.
nocturnal drinking s.
nocturnal eating s.
non-24-hour sleep-wake s.

NOTES

syndrome *(continued)*
nonpsychotic posttraumatic brain s.
nonpsychotic psychoorganic s.
nonsense s.
nonspecific s.
nonspecific neurotic s. (NNS)
Nothnagel s.
obsession s.
obsessional s.
obstructive sleep apnea s. (OSAS)
obstructive sleep apnea-hypopnea s. (OSAHS)
old-sergeant s.
olfactory reference s.
opiate abstinence s.
Oppenheim s.
orbitomedial s.
organic affective s.
organic amnestic s.
organic brain s. (OBS)
organic hallucinosis s.
organic mental s. (OMS)
organic mood s. (OMS)
organic personality s.
oriental nightmare death s.
orofaciodigital s.
oromotor apraxia s.
Othello s.
pain dysfunction s. (PDS)
pain, touch and stroke psychiatric s.
pallidal s.
paranoia and delusions psychiatric s.
paranoid-type psycho-organic s.
s. pattern
Pepper s.
persecution s.
Persian Gulf War s.
personality s.
phantom lover s.
phencyclidine mixed organic brain s.
phobic s.
piblokto s.
Pick s.
pickwickian s.
Pinel-Haslam s.
Pisa s.
polysymptomatic s.
pontocerebellar angle s.
postabortion s.
postadrenalectomy s.
post concentration camp s.
postcontusion s.
postencephalitic s.
posteroinferior cerebellar artery s.
postleukotomy s.
postlobotomy s.
postpartum s.
postrape s.
posttraumatic amnestic s.
posttraumatic brain s.
posttraumatic stress s.
post-Vietnam psychiatric s. (PVNPS)
POW s.
premenstrual s. (PMS)
premenstrual tension s. (PMTS)
premotor s.
prisoner-of-war s.
professional patient s.
protracted withdrawal s.
proxy-for-deficit s.
pseudocyesis s.
psychiatric s.
psychic shock s.
psychoactive substance-induced organic s.
psychogenic effort s.
psychogenic nocturnal polydipsia s.
psychogenic purpura s.
psychological s.
psychomimic s.
psychoorganic brain s.
psychotic posttraumatic brain s.
punch-drunk s.
purple people s.
rape trauma s.
rapid time zone change s.
rapture-of-the-deep s.
Rapunzel s.
Renpenning s.
restless leg s.
retirement s.
Rett s.
reversible affective disorder s.
revolving door s.
Richardson-Steele-Olszewski s.
Richards-Rundel s.
rigid akinetic s.
Riley-Day s.
Rosenthal s.
Rubinstein-Taybi s.
rumination s.
Russell s.
Sanfilippo s.
Saunders-Sutton s.
schedule for Tourette syndrome and other behavioral s.'s
Scheid cyanotic s.
Schirmer s.
schizoaffective s.
schizophrenia s.
schizophrenic s.
school refusal s.
seasonal affective disorder s.
seasonal energy s.

Seckel s.
second impact s.
senile brain s.
sensory deprivation s. (SDS)
sensory dissociation s.
serotonin s.
shock s.
silver cord s.
sleep phase s.
sleep-related abnormal swallowing s.
sleep-related myoclonus s.
Smith-Lemli-Opitz s.
smoker's s.
social breakdown s. (SBS)
social deprivation s.
social disability s.
social isolation s.
solitary hunter s.
Sotos s.
spasmodic laughter s.
spasmodic winking s.
specific neurotic s. (SNR)
spiritual emergence s.
startle s.
steroid withdrawal s.
Stewart-Morel s.
Stockholm s.
stress-related s.
stress response s.
subacute psychoorganic s.
subclavian steal s.
subclinical s.
substance-induced s.
substance-related s.
sudden infant death s. (SIDS)
Sudeck s.
suicide survivor s.
sundown s.
sundowner s.
sunrise s.
survivor s.
tabagism s.
Taijin-Kyofusho s.
Tapia s.
tardive Tourette s.
tea-and-toast s.
temporal lobe s.
teratogenic s.
testicular feminization s. (TFS)
time zone change s.
Todeserwartung s.
Tolosa-Hunt s.
Tourette s. (TS)
trait-like s.
trisomy s.
vasovagal s.
vibration s.
victim s.
Vietnam s.
VIP s.
visual hallucination s.
visual hallucination denial s.
vulnerable child s.
Wernicke s.
Wernicke-Korsakoff s.
Werther s.
Westphal-Leyden s.
wet brain s.
white-out s.
Wilson s.
Windigo culture-specific s.
winking spasmodic s.
withdrawal s.
Wittmaak-Ekbom s.
wounded victim s.
Wyburn-Mason s.
Zange-Kindler s.
Zanoli-Vecchi s.
Zappert s.

syndromic
s. depression
s. pattern

synergetic

synergic
s. control
s. marriage

synergism
sexual s.

synergistic

synergy

synesthesia
s. algica
auditory s.
auditory-visual s.

synesthesialgia

synesthetic stimulation

synkinesis, synkinesia

synkinetic motor movement

synonymous

synostosis

syntactic
s. aphasia
s. category
s. complexity

NOTES

syntactic *(continued)*
s. language structure
s. rule
syntality
syntaxic
s. language
s. mode
s. mode of experience
s. thought
synthesis, pl. **syntheses**
analysis by s.
analysis and s.
distributive analysis and s.
dopamine s.
illegal drug s.
illicit drug s.
perceptual s.
synthesizing ability
synthetic
s. drug dependence
s. function
s. heroin dependence
s. method
syntone
syntonic
s. personality
syntropic
syntropy
syphilis
cerebral s.
CNS s.
meningovascular s.
primary s.
psychosis of s.
s. screen
secondary s.
tertiary s.
syphilitic
s. alopecia
s. cirrhosis
s. encephalitis
s. meningitis
s. meningoencephalitis
s. paralytic dementia
s. progressive dementia
syphilitica
alopecia s.
syphilology
syphilomania
syphilopsychosis
syringe
syringobulbia
syringoid
syringomyelia
syringomyelic
syringomyelus
syringopontia
system
action s.
activity s.
Act & React test s.
ADAM s.
adaptive control of thought s.
adolescent support s.
alcohol metabolizing s.
antireward s.
ascending neurotransmitter s.
ascending reticular activating s.
auditory s.
autonomic nervous s. (ANS)
5-axis s.
behavior s.
behavioral activation s. (BAS)
behavioral inhibition s. (BIS)
biomedical monitoring s. (BMS)
biophysical s.
Bleuler diagnostic s.
boarding-out s.
brain dopaminergic s.
Brown School Behavioral Health S.
categorical s.
central nervous s. (CNS)
cerebrospinal s.
circadian s.
classification s.
closed-loop feedback s.
community support s.
conceptual nervous s.
criminal justice s.
CYP 1A2 cytochrome s.
cytochrome P450 s.
decision support s.
Delis-Kaplan executive function s. (DKEFS)
delusional s.
dimensional s.
direct motor s.
disposition s.
dopamine s.
dopaminergic s.
drug risk analysis message s. (DRAMS)
dyadic parent-child interaction coding s.
dysfunctional dopamine s.
enteric nervous s.
epicritic s.
ergotropic s.
esthesiodic s.
expert s.
external support s.
extrafamilial s.
extrapyramidal s. (EPS)
extrapyramidal motor s.
facial action coding s. (FACS)
family support s.
feedback s.
feeding s.

first-signal s.
fixed delusional s.
focus of delusional s.
foster care s.
haptic s.
hemodynamic s.
honor s.
hypothalamic-pituitary-adrenocortical s.
immune s.
incentive s.
indirect motor s.
innate response s.
integrated ECT s.
interactive voice response s.
internal second messenger s.
intracellular second messenger s.
IS900 VET tracking s.
justice s.
juvenile justice s.
kinship s.
knowledge information processing s. (KIPS)
Kraepelin diagnostic s.
life support s.
limbic s.
malevolent thought s.
man-machine s.
medial temporal memory s.
medical value s.
memory s.
mental health information s.
miniature s.
mnemonic s.
mood control s.
motor s.
multiaxial classification s.
multistate information s. (MSIS)
National Association of Psychiatric Health S.'s (NAPHS)
nervous s.
neural s.
neurotransmitter s.
nicotine inhalation s.
nicotine transdermal s.
nonspecific s.
noradrenergic s.
norepinephrine neurotransmitter s.'s
paranoid belief s.
parasympathetic nervous s. (PNS)
peripheral nervous s. (PNS)
persecutory delusional s.
personality assessment s. (PAS)
Pinel s.
s. to plan early childhood services (SPECS)
preferred representational s.
pride s.
private belief s.
psi s.
psychodynamic cerebral s.
psychological defense s.
psychological information, acquisition, processing, and control s. (PIAPACS)
quota s.
ReaCTor s.
reality s.
religious value s.
representational s.
response s.
reticular activating s. (RAS)
reticuloendothelial s.
review of s.'s (ROS)
reward s.
school support s.
second-messenger s.
second signaling s.
sensorimotor s.
serotonergic s.
serotonin s.
sleep-wake s.
somatosensory s.
somesthetic s.
specific s.
speech perception s.
stereotaxic coordinate s.
support s.
sympathetic nervous s. (SNS)
thalamic reticular activating s.
theoretical s.
thermoregulatory s.
third nervous s.
thought s.
transmitter s.
value s.
vegetative nervous s.
ventricular s.
villa s.
visceral nervous s.
welfare s.
well-systematized delusional s.

systematic

s. comparison
s., complete, objective, practical, empirical (SCOPE)

NOTES

systematic *(continued)*
s. desensitization
s. drug administration
s. family therapy
s. followup
s. inquiry (SI)
s. method
s. process
s. quantitative observation
s. rational restructuring (SRR)
s. reinforcement
s. review
s. schizophrenia
s. study
s. vertigo
systematica
paraphrenia s.
systematique
délire chronique à évolution s.
systematization
systematized
s. amnesia
s. assertive therapy (SAT)
s. delusion
systemic
s. assertive therapy
s. delusion
s. desensitization
s. family
s. impact
systems-based learning
systolic pressure (SP)
SZ
schizophrenia

T

T group
T ratio
T score

TA

test age
transactional analysis

TAB

therapeutic abortion

tabagism syndrome

tabes

juvenile t.
peripheral t.
t. spasmodica
t. spinalis

tabetic

t. crisis
t. cuirass
t. psychosis

tabetic-form paralytic dementia

tabetiform

tabic

tabid

table

life t.
somatron t.
under the t.

tablet

DDAVP t.
Methylin chewable t.

taboo, tabu

cultural t.
t. emotion
incest t.
social t.
virginity t.

taboparesis

tabula rasa

tabular index

tabulation

tache

tachistoscope

tachycardia

psychogenic paroxysmal t.

tachylalia

tachylogia

tachyphagia

tachyphasia

tachyphemia

tachyphrasia

tachyphrenia

tachyphylaxis

tachypnea

tachypneic

tachypragia

tachypsychia

tachytrophism

tactic

diversionary t.
guerrilla t.'s

tactical maneuver

tactile

t. agnosia
t. alexia
t. amnesia
t. anesthesia
t. anomia
t. aphasia
t. aphonia
t. extinction
t. feedback
t. genital stimulation
t. hallucination
t. hyperactivity
t. hyperesthesia
t. illusion
t. image
t. imagery
t. perception
t. sensation
t. sense
t. sensory difficulty
t. sensory modality
t. stimulus

tactile-perceptual disorder

tactility

tactometer

tactual hallucination

tadalafil

Tadoma method

tae kwon do

tag

medical identification t.

tagger

graffiti t.

tai chi

Taijin-Kyofusho syndrome

tailor's

t. cramp
t. spasm

taint

Taiwanese

take

t. advantage
t. charge
double t.
t. down
t. for granted
t. heart

T

take *(continued)*
t. issue
t. out
take-home pay
taken out of context
taker
risk t.
taking control
talbutal
tale
tall t.
tell a t. (TAT)
talent
creative t.
grandiose delusion of exceptional t.
inflated appraisal of t.
special t.
Talented
Arizona Association for the Gifted and T. (AAGT)
Austin Association for the Gifted and T. (AAGT)
talion
t. dread
t. law
t. principle
talionis
lex t.
talipes spasmodicus
talisman
talk
baby t.
back t.
t. down
t. down from overdose
facial t.
t. out
t. over
pep t.
small t.
street t.
suicide t.
t. therapy
unwanted sexual t.
t. up
talkative
appropriately t.
talkativeness
excessive t.
talk-down
supportive t.-d.
talking
t. back behavior
t. cure
excessive t.
t. fear
t. it out
tall tale
Tamil refugee
tampering
data t.
tandem reinforcement
tangent
tangential
t. association
t. information
t. layer
t. speech
t. thinking
tangentiality
tangere
noli me t.
tangle
neurofibrillary t.
tannate
Tanner stage in adolescence
tantalize
tantamount
tantra
tantric yoga
tantrum
temper t.
taoism
taoist
tap
glabellar t.
spinal t.
taper
double t.
slow double t.
tapering
drug t.
medication t.
tapeworm fear
taphophilia
Tapia syndrome
tapping compulsion
TaqIA
Taractan
tarantism, tarantulism
Tarasoff
T. case
T. decision
T. principle
T. rule
T. warning
Tarchanoff phenomenon
tarda
tardive
t. dementia
t. dyskinesia
t. dysmentia
t. dystonia
forme t.
t. tic
t. Tourette syndrome
tardy epilepsy

target
t. of aggression
t. behavior
bullying t.
t. language
t. multiplicity
t. organ
t. patient
t. population
potential t.
t. response
t. stimulus
t. symptom
therapeutic t.
t. of threat
t. weight
targeted
t. approach
t. intervention
t. medication
tarot card
tartrate
TAS
turning against self
task
auditory continuous performance t.
Benton word generation t.
category retrieval t.
cognitive t.
t. completion
developmental t.
dichotic listening t.
digit-symbol coding t.
dot-probe t.
drawing t.
t. of emotional development (TED)
t. force on electroconvulsive therapy
t. of independent living
instrumental t.
learning t.
t. management
manipulatory t.
memory t.
necessary t.
neuropsychologically relevant t.
nonverbal t.
organizing t.
particular t.
t. performance
t. performance and analysis
persistence t.
practiced t.
primary t.
problem-solving t.
procedural learning t.
required t.
retrieval t.
simple t.
spatial t.
stay on t.
3-step t.
stopping t.
stop signal t.
structured t.
theory of mind t.
unemotional learning t.
visuomotor t.
work-related t.
task-accuracy
continuous performance t.-a. (CPT-ACC)
task-efficiency
continuous performance t.-e. (CPT-EFF)
task-oriented
t.-o. approach
t.-o. assessment
t.-o. group
t.-o. reaction
task-specific routine
task-switching paradigm
taste
t. aversive conditioning
t. blindness
color t.
t. fear
t. imagery
t. sensation
t. threshold
TAT
tell a tale
tattered clothing
tattle
tattletale
tattoo
tau
t. processing
t. protein
t. protein peptide
taunt
taurine
taut facial skin
tautological
tautologous
tautology

NOTES

tautophone
taxing
emotionally t.
taxometric analysis
taxonic
taxonomic research
taxonomy
t. of anger disorder
biologic t.
personality disorder t.
t. of problematic social situations (TOPS)
t. of problematic social situations for children
taylorism
Taylor series linearization method
TBI
traumatic brain injury
TBRS
timed behavioral rating sheet
TC
therapeutic community
TCA
tricyclic antidepressant
tricyclic antipsychotic
TCAD
tricyclic antidepressant drug
T-cell proliferation
TCET
transcerebral electrotherapy
TCI
total cerebral ischemia
TCP
teacher-child-parent
TCSW
thinking creatively with sounds and words
TD
threshold of discomfort
TDE
thiamine deficiency encephalopathy
TDF
thinking disturbance factor
T&E
testing and evaluation
Te
tetanic contraction
tea-and-toast syndrome
teacher
teacher-child-parent (TCP)
teacher-student
t.-s. model
t.-s. relationship
teaching
clinical t.
diagnostic t.
t. hospital
religious t.
remedial t.
team
t. building
crisis t.
interdisciplinary t. (IDT)
t. leader (TL)
t. member (TM)
mobile crisis outreach t.
pain management t.
2-person interview t.
t. player
psychiatric emergency t. (PET)
psychiatry emergency t.
support t.
treatment t.
teammate
teamwork
tear
t. at
t. away
crocodile t.'s
t. down
t. gas
t. up
teardrop
tearfulness
breakthrough t.
momentary t.
unexplained t.
tearful outburst
technicality
technical limitation
technician
emergency medical t. (EMT)
psychiatric t.
technique
abortion t.
activation t.
active daydream t.
adaptive t.
anxiety control t.
arousal reduction t.
ascending t.
assets-liabilities t.
average evoked response t.
backward-making t.
ballet t.
Bayesian t.
behavioral t.
bell-and-pad t.
blind matching t.
breathing t.
brief stimulus t.
capping t.
clinical monitoring t.
cognitive t.
cognitive-behavioral t.
compensatory t.
corrective t.
crisis intervention t.

critical incident t.
deescalation t.
descending t.
dieting t.
differential diagnostic t.
effective t.
effort-shape t.
empty chair t.
fast gradient-recalled spectroscopic imaging t.
feeding t.
functional imaging t.
glissando t.
graphomotor t.
Hartel t.
head turn t.
homogenate t.
hot-seat t.
interview t.
interviewing t.
kinesthetic t.
Luria t.
manipulative t.
microelectrode t.
mirror t.
monitoring t.
morphometric t.
multiple regression t.
multivariate t.
observation t.
paradoxical t.
picture-in-picture t.
plain-folks t.
plateau masking t.
play t.
positron emission tomography t.
postmortem t.
projective t.
psychoanalytic t.
psychological t.
Q t.
Q-Sort t.
quantitative morphometric t.
reattribution t.
relapse prevention t.
relaxation t.
replacement t.
rest-cure t.
Rorschach projective t.
self-control t.
self-soothing t.
shadow mask t.
shift masking t.
short-term psychotherapy t.
squeeze t.
standardized cognitive assessment t.
startle t.
state-of-the-art analysis t.
stop-and-think t.
stop-start t.
sucking t.
threshold shift masking t.
time-out t.
unconscious mental t.
uncovering t.
utilization t.
verbal t.
word association t.

technological
t. detection of deceit
t. disaster
t. illiteracy
t. limitation

technology
genetic t.
information t.

technostress

tecum
subpoena duces t.

TED
task of emotional development

tedious

tedium

teen
frightened t.
t. killer
rebellious t.
t. silence
t.'s in crisis
troubled t.
victimized t.
t. violence

teenage
t. father
t. smoking behavior
t. suicide
t. violence

teenager
antisocial t.

teeth
clenched t.

teetotaler, teetotalist

teetotalism

tegmental

teichopsia

telalgia

NOTES

telangiectasia
teleceptor
telegnosis
telegrammatism
telehealth
telekinesis
telemnemonike
telencephalic
t. fusion
t. sleep
telencephalization
teleoanalysis
teleologic
t. hallucination
t. regression
teleological
teleology
teleonomic
teleonomy
telepathic dream
telepathy
telephone
t. counseling
t. scatologia
t. sex
teleplasm
telepsychiatry
telergy
telescopia
telesis
telesthesia
teletactor
television
closed-circuit t. (CCTV)
sexually charged t.
t. violence
violent acts on t.
telling
diagnostic truth t.
principle of truth t.
tell a tale (TAT)
telltale sign
telomere length
temerarious
temerity
temper
t. display
t. dyscontrol
evil t.
explosive t.
hot t.
t. outburst
short t.
t. tantrum
violent t.
volatile t.
temperament
affective t.
angry t.
demanding t.
hyperesthetic variant of schizoid t.
hyperthymic t.
irritable t.
manic t.
t. trait
temperamental
t. behavior
t. characteristic
temperance
temperate
temperature
ambient t.
basal t.
t. biofeedback
core body t.
t. effect
t. eroticism
t. fluctuation
t., pulse, respiration (TPR)
t. regulation
t. sensation
t. sense
t. spot
tempestuous course
template
diagnostic t.
temple
tempo
conceptual t.
temporal
t. association
t. characteristic
t. contiguity
t. cortex
t. course
t. dynamic
t. hallucination
t. headache
t. integration deficit
t. lobe
t. lobectomy
t. lobe epilepsy (TLE)
t. lobe illusion
t. lobe seizure
t. lobe status
t. lobe syndrome
t. neocortical association area
t., occipital, parietal (TOP)
t. organization
t. orientation
t. pattern
t. perspective
t. relationship
t. resolution
t. speech region
t. sulcus
t. tissue

temporale
planum t.
temporal-perceptual disorder
temporarily disabled
temporary
t. admission
t. commitment
t. deafness
t. disability
t. epilation
t. habit
t. personality disorder
t. stress
t. threshold shift (TTS)
temporizer
Temposil
temptation
fit of horrific t.
horrific t.
tempting
tenable
tenacious
tenacity
tenancy
tendency, pl. **tendencies**
acting-out t.
t. of action
anagogic t.
antisocial t.
central t.
cognitive t.
coping t.
deceit t.
dependence t.
destructive t.
dissociative t.
evasive t.
excitement-seeking t.
familial t.
final t.
hypomanic t.
impulsive t.
introversive t.
iterative t.
manipulation t.
measure of central t.
narcissistic t.
paranoid t.
repeat t.
seductive t.
self-absorbed t.
sleep t.
somatization t.
suicide t.
tender-minded t.
tough-minded t.
t. toward amelioration
t. wit
tendentious apperception
tender
t. loving care (TLC)
t. point
t. years presumption
t. zone
tenderhearted
tender-minded tendency
tenderness
tendinum
subsultus t.
tremor t.
tenement
tenens
locum t.
tenesmus penis
tenet
t. of faith
religious t.
tense gaze
tenseness
tensile
tensiometer
tension
combat t.
conjugal t.
emotional t.
inner t.
instinctual t.
marked t.
mental t.
t. migraine
t. migraine headache
motor t.
muscle t.
muscular t.
nervous t.
physical t.
premenstrual t.
t. reduction
t. reduction therapy
sexual t.
social t.
t. state
t. state psychoneurotic reaction
stimulus t.
t. vascular headache
tension-reduction theory

NOTES

T

tensity
tentative
t. diagnosis
t. finding
tenuous
tenure
job t.
teonanactl
tephromalacia
tephrylometer
teratogen
teratogenicity
behavioral t.
morphologic t.
teratogenic syndrome
teratologic defect
teratology
mammalian t.
terephthalate
tergiversate
tergiversation
tergo
coitus a t.
term
abstract t.
coin new slang t.
general value t.'s
intellectualized t.'s
interaction t.
jail t.
psychometric t.
terminal
axon t.
délire t.
t. dementia
t. insomnia
t. lag
t. neuronal field
t. region
t. reinforcement
t. reinforcement psychotherapy
t. sulcus
t. tremor
video lottery t. (VLT)
terminalis
stria t.
terminally ill
terminate relationship
termination
t. issue
t. of pregnancy
t. of therapy
terminological obfuscation
terpin
terrestial
terrifying
t. experience
t. stimulus
territorial
t. aggression
t. dominance
territoriality
territorialize
territory
interaction t.
vascular t.
terror
current night t.'s (CNT)
t. dream
night t.
reign of t.
sleep t.
terrorism
t. behavior
fear of t.
mass t.
psychiatric sequela of t.
war on t.
terrorist
t. act
t. attack
t. profile
t. profiling
t. violence
terrorize
terse
tertiary
t. amine tricyclic antidepressant drug
t. care
t. circular reaction
t. gain
t. intervention program
t. prevention
t. process thinking
t. stress
t. syphilis
test
t. age (TA)
air conduction t.
t. anxiety
blood screen for drug t.
t. case
t. condition
could not t. (CNT)
t. of criminal responsibility
Denver developmental screening t. II
glucose t.
t. interpretation
laboratory t.
liver function t. (LFT)
t. object
t. orientation procedure (TOP)
t. protocol
t. of significance

urine t.
visual distortion t. (VDT)
testamentary capacity
testicular
t. feminization mutation (TFM)
t. feminization syndrome (TFS)
t. hypofunction
testimonial privilege
testimony
expert t.
psychiatric t.
t. therapy
testing
adaptive t.
American College of T. (ACT)
attention t.
cognitive t.
continuous cognitive t.
cortical t.
cross-cultural t.
cultural t.
demarcation in sensory t.
diminished reality t.
t. and evaluation (T&E)
formal t.
functional gain t.
gross impairment of reality t.
hypothesis t.
mental t.
motivation analysis t.
multiple-choice t.
neurophysiological t.
neuropsychologic t.
t., orientation, and work
t., orientation, and work evaluation for rehabilitation (TOWER)
package t.
psychological t.
psychometric t.
random urine t.
reality t.
reality ability t.
school-age t.
testis
irritable t.
testosterone
serum t.
t. therapy
test-retest
t.-r. reliability
t.-r. reliability coefficient
testy
tetania
t. parathyreopriva
t. rheumatica
tetanic
t. contraction (Te)
t. convulsion
t. seizure
t. stimulation
tetaniform
tetanigenous
tetanilla
tetanism
tetanization
tetanode
tetanoid
t. chorea
t. epilepsy
t. paraplegia
tetanometer
tetanomotor
tetanus
benign t.
cephalic t.
cerebral t.
drug t.
extensor t.
flexor t.
head t.
imitative t.
t. neonatorum
t. posticus
Ritter opening t.
toxic t.
tetany
t. of alkalosis
duration t. (DT)
hyperventilation t.
infantile t.
latent t.
manifest t.
postoperative t.
tetchy
tete-a-tete
tetrabenazine
tetrachloride
carbon t.
tetracyclic
tetrad
narcoleptic t.
tetrahydrobiopterin
tetrahydrocannabinoid (THC)
tetrahydrocannabinol (THC)
t. dependence

NOTES

T

tetraparesis
tetrapeptide
tetraplegia
tetrasomy
teutonomania
text
t. blindness
pragmatic t.
textbook case
textual description
texture
causal t.
t. response
TF
transvestic fetishism
TFM
testicular feminization mutation
TFS
testicular feminization syndrome
TGA
transient global amnesia
thalamic
t. dementia
t. epilepsy
t. region
t. response
t. reticular activating system
thalamocortical activity
thalamotomy
thalamus
anterior nucleus of t.
t. overactivity in OCD
pulvinar nucleus of t.
t. tissue
thalassomania
thalassoposia
thallium poisoning
thanatobiologic
thanatognomonic
thanatography
thanatology
thanatomania
thanatopsis
thanatopsy, thanatopsia
thanatos
thank-you theory
thaumaturgic
thaumaturgy
THC
tetrahydrocannabinoid
tetrahydrocannabinol
THC dependence
The
T. American Academy of Psychoanalysis
T. Center for Mental Health Services
T. Centre for Mental Health Solutions
T. Mental Health Bill of Rights
T. Philippines
T. Systematic Treatment Enhancement Program for Bipolar Disorder
Theater of Spontaneity
theatric
theatrical
theatricalism
theatromania
theft
drug t.
fear of t.
opportunity for t.
petty t.
theism
thematic
t. paralogia
t. paraphasia
t. paraphrasia
t. role
thematically related groups
theme
central t.
common t.
core conflictual relationship t.
cultural t.
death t.
depressed mood t.
deserved punishment t.
disease t.
grandiose t.
guilt t.
identity t.
inflated worth t.
t. interference
knowledge t.
manic mood t.
mood-congruent t.
mythological t.
nihilism t.
persecution t.
persecutory delusional t.
personal inadequacy t.
power t.
recurring t.
religious t.
self-derogatory t.
special relationship to deity t.
special relationship to famous person t.
typical t.
violent t.
themomatic paralogia
theocracy
theologian
theologic
t. issue
t. matter

theologize
theology
natural t.
theomania
theonomous
theophany
theorem
central limit t.
theoretical
t. assumption
t. implication
t. meaningfulness
t. orientation
t. system
t. understanding
theorist
defect t.
theorize
theory
abstract t.
adaptation level t.
addiction t.
Adler t.
adlerian t.
affective arousal t.
aggressive behavior t.
aging t.
Allport group relations t.
Allport personality trait t.
alter ego t.
t. of anxiety
anxiety-sensitivity t.
arousal t.
attachment t.
attitude t.
attribution t.
balance t.
behavioral t.
behavior-constraint t.
biofeedback t.
biolinguistic language t.
biologic t.
biosocial t.
Burn and Rand t.
Cannon t.
Cannon-Bard t.
catastrophe t.
causal-attributional t.
chaos t.
classical psychoanalytical t.
clinical t.
cloacal t.
t. of cognition
cognitive dissonance t.
cognitive learning t.
color t.
communication t.
3-component t.
compulsive loser t.
t. of constitutional bisexuality
constitutional bisexuality t.
continuum t.
crisis t.
cross-linkage t.
cybernetic t.
decay t.
decision t.
degeneracy t.
deontologic t.
developmental t.
dialectical behavior t.
dietary t.
ding-dong t.
double-blind t.
drive reduction t.
dual-instinct t.
dual-process t.
emergency t.
emotive t.
empiricist t.
environmental learning t.
environmental load t.
environmental stress t.
epigenetic t.
equity t.
ERG t.
etiology t.
evolution t.
exclamation t.
existential-humanistic t.
expectancy t.
factor t.
family system t.
field t.
Flourens t.
focal conflict t.
Freud t.
freudian t.
game t.
gate t.
gate-control t.
gating t.
general systems t.
genetic t.
gestalt t.
group relations t.

NOTES

theory *(continued)*
hearing t.
Hilgard neodissociation t.
humanistic t.
human motivation t.
humoral t.
ice block t.
immanence t.
implicit personality t.
incentive t.
information t.
innateness t.
interference t.
interpersonal t.
item response t. (IRT)
James-Lange-Sutherland t.
Jung t.
jungian t.
Klein suffocation alarm t.
labeling t.
lamarckian t.
language t.
leadership t.
learning t.
libido t.
life-cycle t.
life-event stress t.
mass action t.
memory t.
Meyer t.
miasma t.
mind t.
t. of mind
t. of mind task
mixture t.
mnemic t.
mnemism t.
moral t.
nativist t.
object relations t.
observational learning t.
pavlovian t.
periodicity t.
personal construct t.
personality trait t.
person-centered t.
phonatory t.
place t.
psychoanalytic t.
psychodynamic t.
psycholinguistic t.
psychological t.
quantum t.
rankian t.
rapid-change t.
rapid-smoking t.
ratification t.
response t.
rival normative t.
rogerian t.
role-enactment t.
Semon-Hering t.
sensorimotor t.
sexuality t.
social causation t.
social dominance t.
t. of social dominance
social learning t.
social selection t.
societal reaction t.
Spearman 2-factor t.
steppingstone t.
stimulus-response t.
stress t.
structural t.
stuttering block t.
tension-reduction t.
thank-you t.
topographic t.
topographical t.
total composite t.
trace decay t.
trait t.
understimulation t.
Urning t.
utilitarian t.
violence t.
vulnerability t.
watchspring t.
Wollaston t.
X-bar t.

theosophist

theosophy

theoterrorism

theotherapy

therapeusis

therapeutic
t. abortion (TAB)
t. advantage
t. agent
t. alliance
t. approach
t. atmosphere
t. blood level
t. botulinum neurotoxin
t. communication
t. community (TC)
t. connection
t. contract
t. contribution
t. crisis
t. dose
t. dose dependence
t. drug holiday
t. drug monitoring
t. effect
t. efficacy
t. electric stimulation

t. environment
t. exercise
t. exploration
t. failure
t. gender neutrality
t. goal
t. group analysis
t. impasse
t. index
t. insight
t. intervention
t. malaria
t. matrix
t. measure
t. milieu
t. modality
t. nihilism
t. optimism
t. option
t. outcome
t. pessimism
t. play group (TPG)
t. process
t. profile
t. program
t. range
t. reaction (TR)
t. recreation
t. relationship
t. relaxation
t. response
t. role
t. safety
t. school placement
t. strategy
t. success
suggestive t.'s
t. target
t. trial
t. trial visit (TTV)
t. vocational placement
t. window

therapeutically justified
therapeutist
therapia (*var. of* therapy)
therapist

active t.
activities t.
activity t.
t. authentication
auxiliary t.
corrective t.
educational t.
female t.
group t.
individual t.
language t.
licensed marriage and family t.
male t.
monkey t.
movement t.
t. obligation
occupational t. (OT)
passive t.
physical t.
registered recreation t. (RRT)

therapist-guided therapy
therapist-patient relationship
therapy, therapia (Rx)

aboriginal t.
acceptance and commitment t.
active t.
activity group t. (AGT)
acute t.
adaptation-promoting t.
adjunctive t.
adjustment t.
adjuvant t.
administrative t.
adolescent group t.
adult group t.
agonist t.
alternative t.
American Association for Marriage and Family T. (AAMFT)
anaclitic t.
analytic t.
analytical play t.
animal-assisted t.
antiandrogen t.
antidepressant t.
antiinflammatory t.
antioxidant t.
antipsychotic drug t.
apotreptic t.
art t.
assertion-structured t.
assignment t.
Association for Advancement of Behavior T. (AABT)
Association for the Advancement of Gestalt T. (AAGT)
atropine coma t.
attitude t.
aversion t.
aversive t.

NOTES

therapy *(continued)*
avoidance t.
ballet t.
behavior t.
behavioral couples group t.
behavioral marital t. (BMT)
behavior modification t.
bereavement group t.
bioenergetic t.
biologic t.
biomedical t.
body t.
branching steps in t.
brief group t.
brief stimulus t. (BST)
carbon dioxide t.
chelation t.
chemical aversion t.
child group t.
child guidance t.
cholinergic t.
clay-modeling t.
client-centered t.
cloaca t.
cognitive analytic t. (CAT)
cognitive behavior t. (CBT)
cognitive-behavioral t. (CBT)
cognitive-behavioral group t. (CBGT)
cognitive enhancement t.
cognitive-physiological t.
cognitive remediation t.
collaborative t.
color t.
coma t.
combination t.
combined t.
common sense t.
communication t.
compensated work t.
compliance t.
computer-aided t.
computer-guided t.
concurrent t.
conditioned reflex t.
conditioning t.
conjoint t.
constraint-induced t.
contextual t.
continuation t.
continuous sleep t.
contract t.
convulsive t.
convulsive shock t.
cooperative t.
COPE computer software program for depression t.
3-cornered t.
corrective t. (CT)
corticoid t.
counselor-centered t.
couples t.
couples group t.
couples sex t.
crisis t.
dance t.
delayed t.
deliberate t.
dependence on t.
depot medication injection t.
depth t.
deterrent t.
diagnostic t.
dialectical behavior t. (DBT)
directed group t.
diversional t.
divorce t.
drug t.
dual-sex t.
dual transference t.
ego-oriented individual t.
ego-state t.
elective t.
electric shock t.
electroconvulsive t. (ECT)
electroconvulsive shock t. (ECST)
electroshock t. (ECT, EST, est)
electrosleep t.
electrotherapeutic sleep t.
emotional control t.
emotional release t.
emotive t.
endocrine t.
environmental t.
estrogen replacement t.
exercise t.
existential-humanistic t.
experiential t.
experimental t.
exploratory t.
explosive t.
exposure-based cognitive behavior t.
expressive t.
extended family t. (EFT)
family group t.
family member t.
family unit t.
FearFighter computer program tailored for specific fear t.
filial t.
first-line t.
fluency shaping t.
focused expressive t.
food t.
gestalt t.
t. goal
goal-limited adjustment t.
goal setting in couples t.

graphic-arts t.
grief t.
group t.
group adjustment t. (GAT)
helper t.
Heroin Antagonist and Learning T. (HALT)
humanistic t.
imagery t.
implosion t.
implosive t.
inadequate t.
indirect method of t.
individual t. (IT)
individual marital t.
industrial t.
insight t.
inspirational group t.
instigation t.
insulin coma t.
integrated psychological t.
interaction-oriented group t.
interpersonal t. (IPT)
interpretive t.
interview t.
irritation t.
LAAM maintenance t.
language t.
language enrichment t. (LET)
leaderless group t.
light t.
long-term t.
magnetic seizure t.
maintenance drug t.
major role t. (MRT)
marital group t.
marriage t.
mass t.
megavitamin t.
methadone maintenance t.
Metrazol shock t.
milieu t.
minimum-change t.
modified ECT t.
Morita t.
morning bright light t.
motivational enhancement t.
movement t.
multidimensional family t.
multimodal behavior t.
multiple-family t.
multisystemic t. (MST)
music t. (MT)
musical t.
narrative t.
network t.
nicotine replacement t.
nonconfrontive t.
nondirective t.
nonphobic anxiety behavior t.
nutritional t.
occupational t. (OT)
old-age t.
online t.
operant t.
opioid replacement t.
organic t.
orgone t.
outcome-based t.
oxygen t.
paradoxical t.
paraverbal t.
parent-child group t.
passive immunization t.
persuasion t.
physical t.
pineal t.
planned behavioral t.
plastic arts t.
play t.
play group t. (PGT)
positive reinforcement t.
postelectroconvulsive t.
precision t.
primal scream t.
programmed t.
prolonged sleep t.
psychedelic t.
psychiatric somatic t.
psychoanalytic t.
psychodrama group t.
psychoeducational group t.
psychohormonal t.
psychologic programming t.
psychopharmacological t.
psychotherapeutic t.
quadrangular t.
radical t.
rational t. (RT)
rational emotive t. (RET)
reality-oriented t.
reconditioning t.
reconstructive t.
recreational t. (RT)
reeducative t.
reflex t.

NOTES

therapy *(continued)*
relationship t.
relaxation t.
release t.
reminiscence t.
replacement t.
restitutive t.
restraining t.
restricted environment stimulation t. (REST)
rhythmic sensory bombardment t. (RSBT)
rogerian group t.
role t.
sabotage of t.
second-line t.
self-control t.
self-exposure t.
semantic t.
sensate focus-oriented t.
t. session
sex t.
sexuality conversion t.
shame-aversion t.
shock t. (ST)
short-term t.
simulated presence t.
situational t.
sleep t.
sleep-electroshock t.
social interaction t.
social learning group t.
social network t.
socioenvironmental t.
solution-focused t.
somatic t.
sound t.
spectator t.
speech t.
standard antipsychotic t.
stimulant t.
stimulus t.
strategic family t.
structural family t.
structural strategic t.
subcoma t.
subshock t.
substitutive agent t.
suggestion t.
supportive group t.
suppressive t.
symptomatic t.
systematic family t.
systematized assertive t. (SAT)
systemic assertive t.
talk t.
task force on electroconvulsive t.
tension reduction t.
termination of t.
testimony t.
testosterone t.
therapist-guided t.
theta-criterion t.
third-force t.
third-line t.
thought field t.
time-consuming t.
time-extended t.
timeline t.
time line t.
total push t.
trauma-focused t.
triadic t.
understimulation t.
unmodified ECT t.
validation t.
verbal aversion t.
video t.
virtual reality t.
vitamin t.
4-way t.
weight loss t.
Weir Mitchell t.
will t.
work t.
Zen t.

therapy-relevant behavior
there-and-then approach
theriomorphism
thermal
t. anesthesia
t. drive
t. sense
t. stimulus

thermalgesia, thermoalgesia
thermalgia
thermanalgesia, thermoanalgesia
thermanesthesia (*var. of* thermoanesthesia)
thermesthesia
thermesthesiometer (*var. of* thermoesthesiometer)
thermic sense
thermoalgesia (*var. of* thermalgesia)
thermoanalgesia (*var. of* thermanalgesia)
thermoanesthesia, thermanesthesia
thermocoagulation
thermoeffector
t. activity
antagonistic t.
t. function
t. response

thermoesthesiometer, thermesthesiometer
thermogenesis
catecholamine-induced t.
nonshivering t.
normal t.

shivering t.
sympathomimetic-induced t.
thermogenic
t. action
t. component
t. effect
t. mechanism
t. tissue mass
thermohyperalgesia
thermohyperesthesia
thermohypesthesia, thermohypoesthesia
thermometer
fear t.
thermoneurosis
thermoplastic
thermoreceptor
thermoregulation
thermoregulatory
t. function
t. property
t. response
t. system
thermosensory
t. information
t. property
theroid
theta
t. criterion
t. index
t. level
t. rhythm
t. wave
theta-criterion therapy
theurgist
theurgy
thiamine, thiamin
t. deficiency
t. deficiency encephalopathy (TDE)
thick-headed
thick-skinned
thick-witted
thief
thigmesthesia
thin
desire to be t.
thinking
t. ability
abnormal t.
abstract logical t.
adolescent t.
allusive t.
animistic t.
archaic paralogical t.
t. aside
assessment of bizarre idiosyncratic t.
associative t.
asyndetic t.
autistic t.
black-and-white t.
categorical t.
circular t.
clear t.
clinical t.
combinative t.
t. compulsion
conceptual t.
concrete t.
concretistic t.
convergent t.
creative t.
t. creatively with sounds and words (TCSW)
critical t.
delusional t.
dereistic t.
dichotomous t.
directed t.
t. disorder
disordered t.
disorganized t.
distorted inferential t.
distortion of inferential t.
t. disturbance factor (TDF)
disturbance in form of t.
divergent t.
eccentric t.
egocentric t.
either-or t.
erratic t.
externally oriented t. (EOT)
t. fear
fragmentation of t.
futuristic t.
hypothetical deductive t.
idiosyncratic t.
illogical t.
impaired abstract t.
impoverishment in t.
incomprehensible t.
inferential t.
janusian t.
magic t.
magical t.
marginal t.
normal t.

NOTES

thinking *(continued)*
numerical t.
obsessional t.
oppositional t.
overinclusive t.
paranoid t.
perverted t.
physiognomic t.
prearchaic t.
precausal t.
preconscious t.
predicate t.
prelogical t.
preoperational t.
primary process t.
process t.
productive t.
psychotic t.
realistic t.
ritualistic t.
secondary process t.
self-defeating t.
slowed t.
stress effect on adult t.
suicidal t.
symbolic t.
syncretic t.
tangential t.
tertiary process t.
t. through
trouble t.
t. type
undirected t.
vague t.
wishful t.
thinner
paint t.
thin-skinned
thioridazine
third
t. degree
t. ear
t. nervous system
t. sex
third-force therapy
thirdhand information
third-line therapy
third-party administrator
third-person
t.-p. attitude
t.-p. auditory hallucination
third-rate
thirst
t. drive
insensible t.
morbid t.
subliminal t.
twilight t.
Thorndike
T. law of effect
T. trial-and-error learning
Thorndike-Lorge criteria
thoroughness, reliability, efficiency, analytic ability
thought
abstract logical t.
adaptive control of t. (ACT)
aggressive t.
alien t.
anxious t.
archaic t.
audible t.
automatic t.
avoidance of t.'s
blasphemous t.
t. blockade
t. blocking
t. broadcasting
t. broadcasting delusion
categorical t.
characteristic pattern of t.
children's development of moral t.
coherent stream of t.
compulsive t.
considered t.
t. constraint
constraint of t.
constriction of t.
t. content
content of t.
t. control
t.'s of death
t. deletion
delusional t.
t. deprivation
t. derailment
difficulty with t.
diminution of t.
disconnected t.
t. disorder
t. disorder index
t. disorganization
t. disorientation
distressing t.
t. disturbance
disturbance in content of t.
disturbing t.
t. echo
t. echoing
emotional t.
errant t.
evil t.
t. fear
fear-related t.
t. field therapy
fluency of t.
focus of t.

t. form
free t.
gambling t.
t. hearing
homicidal t.
imageless t.
impoverished t.
inappropriate t.
incessantly reiterated t.'s
incomprehensible t.
increased speed of t.
inelasticity of t.
inner t.
t. insertion
t. insertion delusion
interruption of t.
intrusive t.
latent t.
logical analysis of automatic t.
lost in t.
maladaptive t.
maladaptive pattern of t.
moral t.
motor theory of t.
multifocal t.
obsessional t.
obsessive t.
t. obstruction
omnipotence of t.
operational t.
t. out
painful t.
passive suicidal t.
t. pattern
t. period
persistent t.
phenomenalistic t.
phenomenistic t.
poverty of t.
preoccupation of t.
preoperational t.
pressing t.
t. pressure
t. process
productivity of t.
t. provoking
psychopathologic t.
racing t.'s
rambling flow of t.
reactive t.
t. reading
recurrent t.
t. reform
t. rehearsal
reinforced t.
ruminative t.
school of t.
second t.
self-assuring t.
self-deprecating t.
self-related t.
sexual t.
sick t.
slowness of t.
speed of t.
stimulus-independent t.
t. stopping
stream of t. (SOT)
substituting t.
suicidal t.
t. of suicide
supervalent t.
t. suppression
symbolic t.
syncretic t.
syntaxic t.
t. system
train of t.
t. transfer
t. transference
t. transfer experience
t. transfer phenomenon
trend of t.
unacceptable t.
uncontrollable t.
unemotional t.
unrelated t.
unsocialized disturbance of t.
verbal t.
violent t.
wandering t.
wide circles of t.
t. wit
t. withdrawal
worrisome t.

threadbare

thready

threat

acute suicide t.
death t.
t. of death
direct t.
disruptive verbal t.
t. of imminent suicide
t. of job loss
t. to life

NOTES

threat *(continued)*
suicide t.
target of t.
veiled t.
t. of violence
voicing t.
t. of war
threatened death
threatening
t. behavior
t. comment
t. hallucination
t. message
t. remark
t. speech
t. violence
t. voice
threat-related word
threctia
three strikes law
threshold
absolute t.
acoustic reflex t.
auditory t.
awareness t.
blackout t.
brightness t.
t. of consciousness
convulsant t.
detectability t.
detection t.
t. differential
differential t.
discomfort t.
t. of discomfort (TD)
double-point t.
electroshock t. (EST, est)
false t.
intelligibility t.
low anger t.
motor t.
pain intensity t.
reflex t.
relational t.
t. of responsiveness
sedation t.
seizure t.
sensory t.
t. shift masking technique
speech reception t. (SRT)
t. stimulus
stimulus t.
t. symbolism
taste t.
vibrotactile t.
vulnerability t.
thriftless
thrive
failure to t. (FTT)
throat
lump in t.
t. slashing
throaty
throbbing
through
carry t.
fall t.
muddle t.
thinking t.
working t.
throw
t. off
t. out
t. over
t. in the towel
t. up
throwback
thrust
extensor t.
thrusting
pelvic t.
thug
thumb
cerebral t.
rule of t.
t. sucking
thunder
thwart
thymogenic
thymonoic reaction
thyroid
t. augmentation
t. delirium
t. disorder
t. response element (TRE)
thyroid-stimulating hormone (TSH)
thyrotoxic
t. coma
t. encephalopathy
thyrotoxicosis
apathetic t.
thyrotropin-releasing
t.-r. hormone (TRH)
t.-r. hormone stimulation
thyrotropin-stimulating hormone (TSH)
tiagabine
tibiarum
anxietas t.
tickling
tic-like
t.-l. behavior
t.-l. facial grimace
tic-related obsessive-compulsive disorder
ties
breaking of family t.
incestuous t.
reality t.
t. with reality

tight-lipped
tight-mouthed
tightrope
tilt
  head t.
  head-up t.
timbromania
time
  abuse of leave t.
  adaptation t.
  t. agnosia
  association reaction t.
  attention t.
  biologic t.
  central reflex t.
  t. confusion
  t. consciousness
  t. consuming
  t. context
  t. of death
  t. deixis
  t. disorientation
  t. distortion
  t. dominance
  dream t.
  t. error
  t. faction
  t. fear
  inertia t.
  t. interval
  t. killer
  leisure t.
  t. line therapy
  losing t.
  t. of maximum concentration
  t. and motion studies
  one day at a t.
  oriented to person, place, and t.
  t. out
  t. out from reinforcement
  t. perception
  t. periods of satisfactory relating
  t., place, and person (TP&P)
  t. point
  t. pressure
  processing t.
  quality t.
  reaction t. (RT)
  recognition t.
  reflex t.
  relaxation t.
  respite t.
  response processing t.
  t. and rhythm disorder
  sensation of slowed t.
  t. sense
  sleep t.
  t. splitting
  survival t.
  total sleep t. (TST)
  wake t.
  t. zone
  t. zone change syndrome
time-consuming therapy
timed behavioral rating sheet (TBRS)
time-extended therapy
timeless
time-limited psychotherapy (TLP)
timeliness
timeline therapy
timely death
time-motion study
time-out
  involuntary t.-o.
  t.-o. procedure
  t.-o. technique
  voluntary t.-o.
time-series design
time-specific event
timid
timidity
timing
  circadian t.
timorous
tingling sensation
tinnitus
tiotixene
tip of iceberg
tip-off
tip-of-the-tongue (TOT)
  t.-o.-t.-t. phenomenon
tipsy
tiqueur
tirade
tiredness upon awakening
tireless
tissue-type metabolic response
titillate
titillating
titration
  dose t.
titubation
tizzy
TL
  team leader
  tolerance level

NOTES

TLC
tender loving care
TLE
temporal lobe epilepsy
TLP
time-limited psychotherapy
TM
team member
transcendental meditation
TMA-2
2,4,5-trimethoxyamphetamine
TMH
trainable mentally handicapped
TMR
trainable mentally retarded
TMS
transcranial magnetic stimulation
to
face up to
to a fault
to the point
to-and-fro tremor
tobacco
t. abuse
t. addiction
t. amblyopia
t. dependence
t. smoker
t. usage
t. use
t. use disorder
t. user
t. use reduction
t. withdrawal
tobaccoism
tobacism
tobacosis
tobagism
tocomania
toddler
t. negativism
t. stage
Todeserwartung syndrome
toe
t. clonus
t. drop
t. phenomenon
toe-walking
together
fraternal twins raised t.
hang t.
live t.
togetherness need
toilet training
token economy reward
tolerability
tolerance
acute t.
t. to alcohol
alcohol dependence with t.
ambiguity t.
anxiety t.
barbiturate t.
benzodiazepine t.
caffeine t.
distress t.
t. dose
drug t.
frustration t.
t. level (TL)
level of pain t.
low frustration t.
metabolic t.
opioid t.
pain t.
pharmacodynamic t.
t. potential
t. range
social t.
stimulant t.
substance t.
zero t.
tolerant
tolerate
toll
psychological t.
Tolman purposive behaviorism
Tolosa-Hunt syndrome
toluene dementia
toluidine blue stain
Tom
peeping T.
TOMAL
test of memory and learning
TOMAL facial memory
tomboy behavior
tomboyish
Tomism
Uncle T.
tommy gun
tomography
computed axial t. (CAT)
tomomania
tonaphasia
tone
affective t.
belligerent t.
biofeedback t.
complex t.
t. deafness
depressed t.
dopaminergic t.
emotional t.
episodic bilateral loss of muscle t.
t. of feeling
fundamental t.
heightened emotional t.
hostile t.

hyperattentiveness to voice t.
inhibitory t.
muscle t.
reduced body t.
t. of voice

toner
psychological t.

tonetic

tongue
t. clucking
forked t.
t. kiss
t. mobility
t. phenomenon
t. protrusion
t. stiffness
t. twisting
vermicular motion of t.

tongue-lash

tongue-tied

tonic
t. convulsion
t. epilepsy
t. inhibitor control
t. pupil
t. seizure
t. spasm
t. tic

tonic-clonic
t.-c. conversion
t.-c. movement
t.-c. seizure

tonicity

tonoclonic spasm

tonogenic

tonogeny

tonotopic

tonus
plastic t.

tool
BRAINSTRIP semiautomated brain extraction t.
communication t.
genetic t.
relationship t.

tool-using behavior

tooth
t. decay
t. fear
t. grinding
t. spasm

TOP
temporal, occipital, parietal
test orientation procedure

topagnosis

topalgia

top-down
t.-d. organization of memory
t.-d. regulation

topesthesia

topic
change of t.
emotionally laden t.
t. shifting

topiramate

topoanesthesia

topographagnosia

topographic
t. hypothesis
t. mapping
t. theory

topographical
t. agnosia
t. disorientation
t. organization
t. psychology
t. theory

topography
mental t.

topological psychology

topology

toponarcosis

toponeurosis

toposcope

TOPS
taxonomy of problematic social situations

Toradol

torment

tormented
being t.

tornado epilepsy

Toronto
Tower of T.

torpedoing

torpent

torpid
t. idiocy
t. idiot

torpillage

torpor

torrid

torsion dystonia

tort

NOTES

T

torticollis
hysterical t.
psychogenic t.
spastic t.
tortuosity
tortuous
torture
complexity of t.
exposure to t.
t. method
psychological sequela of t.
t. survivor
tortured refugee
TOT
tip-of-the-tongue
total
t. abstinence
t. AIMS score
t. aphasia
T. Army Injury and Health Outcomes Database
t. battery composite
t. brain volume
t. cerebral ischemia
t. communication
t. composite theory
t. disability
t. emotional memory score
t. neuroleptic dosage
t. parenteral nutrition (TPN)
t. phobic anxiety (TPA)
t. push therapy
t. recall
t. response (lz R)
t. response index (TRI)
t. sleep time (TST)
t. symptom
t. symptom score
t. weighted sum score
totalis
alopecia t.
totalism
totality of possible events
totally disabled
totem
totemism
totemistic
toto
pars pro t.
touch
t. off
out of t.
t. perception
t. sensation
t. sense
soft t.
t. spot
toucher
délire de t.
toucherism
touching
t. communication pattern
genital t.
inappropriate t.
t. ritual
sexual t.
unwanted sexual t.
touch-me-not
tough
hang t.
t. love
t. poise
tough-minded tendency
Tourette
T. disorder
T. syndrome (TS)
T. tic
towel
throw in the t.
TOWER
testing, orientation, and work evaluation for rehabilitation
tower
T. of Hanoi
T. of Hanoi puzzle
ivory t.
T. of Toronto
town
skip t.
tox
toxicology
tox screen
toxemia-related personality change
toxic
t. action
t. amaurosis
t. amblyopia
t. cirrhosis
t. confusional state
t. convulsion
t. delirium
t. dementia
t. disorder
t. dose
t. drug state
t. edema
t. effect of alcohol
t. encephalopathy
t. gas exposure
t. hypoxia
t. ingredient
t. injury
t. insanity
t. level
t. metal exposure
t. myocarditis
t. neuritis
t. nystagmus

t. psychosis
t. reaction
t. schizophrenia
t. side effect
t. substance
t. tetanus

toxica
alopecia t.

toxic-infectious psychosis

toxicity
acute drug t.
alcohol t.
behavioral t.
caffeine t.
drug t.
social t.
trichloroethylene t.

toxicological analysis

toxicology (tox)
t. screen
t. screening
urine t.

toxicomania

toxin
dietary t.
environmental t.
exposure to t.

toxin-provoked amnesia

toy
sex t.

TPA
total phobic anxiety

TPG
therapeutic play group

TPN
total parenteral nutrition

TP&P
time, place, and person

TPR
temperature, pulse, respiration

T-Quil

TR
therapeutic reaction

trace
t. conditioned reflex
t. conditioning
t. decay theory
memory t.
mnemonic t.
perseverative t.

tracer
biochemical t.
flow t.

tracing
abnormal EEG t.
dipole t. (DT)
EEG t.
I t.
interrupted t.

track
fast t.
needle t.

tracking
eye t.
saccadic t.
speech t.
visual t.

1-track mind

tract
census t.
cholinergic t.
dopaminergic t.
extrapyramidal t.
mesolimbic-mesocortical t.
serotonergic t.

tractable

traction alopecia

trading
day t.
drug t.
sex t.
t. sex

tradition
childhood t.
cultural t.
t. directed
meditative t.
religious t.

traditional
t. antipsychotic
t. antipsychotic agent
t. belief
t. counseling
t. healing
t. indemnity insurance
t. lifestyle
t. limbic circuit
t. marriage
t. neuroleptic
t. neuroleptic agent
t. phonetic analysis
t. practice
t. psychoanalytic concept
t. psychotherapy
t. society

NOTES

T

traditional *(continued)*
t. treatment
t. value
traditionalism
traditionalist
traditionalize
traditionally defined autism
traffic
t. court
drug t.
trafficker
trafficking
drug t.
Trager method
tragic
trailing
t. image
t. phenomenon
train
t. fear
orphan t.
t. of thought
trainability
trainable
t. mentally handicapped (TMH)
t. mentally retarded (TMR)
trained reflex
trainer
training
aggression replacement t.
alpha-wave t.
American Association of Directors of Psychiatric Residency T. (AADPRT)
t. analysis
anxiety control t. (ACT)
anxiety management t. (AMT)
assertive t.
assertiveness t.
attention t.
audiovisual t.
auditory t.
autogenic t.
aversive t.
avoidance t.
biofeedback t.
biologic t.
bladder t.
bowel t.
clinical t.
cognitive self-hypnosis t.
communication skills t.
cooperative t.
cultural t.
delayed toilet t.
t. discrimination
emotion regulation t.
Erhardt seminar t.
escape t.
evaluation of t.
general relaxation t.
t. group
habit t.
habit reversal t. (HRT)
human relations t.
hypnotic relaxation technique t.
improvement t.
inappropriate religious t.
interviewer t.
laboratory t.
leadership t.
memory t.
metacognitive t.
neurofeedback t. (NT)
occupational skills t.
parent effectiveness t.
perceptual t.
personnel t.
primary and secondary control enhancement t. (PASCET)
problem-solving skills t.
relaxation technique t.
retention control t.
self-reliance t.
sensitivity t.
skill t.
social skills t. (SST)
spontaneity t.
stress inoculation t. (SIT)
toilet t.
trait factor t.
transfer of t.
t. transfer
t. unit
visual t.
vocational t.
train-of-four stimulus
train-then-place philosophy
trait
abnormal t.
anger-related personality t.
t. anxiety
anxious-neurotic personality t.
atypical personality t.
cardinal t.
t. carrier
central t.
character t.
t. characteristic
cluster B t.
cognitive personality t.
common t.
compensatory t.
complex psychological t.
coping t.
culture t.
dependence t.
t. dependent

dominant t.
environmental mold t.
t. factor
t. factor training
genetic t.
harm-avoidant t.
identified t.
impulsive-aggressive t.
inflexible personality t.
interpersonal personality t.
intrapsychic personality t.
introversive t.
maladaptive personality t.
novelty-seeking t.
t. organization
paranoid t.
passive-dependent t.
pathologic t.
peculiar personality t.
personality t.
pervasive and persistent maladaptive personality t.'s
polygenic t.
premorbid personality t.
primary personality t.
t. profile
psychological t.
psychopathic t.
t. rating
recessive t.
schizoid t.
secondary personality t.
self-defeating t.
sensation-seeking t.
temperament t.
t. theory
unique t.
t. variability

trait-level region abnormality

trait-like

t.-l. feature
t.-l. syndrome

trajectory

behavioral t.
cognitive t.
developmental t.
emotional t.
treatment response t.

trance

amnesia after t.
t. coma
death t.
deep t.
dissociative t.
ecstatic t.
hypnotic t.
hysterical t.
induced t.
involuntary state of t.
light t.
t. logic
medium t.
possession t.
somnambulistic t.
t. state

trancelike

t. behavior
t. state

trance-possession disorder

tranquilization

rapid t.

tranquilizer

t. abuse
t. chair
t. drug dependence
major t.
minor t.

transaction

ulterior t.

transactional

t. analysis (TA)
t. evaluation
t. pattern
t. psychotherapy
t. theory of perception

transaminase

transcend

transcendence

ego t.
t. need

transcendental

t. meditation (TM)
t. state

transcendentalism

transcendent reality

transcerebral electrotherapy (TCET)

transcortical

t. aphasia
t. apraxia

transcranial magnetic stimulation (TMS)

transcultural psychiatry

transderivational search

transdermal

t. absorption
t. nicotine patch

transduce

NOTES

transduction
chemical-mechanical t.
postreceptor information t.
transfer
bilateral t.
correctional t. (CT)
custody t.
t. of custody
general t.
t. by generalization
interhemispheric t.
intersensory t.
t. of learning
memory t.
positive t.
t. of principles
thought t.
training t.
t. of training
transference
affectionate t.
aim t.
alter ego t.
analysis of t.
t. behavior
collective t.
t. cure
t. dilution
erotic t.
extrasensory thought t.
t. feeling
floating t.
hostile t.
idealizing t.
identification t.
t. improvement
institutional t.
libidinal t.
t. love
mirror t.
mirroring t.
narcissistic t.
negative t.
t. neurosis
t. paradigm
t. phenomenon
positive t.
t. reaction
t. relationship
t. remission
t. resistance
self-object t.
thought t.
traumatic t.
twinship t.
transference-countertransference
transferential
transferred
t. meaning
t. sensation
transformation
t. of affect
perceptual t.
t. theory of anxiety
Z-score t.
transformational
T. Leadership Development Program
t. rule
transformationally related
transforming agent
transfusion
blood t.
transgender
transgenderism
transgenerational
t. role of giving
t. transmission of trauma
transgress
transgression
behavioral t.
imagined t.
transience
transient
t. auditory hallucination
t. auditory illusion
t. blindness
t. channel activation
t. depressive reaction
t. distortion
t. ego ideal
t. emotional disturbance
t. emotional stress
t. global amnesia (TGA)
t. group
t. hallucinatory experience
t. hypersomnia
t. ideas of reference
t. image
t. insomnia
t. organic psychosis
t. phenomenon
t. postictal confusional state
t. situational disturbance
t. situational personality disorder
t. state of anger
t. stress-related paranoid ideation
t. tactile hallucination
t. tactile illusion
t. tic disorder
t. tic disorder of childhood
t. tremor
t. visual hallucination
t. visual illusion
transilluminate

transition
age t.
high-intensity t.
life-cycle t.
midlife t.
normal t.
t. process
role t.
sleep-wake t.
t. zone
transitional
t. change
t. employment workshop
t. halfway house
t. Lewy body dementia
t. object
t. probability
t. program
t. sleep (TS)
transitivism
transitivity
transitory
t. anoxia
t. mania
t. psychosis
translation
translocation
chromosomal t.
translucent
transmigrate
transmissible
t. agent
t. virus dementia (TVD)
transmission
cholinergic t.
cultural t.
duplex t.
familial t.
genetic t.
indirect genetic t.
intergenerational t.
neurohumoral t.
parent-child t.
synaptic t.
vertical t.
transmitter
chemical t.
t. system
transmutation
transorbital
t. lobectomy
t. lobotomy
transosseous
transpersonal psychology
transpicuous
transplantation
organ t.
t. reaction
t. shock
transport
active t.
passive t.
transportation barrier
transporter
dopamine t.
drug t.
norepinephrine t.
serotonin t. (SERT)
transposition of affect
transracial adoption
transsexual (TS)
nuclear t.
t. voice
transsexualism
transsynaptic
transtentorial
transverse
t. hermaphroditism
t. orientation
transvestic
t. fetishism (TF)
t. phenomenon
transvestism, transvestitism
t. paraphilia
transvestite
marginal t.
nuclear t.
Transylvania effect
trap
death t.
social t.
trauma, pl. **traumata, traumas**
acoustic t.
acute head t.
aftermath of t.
amnesia for t.
anal t.
betrayal t.
birth t.
brain t.
cerebral t.
t. characteristic
child abuse-specific treatment of t. (CASTT)
childhood t.
civilian t.

NOTES

trauma *(continued)*
closed head t.
CNS t.
combat t.
combat-related t.
t. cue
dementia due to head t.
disaster t.
early medical t.
effect of t.
emotional t.
exposure to t.
extreme t.
family war t.
genital t.
head t.
individual war t.
intensity of t.
intergenerational t.
late-age t.
long-term effects of t.
occult head t.
original t.
physical t.
premorbid t.
primal t.
principal t.
psychic t.
psychological t.
race-related t.
recollection of t.
reexperienced t.
refugee t.
repressing emotional t.
resolving emotional t.
self-inflicted t.
severe t.
sexual t.
sexual exposure t.
t. spectrum disorder
subsequent t.
t. survivor
transgenerational transmission of t.
type 1, 2 t.
trauma-focused therapy
trauma-induced delirium
trauma-related
t.-r. repetition
t.-r. stress
trauma-specific
t.-s. anxiety
t.-s. reenactment
traumasthenia
traumata (*pl. of* trauma)
traumatic
t. alopecia
t. amblyopia
t. amnesia
t. anesthesia
t. anxiety
t. aphasia
t. asphyxia
t. bereavement
t. brain injury (TBI)
t. brain injury-associated mania
t. childhood abuse
t. death
t. defect state
t. delirium
t. dementia
t. epilepsy
t. experience
t. grief
t. headache
t. idiocy
t. injury
t. life event
t. memory
t. mutism
t. neurasthenia
t. neuritis
t. neurosis
t. progressive encephalopathy
t. pseudocatatonia
t. psychosis
t. scene
t. seizure
t. separation
t. stress
t. stressor
t. suffocation
t. transference
traumatica
amnesia t.
traumatism
traumatization of libido
traumatize
traumatized
t. adolescent
t. child
t. elderly patient
t. refugee
traumatology
traumatophilia
trauma-type symptom
travail
traveling
traverse jury
travesty in wit
TRD
treatment-resistant depression
TRE
thyroid response element
treacherous
tread
treason
treated
ineffectively t.

treatise
treatment
achievement through counseling and t. (ACT)
acidification t.
active t.
acute t.
acute intensive t. (AIT)
acute-phase t.
addiction t.
adequate t.
adjunct to t.
adjunctive t.
T. for Adolescents with Depression Study
t. alliance
alternative t.
amenable to t.
analytic t.
antidepressant t.
antipsychotic t.
antipsychotic drug t.
appropriate t.
assertive community t.
t. authorization
behavioral t.
Buddhist t.
Center for Substance Abuse T. (CSAT)
t. change
t. choice
coerced t.
coercive t.
cognitive-behavioral t.
cognitive-linguistic t.
cold-pack t.
communication/cognition t.
community-based mental health t.
t. completion
t. completion rate
t. compliance
t. compliance monitoring
comprehensive t.
t. condition
conservative t.
t. consideration
continuation t.
continuous antipsychotic drug t.
continuous bath t.
conventional neuroleptic t.
t. cost
course of t.
court-mandated t.
court-ordered involuntary outpatient t.
daycare residential t.
t. decision
definitive t.
depression t.
Depression: Awareness, Recognition, and T. (D/ART)
T. of Depression Collaborative Research Program
diet t.
direct t.
disrespectful t.
t. driven
t. dropout
drug-induced t.
drug maintenance t.
drug-responsive t.
t. duration
duration of t.
early t.
early and periodic screening, diagnosis, and t. (EPSDT)
educational t.
t. effect
effective t.
t. effectiveness
electric shock t.
electroconvulsive shock t. (ECST)
electroshock t. (EST, est)
emergency t.
t. emergent
empiric drug t.
enforced t.
enhanced methadone maintenance t.
ethanol t.
t. evaluation strategy
evening t.
exercise t.
t. experience
experimental t.
t. facility
family t.
feasible alternative t.
fluoxetine t.
forced t.
format t.
former t.
frequency of t.
t. gap
general medical t.
group t.
habit t.

NOTES

treatment *(continued)*
hazardous t.
high-potency neuroleptic t.
holistic t.
hormone t.
humane t.
inadequate t.
individual t.
ineffective t.
inhalation convulsive t.
t. initiation
inpatient drug t.
insight-oriented t.
insulin coma t.
insulin shock t.
t. intensity
t. intensity parameter
t. intensity by time interaction
t. interference
intravenous t.
intrusive t.
invasive t.
involuntary t.
t. issue
light t.
long-term maintenance t.
low-dose t.
lower-intensity t.
maintenance t.
mandatory t.
medical t.
medication t.
mental health t.
methadone maintenance t. (MMT)
Metrazol shock t.
Mitchell t.
t. modality
t. model
moral t.
multicomponent behavioral t.
multimonitored electroconvulsive t. (MMECT)
neuroleptic t.
new t.
noncompliance with medical t.
nutrition t.
obesity t.
office-based opioid t.
ongoing neuroleptic t.
optimal t.
t. option
t. outcome
outpatient t.
overly stimulating t.
t. package strategy
t. period
pharmacologic t.
t. phase
t. philosophy
t. plan (TRPL)
t. planning
prefrontal sonic t. (PST)
prescribed t.
previous t.
t. program
program of assertive community t. (PACT)
t. progress
prolonged sleep t.
prophylactic t.
t. protocol
psychiatric t.
psychodynamic interpretation and t.
psychopharmacological t.
psychoprophylactic t.
psychosocial t.
psychotherapeutic t.
t. refractory
t. refusal
t. regimen
regressive electroshock t. (REST)
rehabilitation t.
residential t.
t. resistance
t. resistant
t. response
t. response rate
t. response trajectory
t. responsive
t. responsivity
retention in t.
right to refuse t.
school-based child-and-parent-focused psychosocial t.
scope of t.
t. services review
shock t.
short-term t.
silent t.
sleep t.
social support after t.
social support during t.
somatic antidepressant t.
somatized plea for t.
specialty mental health t.
t. specificity
stimulant t.
suboptimal t.
substance abuse t.
symptomatic t.
t. team
traditional t.
unilateral ECT t.
t. unit
Weir Mitchell t.

treatment-emergent
t.-e. adverse event
t.-e. akathisia

t.-e. asthenia
t.-e. extrapyramidal side effect
t.-e. hypertonia
t.-e. hypokinesia
t.-e. hypomania
t.-e. somnolence
treatment-intolerant patient
treatment-refractory
t.-r. catatonia
t.-r. depression
t.-r. patient
t.-r. schizophrenia
treatment-relevant issue
treatment-resistant
t.-r. depression (TRD)
t.-r. schizophrenia
t.-r. schizophrenic
t.-r. symptom
treble safeguard principle
tree
chaste t.
decision t.
family t.
maidenhair t.
tremblant
délire t.
trembling
t. abasia
t. palsy
t. voice
tremens
delirium t. (DT, DTs)
tremogram
tremograph
tremolo massage
tremor
action t.
acute cerebral t.
alcoholic withdrawal t.
alcohol-related t.
alternating t.
anxiety-related t.
arsenic-induced t.
benign essential t.
beta adrenergic medication-induced postural t.
cerebellar t.
cerebral outflow t.
coarse t.
continuous t.
counting money t.
cycles-per-second t.
dopaminergic medication-induced postural t.
dystonic t.
emotional stress precipitating t.
endpoint t.
essential t. (ET)
facial t.
familial t.
fibrillary t.
fine postural t.
fine resting t.
flapping t.
flopping t.
hand t.
head and neck t.
hepatic encephalopathy t.
heredofamilial t.
hysterical t.
intention t.
intentional t.
kinetic t.
medication-induced t.
mercurial t.
metabolic t.
metallic t.
neuroleptic-induced postural t.
non-neuroleptic-induced t.
no-no t.
nonparkinsonian t.
nonpharmacologically induced t.
oscillating t.
passive t.
perioral t.
persistent t.
physiologic t.
pill-rolling t.
positional t.
postural t.
precipitating t.
preexisting t.
progressive cerebellar t.
psychogenic t.
psychologic t.
rapid t.
rest t.
resting t.
rhythmic t.
senile t.
shaking t.
small-amplitude rapid t.
static t.
stimulant-induced postural t.
stress-precipitating t.

T

NOTES

tremor *(continued)*
striatocerebral t.
substance withdrawal t.
t. tendinum
terminal t.
to-and-fro t.
transient t.
volitional t.
wing-beating t.
withdrawal t.
writing t.
yes-yes t.
tremorgram
tremulous
t. movement
t. speech
tremulousness
alcoholic t.
alcohol withdrawal t.
trench
t. lung
t. warfare
trend
age-related t.
amoral t.
death t.
diverging t.
global sociocultural t.
malignant t.
mortality t.
nonsignificant t.
paranoid t.
pernicious t.
phobic t.
psychiatric t.
sadomasochistic t.
secular t.
significant t.
sociocultural t.
statistical t.
t. of thought
trendsetter
trephination, trepanation
trephine, trepan
trepid
trepidans
abasia t.
trepidant
trepidation
TRH
thyrotropin-releasing hormone
TRI
total response index
triable
triad
Charcot t.
cognitive t.
female athlete t.
oral t.
Sandler t.
triadic
t. symbiosis
t. therapy
triage situation
trial
t. analysis
clinical t.
competent to stand t.
controlled medication t.
t. court
t. and error
t. examiner
failure of drug t.
Group ROI Analysis T. (GRAT)
head-to-head clinical t.
t. identification
t. jury
t. lawyer
t. lesson
t. marriage
medication t.
murder t.
open-label t.
placebo-controlled t.
placebo medication t.
randomized clinical t. (RCT)
randomized controlled t. (RCT)
t. run
t. separation
therapeutic t.
t. visit
trial-and-error learning
triangle
tribade
tribadism
tribalism
tribe
tribesman
tribulation
tribunal
trichloroethylene toxicity
trichoesthesia
trichologia
trichology
trichomania
trichomoniasis
trichophagia
trichophagy
trichorrhexis nodosa with mental retardation
trichorrhexomania
trichosis sensitiva
trichotillomania (TTM)
trichotillomania-induced alopecia
triclofos
tricyclic
t. antidepressant drug (TCAD)

t. antipsychotic (TCA)
t. drug
t. effect
t. secondary amine
t. tertiary amine
tridimensional theory of feelings
trigeminal
t. decompression
t. nerve
t. neuralgia
trigger
active t.
t. for anger
anticipation of t.
t. area
disease t.
electromagnetic t.
emotionally salient t.
exposure to t.
t. finger
t. point
t. reaction
situational t.
t. zone
trigger-happy
triggering
t. event
t. mechanism
t. situation
t. stimulus
triggerman
trigram
Trihexy-2, -5
trilogy
2,4,5-trimethoxyamphetamine (TMA-2)
triolist
triorchid
trip
bad t.
drug t.
ego t.
triphosphate
triple insanity
tripped out
trisexuality
trismic
trismoid
trisomy
autosomal t.
chromosome 13, 18, 21 t.
E t.
t. syndrome
triste
postcoitum t.
tristful
tristimania
trite
trivial act
triviality
trochaic stress
trois
folie à t.
menage à t.
tromomania
troops
shock t.
trophesic
trophesy
trophic change
trophicity
trophism
trophoneurotic
trophopathy
trophotropic zone of Hess
tropism
trouble
t. concentrating
t. thinking
troubled
t. adolescent
t. child
t. children
t. conscience
t. marriage
t. relationship
t. teen
troublemaker
troubleshooter
troublesome
t. adolescent
t. symptom
troubling
t. behavior
t. experience
Trousseau
T. point
T. spot
trovato
ben t.
TRPL
treatment plan
truancy
school t.
socialized childhood t.
unsocialized childhood t.

NOTES

truant
truce
truculence
truculent
true
t. addiction
t. amnesia
t. anosmia
t. anxiety
t. aphasia
t. belief
t. chancre
t. communication stage
t. component
t. difference
t. epilepsy
t. hermaphroditism
t. insight
t. intersex
t. motivation
t. negative
t. perception
t. positive
t. self
t. symbolism
t. vertigo
trumped-up
trumpet
angel's t.
truncate
trunk ataxia
trust
atmosphere of t.
basic t.
blind t.
interpersonal t.
mutual t.
sense of t.
t. vs mistrust
trusting physician-patient relationship
trustworthiness
doubts of t.
unjustified doubts of t.
trustworthy
truth
t. disclosure
moment of t.
obscuring fundamental t.
t. serum
support, empathy and t. (SET)
tryptophan hydroxylase gene
tryst
TS
Tourette syndrome
transitional sleep
transsexual
T-score elevation
TSH
thyroid-stimulating hormone
thyrotropin-stimulating hormone
TST
total sleep time
TTM
trichotillomania
TTS
temporary threshold shift
TTV
therapeutic trial visit
tube
feeding t.
tuberculomania
tuberosa
tubulization
tularemic chancre
tulipmania
tumefacient
tumefaction
tumescence
nocturnal penile t. (NPT)
penile t.
tumescent
tumultuous
t. growth
t. life
tunnel vision
turbulence
chronic psychosocial t.
family t.
marital t.
psychosocial t.
turbulent
turf
turgid
turkomania
turmoil
adolescent t.
depressive t.
emotional t.
turn
t. around
t. away
t. back
t. in
turnabout
turned-on
turning
t. against self (TAS)
t. aggression against self
turpitude
moral t.
turricephaly
tussive
TVD
transmissible virus dementia
twice-born

twilight
t. attack
t. confusional state
t. epilepsy
t. sleep
t. thirst
t. vision
twin
biovular t.'s
t. concordance
conjoined t.'s
dizygotic t.'s
fraternal t.'s
identical t.'s
t. language
monozygotic t.'s (MZ)
t. research
same-sex t.'s
t. separation
Siamese t.'s
t. studies
twinship transference
twirling of object
twisted mouth
twisting
tongue t.
twitch
facial t.
focal t.
involuntary t.
muscle t.
rhythmic t.
twitching
muscle t.
two-faced
two-timer
type
t. A, B behavior
t. A, B personality
actively aggressive reaction t.
adenoid t.
affective reaction t.
aggressive predatory t.
apoplectic t.
asthenic constitutional t.
athletic constitutional t.
attention deficit disorder, residual t.
attention deficit hyperactivity disorder, combined t.
attention deficit hyperactivity disorder, predominantly hyperactive-impulsive t.
attitude t.
attitudinal t.
basic personality t.
behavior t.
blood t.
body t.
bulimia nervosa, nonpurging t.
bulimia nervosa, purging t.
character t.
choleric t.
chronic t.
circumplex of premorbid personality t.'s
complex t.
constitutional t.
conversion disorder, mixed t.
conversion disorder, motor t.
conversion disorder, seizure t.
conversion disorder, sensory t.
dementia of Alzheimer t. (DAT)
depressed t.
t. 1, 2 diabetes
Don Juan t.
dysplastic constitutional t.
ectomorphic constitutional t.
eidetic t.
endomorphic constitutional t.
erotic t.
erotomanic t.
explicit t.
exploiting t.
extroverted t.
family t.
functional t.
grandiose t.
hypochondriasis with poor insight t.
idiotropic t.
t. I, II alcoholic
t. I, II error
t. indicator
introverted t.
intuitive t.
irrational t.
jealous t.
Kretschmer t.
libidinal t.
linear t.
melancholic constitutional t.
mesomorphic constitutional t.
mixed t.
noradrenaline dementia of Alzheimer t.

NOTES

type *(continued)*
nosotropic drug dementia of Alzheimer t.
objective t.
obsessional t.
obsessive-compulsive disorder with poor insight t.
paranoid reaction t.
persecutory t.
personality change due to general medical condition, aggressive t.
personality change due to general medical condition, aphasic t.
personality change due to general medical condition, disinhibited t.
personality change due to general medical condition, labile t.
personality change due to general medical condition, paranoid t.
phlegmatic constitutional t.
physique t.
primary degenerative dementia of Alzheimer t. (PDDAT)
primary hypersomnia, recurrent t.
pyknic constitutional t.
reaction t.
reactive attachment disorder of infancy or early childhood, disinhibited t.
reactive attachment disorder of infancy or early childhood, inhibited t.
receiving t.
restricting t.
sanguine constitutional t.
schizoaffective disorder, bipolar t.
senile dementia of Alzheimer t. (SDAT)
social t.
somatic t.
t. specifier
substitutive reaction t.
thinking t.
t. 1, 2 trauma
undersocialized conduct disorder, aggressive t.
undersocialized conduct disorder, nonaggressive t.
unspecified t.
working t.

typhomania

typical
t. absence
t. absence seizure
t. age
t. antipsychotic
t. antipsychotic agent
t. behavior
t. neuroleptic
t. presentation
t. theme

typical-onset case

typify

typing
genetic t.
sex t.

typology
anxiety t.
personality disorder t.
t. of values

typomania

tyramine-rich food

tyrannical
t. behavior
t. decision making

tyrannism

tyranny of silence

tyrant
evil t.

tyrosine hydroxylase

UA
unauthorized absence
ubiquitin protein
ubiquitous
ubiquity
UCR
unconditioned reflex
unconditioned response
UCS
unconditioned stimulus
ugliness
imagined u.
Uhthoff sign
UL
unauthorized leave
ulcer
u. personality
psychogenic duodenal u.
psychogenic gastric u.
psychogenic peptic u.
ulegyria
Ullmann line
ulterior
u. motive
u. transaction
ultradian rhythm
ultradistant
ultrafastidious
ultrafeminine
ultraism
ultraliberal
ultramarginal zone
ultramasculine
ultrarapid metabolizer
ultrashort-acting barbiturate
ultrastructural study
ultraviolent
ultromotivity
ululation
umbrage
umbrageous
unabashed
unable
u. to follow instructions
u. to listen
unacceptable
u. action
u. behavior
u. feeling
u. impulse
u. thought
unaccompanied adolescent asylum seeker
unacknowledged victim
unadulterated
unaffective
unaggressive
u. conduct disorder
u. undersocialized reaction
unaided augmentative communication
unalterable, inalterable
unaltered drug
unambiguous measure
unanalyzable
unanswered question
unanticipated crisis
unapproachable
unarmed
unarousable
unassertive
u. aggression
u. expression
unattached
unattained goal
unattended death
unattractive
unauthorized
u. absence (UA)
u. leave (UL)
unavailable
emotionally u.
unavoidable placement
unawareness of environment
unbearable
unbecoming
unbelievable storytelling
unbendable
unbiased
u. evaluation
u. information
unblinking stare
uncanny emotion
uncertain biological status
uncertainty
u. factor
fear of u.
u. level
uncertainty-arousal factor
uncharacteristic
u. behavior
u. outburst
uncharacteristically
uncinate
u. attack
u. convulsion
u. epilepsy
u. fit
u. seizure
uncivil
uncleanliness

U

unclear
u. diagnosis
u. etiology
Uncle Tomism
unclothed
uncluttered
uncomfortable feeling
uncomplaining
uncomplicated
u. alcohol withdrawal
u. arteriosclerotic dementia
u. arteriosclerotic psychosis
u. bereavement
u. presenile dementia
u. recovery
u. sedative, hypnotic, or anxiolytic withdrawal
u. senile dementia
uncomprehending
uncompromising
unconcernedness
unconditional positive regard
unconditioned
u. reflex (UCR)
u. response (UCR)
u. stimulus (UCS)
unconscionable
unconscious
u. cerebration
collective u.
u. concern
u. conflict
u. distress
u. emotion
u. factor
familial u.
u. fantasy
u. guilt
u. homosexuality
impersonal u.
u. instinctual impulse
u. memory
u. mental technique
u. motivation
u. need for punishment
personal u.
u. process
u. processing
u. rage
u. resistance
superpersonal u.
unconsciousness
absolute u.
conversion u.
u. conversion
unconsolable
unconsummated marriage
uncontrollability
stressor u.
uncontrollable
u. action
u. anxiety
u. compulsion
u. crying
u. laughter
u. quality
u. sleep attack
u. thought
uncontrolled
u. laughter
u. worry
unconventional
uncooperative patient
uncoordinated
u. gait
u. motor skill
uncovering technique
uncriticalness
uncued
u. behavior
u. panic attack
undauntable
undeniable
under
u. the counter
knuckle u.
u. the skin
snow u.
u. the table
underachievement disorder
underachiever
underage gambling
underarousal
underclass
undercontrolled
undercover
undercurrent
undercutting
underdeveloped
underdiagnosed sequela
underdog
undereducated
underestimate
underestimating
u. danger
u. risk
underestimation
underfocused
undergraduate education
underhanded
underinsured
underlie
underload
information u.
underlying
u. condition
u. depression
u. emotional issue

u. medical illness
u. organic etiology
u. psychological manifestation
u. structure
undermine
undermining
undernourished
undernutrition
underpayment
underprepared
underprivileged
underproductive speech
underrate
underreact
underreporting
underrepresented minority
underscore
undersexed
undersocialized
u. aggressive reaction
u. conduct behavior
u. conduct disorder, aggressive type
u. conduct disorder, nonaggressive type
u. disorder
u. nonaggressive reaction
u. runaway reaction
u. socialized disturbance
understandable
understanding
clinical u.
consensual u.
core consensual u.
empathic u.
shared u.
theoretical u.
word u.
understatement
understimulation
u. theory
u. therapy
understood
understudy
undertake
undertone
undertreated
undesirable
social u.
undetermined origin (UO)
undeviating
undifferentiated
u. attention-deficit disorder
chronic u.
u. effect
u. schizophrenia
schizophrenic reaction, acute u. (SR/AU)
schizophrenic reaction, chronic u. (SR/CU)
u. somatoform disorder
u. wholeness
undifferentiated-type
u.-t. conduct disorder
u.-t. schizophrenia
u.-t. schizophrenic disorder
undinism
undirected
u. aggression
u. thinking
u. violent fantasy
undisciplined self-conflict
undisturbed nocturnal sleep
undoing defense mechanism
undoubtedly
undressed
undressing
paradoxical u.
undue social anxiety
unduly
unearned
unease
unemotional
u. learning task
u. thought
unemployable
unemployment
u. insurance
u. problem
unencapsulated joint receptor
unencumbered
unendurable psychological pain
unequal distribution
unequivocal change in functioning
unethical behavior
unexpected
u. behavior
u. panic attack
u. reaction
u. response
unexplainable
unexplained
u. absence from work
u. bruising
u. pain
u. pain complaint

NOTES

unexplained *(continued)*
u. skin lesion
u. tearfulness
unexpressive
unfaithful
unfaltering
unfamiliar
u. face
u. place
unfathered
unfathomable
unfavorable
unfazed
unfeeling
unfinished
unfit
unflappable
unfocused delirium
unforgiving
unformed
u. auditory hallucination
u. image
u. visual hallucination
unformism
unforthcomingness
unfounded complaint
unfriendly
ungiving parent
ungodly
ungrateful
unhappiness
u. and misery disorder
pattern of pervasive u.
pervasive u.
unhappy
u. facial expression
u. love affair
u. memory
unhealthy
unhinge
unhygienic
u. bathroom habit
u. grooming
unifactorial approach
unifamilial
unification in wit
uniformly progressive deterioration
unifying force
unilateral
u. abductor paralysis
u. adductor paralysis
u. anesthesia
u. brief pulse ECT
u. decision
u. ECT treatment
u. focus
u. hermaphroditism
u. migraine
u. migraine headache
u. nondominant-hemisphere ECT
u. organic neglect
u. seizure
u. sine wave ECT
u. spatial neglect
u. visual neglect
unimaginable
unimportant
unimproved
uninhibited
u. behavior
u. motor planning
u. neurogenic bladder
uninsured patient
unintelligible speech
unintended
u. effect
u. sleep
unintentional
u. daytime sleep episode
u. death
unintentionally produced symptom
uninterested
uninterrupted episode
unio mystica
union
American Civil Liberties U. (ACLU)
mystic u.
uniparental disomy
unipolar
u. chronic depression
u. disorder
u. major depression
u. mania
u. manic-depressive psychosis
u. patient
u. recurrent depression
unique
u. characteristic
u. lexicon
u. pedigree structure
u. trait
u. vocabulary
uniqueness
sense of u.
unisex
Unisom
U. Nighttime Sleep Aid
U. with Pain Relief Sleep Aid
unit
acute adolescent inpatient u.
acute care u. (ACU)
addictive disease u. (ADU)
adolescent inpatient u.
adult u.
California drug-endangered children's u.
child inpatient u.

communication u.
day treatment u.
delirium u.
emergency u. (EU)
family u.
inpatient u.
intensive care u. (ICU)
intensive treatment u. (ITU)
life change u. (LCU)
locked hospital u.
maximum-security u.
memory for symbolic u. (MSU)
polysensory u.
psychiatric u.
psychiatric intensive care u. (PICU)
relational u.
u. restriction
state hospital children's u. (SHCU)
training u.
treatment u.
work-for-pay u.

unitary
u. consciousness
u. disorder

United
U. Nations Office on Drugs and Crime
U. States (US)
U. States Pharmacopeia (USP)
U. States Public Health Service (USPHS)
U. States-United Kingdom Study
U. States vs. Brawner

unitization

unity
functional u.
u. and fusion

universalis
alopecia u.

universalism

universality

universalization

universals
substantive u.

universal symbol

unjustified
u. doubt of loyalty
u. doubts of trustworthiness

unkempt
u. appearance
u. manner

unkindly

unknowing

unknown
u. language
u. meaning
u. substance-induced mood disorder

unlawful behavior

unlearning

unlicensed handgun

unlocked seclusion

unloved

unmarried

unmedicated patient

unmentionable

unmerciful

unmet
u. dependence
u. dependency need

unmistakable

unmitigated echolalia

unmodified ECT therapy

unmotivated

unnatural
u. cheerfulness
u. motor behavior

unnecessarily

unnecessary
u. medication
u. sedation

unnerve

unobtrusive measure

unorganized

unpalatable

unpardonable

unplanned pregnancy

unpleasant
u. dream
u. hallucination
u. mood
u. withdrawal symptom

unpleasantness
relative u.

unpleasure

unpredictability

unpredictable
u. act of violence
u. agitation
u. mood change
u. parenting

unprepared

unpretentious

unprincipled

unproductive mania

unprofessional

unpromising

NOTES

unprotected
u. intercourse
u. sex
unpunished
unpurposeful behavior
unquestionable
unquiet
unravel
unrealistic
u. expectation
u. worry
unreality
feeling of u.
idea of u.
unreasonable
u. belief
u. compulsion
u. demand
u. fear
u. idea
unreasoning
unrecognized
unrefined motor skill
unrelated
u. diagnosis
u. thought
unrelenting pain
unreliability
unreliable
unrelieved agitation
unremitting
unresolved
u. bereavement
u. conflict
u. grief
u. loss
unresponsive
u. patient
u. state
unresponsiveness
emotional u.
unrest
unrestricted diet
unruffled
unruly child
unsafe sexual behavior
unsanctioned
culturally u.
u. response
unsanitary drug administration
unsatisfactory relationship
unsavory
unsayable
unscientific
unscrupulous
unseasonable
unseen reality
unselective observation
unselfish
unsettled
unshakable
u. belief
u. preoccupation
unshaven
unsightly
unskilled
unsociable
unsocialized
u. aggressive disorder
u. aggressive reaction
u. childhood truancy
u. disturbance of thought
unsophisticated
unsound business venture
unspeakable
unspecified
bipolar I disorder, most recent episode u.
u. depression
u. mental disorder
u. mental disorder, nonpsychotic
u. mental retardation
mental retardation, severity u.
u. mood episode
u. psychological factor
u. schizophrenia
u. substance dependence
u. type
unspecified-type
u.-t. delusion
u.-t. dyssomnia
unstable
u. affect
u. attachment
u. behavior
emotionally u.
u. interpersonal relationship
u. lifestyle
u. mood
u. personality
u. self-image
stably u.
unsteadiness
postural u.
unsteady gait
unstoppable flow of speech
unstructured
u. interview
u. verbal information
u. verbal material
unsuccessful
unswerving
unsympathetic attitude
unsystematized delusion
untenable
unthinkable
untimely
u. death

u. demise
u. pregnancy
untiring
untouchable
untouched
untoward
u. cholinergic effect
u. outcome
untreated
u. episode
u. psychiatric illness
u. psychosis
u. sequela
untriggered agitation
untroubled
untrue
untruthful
unusual
u. behavior
u. detail response (Dd)
u. dressing
u. facial expression
u. fatigue
u. hand movement
u. language
u. manner
u. perceptual experience
u. personality
u. punishment
u. rare detail response (dr)
u. sleep posture
u. thought content
unveiling
unwanted
u. anal sex
u. child
u. oral sex
u. pregnancy
u. sexual advance
u. sexual attention
u. sexual contact
u. sexual talk
u. sexual touching
u. vaginal sex
unwarranted idea
unwieldy
unwilling
unwise dieting
unwitting
unwonted
unworldly
unworthiness
feeling of u.
unworthy
unyielding
UO
undetermined origin
up
act up
acting up
ball up
up in clouds
damming up
difficulty waking up
dream up
drum up
dry up
face up
fed up
frame up
gang up
knocked up
mixed up
open up
rub up
send up
shut up
speak up
talk up
tear up
throw up
washed up
upbeat
upbringing
religious u.
update
up-front
upheaval
emotional u.
uphill
uphold
uplift
upper
u. abdominal periosteal reflex
u. bound
u. crust
u. hand
u. motor neuron
upper-class
uppity
up-regulated
up-regulation
receptor u.-r.
up-regulation/down-regulation hypothesis
uproar
uproot

NOTES

uprooted psychology
uprooting neurosis
ups and downs
upset
emotional u.
emotionally u.
excessively u.
gastrointestinal u.
mental u.
upsetting
upstanding
upswap
uptake site
uptight
up-to-date medication
upward
u. masking
u. mobility
upwardly mobile
UR
utilization review
uranism
uranoplasty
urban
u. crisis
u. psychiatry
urbanite
urbanization
urchin
ur-defense
uremia
uremic
u. convulsion
u. encephalopathy
u. seizure
urethral
u. anxiety
u. eroticism
u. phase
u. stage
urge
anomalous sexual u.
craving-related u.
ego-syntonic gambling u.
u. to gamble
gambling u.
inappropriate u.
u. incontinence
intense sexual u.
intrusive u.
involuntary premonitory u.
masochistic sexual u.
mental u.
premonitory u.
self-destructive u.
sexual u.
urgency
urinary
u. continence
u. incontinence
urinate
urine
dirty u.
drug-negative u.
u. drug screen
U. Luck adulterant for urine drug screen
opioid-positive u.
u. test
u. toxicology
u. toxicology screen
white turbid u.
uriposia
Urning theory
uroclepsia
urocrisia, urocrisis
urogenital reflex
urolagnia
urophilia
urticaria
giant u.
psychogenic u.
US
United States
US Air Force
US Army
US Coast Guard
US Marines
US Navy
Sex Information and Education Council of the US (SIECUS)
usage
idiomatic u.
tobacco u.
use
adjunctive u.
adolescent alcohol u.
adolescent drug u.
alcohol u.
u. of alias
caffeine u.
chemical of u.
chronic u.
clinical u.
compulsive substance u.
employee drug u.
excessive drug u.
excessive laxative u.
u. of expletives
fatal complications of illicit drug u.
frequency of drug u.
general medical u.
hard-drug u.
history of tobacco u.
illegal drug u.

illicit drug u.
illicit opiate u.
intranasal cocaine u.
intravenous drug u.
IV drug u.
long-term heavy u.
medical u.
neuroleptic u.
nicotine u.
nonpathological substance u.
opioid u.
parental alcohol u.
past month alcohol u.
pathological Internet u.
pathologic substance u.
potentially fatal complications of illicit drug u.
prenatal illicit drug u.
problematic Internet u.
u. of profanity in public
psychoactive substance u.
recreational drug u.
routine u.
substance u.
tobacco u.

user
caffeine u.
chronic cocaine u.
chronic ethanol u.
cocaine u.
drug u.
ethanol u.
heroin u.
injecting drug u. (IDU)
intravenous drug u.
juvenile drug u.
needle u.
nicotine u.
regular caffeine u.
regular drug u.
tobacco u.

USP
United States Pharmacopeia

USPHS
United States Public Health Service

usual
u. behavior
u. childhood illness
u. mood

usurp

utilitarian
u. principle
u. theory

utilitarianism
act u.
hedonistic u.
negative u.
pluralistic u.
rule u.

utility
expected u. (EU)

utilization
u. behavior
evaluation u.
medical u.
u. review (UR)
u. review committee
u. technique

utilizer
high u.

Utopia

utricular reflex

utterance

uxorial

uxoricide

uxorious

NOTES

v, vs
versus
VA
Veteran's Administration
vacant
v. spell
v. stare
vaccination
vache
coitus à la v.
vacillate
vacuo
hydrocephalus ex v.
vacuous affect
vacuum
v. activity
existential v.
v. headache
vagabondage
vagabond neurosis
vagal attack
vagarious
vagina, pl. **vaginae**
v. dentata
vaginal
v. envy
v. father
v. hypesthesia
v. orgasm
v. penetration
v. plethysmograph
vaginam
per v.
vaginate
vaginism
vaginismus, vaginism
lifelong-type v.
psychic v.
vagolysis
vagolytic
vagomimetic
vagotomy
vagotonia
vagotropic
vagovagal
vagrancy
vagrant
vague
v. communication
v. complaint
nouvelle v.
v. perplexity
v. speech
v. thinking
vagueness
vagus
v. nerve
v. nerve stimulation (VNS)
vail
vain
vainglorious
vainglory
Valdoxan
valence
emotional v.
normal v.
positive v.
valerate
amyl v.
valerian
valetudinarian
valetudinary
valid
v. consent
v. diagnosis
v. information
validating variable
validation
v. communication pattern
consensual v.
v. strategy
supportive v.
v. therapy
validity
clinical v.
v. coefficient
concurrent v.
construct v.
content v.
convergent and divergent v.
criterion v.
criterion-related v.
descriptive v.
discriminant v.
ecological v.
empirical v.
etiological v.
external v.
face v.
factorial v.
v. indicator profile
internal v.
internalized v.
intervening v.
item v.
known group v.
predictive v.
psychometric v.
Valleix point
valor

valuable
value
- acculturation problem with expression of political v.
- acculturation problem with expression of religious v.
- aesthetic v.
- affective v.
- Allport-Vernon-Linzey study of v.'s
- being v.
- confusion of v.'s
- core v.'s
- critical v.
- cultural v.
- educational v.
- face v.
- fluidity v.
- foreign v.
- v. history
- idealized v.
- internal v.
- v. judgment
- moral v.
- nontrivial v.
- p v.
- parental v.
- personal v.
- political v.
- predictive v.
- prognostic v.
- religious v.'s
- self-reference v.
- sentimental v.
- sharing of v.'s
- social v.
- spiritual v.
- status v.
- Study of V.'s (SV)
- symbolic v.
- v. system
- traditional v.
- typology of v.'s
- Wilder law of initial v.

value-laden comment
valve
- safety v.

vamp
vampirism
- parasitic v.

vandal
vandalism
- sexual v.

vandalize
van der Kolk law
vanillylmandelic acid (VMA)
vaniteuse
- folie v.

vanity
Vantaa depression study (VDS)
vantage
vapor
- chemical v.

variability
- behavioral v.
- drug concentration v.
- metabolic v.
- trait v.

variable
- antecedent v.
- antecedent-consequence v.
- autochthonous v.
- v. behavior
- biopsychosocial v.
- clinical v.
- cognitive v.
- continuous v.
- criterion v.
- demographic v.
- dependent v.
- dynamic v.
- experimental v.
- health-related v.
- independent v.
- index v.
- v. interval (VI)
- intervening v.
- memory v.
- moderator v.
- organic v.
- organismic v.
- outcome v.
- predictor v.
- psychiatric v.
- quantitative v.
- random v.
- v. ratio (VR)
- v. reinforcement
- situational v.
- sleep continuity v.
- sociodemographic v.
- validating v.

variable-interval reinforcement schedule
variance
- analysis of v. (ANOVA)
- between-group v.
- v. components analysis
- error v.

variant
- bizarre v.
- emotional v.
- epileptic v.

variate
variation
- cerebral hemodynamic v.
- chance v.
- circadian v.
- coefficient of v. (CV)
- conative negative v. (CNV)

contingent negative v. (CNV)
cultural v.
diurnal mood v.
interindividual v.
negative v.
physiologic functional v.
reverse diurnal v.
situational tic v.

varices
gastric v.

variety of sexual behaviors
varimax rotation
vascular
v. dementia
v. dementia with delirium
v. dementia with delusions
v. dementia with depressed mood
v. depression
v. headache
v. muscle
v. neurosyphilis
v. territory

vasculogenic loss of erectile functioning
vase
Rubin v.

vasectomy
vasoactive intestinal peptide (VIP)
vasoconstriction
caffeine-induced v.
sympathetic nervous system-medicated v.

vasoconstrictive action
vasogenic shock
vasomotor
v. absence
v. component
v. epilepsy
v. headache
v. imbalance
v. instability
v. spasm
v. syncope

vasoneurosis
vasopressor syncope
vasoreflex
vasostimulant
vasovagal
v. attack
v. attack of Gowers
v. epilepsy
v. syncope
v. syndrome

vaunt
VBR
ventricle-to-brain ratio

VC
visual communication

VD
venereal disease

VDR
vitamin D receptor

VDS
Vantaa depression study

VDT
visual distortion test

vécu
déjà v.

veganism
vegan vegetarian diet
vegetarian diet
vegetarianism
vegetate
vegetative
v. level
v. life
v. nervous system
v. neurosis
v. retreat
v. sign
v. state
v. symptom

vehemence
vehement
vehicle
v. for communication
v. fear

veil
aqueduct v.

veiled threat
velar assimilation
velars
backing to v.

velleity
vellicate
vellication
velnacrine
velocity
nerve conduction v.

vendetta
venereal
v. bubo
v. disease (VD)
v. sore

venereophobia
veneris ardor
vengeance

NOTES

vengeful
venial sin
venipuncture
stigma of v.
venomous
venter
abactus v.
ventilate concern
ventilation of feelings
ventilatory
ventral
v. amygdala fugal pathway
v. amygdaloid fugal projection
v. paralimbic region
ventricle
lateral v.
v. size
ventricle-to-brain ratio (VBR)
ventricular
v. arrhythmia
v. dysphonia
v. system
v. widening
ventriculi (*pl. of* ventriculus)
ventriculitis
ventriculography
ventriculoscopy
ventriculus, pl. **ventriculi**
ventromedial
v. cortex
v. hypothalamus
v. prefrontal cortex of brain
venture
unsound business v.
venturesome
VEP
visual evoked potential
VER
visual evoked response
vera
melancholia v.
neuralgia facialis v.
veracious
veracity
verbal
v. abuse
v. aggression
v. agitation
v. agnosia
v. agraphia
v. alexia
v. amnesia
v. aphasia
v. apraxia
v. assault
v. association
v. automatism
v. aversion therapy
v. behavior
v. communication
v. comprehension factor
v. comprehension index
v. conceptualization ability
v. cue
v. deficit
v. expression
v. fluency
v. generalization
v. information
v. insult
v. intellectual functioning
v. intelligence
v. intervention
v. language quotient
v. leakage
v. learning
v. masochism
v. material
v. mediation
v. memory exercise
v. memory impairment
v., numerical, and reasoning (VNR)
v. outburst
v. paired associates
v. paraphasia
v. perceptual speed
v. perseveration
v. play
v. reasoning
v. redirection
v. regression
v. reinforcement
v. slur
v. suggestion
v. technique
v. thought
v. weighted sum score
v. working memory
verbal-auditory agnosia
verbalis
asemasia v.
verbalism
verbalization of feelings
verbalize
verbalizing
inappropriate v.
verbally dramatic
verbal-visual agnosia
verbatim recall
verbiage
verbicide
verbigerate
verbigeration
hallucinatory v.
verbochromia
verbomania
verborum
verbose

verboten
verbous
verdict
guilty v.
veridical dream
verifiable
veritable
verity
vermicular
v. motion of tongue
v. movement
verminous
vermis
anterior v.
verna
Amanita v.
vernacular
veroomania
versatile
versatility
Versed
versenate
version
episode v.
versus (v, vs)
vertebral cervical instability
vertebrobasilar insufficiency
vertical
v. conflict
v. mobility
v. nystagmus
v. transmission
v. vertigo
vertiginosa
epilepsia v.
vertiginosus
status v.
vertiginous
v. epilepsy
v. seizure
vertigo
Charcot v.
chronic v.
endemic paralytic v.
epileptic v.
essential v.
galvanic v.
height v.
horizontal v.
hysterical v.
laryngeal v.
lateral v.
mechanical v.
nocturnal v.
objective v.
organic v.
paralyzing v.
postural v.
psychogenic v.
rotary v.
sham movement v.
subjective v.
systematic v.
true v.
vertical v.
voltaic v.
vesania
vesicle
synaptic v.
vestibular
v. hallucination
v. migraine
v. movement
v. nerve
vestibuloequilibratory control
vestibulospinal
veteran
Bosnian army v.
combat v.
Desert Storm v.
Iraq v.
Korean War v.
psychotic v.
Vietnam v.
Vietnam-era v.
war v.
women v.'s
Yom Kippur War v.
Veteran's Administration (VA)
vex
vexatious
VI
variable interval
visual imagery
viable
v. alternative
v. synapse
Viagra
vial
vibrant
vibration
forced v.
v. syndrome
vibrator
electrical v.

NOTES

V

vibratory
v. massage
v. sensibility
vibrotactile
v. response
v. threshold
VIBS, vibs
vocabulary, information, block design, similarity
VIC
visual communication
vicarious
v. conditioning
v. function
v. learning
v. liability
v. living
v. trial and error (VTE)
v. violence
vice
vice-like pain
vicious
v. circle
v. cycle
vicissitude
instinctual v.
v.'s of life
victim
v. abuse
accident v.
acknowledged v.
crime v.
v. of criminal violence
cyberstalking v.
depressed suicide v.
disaster v.
v. of domestic violence
v. empathy
female v.
home invasion v.
intended v.
land mine v.
male v.
potential suicide v.
primary v.
v. psychology
rape v.
v. recidivism
v. role
stalking v.
suicide v.
v. syndrome
unacknowledged v.
victimization
multiple v.'s
victimize
victimized teen
victimology in abuse
victorianism
video
v. feedback
v. game violence
v. lottery terminal (VLT)
v. lottery terminal gambling
v. therapy
videoconferencing
videotape
Vienna Psychoanalytic Society
Viet Cong
Vietnam
V. syndrome
V. veteran
V. War
Vietnam-era veteran
Vietnamese refugee
view
point of v.
Pollyanna-like v.
stilted v.
viewing
viewless
viewpoint
alternative v.
biologic v.
economic v.
genetic v.
health v.
vigil
coma v.
fatiguing v.
vigilambulism
vigilance
v. deficit
perceptual v.
visuomotor v.
vigilant
vigilante
vigility of attention
vignette
vigor
vigorous
vile
vilification
vilify
villainous
villa system
vincible
vindicate
vindictive
vine
matrimony v.
violate
violated
sexually v.
violating behavior
violation
boundary v.
civil rights v.

ethics v.
nonsexual boundary v.
probation v.
restraining order v.
v. of rules
sexual boundary v.

violator
norm v.

violence
act of v.
activity of v.
adolescent risk for v.
alcohol-related risk for v.
alleviating v.
American Academy of Pediatrics Task Force on V.
antecedent of v.
arrest for v.
cognitive v.
community v.
crime of v.
dating v.
domestic v. (DV)
drug-related v.
exposure to v.
extreme act of v.
extreme level of v.
family v.
good kid v.
graphic v.
history of v.
impending v.
inpatient v.
intimate partner v.
juvenile v.
likelihood of v.
manifestation of v.
marital v.
mass v.
media v.
motion picture v.
National Resource Center on Domestic V.
occupational v.
origin of v.
pathogen of v.
peer support for v.
perpetrator of v.
personalizing v.
v. potential
predatory v.
v. prediction
predisposing socioculture factors for v.
preemptive v.
v. prevention
prior v.
random act of v.
recent v.
repetitive v.
v. risk
risk factor for v.
sexual v.
sign of impending v.
v. in stalking
teen v.
teenage v.
television v.
terrorist v.
v. theory
threat of v.
threatening v.
unpredictable act of v.
vicarious v.
victim of criminal v.
victim of domestic v.
video game v.
witness to repetitive v.
workplace v.
youth v.

violence-promoting factor

violent
v. act
v. acting out
v. acts on television
v. adolescent
v. agitation
v. child
v. command hallucination
v. conduct disorder
v. crime
v. criminal behavior
v. death
v. delinquent
v. fantasy
v. figure
v. history
v. ideation
v. intent
v. media
v. offender
v. offense
v. outburst
v. past
v. pediatric patient

NOTES

violent *(continued)*
v. personal assault
v. rearing
v. resistance
sexually v.
v. stalker
v. temper
v. theme
v. thought
VIP
vasoactive intestinal peptide
voluntary interruption of pregnancy
VIP syndrome
viraginity
viral hepatitis
virgin
v. cleansing
v. fear
V. Mary vision
virginal anxiety
Virginia Adult Twin Study of Psychiatric and Substance Use Disorders
virginity
v. scruple
v. taboo
virgophrenia
virile
molimen climacteriuhm v.
virilescence
virilia
virilism
virility
virilization
virtuality
virtual reality therapy
virtue
cardinal v.
easy v.
v. ethics
virtuous
virulence
virulent
virus
Epstein-Barr v. (EBV)
herpes simplex v.
human immunodeficiency v. (HIV)
slow v.
VIS
vocational interest schedule
visage
scanning v.
visceral
v. anesthesia
v. disorder
v. emotional state
v. epilepsy
v. hallucination
v. learning
v. nervous system
v. neurosis
v. sense
visceromotor pathway
viscerotonia
viscosity
v. of libido
v. personality
social v.
visibility
visible agitation
visile
vision
altered v.
beatific v.
binocular v.
blurred v.
blurring of v.
central v.
darkening v.
v. disparity
double v.
entopic v.
field of v.
foveal v.
hemifield of v.
hypnagogic v.
impaired v.
inner v.
patterning v.
phantom v.
photopic v.
stereoscopic v.
subjective v.
tunnel v.
twilight v.
Virgin Mary v.
visionary
visionism
visionless
visit
baseline v.
clinical v.
conjugal v.
followup v.
home v.
postbaseline v.
reason for v.
therapeutic trial v. (TTV)
trial v.
weekend v.
visitant
visitation
conjugal v.
v. rights
visiting nurse
vista response
visual
v. accommodation

v. acuity
v. agnosia
v. aid
v. alertness
v. alexia
v. amnesia
v. aphasia
v. association cortex
v. attention
v. aura
v. center
v. closure
v. communication (VC, VIC)
v. cortical area
v. cue
v. discrimination
v. disorientation reaction
v. distortion
v. distortion test (VDT)
v. epilepsy
v. evoked potential (VEP)
v. evoked response (VER)
v. extinction
v. field
v. field construction
v. field cut
v. field defect
v. field disturbance
v. hallucination
v. hallucination denial syndrome
v. hallucination syndrome
v. hearing
v. illusion
v. image
v. imagery (VI)
v. inattention
v. letter dysgnosia
v. literacy
v. memory impairment
v. neglect
v. number dysgnosia
v. obstruction
v. pattern recognition
v. perception
v. perceptual deficit
v. perceptual skill
v. perceptual speed
v. processing
v. prodrome
v. pursuit movement
v. radiation
v. region
v. representation strategy
v. reproduction
v. seizure
v. sensation
v. sensory modality
v. stimulation
v. stimulus
v. symptom
v. tracking
v. training
v. zone

visualization

visualize

visual-kinetic dissociation

visual-motor (*var. of* visuomotor)

visuoauditory

visuoconstructional ability

visuognosis

visuomotor, visual-motor

v. ability
v. coordination
v. impairment
v. problem-solving skill
v. task
v. vigilance

visuoperceptive defect

visuopsychic

visuosensory

visuospatial

v. ability
v. acalculia
v. agnosia
v. attention
v. disorder
v. disorientation
v. distortion
v. functioning
v. memory
v. problem solving
v. processing
v. scratch pad
v. stimulus

visuotopic

vita

la dolce v.

vital

élan v.
v. energy
v. sign (VS)
v. statistic

vitality

vitalize

vitam

intra v.

NOTES

vitamin
v. B, B12 deficiency
v. B12 neuropathy
v. deficiency-associated dementia
v. D receptor (VDR)
v. E
v. therapy
vituperate
vituperative
vivacious
vivid
v. dream
v. dream image
v. dream recall
v. hallucination
v. nightmare
vividness
vivify
Vivitrol
vivo
ex v.
exposure in v.
in v.
inter v.'s
vixen
vizard
VLT
video lottery terminal
VMA
vanillylmandelic acid
VNR
verbal, numerical, and reasoning
VNS
vagus nerve stimulation
vocabulary
active v.
v., information, block design, similarity (VIBS, vibs)
v. language quotient
passive v.
poor v.
v. skill
unique v.
vocal
v. abuse
v. amusia
v. attack
v. band
v., chronic motor, or tic disorder
v. pitch abnormality
v. tic
vocalization
involuntary v.
motor v.
nonrhythmic v.
rapid v.
recurrent v.
repetitive v.
stereotyped v.
sudden v.
vocalize
vocation
vocational
v. achievement
v. adjustment
v. appraisal
v. choice
v. counseling
v. evaluation
v. functioning
v. goal setting
v. guidance
v. identity
v. interest schedule (VIS)
v. maladjustment
v. outcome
v. performance
psychological, social, and v. (PSV)
v. rehabilitation (VR)
v. rehabilitation and education (VR&E)
v. service
v. strain
v. training
vociferate
vociferous
Vogt-Spielmeyer idiocy
voguish
voice
active v.
adolescent v.
altered v.
breathy v.
chest v.
v. commenting
condescending tone of v.
conversational v.
v. conversing
disapproving v.
discordance of v.
v. disorder
esophageal v.
eunuchoid v.
gravel v.
hallucinated v.
hearing v.'s
high-pitched v.
hysterical v.'s
v. inside head
v. intonation
monotone v.
monotonous v.
muted v.
negative v.
v. outside head
panicky v.
pejorative v.

quavering v.
shaking v.
soundless v.
threatening v.
tone of v.
transsexual v.
trembling v.

voiceless

voiceprint

voicing threat

void fear

voiding

inappropriate v.

voilá

vol

monomanie du v.

volatile

v. disposition
v. hydrocarbon
v. personality
v. situation
v. solvent
v. solvent dependence
v. temper

volition

act and v.
derailment of v.
hedonic v.

volitional

v. capacity
v. control impairment
v. drinking
v. movement
v. tremor

volley

voltage-gated

voltaic vertigo

volte-face

volubility

excessive v.

voluble

volume

amygdala v.
blood v.
brain v.
cortical v.
frontal lobe v.
hippocampal raw v.
intracranial brain v.
intracranial raw v.
mean intracranial raw v.
mean normalized whole brain v.
normalized whole brain v.
prefrontal cortical v.
raw v.
total brain v.
whole brain raw v.

volumetric loss

volumetry

MRI v.

voluntarism

voluntary

v. active imagining
v. admission
v. behavior
v. commitment
v. control
v. dehydration
v. euthanasia
v. hospitalization
v. hysterical overbreathing
v. impulse
v. interruption of pregnancy (VIP)
v. motion
v. motor functioning
v. movement peculiarity
v. muscle movement
v. mutism
v. napping phenomenon
v. retention
v. seclusion
v. sensory functioning
v. social withdrawal without psychosis
v. time-out

voluptuous

volupty

vomit

need to v.

vomiting

cyclic v.
cyclical psychogenic v.
v. fear
nausea and v. (N&V)
nervous v.
psychogenic cyclical v.
v. reflex
self-induced v.

vomitory

vomiturition

vomitus

von

v. Domarus principle
v. Graefe sign
v. Hippel-Lindau disease
v. Knorring criterion

NOTES

von *(continued)*
v. Zerssen circumplex model of premorbid personality
voodoo death
voodooism
voodooistic
voracious appetite
vorbeireden
votary
votive
voulu
déjà v.
vow
celibacy v.
marriage v.'s
solemn v.
vowel assimilation
voxel
cerebral v.
contiguous v.
voyeur
voyeurism
adolescent v.
v. paraphilia
voyeuristic
v. activity
v. sexual behavior
v. sexually arousing fantasy
voyeuse
VPCM
vulnerable populations conceptual model
VR
variable ratio
vocational rehabilitation
VR&E
vocational rehabilitation and education
VS
vital sign
vs (*var. of* v)
VTE
vicarious trial and error
vu
déjà vu
jamais vu
vulgaris
acne v.
Artemisia v.
vulgarism
vulgarity
vulgarize
vulgar language
vulnerability
danger-laden schema v.
emotional v.
genetic schizophrenia v.
narcissistic v.
predisposing v.
pretraumatic v.
putative adoptee v.
suicide v.
v. theory
v. threshold
vulnerable
v. child
v. child syndrome
emotionally v.
v. narcissism
v. populations conceptual model (VPCM)
Vulpian effect
vulpine
vulturous
vulvismus

W
whole response
WA
Workaholics Anonymous
waddling gait
wage
w. earner
living w.
wager
wagering
waggish
waif
wail
waiver
wakefulness
w. epoch
full w.
intermittent w.
midpontine w.
primary disorder of w.
quiet w.
resting w.
wakeful state
wake time
waking
w. EEG
w. frequency
w. hypnosis
w. numbness
walking disorder
wallerian
wallflower
wallow
wan
wand
NCP programming w.
wander
wandering
aimless w.
w. attention
w. cell
w. impulse
intrusive w.
w. mind
w. pain
w. thought
wanderlust
wane
wax and w.
wanton
war
w. baby
w. bride
consequences of w.
disabled by w.
w. footing
former prisoner of w.
w. game player
gang w.
w. gas
injury of w.
limited w.
mentally ill from w.
w. of nerves
w. neurosis
not prisoner of w. (NPOW)
nuclear w.
w. on drugs
w. on terrorism
w. power
prisoner of w. (POW)
psychological aspect of w.
threat of w.
w. veteran
Vietnam W.
world w.
World W. I (WWI)
World W. II (WWII)
Yom Kippur W.
w. zone
w. zone exposure
ward
disturbed w.
locked w.
long-stay w.
open w.
psychiatric w.
wardrobe
Wardrop method
warehousing
mental patient w.
warfare
ABC w.
atomic, biological, chemical w.
biologic w.
biologic and chemical w. (BCW)
chemical and biological w. (CBW)
chemical, radiological, and biological w.
gang w.
guerrilla w.
psychological w. (PW)
trench w.
warlike
warlock
warm
w. contact
w. effector
failure to w.
w. sensitivity

W

warmhearted
warm-sensitive neuron
warmth
paradoxical w.
warn
duty to w.
failure to w.
warning
black box w.
Tarasoff w.
warp
warrant
bench w.
death w.
search w.
war-related stress
warrior
wartime
war-wounded refugee
wary
washed
w. out
w. up
washing
repetitive hand w.
Washington Psychiatric Foundation
washout
drug w.
WASP
White Anglo-Saxon Protestant
World Association for Social Psychiatry
waspish
wastage
air w.
wastebasket diagnosis
wasted
wasting
w. palsy
w. paralysis
watchful
watchfulness
frozen w.
watching
repetitive w.
watchspring theory
watchword
water
w. balance
w. balance in schizophrenia
body w.
w. deprivation
w. drinking
w. intoxication
w. on brain
water-seeking behavior
watershed
w. area
w. infarction
waveform
brief pulse w.
early component w.
pulse w.
waveshape
waving
hand w.
waxen
wax and wane
waxy flexibility
way
maladaptive w.
parting of w.'s
set in one's w.'s
1-way mirror
4-way
4-w. session
4-w. therapy
wayward
weak
w. ego
w. ego control
w. parent
w. stress
weak-hearted
weakling
weak-minded
weak-mindedness
weakness
color w.
ego w.
w. fear
localized w.
psychological w.
strengths and w.'s
weak-willed
wealth
delusion of w.
inflated w.
wealthy
wean
weaning
weapon
access to w.
assault w.
assault with a deadly w. (ADW)
attacked with w.
availability of w.
biologic w.
carrying a w.
chemical w.
w.'s hoard
possession of w.
weaponry
wear down
weariless
wearisome
weary
weasling

weathered
weatherworn
weaving
head w.
Web counseling
Weber-Fechner law
wedding
w. night
shotgun w.
Wedensky facilitation
wedlock
out of w.
Wednesday Evening Society
weed
week
drinking days per w.
weekend
w. drinker
w. drinking
w. headache
w. hospital
w. hospitalization
w. neurosis
w. parent
w. pass
w. visit
Weekly
Prozac W.
weeping
overt w.
weepy
we-group
weigh down
weight
beta w.
birth w.
body w.
brain w.
w. concern
decreased brain w.
w. discrimination
failure to gain w.
w. gain
w. gain potential
ideal body w. (IBW)
w. issue
w. liability
w. lifter
w. loss
w. loss maintenance
w. loss therapy
w. maintenance
w. management
w. perception
w. regulation
target w.
W. Watchers diet
weight-control program
weighted-harm principle
weighted sum score
weighting
item w.
weight-loss program
weight-neutral psychotic medication
Weir
W. Mitchell therapy
W. Mitchell treatment
weird behavior
welfare
w. emotion
Health, Education, and W. (HEW)
International Committee on Social W. (ICSW)
live on w.
w. organization
social w.
w. system
well
w. adjusted for age
w. groomed
w. oriented
well-advised
well-articulated speech
well-being
emotional w.-b.
global w.-b.
sense of w.-b.
subjective w.-b.
well-conditioned
well-defined
well-delineated psychiatric disorder
well-formed
w.-f. delusion
w.-f. outcome
well-groomed
well-motivated
wellness
w. principle
sense of w.
well-off
well-read
well-rounded
well-spoken
well-systematized delusional system
well-systemized delusion
well-timed

W

NOTES

well-to-do
welsh
welt
weltmerism
weltschmerz
wench
Werdnig-Hoffmann disease
werewolf
Wernicke
W. aphasia
W. 22, 39, 40 area
W. center
W. cramp
W. dementia
W. disease
W. dysphasia
W. encephalopathy
W. reaction
W. syndrome
Wernicke-Korsakoff
W.-K. encephalopathy
W.-K. syndrome
Werther syndrome
Western
W. diagnosis
W. diagnostic concept
W. ethics
W. medicine
W. subtype
Westphal
W. disease
W. phenomenon
W. pseudosclerosis
W. sign
Westphal-Leyden syndrome
Westphal-Piltz phenomenon
wet
w. behind ears
w. beriberi
w. brain syndrome
w. dream
Wever-Bray
W.-B. effect
W.-B. phenomenon
wheal
Wheatley stress profile
wheel
activity w.
wheelchair sports
whereabouts
whiff
whimper
whine
whinge
whininess
whiplash injury
whipping
whirling
whisper
forced w.
whispered speech
whispering
involuntary w.
whispery
white
W. Anglo-Saxon Protestant (WASP)
w. blood cell
w. knuckling sobriety
w. lie
w. matter
w. matter change
w. matter dementia
w. matter disease
w. matter hyperintensity
w. matter lactate
w. matter lactate level
w. matter pathology
w. matter region
w. matter structure
w. matter tissue
w. noise
w. supremacist
w. turbid urine
white-collar worker
white-headed
Whiteley index
white-out syndrome
whitewash
WHO
World Health Organization
whole
w. brain atrophy
w. brain blood flow
w. brain boundary
w. brain raw volume
detail response elaborating w. (DdW)
w. focus orientation
w. response (W, WR)
wholeness
sense of w.
undifferentiated w.
Wiccan whore
wide
w. circles of thought
w. range
wide-based gait
widening
ventricular w.
widowed status
widowhood crisis
wieldy
wife, pl. **wives**
battered w.
wife-beating
wife-to-husband aggression
wihtiko

wild
- w. behavior
- w. psychoanalysis

Wilder law of initial value
will
- ambivalence of w.
- w. to be oneself
- concept of w.
- w. disturbance
- disturbance of the w.
- w. factor
- free w.
- general w.
- gesture of good w.
- God's w.
- ill w.
- lack of w.
- w. to live
- living w.
- w. to meaning
- w. to power
- w. to surrender
- w. therapy

willed action
willful feigning
willfulness
willingness
- reasonable w.

Willowbrook consent
Wilson
- W. disease dementia
- W. hepatolenticular degeneration disease
- W. syndrome

wind
- w. contusion
- w. effect
- w. fear

windage
Windigo
- W. culture-specific syndrome
- W. psychosis

windmill illusion
window
- therapeutic w.

wine
- electric w.

wing-beating tremor
Wing symbol
Winkelman disease
winking
- w. spasm
- w. spasmodic syndrome

Winkler body
winter depression
wipe out
wise old man
wish
- child-penis w.
- death w.
- w. to die
- w. dream
- w. fulfillment
- fundamental w.
- gratification of dependent w.'s
- id w.
- intense w.
- Klein death w.
- libido w.
- masochistic w.
- penis w.
- recovery w.

wishful thinking
wit
- abstract w.
- allusion in w.
- characterization w.
- displacement w.
- exaggeration in w.
- exhibition w.
- harmless w.
- indirect w.
- naive w.
- nonsense in w.
- obscene w.
- omission in w.
- outdoing w.
- parody in w.
- recognition in w.
- tendency w.
- thought w.
- travesty in w.
- unification in w.
- word w.
- w. work

witchcraft
witch doctor
witchery
withdrawal
- addiction w.
- w. adjustment
- w. adjustment reaction
- amphetamine w.
- anchor sign of w.
- anxiolytic w.
- apathetic w.

NOTES

withdrawal *(continued)*
w. avoidance
barbiturate w.
benzodiazepine w.
caffeine w.
cocaine w.
conditioned w.
w. criteria
w. delirium
delusion of thought w.
w. destructiveness
w. disorder
drug w.
w. dyskinesia
w. dystonia
w. effect
emotional w.
ethanol w.
w. from social affair
w. hallucinosis
hypnotic w.
infant narcotic w.
w. insomnia
interpersonal w.
w. method of contraception
morphine w.
w. movement
narcotic w.
newborn drug w.
nicotine w.
opiate w.
opioid w.
physical w.
w. process
psychoactive substance w.
w. reaction of adolescence
w. reaction of childhood
w. reflex
sedative w.
w. seizure
w. sign
social w.
w. state
substance-specific w.
sympathomimetic w.
w. symptom
w. syndrome
w. syndrome alcoholic psychosis
w. syndrome drug psychosis
thought w.
tobacco w.
w. tremor
uncomplicated alcohol w.
uncomplicated sedative, hypnotic, or anxiolytic w.
withdrawal-based craving
withdrawal-related
w.-r. anger
w.-r. depression
w.-r. mood disorder
withdrawn
w. behavior
w. catatonic schizophrenia
socially w.
withhold
within-family environmental factor
within normal limits (WNL)
witless
witness
w. to assault
character w.
w. credibility
w. to crime
expert w.
w. to murder
w. to repetitive violence
witnessed
w. atrocities
w. incoming fire
w. someone being killed
Wittigo psychosis
Wittmaak-Ekbom syndrome
witzelsucht
primary affective w.
wives (*pl. of* wife)
wizardry
WNL
within normal limits
wolf-man
Wollaston theory
Woltman sign
woman, pl. **women**
women at risk
drug-using w.
freed w.
medicine w.
non-drug-using w.
other w.
phallic w.
physiology of women
psychology of women
women veterans
womanhood
woman's role
womb
w. envy
w. fantasy
women's
w. liberation
w. liberation movement
wonder drug
wont
woodbine
woodrose
wool hwa-byung
woozy

word
- anxiety-related w.
- w. approximation
- w. association
- w. association technique
- w. attack
- base w.
- w. blindness
- w. cathexis
- w. center
- class w.
- w. coinage
- coin new w.
- w. configuration
- w. deafness
- w. debris
- derogatory w.
- dirty w.'s
- w. discrimination score
- w. dumbness
- emotional w.
- empty w.
- feared w.
- w. fluency
- function w.
- grandiose w.
- incessantly reiterated w.'s
- Jonah w.
- last w.
- microcosm of w.'s
- negative w.
- neutral w.
- parroting w.'s
- phonetically balanced w.'s
- phonologically irregular w.'s
- phonologically regular w.'s
- play on w.'s
- positive w.
- w. processing
- w. production
- w. retrieval
- w. retrieval error
- w. rhyming
- w. salad
- w. search
- stimulus w.
- w. stimulus
- thinking creatively with sounds and w.'s (TCSW)
- threat-related w.
- w. understanding
- w. wit

word-attack skill

word-finding
- w.-f. ability
- w.-f. ability disturbance
- w.-f. difficulty
- w.-f. problem
- w.-f. skill

2-word messages stage

word-recognition skill

work
- w. absenteeism
- w. addict
- w. addiction
- Bachelor of Social W. (BSW)
- breath w.
- circadian rhythm sleep disorder, shift w.
- w. cure
- w. decrement
- w. disability
- disaster w.
- dream w.
- w. dysfunction
- w. ethic
- family social w.
- field w.
- fired from w.
- w. force
- gratifying w.
- grief w.
- w. group
- group w.
- inability to finish w.
- w. inhibition
- Master of Social W. (MSW)
- w. motivation
- mourning w.
- overcommitment to w.
- w. paralysis
- w. performance
- w. personality profile
- psychiatric social w.
- w. rehabilitation
- right to w.
- w. schedule
- social w.
- testing, orientation, and w.
- w. therapy
- unexplained absence from w.
- wit w.

workable

Workaholics Anonymous (WA)

NOTES

worker
Academy of Certified Social W.'s (ACSW)
aftercare w.
blue-collar w.
certified social w. (CSW)
childcare w.
clinical social w.
disaster w.
indigenous w.
intake w.
linkage w.
mental health w.
National Association of Social W.'s
pink-collar w.
psychiatric social w.
skilled w.
social w.
white-collar w.
workforce issue
work-for-pay unit
workhorse
working
w. alliance
w. community
w. diagnosis
w. environment
w. memory
w. memory function
w. mother
w. out
w. over
w. relationship
w. through
w. type
workload
mental w.
workmanship
workplace
w. problem
w. psychopath
w. psychopathy
w. safety
w. violence
work-related task
work-release center
workshop
career w.
employment w.
sheltered w.
survival skills w.
transitional employment w.
work-study program
world
W. Association for Social Psychiatry (WASP)
W. Congress of Psychiatry
w. destruction fantasy
dream w.
external w.
W. Federation of Biological Psychiatry
W. Health Organization (WHO)
W. Health Organization Quality of Life-BREF (WHOQOL-BREF)
inner w.
intrapsychic w.
make-believe w.
on top of the w.
W. Psychiatric Association (WPA)
w. soul
W. Trade Center attack
w. war
W. War I (WWI)
W. War II (WWII)
worm
worrier
born w.
worrisome thought
worry
anticipatory w.
w. beads
w. circuit
constant w.
w. control
disabling w.
excessive w.
moral w.
ruminative w.
severity of w.
uncontrolled w.
unrealistic w.
worrying
excessive w.
w. symptom
worsening
symptom w.
worse sleep continuity
worship
ancestral w.
devil w.
hero w.
Satan w.
satanic w.
wort
St. John's w.
worth
comparable w.
inflated w.
worthless
worthlessness
feeling of w.
preoccupation with w.
self-reported w.
wound
gunshot w. (GSW)
invisible w.

multiple stab w.'s (MSW)
psychic w.
self-inflicted w. (SIW)
self-inflicted gunshot w.
self-inflicted stab w.

wounded
w. in action
w. feeling
w. victim syndrome

wounding
narcissistic w.
symbolic w.

WPA
World Psychiatric Association

WR
whole response

wraparound

wretched

wrinkling

wrist
w. clonus
w. cutting
w. drop
w. restraint

wrist-cutting behavior

wristed

writhe

writhing movement

writing
w. ability
w. assignment
ataxic w.
automatic w.
compulsive w.
w. disorder
w. fear
w. hand
mirror w.
pornographic w.
self-directed w.
spirit w.
w. tremor

written
w. command
w. communication
w. expression
w. informed consent
w. language
w. language quotient

wrongdoer

wrongdoing
moral w.

wry neck

WWI
World War I

WWII
World War II

Wyburn-Mason syndrome

NOTES

W

X

X chromosome

X zone

xanomeline

X-bar theory

X-chromosome marker

Xe clearance method

xenoglossophilia

xenon inhalation

xenorexia

xerophagia

xerostomia

X-linkage

X-linked

X-l. dominance

X-l. genetic abnormality

X-negative

xyrospasm

X

yan
yancy
yang
shuk y.
suo y.
yin and y.
yantra
yawning
psychogenic y.
yawn-sign approach
YBR
yellow brick road
Y chromosome
year
y. of birth (YOB)
childhood y.'s
disability-adjusted life y.'s
jail days per y.
quality-adjusted life y. (QALY)
yearbook
yearning
yellow brick road (YBR)
Yerkes-Dodson law
YES
Youth Enjoying Sobriety
yes-no
y.-n. answer
y.-n. question
yes-yes tremor
yin and yang
YOB
year of birth
yoga
Hatha y.
tantric y.
yohimbe
Pausinystalia y.
yohimbine
yoke
yoked control
Yom
Y. Kippur War
Y. Kippur War veteran
yong
York retreat
young
y. adulthood
y. adult psychiatry
y. adult self-report
developmentally appropriate self-stimulatory behaviors in the y.
young-old patient
youngster
rebellious y.
youth
at-risk y.
y. counselor
y. culture
delinquent y.
Y. Enjoying Sobriety (YES)
y. gambling
incarcerated y.
maladaptively aggressive y.
middle-class y.
y. self-report
y. self-support
y. violence
youthful
Yugoslavian refugee

Z
Z code
Z score
Zanarini concept
Zange-Kindler syndrome
zaniness
Zanoli-Vecchi syndrome
Zappert syndrome
zazen
zealot
zealous
zealousness
Zeigarnik
Z. effect
Z. effect phenomenon
zeitgeber
endogenous z.
exogenous z.
social z.
Zeitgeist
zelotypia
Zen
Z. Buddhism
Z. therapy
zeppia
zero-order elimination kinetics
zest
loss of z.
reasonable z.
zimeldine
zoanthropic
zoanthropy
melancholia z.
zodiac
zoetic
zoic
Zollner illusion
zombie-like
zombiism
zonal
zona medullovasculosa
zone
anelectrotonic z.
anterior speech z.
body buffer z.
chemoreceptor trigger z.
color z.
cortical z.
dolorogenic z.
epileptogenic z.
erogenous z.
erotogenic z.
functional deficit z.
genital z.
Head z.
hyperesthetic z.
hypnogenic z.
hysterogenic z.
ictal symptomatic z.
intimate z.
irritative z.
language z.
latent z.
limbic z.
Marchant z.
motor z.
peripolar z.
personal distance z.
polar z.
posterior language z.
primary z.
reflexogenic z.
Rolando z.
social z.
subplate z.
tender z.
time z.
transition z.
trigger z.
ultramarginal z.
visual z.
war z.
X z.
zonesthesia
zonifugal
zonipetal
zooerastia
zooerasty
zoogenic
zoolagnia
zoolatry
zoomania
zoomorphism
zoon politikon
zoophagous
zoophile psychosis
zoophilia
zoophilic
zoophilism
erotic z.
zoopsia
zoosadism
zootic
zoroastrianism
zoster
herpes z.
zosteriform
zosteroid
ZPG
zero population growth

Contents: The Appendices

Appendix 1

Alphabetical Listing of DSM-IV Diagnoses and Codes

Editor's Note: This listing is reprinted with permission from the *Diagnostic and Statistical Manual of Mental Disorders, Fourth Edition, Text Revision* (Copyright 2000, American Psychiatric Association). Please note that the terms in this listing follow APA style, which does not always conform with AAMT or AMA style. NOS = Not Otherwise Specified.

Code	Diagnosis
V62.3	Academic Problem
V62.4	Acculturation Problem
308.3	Acute Stress Disorder
	Adjustment Disorders
309.9	Unspecified
309.24	With Anxiety
309.0	With Depressed Mood
309.3	With Disturbance of Conduct
309.28	With Mixed Anxiety and Depressed Mood
309.4	With Mixed Disturbance of Emotions and Conduct
V71.01	Adult Antisocial Behavior
995.2	Adverse Effects of Medication NOS
780.9	Age-Related Cognitive Decline
300.22	Agoraphobia Without History of Panic Disorder
Alcohol	
305.00	Abuse
303.90	Dependence
291.89	-Induced Anxiety Disorder
291.89	-Induced Mood Disorder
291.1	-Induced Persisting Amnestic Disorder
291.2	-Induced Persistent Dementia
291.2	–Induced Psychotic Disorder
291.5	With Delusions
291.3	With Hallucinations
291.89	-Induced Sexual Dysfunction
291.89	-Induced Sleep Disorder
303.00	Intoxication
291.0	Intoxication Delirium
291.9	-Related Disorder NOS
291.81	Withdrawal
291.0	Withdrawal Delirium
294.0	Amnestic Disorder Due to (indicate the General Medical Condition)
294.8	Amnestic Disorder NOS
Amphetamine (or Amphetamine-Like)	
305.70	Abuse
304.40	Dependence
292.89	-Induced Anxiety Disorder
292.84	-Induced Mood Disorder
	-Induced Psychotic Disorder
292.11	With Delusions
292.12	With Hallucinations
292.89	-Induced Sexual Dysfunction
292.89	-Induced Sleep Disorder
292.89	Intoxication
292.81	Intoxication Delirium
292.9	-Related Disorder NOS
292.0	Withdrawal
307.1	Anorexia Nervosa
301.7	Antisocial Personality Disorder

293.84 Anxiety Disorder Due to (indicate the General Medical Condition)
300.00 Anxiety Disorder NOS
299.80 Asperger's Disorder
Attention Deficit/Hyperactivity Disorder
314.01 Combined Type
314.01 Predominantly Hyperactive-Impulsive Type
314.00 Predominantly Inattentive Type
314.9 Attention-Deficit/Hyperactivity Disorder NOS
299.00 Autistic Disorder
301.82 Avoidant Personality Disorder
V62.82 Bereavement
296.80 Bipolar Disorder NOS
Bipolar I Disorder, Most Recent Episode Depressed
296.56 In Full Remission
296.55 In Partial Remission
296.51 Mild
296.52 Moderate
296.53 Severe Without Psychotic Features
296.54 Severe With Psychotic Features
296.50 Unspecified
296.40 Bipolar I Disorder, Most Recent Episode Hypomanic
Bipolar I Disorder, Most Recent Episode Manic
296.46 In Full Remission
296.45 In Partial Remission
296.41 Mild
296.42 Moderate
296.43 Severe Without Psychotic Features
296.44 Severe With Psychotic Features
296.40 Unspecified
Bipolar I Disorder, Most Recent Episode Mixed
296.66 In Full Remission
296.65 In Partial Remission
296.61 Mild
296.62 Moderate
296.63 Severe Without Psychotic Features
296.64 Severe With Psychotic Features
296.60 Unspecified
296.7 Bipolar I Disorder, Most Recent Episode Unspecified
Bipolar I disorder, Single Manic Episode
296.06 In Full Remission
296.05 In Partial Remission
296.01 Mild
296.02 Moderate
296.03 Severe Without Psychotic Features
296.04 Severe With Psychotic Features
296.00 Unspecified
296.89 Bipolar II Disorder
300.7 Body Dysmorphic Disorder
V62.89 Borderline Intellectual Functioning
301.83 Borderline Personality Disorder
780.59 Breathing-Related Sleep Disorder
298.8 Brief Psychotic Disorder
307.51 Bulimia Nervosa
Caffeine
292.89 -Induced Anxiety Disorder
292.89 -Induced Sleep Disorder
305.09 Intoxication
292.9 -Related Disorder NOS

Cannabis

305.20	Abuse
304.30	Dependence
292.89	-Induced Anxiety Disorder
	-Induced Psychotic Disorder
292.11	With Delusions
292.12	With Hallucinations
292.89	Intoxication
292.81	Intoxication Delirium
292.9	-Related Disorder NOS
293.89	Catatonic Disorder Due to (indicate the General Medical Condition)
299.10	Childhood Disintegrative Disorder
V71.02	Child or Adolescent Antisocial Behavior
307.22	Chronic Motor or Vocal Tic Disorder
307.45	Circadian Rhythm Sleep Disorder

Cocaine

305.60	Abuse
304.20	Dependence
292.89	-Induced Anxiety Disorder
292.84	-Induced Mood Disorder
	-Induced Psychotic Disorder
292.11	With Delusions
292.12	With Hallucinations
292.89	-Induced Sexual Dysfunction
292.89	-Induced Sleep Disorder
292.89	Intoxication
292.81	Intoxication Delirium
292.9	-Related Disorder NOS
292.0	Withdrawal
294.9	Cognitive Disorder NOS
307.9	Communication Disorder NOS

.

Conduct Disorder

312.81	Childhood-Onset Type
312.82	Adolescent-Onset Type
312.89	Unspecified Onset
300.11	Conversion Disorder
301.13	Cyclothymic Disorder
293.0	Delirium Due to (Indicate the General Medicine Condition)
780.09	Delirium NOS
297.1	Delusional Disorder
290.10	Dementia Due to Creutzfeldt-Jakob Disease
294.1	Dementia Due to Head Trauma
294.1	Dementia Due to HIV Disease
294.1	Dementia Due to Huntington's Disease
294.1	Dementia Due to Parkinson's Disease
290.10	Dementia Due to Pick's Disease
294.1	Dementia Due to (Indicate the General Medicine Condition)
294.8	Dementia NOS

Dementia of the Alzheimer's Type, With Early Onset

290.10	Uncomplicated
290.11	With Delirium
290.12	With Delusions
290.13	With Depressed Mood

Dementia of the Alzheimer's Type, With Late Onset

290.0	Uncomplicated
290.3	With Delirium
290.20	With Delusions
290.21	With Depressed Mood
301.6	Dependent Personality Disorder
300.6	Depersonalization Disorder
311	Depressive Disorder NOS

Code	Diagnosis
315.4	Developmental Coordination Disorder
799.9	Diagnosis Deferred on Axis II
799.9	Diagnosis of Condition Deferred on Axis I
313.9	Disorder of Infancy, Childhood, or Adolescence NOS
315.2	Disorder of Written Expression
312.9	Disruptive Behavior Disorder NOS
300.12	Dissociative Amnesia
300.15	Dissociative Disorder NOS
300.13	Dissociative Fugue
300.14	Dissociative Identity Disorder
302.76	Dyspareunia (Not Due to a General Medical Condition)
307.47	Dyssomnia NOS
300.4	Dysthymic Disorder
307.50	Eating Disorder NOS
787.6	Encopresis, With Constipation and Overflow Incontinence
307.7	Encopresis, Without Constipation and Overflow Incontinence
307.6	Enuresis (Not Due to a General Medical Condition)
307.6	Exhibitionism
315.31	Expressive Language Disorder
Factitious Disorder	
300.19	With Combined Psychological and Physical Signs and Symptoms
300.19	With Predominantly Physical Signs and Symptoms
300.16	With Predominantly Psychological Signs and Symptoms
300.19	Factitious Disorder NOS
307.59	Feeding Disorder of Infancy or Early Childhood
625.0	Female Dyspareunia Due to (Indicate the General Medical Condition)
625.8	Female Hypoactive Sexual Desire Disorder Due to (Indicate the General Medical Condition)
302.73	Female Orgasmic Disorder
302.72	Female Sexual Arousal Disorder
302.81	Fetishism
302.89	Frotteurism
Gender Identity Disorder	
302.85	in Adolescents or Adults
302.86	in Children
392.6	Gender Identity Disorder NOS
300.02	Generalized Anxiety Disorder
Hallucination	
305.30	Abuse
304.50	Dependence
292.89	-Induced Anxiety Disorder
292.84	-Induced Mood Disorder
	-Induced Psychotic Disorder
292.11	With Delusions
292.12	With Hallucinations
292.89	Intoxication
292.81	Intoxication Delirium
292.89	Persisting Perception Disorder
292.9	-Related Disorder NOS
301.50	Histrionic Personality Disorder

307.44	Hypersomnia Related to (Indicate the Axis I or Axis II Disorder)
302.71	Hypoactive Sexual Desire Disorder
300.7	Hypochondriasis
313.82	Identity Problem
312.30	Impulse-Control Disorder NOS
Inhalant	
305.90	Abuse
304.60	Dependence
292.89	-Induced Anxiety Disorder
292.84	-Induced Mood Disorder
292.82	-Induced Persisting Dementia
	-Induced Psychotic Disorder
292.11	With Delusions
292.12	With Hallucinations
292.89	Intoxication
292.81	Intoxication Delirium
292.9	-Related Disorder NOS
307.42	Insomnia Related to (Indicate the Axis I or Axis II Disorder)
312.34	Intermittent Explosive Disorder
312.32	Kleptomania
315.9	Learning Disorder NOS
Major Depressive Disorder, Recurrent	
296.36	In Full Remission
296.35	In Partial Remission
296.31	Mild
296.32	Moderate
296.33	Severe Without Psychotic Features
296.34	Severe With Psychotic Features
296.30	Unspecified
Major Depressive Disorder, Single Episode	
296.26	In Full Remission
296.25	In Partial Remission
296.21	Mild
296.22	Moderate
296.23	Severe Without Psychotic Features
296.24	Severe With Psychotic Features
296.20	Unspecified
608.89	Male Dyspareunia Due to (Indicate the General Medical Condition)
302.72	Male Erectile Disorder
607.84	Male Erectile Disorder Due to (Indicate the General Medical Condition)
608.89	Male Hypoactive Sexual Desire Due to (Indicate the General Medical Condition)
302.74	Male Orgasmic Disorder
V65.2	Malingering
315.1	Mathematics Disorder
Medication-Induced	
333.90	Movement Disorder NOS
333.1	Postural Tremor
293.9	Mental Disorder NOS Due to (Indicate the General Medical Condition)
319	Mental Retardation, Severity Unspecified
317	Mild Mental Retardation
315.32	Mixed Receptive-Expressive Language Disorder
318.0	Moderate Mental Retardation
293.83	Mood Disorder Due to (Indicate the General Medical Condition)
296.90	Mood Disorder NOS

Code	Diagnosis
301.81	Narcissistic Personality Disorder
347	Narcolepsy
V61.21	Neglect of Child
995.52	Neglect of Child (if focus of attention is on victim)
Neuroleptic-Induced	
333.99	Acute Akathisia
333.7	Acute Dystonia
332.1	Parkinsonism
333.82	Tardive Dyskinesia
333.92	Neuroleptic Malignant Syndrome
Nicotine	
305.10	Dependence
292.9	-Related Disorder NOS
292.0	Withdrawal
307.47	Nightmare Disorder
V71.09	No Diagnosis on Axis II
V71.09	No Diagnosis or Condition on Axis I
V15.81	Noncompliance With Treatment
300.3	Obsessive-Compulsive Disorder
301.4	Obsessive-Compulsive Personality Disorder
V62.2	Occupational Problem
Opioid	
305.50	Abuse
304.00	Dependence
292.84	-Induced Mood Disorder
	-Induced Psychotic Disorder
292.11	With Delusions
292.12	With Hallucinations
292.89	-Induced Sexual Dysfunction
292.89	-Induced Sleep Disorder
292.89	Intoxication
292.81	Intoxication Delirium
292.9	-Related Disorder NOS
292.0	Withdrawal
313.81	Oppositional Defiant Disorder
625.8	Other Female Sexual Dysfunction Due to (Indicate the General Medical Condition)
608.89	Other Male Sexual Dysfunction Due to (Indicate the General Medical Condition)
Other(or Unknown) Substance	
305.90	Abuse
304.90	Dependence
292.89	-Induced Anxiety Disorder
292.81	-Induced Delirium
292.84	-Induced Mood Disorder
292.83	-Induced Persisting Amnestic Disorder
292.82	-Induced Persisting Dementia
Induced Psychotic Disorder	
292.11	With Delusions
292.12	With Hallucinations
292.89	-Induced Sexual Dysfunction
292.89	-Induced Sleep Disorder
292.89	Intoxication
292.9	-Related Disorder NOS
292.0	Withdrawal
Pain Disorder	
307.89	Associated With Both Psychological Factors and a General Medical Condition
307.80	Associated With Psychological Factors
Panic Disorder	
300.21	With Agoraphobia
300.01	Without Agoraphobia
301.0	Paranoid Personality Disorder
302.9	Paraphilia NOS

307.47 Parasomnia NOS
V61.20 Parent-Child Relational Problem
V61.10 Partner Relational Problem
312.31 Pathological Gambling
302.2 Pedophilia
310.1 Personality Change Due to…(Indicate the General Medical Condition)
301.9 Personality Disorder NOS
299.80 Pervasive Developmental Disorder NOS
V62.89 Phase of Life Problem

Phencyclidine (or Phencyclidine-Like)
305.90 Abuse
304.60 Dependence
292.89 -Induced Anxiety Disorder
292.84 -Induced Mood Disorder
-Induced Psychotic Disorder
292.11 With Delusions
292.12 With Hallucinations
292.89 Intoxication
292.81 Intoxication Delirium
292.9 -Related Disorder NOS

315.39 Phonological Disorder
V61.12 Physical Abuse of Adult (if by partner)
V62.83 Physical Abuse of Adult (if by person other than partner)
995.81 Physical Abuse of Adult (if focus of attention is on victim)
V61.21 Physical Abuse of Child
995.54 Physical Abuse of child (if focus of attention is on victim)
307.52 Pica
304.80 Polysubstance Dependence
309.81 Posttraumatic Stress Disorder
302.75 Premature Ejaculation
307.44 Primary Hypersomnia
307.42 Primary Insomnia
307.42 Profound Mental Retardation
316 Psychological Factors Affecting Medical Condition

Psychotic Disorder due to (Indicate the General Medical Condition)
293.81 With Delusions
293.82 With Hallucinations

298.9 Psychotic Disorder NOS
312.33 Pyromania
313.89 Reactive Attachment Disorder of Infancy or Early Childhood
315.00 Reading Disorder
V62.81 Relational Problem NOS
V61.9 Relational Problem Related to a Mental Disorder or General Medical Condition
V62.89 Religious or Spiritual Problem
299.80 Rett's Disorder
307.53 Rumination Disorder
295.70 Schizoaffective Disorder
301.20 Schizoid Personality Disorder

Schizophrenia
295.20 Catatonic Type
295.10 Disorganized Type
295.30 Paranoid Type
295.60 Residual Type
295.90 Undifferentiated Type

295.40 Schizophreniform Disorder
301.22 Schizotypal Personality Disorder

Sedative, Hypnotic, or Anxiolytic
305.40 Abuse
304.10 Dependence
292.89 -Induced Anxiety Disorder
292.84 -Induced Mood Disorder

292.83	-Induced Persisting Amnestic Disorder
292.82	-Induced Persisting Dementia
	-Induced Psychotic Disorder
292.11	With Delusions
292.13	With Hallucinations
292.89	-Induced Sexual Dysfunction
292.89	-Induced Sleep Disorder
292.89	Intoxication
292.91	Intoxication Delirium
292.9	-Related Disorder NOS
292.0	Withdrawal
292.81	Withdrawal Delirium
313/23	Selective Mutism
309.21	Separation Anxiety Disorder
318.1	Severe Mental Retardation
V61.12	Sexual Abuse of Adult (if by partner)
V62.83	Sexual Abuse of Adult (if by person other than partner)
995.83	Sexual Abuse of Adult (if focus of attention is on victim)
V61.21	Sexual Abuse of Child
995.53	Sexual Abuse of Child (if focus of attention is on victim)
302.79	Sexual Aversion Disorder
302.9	Sexual Disorder NOS
302.70	Sexual Dysfunction NOS
302.83	Sexual Masochism
302.84	Sexual Sadism
297.3	Shared Psychotic Disorder
V61.8	Sibling Relational Problem
	Sleep Disorder Due to (Indicate the General Medical Condition)
780.54	Hypersomnia Type
780.52	Insomnia Type
780.59	Mixed Type
780.59	Parasomnia Type
307.46	Sleep Terror Disorder
307.46	Sleepwalking Disorder
300.23	Social Phobia
300.81	Somatization Disorder
300.82	Somatoform Disorder NOS
300.29	Specific Phobia
307.23	Stereotypic Movement Disorder
307.0	Stuttering
307.20	Tic Disorder NOS
307.23	Tourette's Disorder
307.21	Transient Tic Disorder
302.3	Transvestic Fetishism
312.39	Trichotillomania
300.82	Undifferentiated Somatoform Disorder
300.9	Unspecified Mental Disorder (nonpsychotic)
306.51	Vaginismus (Not Due to a General Medical Condition)
290.40	Uncomplicated
290.41	With Delirium
290.42	With Delusions
290.43	With Depressed Mood
302.82	Voyeurism

Appendix 2
Sample Reports

ACUTE CONFUSION – PSYCHIATRIC DISCHARGE SUMMARY

HISTORY: This gentleman was admitted with a history of having been found wandering around the community and having some paranoid ideas. There is a history of him having sustained some blunt trauma to the head prior to coming to the hospital. This apparently was 10 days before admission.

The investigations, which were done while he was admitted, did not show any obvious cause for the acute confusional state. A noncontrast CT scan of the brain was normal. Electrolytes, urea, creatinine, and his liver function tests as well as calcium, B12, and TSH levels were all within normal range. The only abnormality was an elevated CPK, which came down to 297 prior to discharge. There was some myoglobulin in his urine and that probably explains the elevated CPK.

The house psychiatrist saw the patient during this admission. His impression was that the patient is suffering from a mild form of Alzheimer disease.

The psychogeriatric assessment team also evaluated the patient. We do not have a formal feedback from this assessment as yet.

He was discharged to the care of his family. I have asked him to make followup arrangements with my office in 4 weeks' time and also to follow up with the psychiatrist. He will continue on risperidone, which was initiated on this admission.

DISCHARGE DIAGNOSIS: Acute confusional state, not yet diagnosed.

ALCOHOL ABUSE – PSYCHIATRIC DISCHARGE SUMMARY

DISCHARGE DIAGNOSES

Axis I	Alcohol-induced delirium, major depression, and alcohol abuse, continuous.
Axis II	Dependent personality traits.
Axis III	Lupus and delirium tremens and elevated liver enzymes.
Axis IV	Marital conflict, psychosocial stress.
Axis V	Global assessment of functioning on admission 31 to 40 and on discharge 41 to 50.

Brief History: This is a 53-year-old gentleman with longstanding history of alcohol abuse and apparently was admitted to the hospital following an alcohol binge and that resulted in going into alcohol-related delirium tremens while he was on the medical unit. Since my involvement, we have tried to stabilize him in regards to his delirium tremens and at that time, the patient had significant elevated liver enzymes. He was under the care of internal medicine.

Once his delirium tremens resolved, his electrolytes and enzymes started to get regulated. The patient became more alert and oriented, and a family meeting was held to discuss future treatment plans with this gentleman. From the psychiatric point of view, alcohol has been the main precipitating factor. There has also been a history of depression in the past, probably related to alcohol abuse.

Plans were discussed at the family meeting, which was attended by his wife and his two children, a daughter and a son. During this meeting, the family was to inform me in regards to future goals and treatment options. The patient had been referred to the dual diagnosis program. His attendance date is some time next month. The next plan was how to keep the patient busy in a way to prevent any relapse and as a result of that, a date was obtained to attend a rehabilitation program until he can get into the dual diagnosis program. The patient was then transferred to the psychiatric unit, where all these placement issues, etc., were addressed.

As the patient progressed during this time, antidepressants, including BuSpar for anxiety and Celexa for depression, were introduced. Other medications were slowly tapered and minimized, and my involvement with the patient became a little bit more frequent. Eventually, as the patient progressed, he was given overnight passes with his family.

Another family meeting was held 2 days ago to address his discharge plans, and his concerns were addressed. Eventually, it was decided that the patient will go back home with his wife and get into the rehabilitation program on the appointed date. In the meantime, the patient is instructed to keep calling the rehab facility for any openings prior to his scheduled date. He will continue to see his internist in regards to his medical concerns. A followup appointment with myself in regards to his psychotropic medications and psychiatric concerns will be set prior to his discharge. I will be able to see him every 2 weeks, and he has also been advised to contact me should there be any concerns in between.

Mental Status Examination Upon Discharge: The patient was awake, alert, and oriented to all three spheres. Mesomorphic build with good hygiene and grooming, maintained good eye contact. Affect is constricted, decreased intensity and mood appears to be euthymic. Speech is normal. No formal thought disorders. No psychosis of any kind. Insight and judgment appear to be good. The patient's condition upon discharge is medically and psychiatrically stable. The patient has been instructed to keep himself busy to avoid any relapses. Family involvement is quite active and so that certainly will also help him down the road.

ADDENDUM: The patient's liver enzymes are continuing to drop significantly from the time when he was admitted. I believe his internist will continue to monitor him as an outpatient.

ALCOHOL DEPENDENCE – PSYCHIATRIC DISCHARGE SUMMARY

The patient is a 38-year-old female, working on a part-time basis, in a common-law relationship, referred by her family physician for inpatient care to help her with depression and suicidal ideation. She was admitted to the unit as a voluntary patient for management of the same. However, on obtaining history, it transpired that she was dependent on alcohol for last 28 years and was going through severe withdrawal symptoms.

Her circumstances of admission and history are recorded in admission note. Therefore, I will not be repeating the same.

HOSPITAL COURSE: She settled fairly well on the ward and did not pose any management difficulties. She was initiated on a reducing dose of benzodiazepines. Her withdrawal symptoms have responded favorably to diazepam 5 mg b.i.d. Her sleep improved on temazepam 15 mg to 30 mg at bedtime, which was given on p.r.n. basis. Most of the routine blood work was organized and was within normal limits. Intermittently, she had breakthrough withdrawal symptoms from alcohol despite being on reducing dose of diazepam. Gradually, the dose of diazepam was reduced to 2 mg t.i.d. and subsequently b.i.d. Eventually, she did not take diazepam when she did not experience any acute withdrawal symptoms. Her sleep and appetite improved. Likewise, her mood improved and there was no evidence of any overt psychopathology. She also denied feeling suicidal. She was allowed to go on passes with her common-law husband, which went quite well.

She had connected with the alcohol and drug counselor on the unit. She was willing to continue with outpatient counseling with them. However, alcohol rehab program was suggested, but she declined the same. A note was given to her so she could attend counseling services as an outpatient and recover from dependence on alcohol. She was not inclined to connect with mental health services to help her deal with past sexual abuse.

She was discharged home. Upon discharge, her mental state was stable.

Discharge Diagnoses

Axis I	Alcohol dependence.
Axis II	Deferred.
Axis III	Backache.
Axis IV	Relationship difficulties, financial difficulties, problems with primary support group, past history of child sexual abuse.
Axis V	Global assessment of functioning 65.

I have asked her to continue her followup with her family physician. If needed in the future, she would be making an outpatient appointment with me following referral from her family physician. I have given her a prescription for citalopram 40 mg a.m. for a month. The dose of citalopram was gradually increased to current dosage as an inpatient, which she has tolerated fairly well without any side effects. Her benzodiazepines were completely tapered off. She will continue with her alcohol counselor on outpatient basis. At this stage, we will wait to hear from her if she requires any further services from mental health.

Alcohol Overuse - Psychiatric Discharge Summary

History: The patient was initially admitted here after he had seizures caused by severe alcohol intoxication. The patient initially was assessed on the medical floor, deemed to have no specific brain injury, and then transferred back to the psychiatric unit for admission and further management of his problem.

The patient has a long history of alcohol abuse as well as depression and chronic anxiety. Unfortunately, the patient has had poor treatment in the past for these problems. In-hospital stay was rather uneventful. The patient was started on Celexa. The patient did well on this but felt that he had no specific benefit from the medication. The patient was repeatedly motivated to enlist in a dual diagnosis program near his home by myself and his family physician, as well as his family. At this stage, the patient still does not seem motivated to attend this program. All the necessary information was given, and the patient said he would consider the option. The patient is otherwise stable. No other specific abnormalities.

The plan is to discharge the patient and continue him on Celexa and Haldol at home. He will have followup next week at the clinic to make sure that he gets suitably followed for a full psychiatric assessment and find out about the waiting period for entrance into the dual diagnosis program.

Discharge Diagnoses

1. Alcohol abuse.

2. Depression.
3. Chronic anxiety.
4. Seizures and hypomagnesemia due to alcohol intoxication.

Bipolar, Oppositional Defiant Disorder – Pediatric Psychiatric Discharge Summary

This 12-1/2-year-old boy was admitted on an urgent basis via the emergency department. The patient had a prior admission to the child adolescent psychiatry unit. He was admitted to the regular psychiatry floor on this occasion as the child unit was closed. The presenting history was similar to his last admission. He was residing in the care of his grandmother as his mother was admitted again to hospital. Over the last 3 weeks, he had been taking his medication intermittently and then stopped altogether about a week prior to admission. At the time of his discharge last time, he was making some behavioral gestures in an effort to get readmitted to hospital as he enjoyed his time here.

When assessed on the morning after admission by this writer, he was showing a mild mixed mood state. He was very irritable but reasonably easy to redirect. He showed very poor insight and was stating very loudly that he had no need for medication. He was blaming others for overreacting and denied having any aggressive tendencies or management problem at his grandmother's. He complained that she would not allow him to listen to the music he liked. It was the patient's desire to go back in the foster care as had been arranged when his mother was hospitalized. With some prompting, he agreed to go on medication. He was started on olanzapine 5 mg at bedtime, which he claimed made him sedated the next day. He also started back on lithium 300 mg at bedtime. His olanzapine was reduced to 2.5 mg and the next night he refused to take it at all. He still complained of being tired in the morning although that was not observed in his behavior. He remained somewhat volatile, with some irritability. His previous pressured speech resolved and his mood became more pleasant and agreeable, partly because of the environment offering less stimulation.

No laboratory or other investigations were done while the patient was in the hospital. This writer communicated with his social worker, who was agreeable to have him go back into foster care provided it was okay with his mother. A conversation with his mother confirmed that a lot of his difficulties were behavioral, and the mood component would settle quickly if he were back on his medications.

He was discharged on olanzapine 2.5 mg at bedtime and lithium carbonate 600 mg at bedtime. Followup will be arranged through the mental health clinic. His complaints of headaches from the medication will be followed. Risperdal was not restarted for that reason, but that will be reviewed at his next clinic appointment.

Discharge Diagnoses
1. Bipolar mood disorder, mixed state.
2. Parent-child problem.
3. Oppositional defiant disorder.

Borderline Personality – Psychiatric Pediatric Discharge Summary

History: This 14-year-old girl was admitted on an urgent basis to the psychiatric service. She was admitted following allegations that she had made serious threats regarding wanting to kill her father. The patient had been seen at the mental health clinic on an ongoing basis, and it was at the clinic that she apparently made these allegations.

On the evening of her admission, she was seen by the psychiatrist on call and was threatening to leave. As a result, she was placed under Chapter 51. The patient was initially started on olanzapine on a p.r.n. basis, and her Advair was continued for her asthma symptoms. Celexa 20 mg was restarted as she had been on that. She refused to take that medication, and this writer eventually discontinued Celexa 4 days after admission, as the patient's behavior did not point to any acute underlying mood disorder. There was ample evidence of behavior problems and emerging personality difficulties. Information provided by her community therapist tended to point towards reactive attachment disorder as well. The patient lives with her grandmother, with whom she has had a great deal of conflict. She feels that she is restricted in her social activities, and she can be very stubborn with respect to defining where she goes. She is prone to significant temper outbursts and making statements about wanting to hurt herself or someone else. Her assessment was very much in keeping with an evolving borderline personality structure.

The patient settled into the ward routine quite easily. She had reasonable interaction with peers. She had trouble with sleep, which more or less resolved with trazodone 50 mg at bedtime. A very volatile family meeting was held with the patient and her grandparents. Initially, she refused to allow any information to be exchanged with her grandparents or her father. She did go home for weekend pass and came back with the usual complaints. It was established that most of her difficulties at home are behavioral, and it was left to her caregivers to try to find a suitable arrangement in terms of placement if she could not be managed there. Throughout her stay, she denied making any allegations of wanting to harm anyone. Her status was changed and she was allowed to go on a weekend pass, which went reasonably well.

Laboratory investigations in the hospital included a pregnancy test, which was negative, as well as a drug screen for amphetamines and cannabis products, which was also negative.

Although her interaction remained fairly volatile, with exceptionally good days mixed with bad days, she had no indication of an underlying mood basis. She denied any sort of suicidal inclinations, and there was no suggestion that way. It is evident that she needs to learn better stress management tactics.

DISCHARGE MEDICATIONS

1. Trazodone 50 mg at bedtime.
2. Seroquel 25 mg at bedtime p.r.n.

The patient was to continue followup at the mental health clinic.

DISCHARGE DIAGNOSIS: Borderline personality traits.

CLUSTER B PERSONALITY – PSYCHIATRIC DISCHARGE SUMMARY

This 17-year-old girl presented to the emergency department accompanied by her boyfriend. She had been seen at the mental health clinic where there were concerns about her suicidal risk and possible depression. She had presented to the emergency department the night before as well. Her current stressors include recent apprehension about her 1-1/2-month-old baby. She had no fixed address and had complex living arrangements with her boyfriend and a female friend. She reported multiple evictions and numerous crises. She did have a court appearance scheduled for the next day at which family services would make application for an extension of their care of the baby.

Her assessment at the time of admission showed no indication of any depressed mood. She had reactive mood and no indication of any psychosis. She had no suicidal intent. She was found to be very immature and had limited insight. There were very obvious emerging personality problems with mixed cluster B traits, including borderline dependency traits. Because of the court date, she decided that she would be discharged early in the morning in the company of her boyfriend so that they could both attend court. A prescription for Seroquel 25-mg tablets with a very small supply was provided. She was encouraged to seek out psychiatric followup in the community she settled in.

DISCHARGE DIAGNOSES

1. Cluster B personality traits.
2. Dependent personality disorder.

Cyclothymia – Psychiatric Discharge Summary

History and Hospital Course: This 15-year-old girl presented to the emergency department accompanied by her parents late in the evening. Once again, she had a huge behavioral reaction and was destructive and threatening. She had a 2-week stay on the unit in mid October when she was admitted for extensive drug use and an underlying cycling mood disorder. She responded very well to medication treatment. On discharge at that time, she was taking trazodone for sleep and lithium carbonate for mood stability. Shortly after her discharge, she became resistant to taking medication. At the time of this admission, she admitted that she was not taking her medications partly to get revenge against her parents who she felt were restricting her social activities too much.

In the emergency department, her parents felt unable to take her home. As there were no other placement options available through child services, she was admitted to the hospital for stability. Two or three days into her hospital stay, she continued to refuse medication. She was showing all sorts of behavioral maneuvers, including some attempts to get Ritalin or Dexedrine, which were her previous drugs of abuse. My partner took over care for a period in this writer's absence. She agreed to Seroquel and Topamax, which was a change from her previous medications. Lithium was discontinued.

This girl showed no reactive moods or angry outbursts during her hospital stay. Ongoing discussion with her parents improved the awareness of the behavioral component. It was suggested that she be transferred to a group home, and if there were further behavioral problems like this, perhaps we should consider seeing this girl's behavior as not due to an acute psychiatric disorder but as more behavioral and manipulative. She was discharged in the care of her parents, with followup arranged with mental health clinic.

Discharge Diagnoses

1. Cyclothymic mood disorder.
2. Oppositional defiant disorder.

Drug-Induced Psychosis – Psychiatric Discharge Summary

Admission Diagnosis: Drug-induced psychosis, cocaine.

History and Hospital Course: The patient is a 32-year-old male, who was brought here by the police. They stated that he was quite paranoid. He admitted to doing cocaine for the last 3 to 4 months and has been visiting crack houses. He is convinced that there were people out to get him. He denies any thoughts of harming himself or others. He does have a criminal record from the past, which he says he is now over with. However, on this admission it was noted that he has major problems getting along with his mother, who he says has schizophrenia. He gave me permission to talk to his mother and this confirmed that they do not get along. She states that he does not pay his rent, he is eating all the food in the house, and she has no money for that. The patient says that she is mentally unstable.

On the unit, he settled quite well and on discharge there was no evidence of any aggression, aggressive behavior, psychosis or depression. He denied any suicidal or homicidal ideation or plans. I did tell him that he has a drug problem, which he did not have any insight into, and that he should go to outpatient therapy for followup. I suggested olanzapine 5 mg at bedtime for at least 3 months to help him deal with the psychosis, which was drug-induced. He was not very keen on going on any medication. He settled on the unit quite well with diazepam 5 mg. On his way out, he stated that he would be in touch with the drug treatment center and he did say that he would see me after discharge in my office.

MOST RESPONSIBLE DIAGNOSES

Axis I Drug-induced psychosis, cocaine.
Axis II Antisocial personality traits.
Axis III Nil.
Axis IV Stressors with mother, unemployed, finances.
Axis V Global assessment of functioning 65 on discharge.

HALLUCINATIONS – PEDIATRIC PSYCHIATRIC OFFICE VISIT

The patient was reviewed regarding his hallucinations. This boy had initially presented with some ADHD symptoms, and by age 8, was having auditory hallucinations. These included both a man's and a woman's voice calling his name. He was simply monitored, but over a 2-year period he was hearing them every day. They were telling him to do things and they were certainly bothersome at that point. He was thus started on Risperdal and has been on 0.5 mg every night. The voices seem to have settled down. He was still hearing occasional voices last Christmas, but they seem to have completely disappeared now.

I think there is some eagerness to come off medications, so we will try and reduce the Risperdal to 0.25 mg daily for a month, and if there is no change, they can trial off the medication completely. Certainly if the voices come back, he would have to restart his Risperdal. He seems to be doing okay in school and he is receiving some extra help in math, which has been definitely beneficial. His height today is 146.8 cm and weight 42 kg.

MAJOR DEPRESSION – PSYCHIATRIC DISCHARGE SUMMARY

DISCHARGE DIAGNOSES

Axis I	Major depression, recurrent, acute exacerbation.
Axis II	Mixed cluster B and C traits.
Axis III	Status post pulmonary embolism, on Coumadin, radial palsy, and skin lesions questionable.
Axis IV	Excessive psychosocial stressors, especially dealing with her daughter.
Axis V	Global assessment of function on admission 31 to 40, on discharge 41 to 50.

BRIEF HISTORY: This is a 54-year-old woman who apparently began to feel hopeless and helpless and was not sleeping. This added to her stress levels, mostly brought on by her daughter who has been in and out of the hospital, has been missing for a while and is being very impulsive with several suicidal ideations in the past. This led the patient to become excessively worried and unable to handle work and stress around her. She was admitted to the medical unit, taking into account her occupation in the hospital.

HOSPITAL COURSE: Upon admission, she was reassessed. Medications were resumed. Initially, we gave her a trial with chloral hydrate and Serax to target her insomnia, and along with that we also introduced Remeron. She was on Celexa 10 mg to continue that for a short period of time before discontinuing it. To target anxiety, we introduced clonazepam 0.5 mg twice a day. We also resumed her other medications, including Coumadin 2 mg alternating with 3 mg daily. Dr. Blank was consulted in regard to her codeine and Tylenol #3 use along with Dalmane, and he decreased the dose of her codeine from 100 mg to 50 mg. We also introduced Seroquel, initially at 25 mg and increased it to 50 mg to address some of her questionable delusions that she was experiencing in regard to the skin lesions and also because its sedating effect helped her with insomnia. Internal medicine was consulted as she was on Coumadin and they graciously followed her during her stay in the hospital.

INR initially was a little elevated and subsequently with repeated testing it came down to normal limits. Her hematology was normal. Differential did show a decrease in neutrophils and elevation in lymphocytes that could be secondary to her skin lesions. General blood chemistry showed a slight increase in GGT. TSH was normal. INR, as mentioned earlier, initially was 2.8; however, with subsequent repeating, it did return to normal range of 2.0.

The patient was given day passes during the week, and she was given a weekend pass as things began to settle down. Her sleep did turn around. She felt more rested. Her affect was brighter. Symptoms of depression still present were mild. There was no indication of any suicidal or homicidal ideation, and the decision was made to discharge the patient and follow her as an outpatient.

MENTAL STATUS EXAMINATION: Upon discharge, the patient was awake, alert, and oriented to all three spheres. She had an ectomorphic build with good hygiene and grooming, maintained good eye contact. Affect was reactive and related, mood euthymic. Speech was normal. No formal thought disorders. No psychosis of any kind other than a questionable skin lesion that could be delusional, as we were still waiting for the pathology report on the specimens sent. Her insight and judgment appeared to be good. There was no indication of suicidality.

The patient's condition upon discharge was improving. Discharge plans will be for outpatient followup with myself and for her medical concerns with Dr. Blank. We also discussed a partial return-to-work program with 3 to 4 weeks of recuperating time. She is also agreeable that we discuss shift work as that could again interfere with her sleep cycle and we will do our best to avoid that. The patient's condition upon discharge was much improved and continued to improve.

Her psychotropic medications include chloral hydrate 1000 mg at bedtime, Seroquel 50 mg at bedtime, Remeron 30 mg at bedtime, clonazepam 0.5 mg in the morning and p.m. Dr. Blank also has her on other medications that include codeine 50 mg twice a day, Tylenol #3 one to two q4h. p.r.n. not to exceed 6 tablets in a 24-hour period. She is also using calamine and menthol and phenol lotion topically on her skin lesions. Her other medications also include Dalmane 30 mg and Lasix 40 mg p.r.n., which she usually takes 2 times a week for edema. She is also on clonidine 0.1 mg twice a day and Coumadin 2 mg alternating with 3 mg daily. Dr. Blank will be monitoring these medications.

MAJOR DEPRESSION/OVERDOSE – PSYCHIATRIC DISCHARGE SUMMARY

HISTORY: This 29-year-old woman was admitted to the hospital yesterday. She had taken a significant overdose of doxepin. She has been depressed for quite some time and was out driving around in a car, ran into a median, blew two of her tires and probably damaged the rims of her wheels. Following this, she went home and impulsively overdosed. This was not a carefully planned out suicide effort but rather impulsive with the above-described incident serving as the "final straw."

This woman has led a life characterized by neglect and loss. She has issues around loss of father, loss of mother, loss of relationship with sister, sexual assault x 3, and

2 or 3 years of a severely abusive relationship. She now is living on her own with poor support. She sees a local psychiatrist. She has been difficult to engage in therapy from what I can understand.

HOSPITAL COURSE: She remained in hospital for 24 hours. When I initially assessed her, she had been in hospital for about 1 day. I did not find her to be suicidal, but felt she was still somewhat cognitively impaired from her overdose. She reluctantly agreed to stay in hospital overnight, and seeing her tonight she is now clear. Cognitively, she continues to be not suicidal. She is depressed. She has social anxiety disorder and refuses to stay in the hospital.

We had a long talk about the need for followup, the need for psychotherapy, and the need to get involved in something other than simply trying to take medications.

On her insistence, she was therefore discharged. She will follow up with her local psychiatrist and with her therapist in mental health services.

DISCHARGE DIAGNOSES

1. Major depression.
2. Social anxiety disorder.
3. Ingestion.
4. Asthma.

MAJOR DEPRESSIVE DISORDER – PEDIATRIC PSYCHIATRIC DISCHARGE SUMMARY, #1

HISTORY: This 13-year-old girl was seen on an emergent basis in the mental health clinic 4 days prior to admission. She presented there with persistent auditory hallucinations over the last 2 months. She described a male voice that was outside of her head and giving her directions to do “bad things.” For example, the voice commanded her to kill herself or to kill her sister because her sister makes her angry. She reported that she was having trouble resisting this voice. At that time, she was placed on Seroquel at an eventual dose of 75 mg.

At the time of admission, she reported slight improvement in the voices. Admission assessment revealed a very depressed teenage girl who was quite willing and agreeable. She was grateful for the improvement in her sleep and the quieting of her voices as a result of medication. She still described voices with very negative content.

Laboratory investigations included CBC and differential which were negative, with the exception of mildly elevated eosinophils at 0.6. Electrolytes, fasting blood sugar, urea, creatinine, AST, and ALT were all normal. Serum beta HCG was less than 6.

Internal medicine was consulted regarding some painful lesions on her legs. Soaks and gauze dressing as well as Bactroban ointment were recommended. The culture of these lesions revealed 2+ beta-hemolytic Streptococcus group A. There was indication that these were improving, and no oral antibiotics were started.

The patient was complaining of dry mouth and headache on Seroquel 100 mg at bedtime. Subsequently this was reduced to 75 mg. She was started on fluoxetine at an eventual dose of 20 mg each morning. She had successful weekend passes and engaged well in the activities on the unit. Her mood and affect improved noticeably. It became evident that the patient had some significant behavioral problems. She enjoyed her stay in the unit and at the time of discharge was protesting that she had to leave her good friends. She had no indication of any ongoing acute mood disorder and there was no suicidal intent. Her voices had essentially disappeared, although she could call on them on occasion. She was discharged with close followup arrangements made at the mental health clinic.

DISCHARGE MEDICATIONS

1. Seroquel 75 mg at bedtime.
2. Fluoxetine 20 mg each morning.

MOST RESPONSIBLE DIAGNOSIS: Major depressive disorder with psychotic features.

MAJOR DEPRESSIVE DISORDER – PEDIATRIC PSYCHIATRIC DISCHARGE SUMMARY, #2

DISCHARGE DIAGNOSES

Axis I	A. Major depressive disorder, recurrent, moderate.
	B. Attention deficit hyperactivity disorder.
	C. Oppositional defiant disorder, conduct disorder.
Axis II	Deferred.
Axis III	History of viral meningitis at age 3 months, heart condition under 1 year, may have organic damage secondary to both conditions.
Axis IV	Conflict with stepfather, social difficulties.
Axis V	Global assessment of functioning 55 at the time of discharge.

HOSPITAL COURSE: The patient was admitted following ingestion of 4 tablets of Paxil and threatening suicide. She was admitted to an outside hospital over the weekend and sent home with her mother under her supervision. She was seen on an urgent basis, was continuing to report suicidal thoughts, and was not guaranteeing her safety, following which she was admitted to the hospital.

Her medications were changed from Paxil CR 25 mg up to Paxil 30 mg at night, and risperidone 0.5 mg at bedtime was also added to induce sleep and to control her agitation and aggressive behavior at home. She improved dramatically over the next 2 days, reported not being suicidal and was guaranteeing her safety.

She has been upset with her stepfather, who has been drinking and smoking in the house. Now that she is calm and willing to be discharged, a second opinion was arranged with my colleague the following day before discharging her, but he could not see her. As she was not threatening any suicidal ideations, she was discharged home with her mother. She was not overall pleased with her quick discharge, as she wanted to stay with other kids up here on the unit. Her mother was okay with her discharge.

Discharge Medications and Instructions

1. She was discharged on Paxil 30 mg at night and risperidone 0.5 mg bedtime.
2. She was advised to contact mental health therapist for support and followup.
3. Followup with writer in 10 days for medication review.
4. To use strategies and coping skills to deal with her symptoms of depression and suicidal thoughts.

Medication Adjustment – Psychiatric Discharge Summary

Axis I	None.
Axis II	Deferred.
Axis III	Morbid obesity.
Axis IV	Relationship difficulty with siblings, conflict with father.
Axis V	Global assessment of functioning 55 at the time of discharge.

Hospital Course: The patient was admitted electively for an assessment and further treatment recommendations. She had numerous diagnoses ranging from schizoaffective disorder, bipolar disorder, Asperger disorder, ADHD, etc. She underwent routine lab work and nothing abnormal was detected. She was unconcerned about her obesity and did not want to see the dietician. My partner gave a second opinion and suggested that her medication be changed. She was on lamotrigine, Celexa, Zyprexa, and Neurontin. Her psychological assessment showed IQ of 98, and she appeared to be very cognitively dull and socially inept. Overall, she presented with a picture of schizoaffective disorder and her treatment was changed accordingly. A referral was also sent for long-term hospitalization and rehabilitation.

While waiting for the referral to go through, the writer took it upon himself to take her off her medication gradually considering it to be the effect of medication. She was first taken off her Zyprexa, and there was no emergence of any psychotic symptoms. She was taken off Celexa as well and had no emergence of depressive symptoms. Finally, she was taken off her two mood stabilizers, Neurontin and lamotrigine. She immediately showed brightening of her mood and affect. She did not display any manic or psychotic symptoms. She was found to be somewhat socially inappropriate, but otherwise she participated fully in the program and was also able to work in school as well. She was observed for a few days, and there was no emergence of any psychiatric symptomatology. So, it was inferred that her flat affect and cognitive dulling were probably related to medication. A case conference was done with her father, and he was updated about her treatment in the past few weeks. She was sent home on passes, which went well, and finally she was discharged on no medication.

DISCHARGE INSTRUCTIONS: She was instructed to follow up with her counselor to work on some of the social skills and other coping mechanisms to deal with other kids teasing her both at home as well as at school. The writer also arranged for followup appointment the following week in mental health clinic to assure that she does not decompensate at home. No further followup is required except with her mental health therapist.

OPPOSITIONAL DEFIANT DISORDER – PEDIATRIC PSYCHIATRIC DISCHARGE SUMMARY

HISTORY: This almost 10-year-old girl presented to the emergency department accompanied by her grandmother. The patient and her grandmother had had several recent presentations to the emergency department as a result of her out-of-control behavior. She is prone to very angry episodes. Her grandmother is increasingly unable to manage her behavioral outbursts. The police have been involved on a number of occasions, and the patient has had some encounters with children's services. They presented at the emergency department with grandmother pleading for admission or change in medication to try to manage this girl's behavior. The insight into the behavioral aspect of her problems was a bit limited.

Because of the numerous presentations to the emergency department, it was felt prudent to admit the patient to deescalate the crisis and avoid future visits to the ER. This girl was admitted and left on her current medications, which include melatonin 3 mg at bedtime, sertraline 50 mg at bedtime and Seroquel 50 mg at bedtime. In addition, she was placed on Risperdal 0.5 mg every morning. On hospital day #2, her bedtime Seroquel was discontinued and Risperdal was increased to 0.5 mg b.i.d. Mental status exam at the time of admission and on subsequent inpatient visits revealed no indication of underlying mood disorder. There was ample evidence of severe oppositional defiant disorder and complex family problems.

The patient did not have any laboratory or other investigations.

She settled very quickly with respect to her behavior, largely due to the environment with the ability to strictly manage her behavioral episodes. There was some early indication that Risperdal might have been helpful in softening some of her stubborn defiance. I have been aware of the fact that this was a brief crisis intervention admission and she was discharged to her grandmother's care. There was discussion with the grandmother regarding the possible benefit of looking at some other placement for this very challenging child. It was grandmother's impression that she would not be going back to the behavioral school classroom, which she has been attending, and that leaves her schooling a real concern. She might benefit from a stay at a group home facility sponsored by children's services, as they have classroom activities as well as 24-hour behavioral management capability. It seems behavioral management at home is quite broken down.

Discharge Diagnosis: Oppositional defiant disorder (severe).

Paranoia – Psychiatric Discharge Summary

History: This young man was admitted for observation. He had presented to the mental health clinic for consultation where he was felt to have elements of significant characterological disorder and possible adult-form ADD and possible hypomania.

Hospital Course: In the hospital, he was observed for about 10 days. He was given the MMPI and the Millon as well as the WAIS. He also did an attention deficit checklist and was interviewed on a regular basis. At the end of his stay, the psychodiagnostic testing and clinical observations suggested his problems were primarily in the area of characterological disturbance, more specifically narcissistic and paranoid characterological disorder, and there was some suspicion that he may well have attention deficit on a smaller and less significant degree.

In the hospital, he was not treated with medication.

He was floridly inappropriate on number of occasions being loud and very inappropriately sexual on the telephone and in the public area. He was threatening and extremely aggressive over the telephone in the public area and expressed a number of concerning thoughts, such as his right to go about breaking peoples' legs because the police, after all, were not doing their job.

He is presently facing some criminal charges, which he was not willing to discuss in detail except to insist on his innocence.

On the night before discharge, he created a very significant disturbance on the unit. He had discovered that his girlfriend was spending a bit of time with some fellow that he did not like, and on the phone he became very, very loud and then very, very aggressive and was told to desist. Eventually security and later the police were called.

This morning he was discharged as our period of observation required for diagnosis was felt to have concluded, and it was also felt that, particularly in the face of no evidence of significant psychiatric disease, his behavior was inappropriate on the psychiatric ward.

DISCHARGE DIAGNOSIS: Character disorder, with narcissistic and paranoid traits.

SCHIZOPHRENIA – PSYCHIATRIC DISCHARGE SUMMARY

HISTORY: The patient is a 41-year-old single, unemployed man, who was self-referred to the emergency department and admitted to the unit under certification. He claimed to have been experiencing auditory as well as visual hallucinations apart from some paranoid thoughts. He wanted a neurological assessment for a click in his jaw, which would help him with all the hallucinatory experiences as described above. He was assessed in the emergency department and it was deemed he needed inpatient care for further stabilization. I have known him from the outpatient clinic for the last 6 months. He has a history of paranoid schizophrenia and noncompliance with medication.

HOSPITAL COURSE: He settled fairly well on the unit and did not pose any management difficulties. For his own safety, he was put on very close observation in the beginning. Chronically, he has delusional zoopathy; he believes that he is infected with worms, causing neurological symptoms. He described these hallucinatory experiences as visual in nature and sometimes voices telling him to do things but he resisted. He also had delusion of reference. His mood was congruent with psychotic phenomenon as described above. Initially, the second certificate was completed on the grounds that if he were left untreated, indirectly he would pose a threat of harming himself or others. He was initiated on olanzapine 5 mg b.i.d. and at bedtime. His risperidone 1 mg b.i.d. was discontinued.

He was also initiated on haloperidol 5 mg to 10 mg any form p.r.n. up to t.i.d., lorazepam 1 mg to 2 mg any form p.r.n. up to t.i.d. as well. He was given Cogentin 2 mg p.r.n. up to b.i.d. for any symptoms of acute paranoid schizophrenia.

On the above medication, he was more amenable for reason and he agreed to comply with inpatient treatment. Nevertheless, he continued to experience the above-described psychotic phenomenon in the background. A second opinion was sought with regards to the certification. However, it was decided that he no longer fulfilled the criteria for certification and therefore it was revoked.

Once he was a voluntary patient, he wanted to return home on a pass to pay some bills and come back to the unit. However, he never returned to the unit following this pass, despite making phone calls to his home and requesting him to come back to the hospital but he declined the same; therefore, he was considered to be discharged against medical advice.

DISCHARGE DIAGNOSES

Axis I	Paranoid schizophrenia.
Axis II	Deferred.
Axis III	Asthma.
Axis IV	Poor social and family support, unemployed and financial difficulties.
Axis V	Global assessment of functioning 50.

At this stage, we will wait to hear from him if he requires any further services from us. However, his family physician will be notified about his AMA discharge and if possible to have a followup on him. The patient was also encouraged to connect with his counselor and maintain outpatient followup with me.

SUICIDAL GESTURES, OPPOSITIONAL DEFIANT DISORDER – PEDIATRIC PSYCHIATRIC DISCHARGE SUMMARY

HISTORY: This 12-year-old boy was admitted to the child adolescent psychiatric unit, following transfer from his home community. He had made a previous trip to the emergency department days before where his problems were felt to be more behavioral. Because of his threats of suicide, he was admitted on this occasion for assessment and safety purposes. His care was transferred to this writer 2 days after admission.

Assessment at that time revealed a rather reluctant youngster who was not very forthcoming. He tended to downplay his responsibility and problems. He said he was threatening suicide because his mother was angry with him for getting kicked out of school. He stated that he had damaged some school property (toilets) and was now being expelled. He claimed that he was picked on by kids at that school and felt that he was not dealt with fairly by administrators. He was refusing to go back. The patient described some past symptoms of anxiety. There was information that he had been abused earlier in his life and that his behavioral problems had been ongoing throughout his elementary school years. He reported that he had been on Paxil in the past and that was recently restarted at a dose of 10 mg at bedtime. He was claiming that he was now feeling better and making a strong argument to go home.

The patient had a routine urinalysis while admitted and that was normal. His vitals and activity level were recorded as normal. Mental status exam, initially and ongoing, was more suggestive of behavioral problems with some occasional anxiety than mood-based problems. Paxil was discontinued to allow for a review of medications. Celexa was going to replace the medication but was never initiated, as there was not evidence to support an underlying mood problem.

During his hospital stay, his mother was taking steps to find him another school, thinking of one where his sibling goes and has good success. During his hospital stay, he did not show any indication of suicidal intent or underlying mood disorder. There was nothing suggesting any psychotic thought processing. He did display fairly severe behavioral problems with a lot of attention-seeking behavior. It was thought that some of his behavioral problems arise from the inconsistencies at home, with a significant contribution likely coming from past abuse that has not fully resolved. He was discharged in the care of his mother on no medications with followup recommended through his previous mental health clinic contacts.

DISCHARGE DIAGNOSES
1. Suicidal gestures.
2. Oppositional defiant disorder.
3. Question evolving conduct disorder.

SUICIDAL IDEATION – PEDIATRIC PSYCHIATRIC DISCHARGE SUMMARY

HISTORY: This 14-year-old girl presented to the emergency department, accompanied by her mother. The patient was complaining of a re-emergence of auditory hallucinations commanding her to harm herself. She did not feel safe. Although there were some inconsistencies in her account of hearing voices, earlier in December she took a very serious overdose, apparently in response to these voices. At the time of her assessment in emergency, neither the patient nor her mom felt safe in having her go home. She had been admitted because of that overdose, stabilized on pediatrics and then was in the pediatric psychiatry unit for 1 day. At that time, her mood was bright, and there was no indication of ongoing hallucinations or suicide risk.

The patient's mother indicates that this girl has been having trouble for approximately 4 months. She has had numerous fainting spells at school necessitating ambulance rides. She is in the middle of a workup, including a neurology appointment later this month.

In the hospital, this girl showed no indication of acute psychiatric disturbance. She reported the next morning that her voices were completely gone and could not explain how they went away. Her affect of expression was quite buoyant and upbeat. There was a significant element of attention-seeking behavior in her interaction. There was nothing suggesting psychotic thought processing. She was very vague in her description of voices and seemed unable to provide any details. The morning after her admission, there was no indication of suicidal inclinations and she was quite eager to go home.

A meeting with her mother on the evening of discharge, 24 hours after admission, concluded that it was best for her to go home. There are a number of indicators that this has an underlying histrionic personality basis to it. Close followup has already been arranged at the mental health clinic in her community. Her Celexa was discontinued because there was no evidence of depression and her Seroquel was increased from 25 mg to 50 mg. Followup will be arranged through the mental health clinic.

Discharge Diagnoses

1. Suicidal ideation.
2. Question of histrionic personality traits.

Tourette Syndrome – Pediatric Psychiatric Discharge Summary

History: This 12-year-old seventh grade student was admitted on an elective basis for a review of her medications. The patient has longstanding Tourette syndrome, accompanied by a lot of anxiety and obsessive-compulsive traits. She has been maintained on fairly high doses of SSRI medication and Risperdal for some time. There was indication that this was losing its effectiveness. The patient's concentration had been an ongoing problem. Treatment with Dexedrine seemed to worsen some of her other symptoms and a comprehensive review was indicated.

On admission, this girl showed very poor concentration. She has excellent insight. Her anxiety is very high. There is no indication of acute depression, but she is at risk for that. There are no indications of any psychotic thought processing. Normal laboratory investigations included CBC and differential, TSH, prolactin at 21.3, and

FSH at 5.3. In addition, LH was normal at 4.4 and HCG was less than 6. ECG was also normal.

The patient was initially maintained on low-dose citalopram, which was discontinued on hospital day #2. Her Risperdal was reduced to her eventual dose of 1.5 mg at bedtime. The 1 mg she was taking in the evening was discontinued. She was placed on Prozac at an initial dose of 10 mg, which was then increased to 20 mg each morning. The patient's mood brightened. She was very enthusiastic about the reduction in her obsessive ideation. She was eager to get back to school, feeling much better with respect to her mood. She had a successful weekend pass which was mostly spent with her father. It was thought prudent to have her try a day or two at school prior to discharge. She did go on an overnight pass, attended school, and the patient, her mother and father were all agreeable with her being discharged to home.

DISCHARGE MEDICATIONS

1. Prozac 20 mg every morning.
2. Risperdal 1.5 mg at bedtime.

She reported that her concentration was much improved on the Prozac, most likely due to better anxiety control. Followup was arranged with her regular psychiatrist and therapist at the mental health clinic.

DISCHARGE DIAGNOSIS: Tourette syndrome.

Appendix 3

Common Terms by Procedure

Acute Confusion – Psychiatric Discharge Summary

paranoid ideas
confusional state
noncontrast CT scan
Alzheimer disease
psychogeriatric assessment
risperidone

Alcohol Abuse – Psychiatric Discharge Summary

alcohol-induced delirium
major depression
alcohol abuse
dependent personality traits
alcohol-related delirium tremens
liver enzymes
dual diagnosis program
BuSpar
Celexa
family meeting

Alcohol Dependence – Psychiatric Discharge Summary

suicidal ideation
withdrawal symptoms
benzodiazepines
diazepam
temazepam
alcohol dependence
child sexual abuse

Alcohol Overuse – Psychiatric Discharge Summary

alcohol abuse
depression
chronic anxiety
dual diagnosis program
Celexa
Haldol

Bipolar, Oppositional Defiant Disorder – Pediatric Psychiatric Discharge Summary

behavioral gestures
mixed mood state
poor insight
foster care
olanzapine
lithium
bipolar mood disorder
parent-child problem
oppositional defiant disorder

Borderline Personality – Pediatric Psychiatric Discharge Summary

Chapter 51
Olanzapine
Celexa
borderline personality structure
behavior problems
reactive attachment disorder
temper outbursts
trazodone
Seroquel

Cluster B Personality – Psychiatric Discharge Summary

suicidal risk
depression
court appearance
cluster B personality traits
dependent personality disorder
Seroquel

Cyclothymia – Psychiatric Discharge Summary

behavioral maneuvers
cyclothymic mood disorder
oppositional defiant disorder
drug use
Seroquel
Topamax
group home

Drug-Induced Psychosis – Psychiatric Discharge Summary

drug-induced psychosis
crack houses
criminal record
diazepam
antisocial personality traits
stressors

Hallucinations – Pediatric Psychiatric Office Visit

auditory hallucinations
occasional voices
Risperdal

Major Depression – Psychiatric Discharge Summary

major depression
psychosocial stressors
mixed cluster B and C traits
skin lesion
clonazepam
chloral hydrate
Coumadin
Seroquel
Codeine
INR

Major Depression/ Overdose – Psychiatric Discharge Summary

cognitively impaired
social anxiety disorder
loss of father
loss of mother
loss of relationship
sexual assault
major depression
social anxiety disorder
ingestion

Major Depressive Disorder – Pediatric Psychiatric Discharge Summary, #1

auditory hallucinations
major depressive disorder
Seroquel
Fluoxetine
2+ beta-hemolytic Streptococcus group A
Bactroban ointment

Major Depressive Disorder – Pediatric Psychiatric Discharge Summary, #2

suicidal thoughts
Paxil
Risperidone
major depressive disorder
attention deficit hyperactivity disorder
oppositional defiant disorder
conduct disorder
social difficulties

Medication Adjustment – Psychiatric Discharge Summary

morbid obesity
schizoaffective disorder
flat affect
relationship difficulty

cognitive dulling
long-term hospitalization
social skills
coping mechanisms

Oppositional Defiant Disorder – Pediatric Psychiatric Discharge Summary

out-of-control behavior
behavioral episodes
melatonin
sertraline
Seroquel
Risperdal
oppositional defiant disorder
group home

Paranoia – Psychiatric Discharge Summary

paranoid characterological disorder
attention deficit
psychodiagnostic testing
clinical observations
inappropriately sexual
floridly inappropriate
narcissistic traits
paranoid traits

Schizophrenia – Psychiatric Discharge Summary

auditory experiences
paranoid schizophrenia
noncompliance
delusional zoopathy
delusion of reference
psychotic phenomenon
haloperidol
lorazepam
Cogentin
certification

Suicidal Gestures, Oppositional Defiant Disorder – Pediatric Psychiatric Discharge Summary

threats of suicide
behavioral problems
anxiety
past abuse
suicidal gestures
oppositional defiant disorder
conduct disorder

Suicidal Ideation – Pediatric Psychiatric Discharge Summary

histrionic personality
suicidal ideation
auditory hallucinations
pediatric psychiatry
affect of expression
attention-seeking behavior

Tourette Syndrome – Pediatric Psychiatric Discharge Summary

Tourette syndrome
Risperdal
Prozac

Appendix 4
Slang Terms

151	crack cocaine
420	a marijuana user
3750	marijuana and crack rolled into a joint
007s	MDMA
10¢ bag	$10 drug supply
10¢ pistol	$10 bag of poisoned heroin that is sold to an informer
24-7	crack cocaine
2-CB	Nexus
2-for-1 sale	crack sales promotion
45-minute psychosis	dimethyltryptamine
49er	a cocaine user
69s	MDMA
714s, 7-14s	methaqualone
a bean	MDMA
a la canona	abrupt withdrawal from heroin
Abe	$5 worth of drugs
abolic	veterinary steroid
a-bomb, atom bomb	marijuana joint, with heroin or opium
a-boot	under the influence of drugs
AC/DC	cough syrup with codeine; one who is bisexual
Acapulco gold	gold-colored Mexican marijuana
Acapulco red	Mexican marijuana
ace	a puff from a cigarette
ace boon coon	a prisoner's best friend
acid	LSD
acid cube	LSD on a sugar cube
acid freak	a heavy user of LSD
acid head	LSD user
action	gambling activity; sexual activity
ad	an addict; PCP
Adam	MDMA/MDA
Adam and Eve	MDMA, MDEA combination
Afghani or Afgani indica	marijuana
Afghanistan black	hashish
African black	marijuana
African bush	marijuana
African woodbine	marijuana cigarette
age out	to reach an age where drugs no longer have the effect they once had

agonies	withdrawal symptoms
a-head	an amphetamine user
ah-pen-yen	opium
AIP	heroin from Afghanistan, Iran, and Pakistan
air blast	inhalant
Al Capone	heroin
alamout black hash	hashish, belladonna
alcopops	flavored alcohol-containing drinks
Alice	LSD or mushrooms
Alice B. Toklas	marijuana brownie
alien sex fiend	strong powdered PCP laced with heroin
alki, alky	alcohol
all day	sentenced to life in prison
all day and a night	life sentence without parole
all star	a user of multiple drugs
all-American drug	cocaine
alley cat	a sexually promiscuous woman
alley juice	methyl alcohol
alligator	a physically attractive male
alpha-ET	alpha ethyltryptamine
ambition	amphetamine
American dream game	the choking game
ames, aimes	amphetamine; amyl nitrite
amidone	methadone
ammo	amobarbital
amoeba	PCP
amp	ampule; amphetamine; marijuana cigarette dipped in formaldehyde or embalming fluid, sometimes laced with PCP
amp head	an LSD user
amped	under the influence of drugs
amped out	fatigue after using amphetamines
amping	an accelerated heartbeat after drug use
AMT	dimethyltryptamine
amys	amyl nitrite
anavar	an oral steroid
angel	PCP
angel dust	PCP
angel hair	PCP
angel mist	PCP
angel poke	PCP
angel tears	liquid LSD
angels in a sky	LSD

Angie	cocaine
angola	marijuana
animal	LSD
animal trank, tranq	PCP
antifreeze	heroin
Anything going on?	Do you have drugs to sell?
Apache	fentanyl
apple jacks	crack
apples	fellow addicts
Archie Bunker	a bigoted person
Are you anywhere?	Do you use marijuana?
Are you holding?	Do you have any drugs?
Aries	heroin
arm	a police officer
aroma of men	isobutyl nitrite
around the turn	has gone through withdrawal
artillery	equipment for injecting drugs
ashes	marijuana
Asian white	cocaine
ass betting	gambling without funds
assassin of youth	marijuana
Astroturf	marijuana
at liberty	unemployed
ate up	one who is always under the influence of drugs
atom bomb	marijuana and heroin
atshitshi	marijuana
attitude	a sudden hostile feeling
Aunt Hazel	heroin
Aunt Mary	marijuana
Aunt Nora	cocaine
Auntie, Auntie Emma	opium
aurora borealis	PCP
Australian	1 ounce; ozzy
author	doctor who writes illegal prescriptions
B	amount of marijuana that fills a matchbox
B-40	cigar laced with marijuana and dipped in malt liquor
babe	drug used for detoxification; a sexually attractive woman
baby	marijuana; minor heroin habit; one who is just getting started on drugs; a prisoner who is used for sex
baby bhang	marijuana

baby boomers	generation of people born immediately following World War II
baby habit	occasional use of drugs
baby slits	ecstasy
baby T	crack cocaine
babysitter	one who guides an individual through the first drug experience
back dex	amphetamine
back door	residue left in a pipe
back to back	smoking crack after injecting heroin, or heroin used after smoking crack
backbreaker	LSD and strychnine
backjack	to inject a drug
backtrack	to gradually inject a drug by pulling back and reinjecting it repeatedly to increase the drug's effect
backup	to prepare a vein for injection
backwards	depressant; to get a habit again
bad	crack cocaine; good
bad bundle	inferior quality heroin
bad go	a bad reaction to a drug
bad paper	a worthless check
bad pizza	PCP
bad rock	crack cocaine
bad scene	uncomfortable or unfriendly surroundings; an unpleasant experience or situation; ugly reverberation
bad seed	peyote; heroin; marijuana; mescaline
bad trip	a frightening reaction after use of a hallucinogen
baddie	a criminal
badge bandit	a police officer
badger game	a method of extortion
bag	a drug container (usually 1 ounce); an unattractive woman; to kill
bag boy	one who sells dope for someone else
bag bride	crack-smoking prostitute
bag lady	a female street person
bag man	a person who transports money; one who has a small habit; a drug dealer
bag; baggage	measurement of marijuana or heroin; condoms
bagging	concentrating vaporized fumes by pouring liquid into a plastic bag, then inhaling and exhaling into the bag; using an inhalant

bake	to smoke marijuana
baked	under the influence of drugs or alcohol
baker (the)	the electric chair
bale	1 pound of marijuana
ball	crack cocaine; a testicle
balling	vaginally implanted cocaine
balloon	heroin supplier; a balloon that contains drugs
ballot	heroin
bam, bamb	depressant; amphetamine
bambalacha	marijuana
bambita, bombita	Desoxyn or amphetamine derivative
bammie, bammy, bammer	inferior quality marijuana
banano	marijuana or tobacco cigarette laced with cocaine
bang	to inject a drug; inhalant; sexual intercourse
banger	a prison-made knife
bangin' it in	shooting heroin via needle
banging	under the influence of drugs; engaging in sexual intercourse
bank	cash flow for buying drugs
bank bandit pills	depressant
bar	marijuana
Barbara Jean	marijuana
Barbies	depressants
barbs	barbiturates; jagged edges on a used hypodermic needle
bareback rider	a man who has sex without using a condom
barf tea	peyote
barfly	a heavy drinker
bark at the moon	under the influence of drugs or alcohol
barr	codeine cough syrup
barrels	LSD
Bart Simpson	LSD
base	to freebase cocaine; crack
base crazies	searching on hands and knees for crack
base head	person who freebases
base house	place for smoking freebase cocaine or crack cocaine
baseball	crack cocaine
based out	one who has lost control over free-basing
bash	marijuana; party
baste (to)	to beat
Bastille by the Bay	San Quentin

basuco (Spanish), bazulco	cocaine; coca paste residue sprinkled on marijuana or tobacco cigarette
bat	marijuana pipe, easily disguised as a cigarette
bathtub crank	poor quality methamphetamine
bathtub speed	methcathinone
Batman	MDMA
Batman and Robin	inseparable
batt	IV needle
batted out	to be arrested
battery acid	LSD
batu	smokable methamphetamine
bazooka	cocaine; crack; crack and tobacco
B-ball	methylphenidate
BC Budd	high-grade marijuana from British Columbia
BD	belladonna
BDMPEA	Nexus
beagle	a detective or investigator
beam me up Scottie	crack dipped in PCP
beamers, beemers	crack users
beaners	drugs
beans	amphetamine; depressant; mescaline
bear	a capsule that contains a narcotic
bear in the air	a police officer in a helicopter
bear trap	a police radar trap
beast	LSD; a prostitute; heroin; an unattractive woman
beat	a counterfeit drug
beat artist	person selling bogus drugs
beat generation	young people of the 1950s and 1960s, known for rejecting conventional social values
beat it	to leave in a hurry
beat off	to masturbate (male)
beat the bricks	to get out of jail or prison
beat the gong	to smoke opium
beat the rap	to go unpunished or be acquitted
beat vials	vials containing sham crack
beautiful boulders	crack
beautiful people (the)	individuals who are stylish and wealthy
Beavis & Butthead	crack cocaine
bebe	crack cocaine
bedazzled	under the influence of drugs
bedbugs	fellow addicts
bee	bong hits

beedies	East Indian cigarettes, resemble joints
been had	arrested; to have had sexual intercourse
beetle crusher	a police officer
behind the iron house	in jail or prison
behind the scale	to weigh and sell cocaine
beiging	cocaine chemically altered to make it appear to be a higher purity
belch	to inform
belly habit	to take a drug orally
belongs	uses drugs
belt	a marijuana cigarette; an alcoholic drink
belted	under the influence of drugs; to rapidly consume an alcoholic drink
Belushi; Belushi cocktail	cocaine and heroin mixture
belyando spruce	marijuana
bender	drug party; rave
benny, bennie(s)	Benzedrine
benz	Benzedrine
Bermuda triangles	MDMA
Bernice	cocaine
Bernie	cocaine
Bernie's flakes	cocaine
Bernie's gold dust	cocaine
Betsy, Betsy, Betsie	a gun
bhang	marijuana, East Indian term
bibs	MDMA
big 8	1/8 kilogram
big bag	heroin
big bloke	cocaine
big C	cocaine
big chief	peyote; mescaline
big D	LSD
big flake	cocaine
big H	heroin
big Harry	heroin
big house	prison
big jab	lethal injection
big John	a police officer
big man	drug supplier
big O	opium
big one	a $1,000 bet
big rush	cocaine
biggy	marijuana

Slang Terms

big-timer	a gambler or risk taker
bike	a motorcycle police officer
biker's coffee	methamphetamine and coffee
biker's speed	methamphetamine
bill	a $100 bill
Bill Blass	crack
billie hoke	cocaine
bimbo	an immature woman; a prostitute
bindle	small packet of drug powder; heroin
bing	enough of a drug for one injection
bingers	crack addicts
bingler	one who sells narcotics
bingo	to inject a drug
bingo house	where addicts go to buy and use drugs
bird cage hype	addicts who have trouble supporting their habits
bird's eye	extremely small quantity of narcotics
birdhead	LSD
birdie powder	heroin; cocaine
birds	marijuana
biscuit	50 rocks of crack
bitch up	to cry
bite	arrest
bite one's lips	to smoke marijuana
biz	equipment for injecting drugs
bizznizzle	business
BJs	crack cocaine
black	tar heroin
black acid	LSD; LSD and PCP mixture
black and white	amphetamine; a patrol car
Black Bart	marijuana
black beauties	depressants; amphetamine
black bombers	amphetamine
black button	dried peyote button
black Cadillacs	amphetamines
black dust	PCP
black ganga	marijuana resin
black gold	high-quality marijuana
black gungi	marijuana from India
black gunion	marijuana
black H	potent Mexican heroin with the consistency of tar
black hash	opium and heroin
black hole	depression associated with ketamine use

black Maria	highly potent marijuana
black mo; black moat; black mote	marijuana that has been cured in sugar or honey, then buried for some time
black Mollies	amphetamines; diet pills
black pearl	heroin
black pill	opium pill
black powder	black hash ground into powder
black rock	crack cocaine
black Russian	hashish mixed with opium
black star	LSD
black stuff	heroin; black tar opium
black sundae	brown heroin cut with cocoa
black sunshine	LSD
black tabs	LSD
black tar	potent heroin
black tootsie roll	black tar heroin
black whack	PCP
blackbird	type of LSD
blackout game	the choking game
blacks	amphetamines
blade	a knife
Blade Queen	a girl who is obsessed with doing blades
blades	after heating 2 knives on an element, one picks up a desired drug with the hot knives and inhales it
blanca (Spanish)	cocaine; heroin
blank	container of non-narcotic powder that is sold as heroin or cocaine
blanket	marijuana cigarette
blanks	inferior quality drugs
blast	to smoke marijuana; to smoke crack; a party; a rave; to shoot with a firearm
blast a joint	to smoke marijuana
blast a roach	to smoke marijuana
blast a stick	to smoke marijuana
blasted	under the influence of drugs or alcohol
blaster	a gunman
blaze	to smoke marijuana
blind munchies	an overwhelming desire for something to eat, usually after smoking marijuana
blind squid	ketamine, belladonna, LSD
bliss out	the mystic daze one is in while under the influence of a guru

Slang Terms

blitzed under the influence of drugs or alcohol
blizzard white cloud in a pipe used to smoke cocaine
block morphine cube; crude opium
blockbusters depressants
blond hash hashish that is gold in color
blond, blonde marijuana
Bloods the name of a well-known street gang
blotter LSD; cocaine; the daily arrest record kept in a police station
blotter acid LSD
blotter cube LSD
blow cocaine or crystal amphetamine; to inhale cocaine; to smoke marijuana
blow a fix to place excessive pressure on a weak or sclerosed vein, causing it to rupture
blow a shot to miss a target one is shooting at
blow a stick to smoke marijuana
blow away to overcome emotionally; to kill with a firearm
blow blue to inhale cocaine
blow Charley to sniff cocaine
blow coke to inhale cocaine
blow grass to smoke marijuana
blow horse to sniff heroin
blow job fellatio
blow off to dismiss or avoid
blow one's mind to soar beyond reality
blow one's roof to smoke marijuana
blow smoke to inhale cocaine; to exaggerate
blow snow to sniff cocaine
blow the joint to leave a place
blow the vein to place excessive pressure on a weak or sclerosed vein, causing it to rupture
blow up crack cut with lidocaine to increase size, weight, and street value; to lose one's temper
blowcaine crack diluted with cocaine
blowing smoke marijuana
blown high on marijuana
blowout crack; a rave; a party at which drugs and alcohol are used to excess
blue depressant; crack cocaine
blue acid LSD
blue and red secobarbital
blue angel amobarbital

blue bag	heroin
blue barrel	LSD
blue boy	amphetamine
blue bullet	depressant
blue cap	LSD
blue cheer	LSD
blue de Hue	marijuana from Vietnam
blue devil	amobarbital
blue doll	amobarbital
blue flag	LSD
blue flick	a pornographic movie
blue fly	LSD
blue hair	a senior citizen
blue heaven	LSD; amobarbital
blue hero	heroin
blue kiss	ecstasy (MDMA)
blue lips	ecstasy (MDMA)
blue madman	PCP
blue meth	methamphetamine
blue microdot	LSD
blue mist	LSD
blue moon	LSD
blue morph	Numorphan (oxymorphone)
blue Nile	MDMA
Blue Nitro Vitality	GBL-containing product
blue sage	marijuana
blue sky	heroin
blue sky blond	high potency Colombian marijuana
blue star	LSD/PCP
blue tips	depressant
blue velvet	paregoric and amphetamine mixture
blue vials	LSD
bluebirds	amobarbital
blued	tattooed
blues	amobarbital; melancholia; police officers; prison clothes
blunt	marijuana inside a cigar or a large rolled joint
blunted out	smoked many blunts of marijuana
bo	marijuana
boat	marijuana laced with PCP
Bob	marijuana
bobo	crack
bobo bush	marijuana

body packer	person who ingests drug vials to transport them or to avoid prosecution
body shake	a skin search for needle marks
body stuffer	person who ingests drug vials to transport them or to avoid prosecution
Bogart	keeping marijuana to oneself
Bogart a joint	to salivate on a marijuana cigarette
bohd	marijuana; PCP
bolasterone	injectable steroid
Bolivian marching powder	cocaine
bolo	crack
bolt	inhalants
bomb	crack; heroin; large marijuana cigarette; high potency heroin
bomb squad	crack-selling crew
bombed out	intoxicated by narcotics
bomber	a large marijuana cigarette
bombido, bombito, bombita	injectable amphetamines and cocaine
bombs away	heroin
bonaroo	a prisoner's best clothes
bone	$50 piece of crack; marijuana; a cigarette
bone crusher	crack
bone shaker	a gambler or risk taker
bones	crack
bong	a device used to smoke marijuana or hashish
Bonita	heroin
boo	marijuana
boo boo bama	100 dose units of LSD
boof	contraband concealed in the rectum
boofing	expelling concealed drugs from your body
booger	cocaine (in the Florida Keys)
boogered up	high on cocaine (in the Florida Keys)
book (a)	a 1-year prison sentence
book (the)	the maximum prison sentence allowed by law
boom	hashish
boom boom	sexual activity
boom-boom girl	a prostitute
boom-boom house	a whorehouse
boomers	psilocybin/psilocin; LSD; baby boomers
boonies	rural area; away from a populated area
boost	to inject a drug; to shoplift
boost and shoot	steal to support a habit
booster	to inhale cocaine

boot	to inject a drug gradually by pulling back and reinjecting repeatedly to increase the drug's effect
boot the gong	to smoke marijuana
booted	under the influence of drugs
booting	drawing blood in and out of a syringe
booty check	rectal search
booty juice	MDMA dissolved in liquid
boppers	inhalants
boss	excellent quality drug
BOT	balance of time (of a prison sentence)
both hands	a 10-year prison sentence
botray	crack
bottles	crack vials; injectable amphetamines
boubou	crack
boulder	$20 worth of crack
boulya	crack
bouncing powder	cocaine
bouncy bouncy	sexual intercourse
bowl	between 1/32 and 1/16 ounce of marijuana; a small pipe used to smoke marijuana
bowling	smoking several marijuana bowls in a row
box man	an expert in breaking into safes
boxcars	sixes on dice
boxed	in jail or prison
boy	heroin
boys uptown (the)	a group of influential criminals
bozo	heroin; an unpleasant, unattractive, or insignificant person
brain bucket	a helmet
brain damage	heroin
brain dead	one who has used drugs for an extended time and has difficulty functioning normally
brain pills	amphetamines
brain ticklers	amphetamines
brand X	inferior quality marijuana
brass (the)	upper ranks of the armed forces
bread	money
break loose	to escape from jail or prison
break night	staying up all night until daybreak
breakdowns	$40 crack rock sold for $20
breakfast of champions	crack
breath play	the choking game

Slang Terms

brew	beer
brewery	place where drugs are made
brick	1 kilogram of crack; marijuana; a carton of cigarettes
brick agent	an FBI agent
brick gum	heroin
bridge up or bring up	ready a vein for injection
bring down	something or someone unpleasant; to cause the downfall of another
Bristol Brown	bad marijuana
britton	peyote
broccoli	marijuana
Brodie	suicide committed by jumping from a high place
broker	go-between in a drug deal
bromo	Nexus
brother	heroin
brown	Mexican heroin, usually light brown
brown bagger	a physically unattractive person
brown bombers	LSD
brown crystal	heroin
brown dots	LSD
brown horse	Mexican heroin
brown noser	a person who flatters in order to gain approval or advantage
brown rhine	heroin
brown sugar	heroin; a dark-skinned prostitute
brown tape	heroin
brownies	brownies laced with marijuana
browns	long-lasting amphetamines
bruiser	a physically fit male
B-ster	low-grade marijuana
bubble gum	cocaine; crack
buck	a physically fit male; $1; a $100 bet
bud(s)	marijuana
Buddha, buda, budda	high-grade marijuana joint laced with opium
buffer	crack smoker; a woman who exchanges oral sex for crack
bufo	5-hydroxy-N,N-dimethyltryptamine, a hallucinogen
bugged	annoyed; to be covered with sores and abscesses from repeated use of dirty needles
build a collar	to gather evidence to make an arrest

bull	a federal narcotics agent; a police officer; a prison guard; exaggeration or untruth
bullet	isobutyl nitrite
bullet bolt	an inhalant
bullion	crack
bullpen	a holding cell in a jail or prison
bumblebee	amphetamine
bummer trip	unsettling and threatening experience from drug intoxication
bump	crack; fake crack; boost a high; small dose of crystal methamphetamine
bundle	twenty-five $5 bags of heroin
bunk	counterfeit drugs
burn	to take money for heroin with no plan to deliver, or by delivering counterfeit bags; to inform on another; to put to death in the electric chair; to kill
burn bag	counterfeit drugs
burn one	to smoke marijuana
burn the main line	to inject a drug
burned	to purchase counterfeit drugs
burned out	to be physically and mentally debilitated from prolonged drug use or stress
burner	the electric chair; a prison-made knife
burnese	cocaine
burnie	marijuana
burning logs	smoking a joint
burnout	heavy abuser of drugs
burnt	one who has smoked too much marijuana
burrito	marijuana
bush	cocaine; marijuana; female genitalia
businessman's high	psilocin/psilocybin mushrooms
businessman's LSD	dimethyltryptamine (DMT)
businessman's special	dimethyltryptamine (DMT)
bust out	to escape from jail or prison
buster	depressant
busy bee	PCP
butler	crack
butt	inferior quality marijuana
butt naked	PCP
butter	marijuana; crack
butter flower	marijuana
buttons	sections of peyote cactus

butu	heroin or crack
buzz bomb	nitrous oxide
buzzed	slightly under the influence of drugs or alcohol
C	cocaine, methcathinone
C&H	cocaine and heroin mixture
C&M	cocaine and morphine mixture
C dust	cocaine
C game	cocaine
C head	a cocaine user
C joint	a place where cocaine can be purchased
CW	completely wrecked (stoned or high on drugs)
CA	cocaine addict
caballo	heroin
cabbage	money
caca	inferior or adulterated heroin, cocaine, or marijuana
cache	a hidden supply of drugs or money
Cacti Joint	a joint of dried and ground-up peyote
cactus	mescaline; peyote
cactus buttons	mescaline; peyote
cactus head	mescaline; peyote
Cad	1 ounce
cadet	a new addict
Cadillac	PCP
Cadillac express	methcathinone
cafeteria	use of various drugs simultaneously
cage	jail or prison cell
caine	cocaine; crack
cake	drugs that are smuggled into a jail, prison or hospital
cakes	round discs of crack
calbo	heroin
California cornflakes	cocaine
California high	the choking game
California sunshine	LSD
California turnarounds	amphetamines
calling card	needle marks
cam trip	high-potency marijuana
Cambodian red, Cam red	reddish-brown Cambodian marijuana
Cambodian trip weed	potent Cambodian marijuana
came	cocaine
campfire boy	an opium addict
can	1 ounce of marijuana

Can you do me good?	Do you have drugs I can buy?
Canadian black	Canadian marijuana
Canadian blues	methaqualone
Canadian quail	methaqualone
canamo	marijuana
canappa	marijuana
canary	Nembutal; an informer
cancelled stick	marijuana cigarette
cancer stick	a cigarette
candied	a cocaine addict
candy	any drug
candy a J	to add another drug to a marijuana cigarette
candy blunt	blunt cigarettes or cigars dipped in cough syrup
candy C	cocaine
candy canes and gumdrops	LSD
candy flip	one hit ecstasy per three hit(s); LSD
candy man	a drug supplier or seller
candy raver	a person who attends raves
canned goods	cans containing drugs
cannon	a huge marijuana cigarette; a gun; a pickpocket
cannon ball	an injection of mixed drugs
canoe	a marijuana cigarette with a hole in its side that looks like a canoe
canvas back	a street person
cap	capsule of drugs; gelatin capsule used to package drugs; packet of heroin
cap up	to transfer drugs from bulk to capsules
capital H	heroin
caps	heroin; psilocybin/psilocin mushrooms; crack
captain	an influential drug distributor
Captain Cody	codeine
carburetor	drug paraphernalia that mixes smoke with air
card	a prepared ration of cocaine, which is weighed on a card
card shark	a card-playing gambler
care bears	MDMA
carga	heroin
carmabis	marijuana
carnie	cocaine
carpet patrol	crack smokers searching the floor for crack
Carrie, Carrie Nation	cocaine
carrier	one who sells drugs as part of a distribution chain

carry, carrying, carry weights	to have drugs in one's possession
cartoon acid	LSD
cartucho	package of marijuana cigarettes
cartwheels	amphetamines
cascade	to move to stronger drugs
cashed	a container of marijuana that has been completely used
cashing a script	getting forged or bogus prescription orders dispensed
Casper the ghost	crack
cast iron horrors	delirium tremens (DTs)
cat	methcathinone
cat killer	ketamine
cat valium	ketamine
cat's pee	crack
catch up	withdrawal process
catcher's mitt	a diaphragm
Catholic aspirin	cross-scored amphetamine tablets
catnip	a marijuana cigarette
cattail	a marijuana cigarette
cattle rustler	one who steals meat and sells it for drug money
caught in a snowstorm	under the influence of cocaine
cave	an abscessed or collapsed portion of a vein
cave digging	searching for a suitable site in which to inject drugs
caviar	combination of cocaine, crack, and marijuana
cavite all star	marijuana
cavities	needle marks
CD	glutethimide
Cecil	morphine
Cecil Jones	a morphine addict
cement	a large quantity of wholesale drugs
cement arm	an addict's heavily scarred arm
cent	$1
cereal	marijuana smoked in a bowl
cess	marijuana
cha cha	an opium pipe
chalk	amphetamine tablets that crumble easily
chalked up	under the influence of cocaine
chalking	chemically altering the color of cocaine so it is white
chamber pipe	a pipe designed to hold a large amount of marijuana

champagne	marijuana and cocaine mixture
chandoo, chandu	Chinese opium
channel	a drug source; the favored vein for injection of drugs
channel swimmer	an addict who takes drugs by injecting into a vein
charas, charash, charras	pure resin of Indian hemp, sometimes mixed with opium
charge	a drug portion
charged up	under the influence of drugs
Charles, Charlie, Charley	cocaine; $1
Charley Cotton	cotton that is used to strain a drug before an injection
Charley goon	a police officer
chase	to smoke cocaine or marijuana
chase the bag	to shop for the best quality of drug
chaser	compulsive crack user
chasing the dragon	inhaling the fumes from heroin or opium through a tube
chasing the nurse	regularly using morphine
chasing the tiger	smoking heroin
chaze	to christen a new bowl or pipe
cheap basing	crack
cheaters	marked playing cards
check	one's personal supply of drugs
check in	a prisoner who is placed in protective custody
check out	a prisoner who is released from protective custody
cheeba	marijuana
cheeo	chewable marijuana seeds
cheese	heroin
chef	one who cooks and prepares opium
chemical	crack
cherry fX bombs	1,4-BD
cherry meth	gamma hydroxybutyrate (GHB)
cherry top	LSD
chestbonz	one taking the biggest bong hit
Chester	a child molester
chewed	severely stoned
chewies	crack; blunt with powdered cocaine inside
chewing the gum	chewing opium
chiba chiba	potent Colombian marijuana

Chicago black	a dark variety of marijuana grown in the Chicago area
Chicago green	a dark green variety of marijuana cured in opium, grown in the Chicago area
Chicago leprosy	scars caused by multiple venous injections
chicharra	mixture of tobacco and marijuana
chick	heroin; an attractive female
chicken hawk	a child molester
chicken head	cocaine addict
chicken powder	powdered amphetamines
chicken scratch	searching floor on hands and knees for crack
chicken-shit habit	a small drug habit
chicle	heroin
chicory	inferior quality opium
chief	peyote; mescaline
chieva	heroin
chill	to ignore or refuse to sell drugs to one suspected of being an informer; to relax; to kill
chill out	to relax
chill pill	a depressant
Chillie Willies	snorting vodka or gin out of a bottle cap
chillum, chillun	equipment used for smoking marijuana
China	opium
China cat	high-potency opium
China girl	fentanyl
Chinatown	fentanyl
China White, Chinese	superior quality Asian heroin
Chinaman on one's back	withdrawal symptoms
Chinese blowing	inhalation of pyrolysate
Chinese connection	Chinese drug smugglers
Chinese cure	gradual drug withdrawal
Chinese molasses	opium
Chinese red	heroin
Chinese saxophone	an opium pipe
Chinese tobacco	opium
Chino	a Chinese drug dealer
chip	drug dose taken in a small enough amount to avoid addiction
chipper	occasional drug user
chippie, chippy	one who takes small amounts of drugs irregularly; a prostitute

chipping	using small amounts of drugs on an irregular basis
chips	marijuana or tobacco cigarettes laced with PCP
chira	marijuana
chiva	heroin
chlorals	chloral hydrate
Cho Mo	a child molester
chocolate	opium; amphetamine
chocolate chip cookies	MDMA with heroin or methadone
chocolate chips	MDMA; LSD
chocolate powder	mescaline
chocolate rock	crack and heroin mixture
chocolate rocket	crack made brown in color by adding powdered chocolate milk during processing
chocolate Thai	marijuana
choke	to dilute drugs
choke out	the choking game
choker	large or powerful hit of crack cocaine
cholly	cocaine
chop	to process heroin or marijuana
Christians	cross-scored amphetamine tablets
Christina	amphetamines
Christine	crystal methamphetamine
Christmas rolls, Christmas trees	different colored barbiturate capsules; amphetamines; dextroamphetamines
chronic	marijuana and crack mixture
Chuck	a white prisoner or officer
chuck a Charley, chuck a dummy	to fake a withdrawal spasm in an attempt to get drugs from a medical practitioner
chuck horrors	voracious craving for food during withdrawal
chuck the habit	to break a drug addiction
chucks	hunger following withdrawal from heroin
chug, chug-a-lug	to quickly drink alcohol
chunky	marijuana
church	LSD paper with cross on it
church key	an opener used to open cans or bottles that contain alcohol
churus	marijuana
cibas (CIBAs)	Doriden
cid	LSD
cigarette papers	packets of heroin
cigarrode crystal	PCP
circles	Rohypnol

circus	faking a withdrawal spasm in an attempt to get drugs from a medical practitioner
citizen	nonuser of drugs
citrol	high-potency Nepal marijuana
CJ, KJ	PCP in crystalline form
clanks	delirium tremens
clarity	MDMA
clay	hashish
clean	one who has ceased using drugs; an addict's arm free of needle marks; not in possession of drugs
clean and manicured	marijuana that is free of stems and seeds
clear light	superior quality LSD in gelatin capsule form
clear up	to cease using drugs
click up	to join a prison gang
clickem, clickum	a marijuana cigarette that has been dipped in embalming fluid and laced with PCP
clicker	crack and PCP mixture
cliffhanger	PCP
climax	butyl nitrite
climb	to ascend to a high from smoking a marijuana cigarette
clink	jail or prison
clip	holder for a marijuana cigarette; to rob
clipped one's wings	arrested
clips	rows of vials heat-sealed together
clocker	an entry-level drug dealer who sells 24 hours a day
clocking paper	money made from selling drugs
closed	a drug source who is not selling because of law enforcement suspicion
closet baser	user of cocaine who prefers anonymity
cloud	smoke created by using pipes
cloud nine	euphoria felt from smoking drugs
clouted	arrested
club	a place to smoke marijuana
cluck	crack smoker
clucker	cocaine addict
Clydesdale	a physically fit or handsome male
coast to coast	long-acting amphetamines
coasting	under the influence of drugs
coca	cocaine
coca paste	a potent form of cocaine

cocaine blues	depression after extended cocaine use
cochornis	marijuana
cock pipe	drug paraphernalia that is shaped like a penis and is used to smoke marijuana
cockle burrs	amphetamines
cocktail	tobacco cigarette mixed with marijuana or dipped in hashish oil
coco rocks	crack cocaine that is made dark brown by adding chocolate pudding during production
cocoa puff	to smoke cocaine and marijuana
coconut	cocaine
cod cock	cough syrup containing codeine
code 21	masturbation
Cody	codeine
coffee	LSD
coffee cups	bags that hold marijuana
coffee dodger	a chain smoker
coffin nail	a cigarette
coke	cocaine; crack
coke bar	a bar where cocaine is openly used
coke blower	one who sniffs powdered cocaine
coke break	a break one takes to use cocaine
coke bugs	sensation that bugs are crawling under the skin after using cocaine
coke crash	severe anxiety or depression following heavy cocaine use
coke freak	a regular cocaine user
coke oven	a place where cocaine is used or sold
coke party, coke time	a gathering in which participants use cocaine
coke whore	one who performs sexual favors in exchange for cocaine
coked up	under the influence of cocaine
cokehead	a habitual cocaine user
cokeroaches	imaginary bugs crawling on one who is high on cocaine
cokie	a cocaine user
cola	cocaine
cold and hot	mixture of cocaine and heroin
cold shake	injection of transiently suspended insoluble particles
cold turkey	an abrupt and complete withdrawal from a habit
coli	marijuana

coliflor tostao	marijuana
collar	a narrow strip of paper that secures a needle to an eyedropper; to make a drug bust; to arrest
collard greens	marijuana
Colombian connection	Colombian drug smugglers
Colombian gold	potent Colombian marijuana
Colombian green	superior quality Colombian marijuana
Colombian roulette	smuggling drugs from Colombia by swallowing packets and excreting them on delivery
Colorado	cocaine
Colorado Kool-Aid	Coors beer
Colorado Rockies	crack cocaine
Columbo	PCP
Columbus black	marijuana grown in the Columbus, Ohio, area
Columbus black tea	marijuana
come back	cocaine that has been adulterated for conversion to crack
come home	to return to reality after an LSD trip
come up	to increase profit made in drug sales
communist M&Ms	red Seconal capsules
comp man	a drug dealer
con	to manipulate by using applied psychology; a convict
conductor	one who guides others through LSD trips
Congo brown	a brown-colored variety of African marijuana
Congo dirt	superior quality African marijuana
connect	to purchase illegal drugs
connection, contact	one who sells or supplies illegal drugs
constitutional	an addict's first injection of the day
contact high	psychological feeling of being high merely from being around a person who is under the influence of drugs or alcohol
contact lens	LSD
convert	one who is recently addicted to drugs
cook	an opium den attendant who prepares opium; to smoke marijuana or hashish
cook down	process in which users liquify drugs
cook up a pill	to prepare a drug for smoking
cooker	a container that is used for heating and dissolving heroin, amphetamines, or cocaine
cookin'	having a good time; process in manufacturing methamphetamines
cooking up	to process cocaine into crack cocaine

cooler	cigarette laced with a drug
coolie	cigarette laced with opium
coolie mud	inferior quality opium
coop	jail or prison
coozie, cozy, couzie, couzy stash	a condom or other parcel of drugs concealed in the vagina
cop	to get anything; to buy dope; a police officer
cop a buzz	to smoke marijuana
cop a deuceway	to purchase a $2 package of narcotics
cop a drag	to draw smoke from a cigarette
cop a feel	to fondle
cop a fix	to obtain a dose of drugs
cop a match	to purchase a matchbox of marijuana
cop a pill	to smoke an opium pellet
cop a sneak	to leave a place
cop and blow	to purchase drugs and quickly leave the scene
cop man	a police officer
cop out	to back out; to inform
co-pilot	amphetamine; sober companion for one who is under the influence of drugs or alcohol
cop-out	an excuse for changing one's mind
copper	a police officer
copping zones	areas where drugs can be purchased
copycat crime	a crime that is committed in imitation of another crime
corals	chloral hydrate
coriander seeds	money
Corinne, Corine	cocaine
cork the air	to inhale cocaine
corn	marijuana
corn dog	a marijuana cigarette laced with cocaine
cornstalk	marijuana cigarette rolled in the shuck of a corn cob, then sealed with honey
cosmic, cozmic	experience on drugs
cosmos, cosmos	PCP
cotics	narcotics
cotton	paper money; OxyContin; the cotton used for straining certain drugs
cotton brothers	heroin, cocaine, morphine
cotton catcher, cotton top	an addict who begs for used straining cotton
cotton fever	fever from infection, allergic reaction, blood poisoning, or other illness contracted after using contaminated straining cotton

cotton freak	one who inhales from straining cotton
cotton shooter	addict who injects residue from straining cotton
cotton shot	water added to cotton in an attempt to get whatever drug is left on straining cotton
cottonhead	one who uses previously used straining cotton as a drug source
cottons	pieces of cotton used to strain dissolved, heated drugs before injecting them
couch doctor	a psychiatrist
count	the purity level of a drug
courage pills	heroin or barbiturates
course note	any bill larger than $2
cowboy	an independent drug seller; a new correctional officer
crack	a purer, more potent form of cocaine, usually mixed with ammonia or baking soda and formed into crystals
crack attack	to crave crack cocaine
crack back	crack and marijuana
crack cooler	crack soaked in a wine cooler
crack dream	vivid or unpleasant dream
crack gallery	a place where cocaine is sold and used
crack house	a gathering place where participants use cocaine
crack kit	glass pipe and copper mesh for use by cocaine users
crack pipe	a pipe used for smoking crack
crack spot	an area where people can purchase or use crack
crack star	a frequent user of crack
crack weed	marijuana laced with crack
cracker	crack cocaine user
cracker jacks	crack smokers
crackers	animal crackers laced with LSD; a mixture of Talwin and Ritalin
crackhead	one who uses crack cocaine
cracking	gesturing as if cracking a whip, used to advertise crack
crank	methamphetamines in powdered form
crank bugs	feeling that bugs are crawling under the skin after heavy amphetamine use
crank freak	one who alternates between amphetamines and barbiturates and tranquilizers
cranking up	to inject a drug
crankster	one who uses and/or manufactures crank

crap	inferior quality heroin; nonsense
crapper dick	a law enforcement agent who patrols public toilets looking for illicit sexual activity and drug deals
crash	to sleep or lose consciousness after drug use; to spend the night
crash pad	a place to recover from a drug trip
crashed	raided by law enforcement agents
crater	a scar of indentation left at a healed abscess site from an injection
crazy coke	PCP
crazy drug	pure form of methamphetamine from Thailand
crazy Eddie	a marijuana or tobacco cigarette dipped in embalming fluid and laced with PCP
crazy weed	marijuana
creamed	alcohol or drug intoxicated
credit card	crack stem
creeper	slow-acting marijuana
creeps	delirium tremens
crib	an addict's dwelling; one's residence
criddy	methamphetamines
crill	a marijuana cigarette laced with cocaine
crimmie	a tobacco cigarette laced with crack
crink	methamphetamines; amphetamines
cripple	a marijuana cigarette laced with a drug
Crips	the name of a well-known street gang
cris	methamphetamine in powdered form
crisco	crystal methamphetamine
crisp	under the influence of drugs
crispo	one who is mentally, socially, and physically burned out from drug use
crispy critter	under the influence of marijuana
crisscrossing	simultaneously snorting heroin in one nostril and cocaine in the other from parallel lines
crissy	crystal methamphetamine
Cristina	methamphetamine
Cristy	smokable methamphetamine
croak	crack and methamphetamine; to die
croaker	a physician
croaker joint	a hospital
crock	an opium pipe; a lie
crocked	intoxicated from alcohol intake
cross tops	cross-scored amphetamine tablets

Slang Terms

cross-country hype	an addict who goes from place to place in search of drugs from medical practitioners
crosses	cross-scored amphetamine tablets
crossroads	cross-scored amphetamine tablets
crow	cocaine
crown crap	heroin
cruise	to drive slowly back and forth along a designated route
crumb snatcher	an addict who steals tiny pieces of crack
crumbs	small rock cocaine particles
crunch & munch	crack
crunk	hip-hop music
crusher	a police officer
crusty treats	crack
crutch	a device used to hold a marijuana cigarette butt
Cruz	opium from Vera Cruz, Mexico
crying weed	marijuana
crypto	methamphetamine
crystal, krystal	crystallized methamphetamine
crystal doe	crystallized methamphetamine
crystal joint, krystal joint	PCP
crystal meth	crystallized methamphetamine
crystal pop	cocaine and PCP
crystal ship	a syringe containing a dissolved crystallized drug
crystal tea, T	LSD
cube	approximately 1 ounce of morphine; LSD on a sugar cube; a person who does not use drugs or alcohol
cube juice	morphine
cubehead	a user who prefers to take LSD in the form of a sugar cube
cubes	sugar cubes that have been laced with LSD
cupcakes	LSD
curbstones	cigarette butts retrieved from gutters
curse	menstrual period
curse of Eve	menstrual period
cushion	vein site for injecting a drug
cut	to dilute a drug by adding some other substance, such as milk, sugar, quinine; to stab someone
cut deck	heroin or morphine diluted with powdered milk
cut loose	to escape from jail or prison

cutting up	prison suicide
cyclones	PCP
D	Dilaudid; LSD; dust
D&D	drunk and disorderly
DA	a drug addict; district attorney
dabble	to use drugs occasionally
dabbler	an occasional drug user
daddy	a homosexual prisoner; a pimp
dagga	South African marijuana
dagga rooker	a smoker of South African marijuana
dagging	trading out for sodomy
daisy chaining	injecting and withdrawing a drug back into a needle for injection by the next user; sexual coupling involving three or more
dai-yen	opium that is prepared for smoking
dals	Dalmane
Dama Blanca	cocaine
Dame DuPaw	marijuana
damps	barbiturates
dance fever	fentanyl
dance hall	chamber in which prisoners are executed
dank	marijuana
dans	oxycodone
date	sex between a John and a whore
dawamesk	marijuana
DD	a deadly dose of drugs
dead	out of drug money; out of drugs
dead on arrival	heroin
deadly nightshade	belladonna
deadwood	an undercover law enforcement agent who is working to trap those involved in drug deals
dealer	one who sells or supplies drugs
deans	codeine
death hit	cyanide, strychnine, battery acid
death trips	LSD mixed with another drug
death wish	PCP
death's head	the Amanita muscaria mushroom
death's herb	belladonna
deazingus	a hypodermic syringe or medicine dropper with a needle attached
debs	MDMA; barbiturates
decadence	MDMA

deck	a pack of cigarettes; folded paper containing heroin
deck up	to fill a packet or envelope with a dose of powdered drugs
deeda	LSD
deens, deines, denes	codeine
dees, Ds	Dilaudid
deferred success	no such thing as failure
Delilah	a prostitute
demis, dems, demies	Demerol
demo	a sample-size quantity of crack
demolish	crack
desert horse	a Camel cigarette
designer drugs	variations of amphetamines, methamphetamines, and heroin
desire	PCP and cocaine mixture
destroyed	heavily drug intoxicated
DET	diethyltryptamine, a hallucinogen
Detroit punk	PCP
deuce	2-year prison sentence; $2 drug purchase
devil	Seconal; crack
devil dust	PCP
devil's apple	jimsonweed
devil's smoke	crack cocaine
devil's dandruff	powdered cocaine
devil's dick	crack pipe
dew	marijuana; hashish; $10 drug purchase
dex, dexies	Dexedrine (dextroamphetamine)
diablo	LSD paper with a devil on it
diambista	marijuana
diamonds	amphetamines; ecstasy
Diane	meperidine
diaper sniper	a child molester
dib & dab	to use drugs intermittently
dice	methamphetamines
dick	a police officer; penis
diddler	a child molester
diddleums	delirium tremens
dids	Dilaudid
dies	Valium
diesel	heroin
digatee	the rush one feels following an injection of a drug

digger	a pickpocket
diggidy	a good herb
digging the bowls	smoking marijuana from a pipe
diggity	heroin
digie	scales used to weigh drugs
dill	Placidyl
dillie, dillies, dilies, dilly	Dilaudid
dimba	marijuana from West Africa
dime	a 10-year prison sentence; a $1000 bet
dime bag	a $10 drug purchase
dime special	crack
dime dropper	an informer
dime's worth	amount of heroin to cause death
dime-store high	glue sniffing
ding	marijuana
ding wing	the area of a prison in which mentally ill prisoners are housed
dingbats	delirium tremens
dingers	equipment for injecting drugs
dinghizen, dingus	a medicine dropper with a needle attached
dinky dow	marijuana
dinosaurs	LSD; baby boomer population who still use illegal drugs
dip	to immerse cigarettes in embalming fluid
dipped	addicted to narcotics
dipper	an opium pipe
dipping out	to take a portion of crack from vials
dirt	marijuana
dirt grass	inferior quality marijuana
dirt nap	to die
dirty arm	scarred arms from needle marks
dirty deed	to inject drugs
dirty joint	marijuana cigarettes laced with another drug
dirty laundry or linen	private matters that have been publicly exposed
dis, dissing	to disrespect
disco biscuits	MDMA; Quaaludes
disco drug	the vapors from butyl nitrite used by some dancers
discorama	inhalants
disease	drug of choice
dispatcher	a killer
ditch	the best vein site for drug injection, usually the inside of the elbow; to get rid of

ditch digger	one who injects drugs
ditch weed	inferior quality marijuana
dithers	delirium tremens
divider	sharing a joint with someone
dizz	a feeling of dizziness following marijuana use
djamba	marijuana
D-man	a federal drug enforcement officer
DMT	N-dimethyltryptamine; a short-duration, fast-acting hallucinogen
DMZ	benactyzine
do a Brodie or Brody	to commit suicide
do a joint	to smoke marijuana
do a line	to snort a drug from a line
do a number	to smoke a marijuana cigarette
do it Jack	to use PCP
do up	to shoot or inject a drug; to smoke marijuana; to place a tourniquet around the arm in preparation for an injection
DOA	PCP; dead on arrival
doctor	MDMA
dodo	a drug addict
does	methamphetamines
dog	weak opium residue
dog biscuits	peyote
dog food	heroin
doggie, dojee, doojee, doogie	heroin
doja	strong marijuana
dollar	$100 worth of drugs
dolls, dollies	depressants; amphetamines; MDMA
dolo	methadone
domes	MDMA; LSD
domestic	marijuana grown in the United States
dominoes	black and white capsules that contain an amphetamine and a barbiturate
Dona Juana, Juanita	marijuana
donjem	marijuana
doobie, dubbe, duby	a marijuana cigarette
dool, dooley	an addict
doormat	a person who is regularly exploited by others
doors and 4s	combination of Doriden and Tylenol 4
dope	habit-forming narcotics
dope daddy	a drug supplier or seller
dope den	a place where users gather to use drugs

dope fiend	a drug-dependent person
dope gun	a hypodermic needle
dope sick	an addict who is in need of drugs
dope smoke	to smoke marijuana
doped up	under the influence of drugs
doper	a drug user or addict
dopium	opium
doradilla	marijuana
dork	an unpleasant, unattractive, or insignificant person
dossing	sleeping after using drugs
dots	mescaline; peyote
doub	$20 rock or crack
double blue	a capsule of Amytal
double breasted dealing	simultaneous dealing of cocaine and heroin
double bubble	cocaine
double crosses	cross-scored amphetamine tablets
double deed	injecting drugs and taking pills
double dome	LSD
double header	2 marijuana cigarettes smoked at the same time
double narky	a double dose of narcotics
double rock	crack diluted with procaine
double trouble	amobarbital and secobarbital
double up	when a dealer delivers extra drugs as a marketing scheme
double ups	a $20 rock that can be broken into two $20 rocks
double yoke	crack
douche	to inject a drug
douche bag	a sleazy person
douse the lamp	to ejaculate during a sexual dream while in a stupor from opium use
dove	base cocaine rock
Dover's deck, powder	opium
downs, downers	sedatives, barbiturates, alcohol, tranquilizers, and narcotics
downtown	heroin
downtown Brown	inferior quality marijuana
dozer	marijuana; depressants
DPT	dipropylphyptamine; a hallucinogen
Dr. Bananas	amyl nitrite
Dr. Feelgood	a physician who will prescribe or sell drugs on request

Dr. White	cocaine
draf weed	marijuana
drag	an unpleasant experience of any kind; puff from a cigarette
drag weed	marijuana
dragged	an anxious state induced by smoking marijuana
draw up	to inject a drug
dread weed	marijuana
dream beads	opium pellets
dream boat	a drug dealer's establishment
dream game	the choking game
dream gum	opium
dream pipe	an opium pipe
dream stick	an opium pipe; a marijuana cigarette
dream, dreamer	morphine; opium; depressants
dreck	heroin
drink	PCP
drink Texas tea	to smoke marijuana
dripper	equipment for injecting drugs, usually an eye dropper
dripping bum	one returning from a cocaine high
drive	a euphoric rush one feels following a drug injection
drivers	amphetamines
droopy	feeling the effects of sedative drugs
drop	to take drugs or pills by mouth
drop a bop	to take drugs in pill form
drop a roll	to take a variety of 3 to 5 pills at once
drop man	one who makes deliveries of substantial amounts of drugs; usually not a user
dropper	to inject a drug
drops	a place to leave drugs after a purchase; point of pick up for drugs
drought	a shortage of drugs
drowsy high	feeling the effects of sedative drugs
drug	to take a large quantity of drugs
drug deal	the exchange of money for drugs
drug store heroin	Dilaudid
drug store Johnson	addiction to drugs usually used as medication
dry high	marijuana
dry out	to stop using drugs for a while
dry spell	when drugs are unavailable; abstinence from drug use

dry up	to stop using drugs for a while
DTs	delirium tremens
dub sack	$20 worth of drugs
dube, dubie, duby	marijuana
duct	cocaine
due	residue of oils remaining in a pipe after smoking base
dugout	veins that are pitted and scarred from multiple injections
duji	heroin
dummies	propoxyphene
dummy	bogus heroin
dummy dust	bogus PCP
dust	heroin; cocaine; PCP mixed with various chemicals
dust a joint	to lace a cigarette with PCP
dust blunt	marijuana and PCP mixture
dust of angels	PCP
dust of Morpheus	morphine
dusted	drug intoxicated
dusted parsley	PCP
duster	heroin and tobacco mixed in a cigarette
dusthead	PCP user
dusting	adding a drug to marijuana
dusty roads	mixture of cocaine and PCP for smoking
dweeb	an unpleasant, unattractive, or insignificant person
dyls	Placidyl
dynamite	heroin and cocaine mixture
dyno, dyno pure	heroin
E	ecstasy
earth	a marijuana cigarette
ease on in	to move slowly so no one knows what you are doing
easing powder	opium; morphine
east side player	crack user
easy lay	one who takes GHB; easy sex
easy score	obtaining drugs or sex easily
eat	to take acid or mushrooms
eater	a user who takes drugs orally
eating	taking a drug orally
E-ball	a type of ecstasy with an eightball on it
E-bomb	MDMA

echoes	LSD trip flashbacks
ecstasy	MDMA/MDA
Edge City	where an addict is when contemplating withdrawal
egg	crack
Egyptian driver	a drug dealer
eight, 8	heroin
eightball	3.5 grams of cocaine or methamphetamine
eighth, eighth piece	1/8 ounce of a drug
eighty-six, 86	to kill
ekies	Mandrax
El Cid	LSD
Elaine	MDMA
elbow	1 pound of marijuana
Eleanor	a narcotic antagonist
electric	hallucinogenic matter
electric butter	marijuana leaves sautéed in butter
electric Kool Aid	LSD
electric wine	wine laced with LSD
elephant flipping	back-and-forth use of ecstasy and PCP
elephant tranquilizer, tranq	PCP
elephants	MDMA
elevator	a regularly used preparation of opium
eleventh finger	penis
Ellis Day	LSD
els, l's	Elavil
Elvis	LSD
embalming fluid	PCP
emergency gun	a safety pin or sewing machine needle used as a substitute for a hypodermic needle
empties	recycled gelatin capsules that are returned to a drug dealer for a discount on a purchase
emsel	morphine
endo	marijuana
ends	money used for drugs
energizer	PCP
enforcer	a strongman for a drug dealer
eng shee	an alcohol extraction of opium residue used for injections
engine	an opium smoking outfit
enhanced	under the influence of drugs
enliven	1,4-BD
enoltestovis	injectable steroid

ephedrone	methcathinone
E-puddle	sleeping after taking ecstasy, or exhaustion after attending a rave
erase	to kill
erth	PCP
esra	marijuana
essence	a variation of amphetamine or methamphetamine; ecstasy
estuffa	heroin
ET	alpha ethyltryptamine
E-tard	person under the influence of ecstasy
euphoria	MDMA, mescaline, and crystal meth
Eve	a variation of amphetamine or methamphetamine; MDEA
Everclear	GHB; Rohypnol
ex	ecstasy
experience	an LSD trip
explorers club	a group of LSD users
exposures	marijuana cigarettes
extasy	ecstasy
eye opener	first narcotcs injection of the day; amphetamines
eyelid movies	images seen during an LSD trip
fachiva	heroin
factory	place where drugs are packaged, diluted, or manufactured
faded	under the influence of marijuana
fainting game	the choking game
fairy	an opium smoker's lamp
fairy dust	PCP
fairy powder	a powdered narcotic
fake	substitute for a hypodermic needle
fake a blast	to pretend to be under the influence of drugs
fake STP	PCP
fall	arrested
fall out	overdose
Fallbrook redhair	marijuana, term from Fallbrook, CA
famine	to be out of drugs
famous dime	crack
fang	a hypodermic needle
fantasy, fantasia	GHB
farmer	one who grows marijuana at home

farm-to-arm	referring to individuals who grow, process, and sell drugs
fart	a foolish or contemptible person
fat bags	bags full of drugs
fat jay	a thick marijuana cigarette
fat pappy	a thick marijuana cigarette
fatty	a thick marijuana cigarette
feathered	under the influence of drugs
fed	a federal law enforcement agent
feebie	an FBI agent
feeblo	a drug addict
feed	drugs; to use drugs
feed and grain man	a drug supplier or seller
feed bag	a package of drugs
feed one's head	to take drugs by mouth
feed store	a place to buy and sell drugs
feeder	a hypodermic needle
Felix the Cat	LSD
fen	fentanyl citrate
fence patrol	escape from prison
fender bender	barbiturate
F-forties, F40s	Seconal tablets that bear the Identi-Code symbol F40
fi-do-nie	opium
fields	LSD
fiend	a drug addict
Fifi	an artificial vagina used for masturbation
fifteen cents, 15¢	drugs worth $15
fifty, 50	LSD
fifty-one, 51	crack; a cigarette laced with crack
figure-8	an addict who feigns a withdrawal spasm in an attempt to get drugs
film can	a container for marijuana
finaject	veterinary steroids
fine stuff	high-quality drugs
finger	a condom or finger cot that is filled with drugs, then swallowed or concealed in the rectum or vagina
finger lid	marijuana
finger wave	digital exam of the rectum or vagina for concealed drugs
fir	marijuana
fire	to inject a drug; crack and methamphetamine

fire it up	to smoke marijuana
firecracker	a marijuana cigarette
fired	marijuana ashes with no active ingredient remaining
firewater	GBL
firing an antiaircraft or ack ack gun	smoking a cigarette that has been laced with heroin
first line	morphine
fish	one who has been arrested; a new prisoner
fish scales	crack
fish slip	the charge brought against an individual who has been arrested
fishbowl	a jail's holding area
fit	equipment used for preparation or use of drugs
five dollar bag	drugs worth $50
five-C note	$500 bill
five-cent bag	drugs worth $5
five-cent paper	powdered drug folded in paper worth $5
five-O	the police
fives	amphetamines
fix	a ration of drugs
fixed up	provided with a ration of drugs
fixer	a drug dealer
fizzies	methadone
flag	appearance of blood in a syringe or medicine dropper, indicating that a needle has entered a vein
flake	cocaine; an eccentric person
flake acid	diluted solution of LSD placed on blotter paper and cut into small servings
flaky	an addict; acting in an eccentric manner
flame cooking	smoking cocaine base with a pipe over a stove flame
flamethrowers	cigarette laced with cocaine and heroin
Flannigan	marijuana
flash	a drug rush; hallucination
flash house	where users congregate to use drugs
flash in the pan	a brief rush after taking heroin cut with quinine
flash out	momentary unconsciousness caused from sniffing an inhalant
flashback	a recurrent hallucination experienced long after an LSD trip
flat blues	LSD

flat chunks	crack cut with benzocaine
flat time	to serve time in prison without parole
flatfoot	a police officer
flatline game	the choking game
flatliner	4-methylthioamphetamine
flats	LSD
flatten the poker	impotence caused from drug use
flattened	alcohol or drug intoxicated
flea powder	drugs of inferior quality
flesh peddler	a pimp; a person who solicits clients for a prostitute
flex	counterfeit crack
flier	a drug user who is always high
flip out	to lose control of oneself as a result of using drugs
flip over	to stop taking drugs temporarily; to become infatuated with a person
flipped	stupefied as a result of drug use
floater	a bit of congealed blood clogging a hypodermic needle; a corpse that is found floating in water
floating	alcohol or drug intoxicated
flogged	alcohol or drug intoxicated
flophouse	a cheap hotel or rooming house
Florida snow	white powdered drugs
flossin'	showing off
flow	to experience euphoria after taking a hallucinogenic drug
flower child	a person who was part of a movement of the 1960s and 1970s that advocated love, beauty, and peace
flower power	morning glory and poppy seeds; peace
flower tops	morning glory and poppy seeds
flowers	morning glory and poppy seeds
fluff	to clean marijuana; to run powdered drugs through a nylon stocking; to chop up dope to make it bulkier and more even in consistency; nonsense; feminine lesbian prisoner
flunk out	to move from occasional drug use to addiction
flunky, flunkey	one who delivers drugs; one who takes foolish risks to obtain drugs; one who is used to perform menial tasks

flush and mush	to flush drugs down the toilet or swallow them so they cannot be found
flushing	injecting and withdrawing a drug back into a needle for injection by the next user
fly	to be intoxicated on drugs
fly Mexican airlines	to smoke marijuana
fly swatter	the muscle man for a drug dealer
fly the coop	to escape from jail or prison
flying	under the influence of drugs
flying saucers	PCP; morning glory seeds
flying triangle	LSD
focus	liquid narcotics
foil	heroin
foilers	smoking cocaine on tin foil
fold up	to become unconscious after alcohol or drug use; to stop selling or taking drugs
following the cloud	searching for drugs
foo-foo stuff	heroin; cocaine
foo-foo dust	powdered drugs
foolish powder	powdered drugs
foon	a pellet of roasted opium
footballs	mixture of amphetamines and dextroamphetamine
fop fops	to fight with fists
foreign mud	opium
foreign smoke	opium
forget-me drug or pill	Rohypnol
forties, 40s	Seconal
fortnighter	one who uses drugs occasionally
forwards	amphetamines
four twenty	marijuana
four ways	LSD, strychnine, methamphetamine, and STP
four-leaf clover	MDMA
fours, 4s	painkillers with codeine in tablets or capsules marked with a 4
4s and doors	Tylenol 4 and Doriden
fourteen	narcotics
fourth degree	withdrawal sickness
four-way hits	cross-scored amphetamine tablets
four-way star	LSD combined with 3 other substances
fraho, frajo	marijuana
frame a twister	feign a withdrawal spasm in an attempt to get drugs

Slang Terms

frantic	in need of drugs
freak	a bizarre-acting person; to experience a bad drug trip; to be afraid
freak house	commune where individuals gather to use drugs
freak out	to have a panic reaction to a drug
freaked out	disturbed or psychotic as a result of previous LSD use
Freddy, Freddie	a stimulant
free trip	a flashback as a result of previous LSD use
freebase	cocaine that has been purified by dissolving it in a heated solvent, such as ether, then separating and drying until it produces vapors for inhalation
freebase rocks	pure form of cocaine
freebie	something for nothing
freeze	refuse to sell drugs to certain individuals; renege on a drug deal
French blues	amphetamines
french fried; fried	under the influence of drugs or alcohol
french fries, fries	crack
Freon freak	one who inhales Freon gas
fresh	PCP
fresh and sweet	recently released from prison; new prostitute; new drug user
fresh kill	to steal someone's drugs
freshman	new drug user or addict
friend	fentanyl
frios	marijuana laced with crack
Frisco special	cocaine, heroin, and LSD mixture
Frisco speedball	cocaine, heroin, and LSD mixture
frisky, frisky powder	cocaine
frog	one who "hops" from place to place in pursuit of drugs
front	to pay money prior to receiving goods or services
frosty	under the influence of cocaine
frozen	under the influence of cocaine
fry stick	a marijuana cigarette laced with embalming fluid or LSD; to be executed in the electric chair
Fu, Fu Manchu	marijuana
fuel	marijuana mixed with insecticides; PCP
fug	a cigarette

full moon	a large portion or the top of peyote cactus
fun joint	a place where individuals gather to use drugs
funky chicken	the choking game
funny paper	marijuana concealed in a newspaper
funny stuff	marijuana
fur	law enforcement agent
future	crystal methamphetamine
fuzz	law enforcement agents
G	a portion of a dollar bill that seals a hypodermic needle onto a medicine dropper; a dollar bill that is rolled up and used for sniffing powdered drugs; $1000; 1 gram of drugs; term for an unfamiliar male; GHB
GB	depressants
gacked	under the influence of amphetamines
gaffel, gaffle	counterfeit cocaine; to handcuff a prisoner
gaffled	arrested
gaffus	an improvised hypodermic needle
gag	heroin
gage, gauge, gauge butt	marijuana; a marijuana cigarette
gagers	methcathinone
gaggler	amphetamines; ecstasy
Gainesville green	marijuana presumably grown near Gainesville, Florida
gak	line of meth or coke
galhead	a drug addict
gallery	a place that sells drugs and equipment for drug users
gallon distemper	delirium tremens
galloping horse	heroin
gamma O	GHB
gammon	1 microgram of LSD
gamot	heroin; morphine
gang bang	rape by a group or a gang
gang jacket	validated as being a gang member
gange	marijuana
gangster	marijuana
gangster pills	barbiturates
ganja, ganga	potent marijuana
gank	counterfeit crack; to steal
gap	yawning and drooling, symptoms of early drug craving
gapper	one who shows early stages of withdrawal

Slang Terms

gar	marijuana rolled in cigar paper
garbage	inferior quality or adulterated drugs; food or meals
garbage freak or garbage head	a person who will take any kind of drug
garbage rock	crack
Garden of Eden	female genitalia
garden variety	middle class citizens
gargoyle	a drug user or addict
garr	large marijuana cigarette
gas	to sniff gasoline fumes; to use nitrous oxide
gash	marijuana; sex
gasket	whatever is used to seal a hypodermic needle onto a syringe
gasper, gasper stick	a marijuana cigarette
gassing	inhaling through a drug-saturated cloth
gate	the vein used to inject drugs
gato	heroin
gazer	a prison officer who watches prisoners take showers
GBL	gamma butyrolactone, used in making GBH
gear	equipment used to inject drugs; drugs in general
gee	opium; paregoric
gee fat	residue of smoked opium pellet which lines an opium bowl
gee gee	an opium pipe
gee head	a paregoric user
gee rag	materials that are used to hold parts of an opium pipe together
gee stick	an opium pipe
gee yen	opium residue
geed up	under the influence of opium
geek	a person who does not fit into the group; marijuana and crack mixture
geek joints	cigarettes filled with marijuana and crack mixture
geeker	a crack user
geeze, geez	to inject drugs
geezer	one who injects drugs
geezin' a bit of dee gee	injecting a drug
gel caps or tabs	form of acid
gelatin	blotter paper soaked in a dilute solution of LSD

generation X	generation following baby boomers, people born in the early 1960s to the late 1970s
generation Y	generation following generation X, people born in early 1980s to the late 1990s
George	heroin
George smack	potent heroin
Georgia home boy	GHB
Georgia home brew	GHB
germs	cigarettes
Geronimo	mixture of alcohol and barbiturates
gestapo	police officers; IRS agents; any oppressive group of people
get a fix	to get drugs
get a gage up	to smoke marijuana
get a gift	receive drugs
get a hit	to take a drug
get behind it	to enjoy or appreciate something
get busy	to rob
get down	to take a drug; to have fun
get high	to be under the influence of drugs
get in the groove	to take a drug
get it on	to take a drug; to engage in sexual activity
get lifted	to be under the influence of drugs
get off	to experience an orgasmic rush after injecting a drug; to come down from a drug trip; to copulate or ejaculate
get off on	to be stimulated by something
get one's nose cold	to snort cocaine
get straight	to relieve a drug craving by taking a dose of a drug; to shake a drug habit
get the wind	to smoke marijuana
get through	obtain drugs
get up	first drug dose of the day
get with it	to inject a drug; to get tasks completed
getting buzzed	getting tattooed
Ghana	marijuana
GHB	gamma hydroxybutyrate; date rape drug
ghost	an opium addict; powdered drugs
ghost busting	smoking cocaine; searching for white particles that may be crack
GHRE	1,4-BD
GI	gang investigator

GI gin	terpin hydrate cough medicine mixed with alcohol
gick monster	crack smoker
gift of the sun, sungod	cocaine
gig	a drug high
giggle smoke	marijuana
giggle weed	marijuana
gigolo	a man who is supported by a woman in return for his attention
gimmicks	equipment used for preparing and injecting drugs
gimmie	crack and marijuana mixture
gin	cocaine
gin mill	a bar
girl, girly	cocaine; crack; heroin
girlfriend	cocaine
gismo	equipment used for injecting drugs
give birth	to defecate hard feces after constipation from prolonged opium use
Give me five.	Put your hand on mine palm to palm.
give someone the go-bye	to refuse to sell drugs to an untrustworthy or undesirable buyer
give up	to inform someone; to stop looking; to let anything go
give wings	inject someone or teach someone to inject heroin
gizzy	marijuana
glacines	heroin
glad stuff	addictive drugs
gladiator school	maximum security prison or penitentiary
glading	using inhalant
glass	hypodermic needle; crystal methamphetamine
glass gun	hypodermic syringe
glasses	a glass pipe
glassy eyes	eyes that resemble glass as a result of being intoxicated from alcohol or drugs
glo	crack
globetrotter	one who moves from place to place in pursuit of drugs; a homeless person who wanders from place to place
glom	to steal drugs
glooch	one whose senses are diminished from prolonged drug use

glory hole	a hole between stalls in a toilet
glory seeds	morning glory seeds
glove	a condom
glue stick	a marijuana cigarette that has been dipped in hashish oil
glued	to be arrested
gluey	a person who sniffs glue
go	amphetamines; ecstasy
go fast	methcathinone; methamphetamines
go faster	amphetamines
go into the sewer	to inject a drug into a vein
go loco	to smoke marijuana
go on a sleigh ride	to use cocaine
go on the boot	a way to inject drugs that allows the user to prolong the rush
go on the wagon	to stop drinking alcohol
go pills	amphetamines; ecstasy
go talk to Al and Herbie	to drink alcohol and smoke marijuana
go to the cathedral	to smoke hashish
go up	to be under the influence of drugs
go with the flow	to deal with adversity
God's drug	morphine
godfather	a marijuana cigarette or cigar that is laced with a drug
God's flesh	psilocybin/psilocin mushrooms
God's medicine	opium
going 90 mph	the peak of a trip
going to the dentist	nitrous oxide
gold	marijuana
gold bud	marijuana, presumably grown in Colombia
gold dust	cocaine
gold duster	one who uses cocaine
gold leaf special	a potent marijuana cigarette
gold star	marijuana
golden dragon	LSD
golden eagle	methamphetamines
golden girl	superior quality cocaine
golden grain	Lebanese hashish
golden leaf	superior quality marijuana
golden spike	a hypodermic needle
golden triangle	boundary areas of Burma, Laos, and Thailand where opium is grown
goldfinger	synthetic heroin

Slang Terms

golf balls	crack
golpe	heroin
goma	opium; black tar heroin
gondola	opium
gong	opium
gong beater	one who uses opium
gong ringer	one who uses opium
gonga smudge	a marijuana cigarette
gongola	an opium pipe
goob	methcathinone
good	PCP
good and plenty	heroin
good butt	a marijuana cigarette
good fella	fentanyl and heroin mixture
good giggles	marijuana
good go	drugs that are good for the amount paid
good H	heroin
good horse	heroin
good lick	good drugs
good stuff	potent drugs
good time man	a drug dealer
good trip	a pleasant experience with hallucinogens
goods	addicting drugs; stolen property
goody-goody	marijuana
goof artist	one who takes unusual drugs
goof balls	barbiturates; amphetamines
goof butt	a marijuana cigarette
goofers	barbiturates
goofing	to be under the influence of a barbiturate; just hanging out
goofy	LSD
goon	PCP
goon dust	PCP
gooney birds	LSD
goop	GHB
gopher	a person who is paid to pick up drugs
goric	paregoric
gorilla	powerfully addicted
gorilla biscuits	PCP
gorilla pills	barbiturates
gorilla tabs	barbiturates
Got any zings?	Do you have amphetamines?
got it going on	a fast sale of drugs

gouch off	to lose consciousness while using drugs
gouger	a marijuana smoker
gow cellar	a place to buy and use opium
gow, ghow	opium
gowhead	an opium user
gowster	an opium user
gozniks	drugs that are addicting
GQ	good quality
grads	amphetamines
graduate	to completely stop using drugs, or to progress to stronger drugs
gram	hashish
granny	to become addicted
granulated orange	methamphetamine
grape parfait	LSD
grapes	prison gossip
grapes of wrath	a wine hangover
grass	marijuana
grass brownies	marijuana
grass mask	a mask with a hose attached to a marijuana pipe
grata	marijuana
gravel	crack
gravy	mixture of heroin and coagulated blood in a hypodermic syringe
Gray Bar Hotel	a prison
gray dust	stale PCP
grease	money
grease pit	a dealer's place of business
greasy	a destitute addict; a severely addicted person; one who is unkempt
greasy bag	a bag in which heroin is kept
great bear	fentanyl
great Scott	an opium pipe
great tobacco	opium
great white hope	crack
greefa, greefo	marijuana
greefer	one who smokes marijuana
green	marijuana that has a low resin content; ketamine
green acorn salad	LSD
green and blacks	Librium
green and clears	Dexamyl
green angelfish	LSD on a blotter stamped with an angelfish

green ashes	usable opium residue from an opium pipe
green beauty	Dexamyl
green bud	home-grown marijuana
green button	a fresh button of peyote
green caps	green LSD capsules
green cigarette	a marijuana cigarette
green dots	LSD
green double domes	LSD
green dragon	LSD on a blotter stamped with a green dragon; LSD combined with another drug
green frog	barbiturates
green goddess	marijuana
green gold	cocaine
green goods	paper money
green hornets	Dexamyl
green hype	a new addict
green leaves	PCP
green light	a target for death
green meanies	amphetamines
green Moroccan	marijuana grown in Morocco
green mud	usable opium residue from an opium pipe
green paint	marijuana
green rot	inferior quality opium
green single domes	LSD
green stuff	paper money
green swirls	LSD combined with another drug
green tea	PCP
green triangles	MDMA
green wedge	LSD
greenies	Dexedrine and amobarbital combination; ecstasy
greens	Dexamyl
greeter	marijuana
Greta	marijuana
grey shields	LSD
griefs	marijuana
grievous bodily harm	GHB
griff, griffa, griffo	marijuana
g-riffick	GHB
grimmy	a marijuana cigarette laced with methamphetamine or crank
grit	crack
groceries	crack

grocery boy	an addict in need of food
G-rock	1 gram of rock cocaine
grogged	under the influence of drugs
groover	a drug user
grooving	alcohol or drug intoxicated; getting to know someone
groovy lemon	a yellow LSD tablet
gross out	to totally repulse
ground control	one who guides a user through a hallucinogenic experience
groupie	a person who follows famous people from appearance to appearance, offering assistance or sexual favors
grower	one who grows marijuana
G-shot	a small amount of liquefied narcotic
G-spot tornado	equal parts of rum and Nyquil
guide	one who guides an LSD user through a trip
gulf	Persian Gulf heroin
gum	opium with MDMA
guma, gumma	opium
gumball	a potent form of heroin; the light bar on top of a police car
gumdrop	Seconal
gun	a hypodermic needle
gungeon	a potent type of marijuana
gungun	marijuana
gunja	marijuana
gunk	morphine
gunny	a potent type of marijuana
gunpowder	raw opium
guns	equipment used for injecting drugs
gunsel	a new prisoner who talks tough
Gunther	a neighborhood drug dealer
guru	one who has experienced an LSD trip and coaches another through it
gutter	the vein inside the elbow used for injecting drugs
gutter hype	a destitute addict
gutter junkie, junky	a destitute addict
guttersnipe	a child who lives on the streets
guy	marijuana
gweebo	an unpleasant, unattractive, or insignificant person

gym candy	steroids
gyve stick	a marijuana cigarette
H	heroin
H&C	heroin and cocaine combination
H&R	hit and run (quick drug purchase and exit)
H bomb	ecstasy mixed with heroin
H caps	powdered heroin in gelatin capsules
hache	heroin
hack	a correctional officer
hail	crack
hair of the dog	a drink of liquor taken in an attempt to cure a hangover
haircut	marijuana
hairy	heroin
half a C	$50 bill
half a football field	50 rocks of crack
half a G	$500
half and half	oral and straight sex
half ass	worthless or near worthless heroin
half bundle	twelve $5 bags of heroin
half kee	fraction of a kilogram
half load	fifteen $3 bags (decks) of heroin
half moons	hashish that is molded into the shape of a half moon; peyote
half piece	1/2 ounce of powdered drugs
half spoon	1/2 spoon of cocaine
half track	crack
halva	illicit drugs
halves	1/2 ounce of heroin
hamburger helper	crack
hammerheading	MDMA used with Viagra
hand-to-hand	delivery that is made by handing drugs to the buyer
hang-up	anything that takes time; a bother; a personal problem
hanhich	marijuana
hanyak	smokable methamphetamine
happy cigarette	a marijuana cigarette
happy dust	powdered drugs
happy grass	marijuana
happy medicine	morphine
happy pills	barbiturates
happy powder	powdered drugs

happy sticks	marijuana cigarettes that are dusted with powdered drugs
happy trails	cocaine
happy-time weed	marijuana
hard candy	heroin
hard hat	a bigoted person
hard line	crack
hard nail	a hypodermic needle
hard rock	a hardened, tough prisoner; crack
hard stuff	morphine; heroin; cocaine; opium; other opiates
hard time	a sentence without parole
hardcore	heavy drug user
hardware	isobutyl nitrite; inhalants
harm reducer	marijuana
harness bulls	uniformed police officers
harpoon	a hypodermic needle
Harry	heroin; morphine
Harry Jones	heroin
harsh	hashish; marijuana
Harvey Wallbanger	STP-LSD combination
hash cannon	a device used to smoke hashish
hash house	a place where hashish is sold or used
hash oil	oil residue from hashish
hashhead	one who smokes hashish
hatchet man	a killer
hats	LSD
have a Chinaman on one's back	to experience withdrawal symptoms; to have a heroin or opium habit
haven dust	cocaine
Hawaiian	potent marijuana
Hawaiian black	marijuana
Hawaiian grass	marijuana, presumably grown in Hawaii
Hawaiian hay	marijuana
Hawaiian pods	a potent hallucinogenic drug
Hawaiian sunshine	LSD
hawk	LSD
hay	inferior quality marijuana
hay burner	a marijuana smoker
hay butt	a marijuana cigarette
hay head	a marijuana smoker
hay puffer	a marijuana smoker
haze	LSD

Hazel	heroin
head	someone who uses drugs; a person who is high much of the time; toilet
head bob	a personal blunt of marijuana
head cleaner	inhalants
head drugs	drugs that affect the mind
head kit	equipment used for smoking or injecting drugs
head running	excessive talking
head rush	the dizziness one experiences after taking a drug
head shop	a shop specializing in drug paraphernalia
head shrinker	a psychiatrist
headlights	LSD
heaped	alcohol or drug intoxicated
hearts	heart-shaped amphetamine tablets
heat	the police; pressure from law enforcement agents
heat wave	a prisoner who is under constant suspicion
heater	a gun
heaven	cocaine
heaven and hell	PCP
heaven dust	powdered drugs
heavenly blue	LSD; morning glory seeds
heavies	addictive drugs
heavy	an altered state of consciousness after drug use; serious
heavy artillery	equipment used for preparing or injecting drugs
heavy biter	one who needs to take more than the usual amount of drugs to feel the effect
heavy joint	a marijuana cigarette that is laced with PCP
heebie jeebies	delirium tremens
heeled	having plenty of money
Helen	heroin
hell	crack
hell dust	powdered heroin or morphine
helpers	amphetamines
he-man	fentanyl
hemp	marijuana
hemp humper	a marijuana smoker
hemp roller	a marijuana smoker
henpecking	searching on hands and knees for crack
Henry	heroin
Henry VIII	1/8 ounce of cocaine

her	cocaine
Herb	a weak prisoner; marijuana
Herb and Al	marijuana and alcohol
Hercules	superior quality PCP
herms	PCP
hero of the underworld	heroin
hero, heroina	heroin
hessle	heroin
hi-fi	mixture of morphine and cocaine
high beams	wide eyes associated with taking crack
high class	hepatitis C
high hat	a prepared opium pellet
high kick	a drug rush
high roller	one who spends money or gambles freely and recklessly
high speed	amphetamines
high tea	a marijuana smoking party
highball	inhalant
hikori, hikuli	peyote; mescaline
hillbilly heroin	OxyContin
him	heroin
Hinkley	PCP
hip layer	an opium smoker
hippie crack	inhalants
hippie flip	mushrooms and MDMA
hiropon, hironpon	smokable methamphetamine
hit	to purchase drugs; to take a drug by snorting, sniffing, injecting, or smoking; an arrest; a dose of drugs
hit it	masturbation; anal sex
hit on	to purchase drugs; to flirt with a person of the opposite sex
hit spike	a substitute for a hypodermic needle
hit the bricks	to be released from prison
hit the flute	to smoke opium
hit the hay	to smoke marijuana
hit the mainline	to inject drugs into a vein
hit the needle	to inject drugs into a vein
hit the pipe	to smoke opium
hit the pit	to inject drugs into a vein
hitch	prison sentence; time in military service
hitch up the reindeer	to prepare to inject or inhale cocaine
hitter	a pipe that is designed for one hit

hitting up	injecting drugs into a vein
ho	a whore
HO	1/2 ounce of marijuana
hocus	liquor that has been laced with drugs; morphine; opium; marijuana
hoe	a whore or prostitute
Hoffman's bicycle	LSD
hog	PCP; one who requires large doses of drugs to sustain a habit; a motorcycle
hog leg	a fat marijuana cigarette
holding	in possession of illicit drugs
hole	solitary confinement; segregation
hole in one	a bullet wound in a body orifice
holy week	menstrual period
hombre	heroin
home	the vein that is the target for an injection
homegrown	marijuana
homicide	heroin cut with scopolamine or strychnine
honey	money
honey blunts	marijuana cigars sealed with honey
honey oil	hashish extract
honeymoon	the stage of drug use before addiction or dependence occurs
hong-yen	heroin in a red pill form
hooch	homemade alcohol; marijuana
hoochie-mamma	a 2-paper marijuana cigarette
hood	neighborhood
hoof	to hide contraband in the rectum
hook	an improvised injection device
hook up	to put an individual in contact with a dealer
hookah	a device used to cool smoke by filtering it through liquid
hooked	addicted or dependent on drugs
hoop	to hide contraband in the rectum
hoosegow	jail or prison
hootchie	a prostitute
hooter	cocaine; marijuana
hop	opium
hop dog	opium addict
hop, hops	opium
hophead	a drug addict
hopped up	under the influence of drugs
horn	to inhale, snort, or sniff a drug; crack pipe

horning	heroin; to inhale cocaine
horror drug	belladonna
horrors	delirium tremens
hors d'oeuvres	Seconal
horse	heroin
horse and buggy	a hypodermic needle and medicine dropper used for injecting drugs
horse bite	heroin
horse heads	amphetamines
horse hearts	Dexedrine
horse tracks	PCP
horsed	under the influence of heroin
horseradish	heroin
hospital heroin	Dilaudid
hot	wanted by the police; stolen items; sexually aroused
hot and cold	mixture of heroin and cocaine
hot box	to fill up a closed area with second-hand marijuana smoke
hot dope	heroin
hot heroin	heroin that has been poisoned with the intent of giving it to a police informant
hot ice	methamphetamine that can be smoked
hot load	lethal injection of a drug
hot rolling	inhaling liquefied methamphetamine from an eye dropper
hot shot	fatal dose; an injection of poison instead of drugs
hot stick	a marijuana cigarette
hotcakes	crack
house	a prison cell
house fee	money paid to enter a house where drugs are being used
housewife's delight	tranquilizers
How do you like me now?	crack
How does your garden grow?	Are you growing marijuana?
hows	morphine
HRN	heroin
huatari	peyote; mescaline
hubba	crack
hubba pigeon	a user looking for crack on the floor after a police raid
huff	an inhalant

huffer	an inhalant abuser
huffing	using an inhalant
hug drug	ecstasy; GHB; Rohypnol
hugs and kisses	methamphetamine and MDMA
hulling	using others to get drugs
Humboldt green	marijuana, presumably grown in Humboldt County, CA
humming	alcohol or drug intoxicated
hungry croaker	a physician who accepts a bribe for prescription drugs
hunk	a small amount of hashish; a physically fit or handsome male
hunter	cocaine
hustle	to make money by drug dealing, gambling, stealing, or prostitution
hydro	a water-cooled marijuana pipe
hygelo	an addict
hyke	cough syrup that contains codeine
hyna	a girlfriend
hype	heroin addict; an addict
hype stick	hypodermic syringe and needle
hyperventilation game	the choking game
I am back.	crack
I'm looking.	Do you have drugs you will sell me?
I'm way down.	I need drugs.
iboga	amphetamines; ecstasy
ice	cocaine; methamphetamine; smokeable amphetamines; ecstasy; diamonds; to kill someone
ice cream	drugs in crystallized form
ice cream habit	an occasional use of drugs
ice cream man	a drug supplier or dealer
ice cube	crack
ice pack	marijuana packed in dry ice to make it more potent
ice tong doc	a physician who will prescribe or sell drugs on request
ice tray	to smoke marijuana from an ice tray covered with foil
ice water doc	a physician who refuses to give drugs to an addict
icicles	crystallized cocaine
icing	cocaine

idiot pills	barbiturates
igloo	MDMA
illies	marijuana cigarettes dipped in PCP
Illinois	marijuana, presumably grown in Illinois
in	connected with drug suppliers
in betweens	a mixture of barbiturates and amphetamines
in flight	under the influence of drugs
in orbit	under the influence of drugs
in the car	prisoners who have formed a tight circle of friends
in the hat	targeted for death
in transit	on an LSD trip
Inca message	cocaine
incense	opium
Indian boy	marijuana
Indian hay	marijuana
Indian hemp	marijuana
Indiana ditch weed	inferior quality marijuana, grown from seeds meant to produce hemp for rope
Indiana hay	marijuana
Indians	mescaline; peyote
indica	species of cannabis, found in hot climates, grows 3.5 to 4 feet
indo	marijuana
Indonesian bud	marijuana; opium
infinity	long-acting drugs
ink	tattoos
ink slinger	one who draws tattoos
instant Zen	LSD
interplanetary mission	travel from one crack house to another in search of crack
iron cure	withdrawal from drugs while imprisoned
isda	heroin
issues	crack
itching	sexually aroused
IZM	marijuana
J	marijuana
J pipe	a pipe used to smoke marijuana
J. Edgar Hoover	police officer; federal agent
jab artist	one who takes drugs by injection
jab joint	where to buy and use drugs
jab stick	a hypodermic needle
jab, job	to inject drugs

jabber	a hypodermic needle
jack	steal someone else's drugs
Jack Ketch	a killer
jack off	to masturbate
jack up	to inject a drug; barbiturate
jackal	an undercover narcotics agent
jacked up	to be under the influence of drugs
jacking off the spike	to release pressure on a syringe before all the liquid has gone into the vein, allowing blood to re-enter the hypodermic syringe
jackpot	fentanyl
jackrabbit parole	to escape from prison after serving a long sentence
jag	a gathering where drugs are used; a prolonged period of drug or alcohol use
jail bait	a female below the legal age of sexual consent
jailbird	a prisoner
jam	amphetamines; cocaine
jam Cecil	amphetamines
Jamaican gold	Jamaican marijuana, gold in color
Jamaican red	Jamaican marijuana, reddish in color
jammed up	an overdose
Jane	marijuana
jar wars	drug testing controversy
jay	marijuana cigarette
jay smoke	marijuana
jazz	heroin
jee gee	heroin
Jeff	methcathinone
Jefferson airplane	a device used to hold a partially smoked marijuana cigarette
jejo	a cigarette
jell	heroin which gels instead of dissolving when heated in water
jellies	barbiturates; ecstasy in gel capsules
jelly	cocaine
jelly babies	amphetamines
jelly beans	amphetamines
jelly roll	sexual intercourse; penis
jerk off	to masturbate
jerks	delirium tremens
Jerry Garcia	MDMA
Jerry Springer	heroin

Jersey green	marijuana thought to grow in New Jersey
jet	ketamine; amphetamines; methamphetamines; dextroamphetamines
jet fuel	PCP
Jezebel	a prostitute
jib	crystal methamphetamine; GHB
jib head	crystal methamphetamine addict
Jif	methylphenidate
Jim Jones	marijuana laced with cocaine and PCP
jim-jams	delirium tremens
jimmies	delirium tremens
Jimmy	a subcutaneous injection of drugs; amphetamines; a condom
Jimmy Valentine	a thief or robber
jimson	a weed containing hallucinogenic substances
jingo	marijuana
jitterbug	juvenile troublemaker
jive	marijuana; dishonest; not trustworthy
jive doo jee	heroin
jive stick	a marijuana cigarette
job pop	to inject drugs
Job's antidote	a hypodermic needle
jockey	an addictive drug
Jody	a prisoner whose wife is cheating on him
Joe Blakes	delirium tremens
john	a prostitute's client; a toilet
Johnny be good	a police officer
Johnny go fast	amphetamines
Johnson	marijuana
Johnson grass	inferior quality marijuana
join the stream	to inject drugs
joint	marijuana cigarette; prison
joint stick	a marijuana cigarette
jojee	heroin
jolly beans	amphetamines
jolly green	marijuana
jolly pop	casual user of heroin
jolt	to inject a drug; strong reaction to drugs
Jones	a heroin habit
joy dust	Vietnamese heroin
joy flakes	heroin
joy juice	chloral hydrate
joy plant	opium

joy pop to inject a drug
joy popping occasional use of drugs
joy powder powdered drugs
joy prick an injection of drugs
joy smoke marijuana
joy stick a marijuana cigarette
joy ride going out and getting high
Js joints
Juan Gomez cocaine-laced marijuana
Juan Valdez marijuana
Juanita marijuana
Judas heroin; a friend who turns on you
juggle to sell drugs to another addict to support a habit
juggler a teen-age street dealer
jugs injectable amphetamines; breasts
juice steroids; alcohol; respect; power; illegally obtained money; gasoline
juice joint a bar; a marijuana cigarette laced with another drug
juiced intoxicated from alcohol
juicehead an alcoholic
ju-ju, juju a marijuana cigarette
jum sealed plastic bag containing crack
jumbos large vials of crack
jump homemade alcohol
jumping out one who turns to crime
jumping the couch losing emotional control
jumpy Stevie one who is jumpy from using drugs
June bug a prisoner who is said to be a slave for others
junk narcotics
junk picker a street person
junk pusher a drug supplier or seller
junk squad narcotics agents
junk tank a jail cell in which addicts are held
junkie an addict
junkie pro a prostitute who sells drugs, or is addicted
juvie juvenile hall
juvies law enforcement agents and social workers who deal with juveniles

K ketamine
K blast PCP
kabayo heroin

kabuki	a crack pipe made from a plastic bottle and a rubber spark plug cover
kaksonjae	smokable methamphetamine
kaleidoscope	LSD
kali	marijuana
kangaroo	crack
Kansas grass	inferior quality marijuana
kaps	PCP
Karachi	heroin
Kate bush	marijuana
katzenjammer	delirium tremens
kaya	marijuana
KB	potent marijuana
keef, keif	inferior quality drugs
keeler	chloral hydrate drops
keep it real	tell the truth
keesh	a fat bag
keister bunny	one who hides contraband in the rectum
keister plant	drugs that are concealed in the rectum or vagina
Keller	ketamine
Kelly's day	ketamine
Ken dolls	barbiturates
Kentucky blue	marijuana thought to be grown in Kentucky
Kentucky fried	alcohol or drug intoxicated
ket	ketamine
ketaset	ketamine
key, kee	kilogram; pack of cigarettes
keyed	high on drugs
keys to the kingdom	LSD
KGB (killer green bud)	marijuana
khat	milder than amphetamines
K-hole, keyhole	ketamine-induced confusion; out-of-body experience
ki	marijuana
Kibbles & Bits	Ritalin and Talwin mixture; crumbs of crack
kick	getting off a drug habit; inhalant
kick it	have sex with someone
kick stick	a marijuana cigarette
kick the clouds	to be under the influence of drugs
kick the engine around	to smoke opium
kicked	to pass out or about to pass out
kicked by a horse	addicted to heroin

kicked out in the snow	drug intoxicated
kicker	OxyContin
kicking it	withdrawing from drug use
kiddie dope	prescription medication
kiff, kif	marijuana
killer weed	potent marijuana
kilo brick	marijuana packed into a brick shape that weighs approximately 1 kilogram
kilter	a marijuana cigarette
kind bud	marijuana
king	cocaine
King Ivory	fentanyl
King Kong	$200 or more a day drug habit
King Kong pills	barbiturates
king of the road	a homeless person who wanders from place to place
king's habit	cocaine
Kipper Lane	urban opium district
kiss ass	to be excessively attentive in order to gain favor
kiss Mary	to smoke marijuana
kiss the fish	to smoke marijuana
kissing	mouth-to-mouth exchange of plastic-wrapped crack rocks
kit	equipment used to prepare or use drugs
kit kat	ketamine
kite	1 ounce of drugs
kitty flipping	to use ketamine and ecstasy back and forth
kitty kitty	female officers
KJ (krystal joint)	PCP
K-land	out-of-body experience
Kleenex	ecstasy
klingon	crack addict
knock off	to kill
knocked out	alcohol or drug intoxicated
knockout drops	chloral hydrate and alcohol
knockout game	the choking game
Kokomo	cocaine addict or user
koller joints	PCP
Kona gold	Hawaiian marijuana
kook	an eccentric person
kools	PCP
kram	to pack a bowl tight with marijuana

krippies	moist marijuana that is smoked out of a bowl or bong
kryptonite	crack
krystal, crystal	crystal methamphetamine; PCP
krystal joint, crystal joint	a marijuana cigarette laced with PCP
kumba	marijuana
kushempeng	marijuana
kutchie	marijuana
KW	PCP
L	LSD
LA	long-acting amphetamine
LA glass	smokable methamphetamine
LA ice	smokable methamphetamine
LA turnabouts	amphetamines
lace	to add a drug or alcohol to ordinary food or drink
lactone	GBL
lady	cocaine
lady caine	cocaine
lady in white	powdered drugs
lady killer	a gigolo
lady snow	cocaine
lady white	powdered drugs
ladyfinger	a marijuana cigarette
lag	a prisoner
lakbay diva	marijuana
lamb's bread	marijuana
Lamborghini	a pipe that is made of a plastic bottle and a rubber spark plug cover
lamp habit	addicted to opium
Latin lettuce	marijuana
laugh and scratch	to inject a drug
laughing gas	inhalant
laughing grass	marijuana
laughing weed	marijuana
lay	a sex partner; to have sexual intercourse
lay back	barbiturates
lay out	to kill
lay up	to stay off the streets after a large drug supply has been obtained
layout	equipment used for injecting drugs
LBJ, LBL	JB-336-N-methyl-3-piperidyl benzilate HCl; a hallucinogen

leaf	marijuana
leak	marijuana and PCP mixture
leaky bolla	PCP
leaky leak	PCP
lean	codeine cough syrup
leap over the wall	escape from jail or prison
leaper	amphetamine
leaping	under the influence of drugs
Leary's	LSD
legal speed	Mini-Thins, an over-the-counter asthma medication
lemon 714	PCP
lemon bowl	an opium pipe that has a lemon rind covering the bowel
lemon drop	methamphetamines of a dull yellow color
lemon wings	Sudafed
lemonade	inferior quality heroin
lemons	methaqualone
lens	LSD
leper grass	potent Colombian marijuana
Let me hold something.	an inquiry from one seeking to buy drugs
let sunshine do	LSD
lethal weapon	PCP
letter biscuit	MDMA
lettuce	money
libs	Librium
lick up a tab	to swallow a tablet or capsule
licorice	opium
lid	approximately 1 ounce of marijuana
lid poppers	amphetamines
lie in state with the girls	to smoke marijuana
lifer	lifetime addict; one serving a lifetime prison sentence
lift pills	amphetamines
light artillery	equipment used for preparing or injecting drugs
light green	inferior quality marijuana
light somebody	to introduce someone to marijuana
light stuff	marijuana; nonaddictive drugs
lightning	amphetamines
lightweight	one who is minimally addicted
lima	marijuana
limbo	Colombian marijuana
lime acid	LSD

line	a vein in the arm; line formed by powdered drugs
line shot	an injection of drugs
liner	one who injects drugs
lint	morphine in fibrous or cotton form
lip	to test whether a drug apparatus is airtight by sucking the air out of it
Lipton Tea	inferior quality drugs
liquid bam	injectable amphetamines
liquid E	ecstasy
liquid ecstasy	GHB
liquid lady	liquid cocaine that is used as a nasal spray
liquid X	GHB
lit, lit up	under the influence of drugs or alcohol
little bomb	amphetamines; heroin; barbiturates
little bowl of Buddha	10-gram bowl of marijuana buds or hashish
little boy blue	a police officer
little D	Dilaudid
little green friend	marijuana
little ones	PCP
little smoke	marijuana; psilocybin/psilocin
live in grass huts	to smoke marijuana
live ones	PCP
live, spit, and die	LSD
load	an injection of drugs; a drug supply; a large drug purchase; bulk sale of heroin
loaded for bear	ready for a fight
loads	glutethimide mixed with codeine
loaf	marijuana
lobo	marijuana
locker room	isobutyl nitrite; inhalants
locoweed	marijuana
locust point	a place from which to buy drugs
log	a marijuana cigarette; an opium pipe
logor	LSD
long draw	a long pull on an opium or marijuana pipe
Looney Toons	LSD
loose	relaxed; sexually promiscuous
loose cannon	a dangerously irresponsible person
loose joint	a single marijuana cigarette
lords	hydromorphone
lorphs	hydromorphone
lotes	butabarbital

loused	covered by sores and abscesses from repeated use of unsterile needles
love	crack
love affair	cocaine and heroin mixture
love blow	marijuana
love boat	marijuana dipped in formaldehyde; PCP
love doctor	ecstasy; GHB; Rohypnol
love drug	ecstasy; GHB; Rohypnol
love flipping	mescaline with MDMA
love nuggets	marijuana
love pearls	alpha ethyltyptamine
love pills	alpha ethyltyptamine; MDMA
love potion # 9	ecstasy
love trip	ecstasy and mescaline
love weed	marijuana
lovelies	marijuana laced with PCP
lovely	PCP
lover's special	MDMA
lover's speed	ecstasy; GHB; Rohypnol
low	in a depressed mood
low rider	a drug addict who is on the skids
LSD	lysergic acid diethylamide
LT	living together
lubage	marijuana
Lucas	marijuana
Lucky Charms	ecstasy
Lucy in the sky with diamonds	LSD
lude out	to take methaqualone and alcohol
ludes	Quaaludes
luggage	LSD
lumber	marijuana stems and waste
lunch box	kids who do drugs
lunch head	alcoholic
lunch money drug	Rohypnol
lunch-hour trip	DMT taken on one's lunch break
lung duster	a cigarette
lush	an alcoholic
M	marijuana; morphine
M&C	morphine and codeine combination
M&M	MDMA/MDA; barbiturates
MJ	marijuana
MO	marijuana
MS	morphine

MU	marijuana
ma'a	Samoan marijuana
machinery	equipment used to prepare and use drug
Machu Picchu	potent Peruvian marijuana
macon	marijuana
mad dog	PCP
mad scientist	someone who makes crank
madman	PCP
Maggie	marijuana
maggot	a cigarette butt
magic	PCP
magic dust	powdered drugs
magic flake	cocaine
magic mushrooms	hallucinogenic mushrooms
magic pumpkin	mescaline
magic smoke	marijuana
mainline	to inject drugs through a vein, usually the median cephalic vein
mainliner	an addict whose habit is to inject drugs
maintain	to keep a certain level of drug effect
make	a person regarded as a sex partner
make a buy	to purchase drugs
make a croaker for a reader	to obtain a prescription drug from a physician
make a spread	to set up equipment for drug use
make it	to have sexual intercourse
make tracks	to leave needle marks on the arm from injecting drugs; to run away
make up	need to find more drugs
mama coca	cocaine
mama's mellow	the effect of taking sedatives
man	one's connection; a police officer
man about town	a gigolo
mandrex	methaqualone
Manhattan silver	marijuana
manicure	to prepare marijuana for use
marathons	amphetamines
marbles	Placidyl
marching dust	powdered drugs
marching powder	powdered drugs
Margie wanna	marijuana
mariholic	a marijuana addict
marimba	marijuana
Marley	marijuana

marshmallow reds	secobarbital
Mary	marijuana
Mary and Johnny	marijuana
Mary Ann	marijuana
Mary Jane	marijuana
Mary Jonas	marijuana
Mary Warner	marijuana
Mary Weaver	marijuana
Mash Allah	opium
matchbox	1/4 ounce of marijuana or 6 marijuana cigarettes
Maui wowie	Hawaiian marijuana
mauve	ketamine
Max	GHB dissolved in water and mixed with amphetamines
maxibolin	oral steroids
mayo	cocaine; heroin
McCoy	pure drugs or alcohol
MDA	methyl diamphetamine
MDM, MDMA	ecstasy
mean	high or superior quality; low or inferior quality drugs
mean green	PCP
meat market	a primarily singles bar where one may look for a sex partner
medical hype	one who is addicted to prescription drugs as a result of legitimate medical care
Medusa	inhalants
Meg, Megg, Meggie	marijuana
mellow	alcohol or drug intoxicated; relaxed
mellow out	to be under the influence of drugs or alcohol
mellow yellows	tranquilizers
melt wax	to smoke opium
melter	morphine
men in blue	male police officers
mepro	meprobamate
Mercedes	MDMA
merchandise	drugs
Merck, Merk	cocaine
mesc	mescaline
mescal beans	mescaline
mescy	mescaline
mess	mescaline

messed up	alcohol or drug intoxicated
messorole	marijuana
metal	a metal pipe
meth	methamphetamine as liquid or in crystalline form
meth freak	a person who uses methamphetamines
meth head	regular user of methamphetamine
meth monster	person who has a violent reaction to methamphetamine
meth speed bass	methamphetamine and heroin mixture
Methlies Quik	methamphetamine
method	marijuana
metros	police officers
Mexican brown	potent marijuana in Mexico, with high resin content
Mexican crack	methamphetamine with the appearance of crack
Mexican green	marijuana grown in Mexico, less potent than Mexican brown
Mexican horse	heroin
Mexican jumping beans	barbiturates manufactured in Mexico
Mexican mud	heroin
Mexican mushrooms	hallucinogenic mushrooms that are grown in Mexico
Mexican red	reddish-brown Mexican marijuana
Mexican reds	secobarbital
Mexican speedballs	crack and amphetamines
Mexican valium	Rohypnol
mezc	mescaline
MFT	Nexus
Michael	chloral hydrate
Michoacan, Mishwacan	potent marijuana, grown in Michoacan, Mexico
Mickey Finn	chloral hydrate and alcohol
Mickey Mouse	blotter impregnated with LSD and stamped with Mickey Mouse as the sorcerer's apprentice
Mickey Mouse ears	the lights and siren on top of a police car
Mickey's	barbiturates
microdot	1 microgram of LSD on a tablet or on blotting paper
mid grade	mediocre marijuana
midget	a young child who is used to run drugs
midnight oil	opium
midnight toker	one who smokes marijuana before bed

Mighty Joe Young	big heroin habit
mighty mezz	marijuana cigarette
Mighty Mite	breed of marijuana plant with huge buds
Mighty Quinn	LSD
mike, mic	1 microgram, usually refers to LSD dose
milk	a marijuana cigarette dipped in embalming fluid and laced with PCP
milk a rush	to inject a drug, then draw blood back into the syringe and dilute it
mind bender	a hallucinogenic drug
mind detergent	LSD
mind spacer	a hallucinogenic drug
ming	a marijuana cigarette made from leftover butts
minglewood	hashish and bud-filled marijuana cigarette or cigar
mini beans	amphetamines
mini bennies	amphetamines
mini white	amphetamines in tablet form
minstrels	amphetamine and barbiturate combination
mint leaf	mint leaves or parsley laced with PCP
mint weed	mint leaves or parsley laced with PCP
Mira	opium
mired in the mud	addicted to opium
miser	a device for holding a marijuana cigarette butt
miss	to miss a vein while attempting to inject drugs, resulting in a subcutaneous or intramuscular injection
Miss Carrie	a stash of drugs carried on one's person
Miss Emma	morphine
Miss Emma Jones	a morphine addict
missile basing	crack liquid and PCP mixture
mission	to go shopping for drugs
missionary	one who attempts to create new addicts
Mississippi marbles	dice
mist	PCP; crack smoke
Mister Blue	hydromorphone
Mister Brownstone	hashish; brown heroin
Mister Natural	LSD
misting	spraying the skin of an individual with LSD
Mitsubishi	ecstasy with the Mitsubishi emblem on it
mohasky	marijuana
mojo	hard drugs; powdered narcotics
Molly	ecstasy

Molotov cocktail	an explosive made by pouring gasoline into a bottle and adding a cloth wick
monkey	a drug habit in which physical dependence is present; morphine; a small heroin habit
monkey bait	a free sample of an addictive drug
monkey drill	a hypodermic needle
monkey dust	powdered drugs
monkey jumps	the disoriented motions and staggering gait of a drug addict
monkey meat	a drug addict
monkey medicine	morphine
monkey on one's back	to be addicted to drugs
monkey pump	a hypodermic needle
monkey talk	the distorted speech of one who is intoxicated
monkey tranquilizer	PCP
monkey wagon	to be addicted to drugs
monolithic	heavily intoxicated by drugs
monos	a cigarette made from cocaine paste and tobacco
Monroe in a Cadillac	mixture of morphine and cocaine
monster	drugs that are powerful enough to affect the central nervous system
monster weed	potent marijuana
monte	marijuana
mooca, moocah	marijuana
mooch joint	a place where drugs are sold
moocher	a drug addict
moody blues	pentazocine mixed with tripelennamine
moon	mescaline; peyote; to show one's bare butt
moon gas	inhalants
moon rock	crack and heroin mixture
moonbeams	PCP
moonshine	illicit liquor
moonstone	a slice of MDMA in a bag of heroin
mooster	marijuana
moota, mutah	marijuana
mooter	a marijuana cigarette
mootie	marijuana
mootos	marijuana
mor a grifa	marijuana
morals	Demerol
more	PCP
morf tab	morphine

morning glory the first injection of an addict's day
morning glory seeds contain lysergic acid amide, related to LSD but only 1/10 as potent
morning shot the first injection of an addict's day
morning wake-up the first drug of the day
morotgara heroin
morph, morf, morpho, morphie morphine
morpho moron a morphine addict
mortal combat potent heroin
moscop morphine and scopolamine combination
mosquito cocaine
mota, moto marijuana
mother a drug dealer
mother dear methadone
mother nature marijuana
Mother of God LSD paper with naked woman on it
Mother's Day the day one receives a welfare check
mother's little helpers tranquilizers
motorcycle crack methamphetamine
mountain dew illicit liquor
mouth habit addiction to drugs taken orally
mouth worker addiction to drugs taken orally
movie star drug cocaine
mow the grass or lawn to smoke marijuana
MPH methylphenidate
MPPP synthetic meperidine
MPTP synthetic drug derived from Demerol
Mr. Lovely marijuana laced with PCP
Mr. Twenty-Six 26-gauge hypodermic needle
Mr. Warner a marijuana smoker
Mr. Whiskers a federal narcotics agent
Mrs. Warren a prostitute
Mrs. White a supplier or seller of white powdered drugs
mu marijuana
mud unprocessed opium; heroin
mud wiggler an opium addict
muff female genitalia
mugger one who attacks and robs a person; a comedian
muggie marijuana
mugglehead a marijuana smoker
muggles marijuana
mule marijuana soaked in whiskey; one who smuggles or carries drugs for a distributor

mule skinner	the person who recruits and supervises people who smuggle or carry drugs
munchies	craving for food after drug use
murder 8	fentanyl
murder one	heroin and cocaine; premediated homocide
muscle pop	to inject a drug intramuscularly because there is not a good vein
mushrooms	innocent bystanders who are wounded or killed in the crossfire of gun battles
musk	psilocybin, psilocin mushrooms
muta, mutah, moota	marijuana
muzzle	heroin
my friend	menstrual period
my man	an addict's drug supplier
nail	a tobacco or marijuana cigarette; to catch
nail in the coffin	a tobacco or marijuana cigarette
nailed	arrested
Nam black	potent black marijuana that is grown in Vietnam or southeast Asia
nanny goat sweat	illicit liquor
nanoo	heroin
narc, nark, narco	an undercover narcotics agent; an informer
narco card	a registration card carried by addicts in order for them to obtain methadone
narcotics bull	a federal narcotics agent
Nazi vitamins	crystal methamphetamine
nebbies	pentobarbital
necessities	drug supplies
needle candy	drugs taken by injection
needle flash	a short high that might come between the time the needle enters the tissue and the drug enters the blood
needle freak	one who enjoys injecting; to get sexual pleasure from injecting
needle park	a public park where users and addicts gather to deal or inject drugs
nembies, nemmies	Nembutal
nemish	Nembutal
Nepalese hash	potent hashish from Nepal
new acid	PCP
New Jack Swing	heroin and morphine
new magic	PCP
newspapers	LSD

Nexus	4-bromo-2,5 diethoxy-phenyethylamine
nice and easy	heroin
nick	1/2 gram
nicked	arrested
nickel	$5 supply of drugs; a 5-year prison sentence
nickel bag	$5 supply of drugs; heroin
nickel deck	$5 supply of drugs; heroin
nickel note	$5 bill
nickelodeons	crack addicts
night on the rainbow	a night spent under the influence of drugs
nighttime	heroin withdrawal
nightingale	an informer
nightshade	belladonna
nimbly, nimble, nimby	Nembutal
nineteen, 19	ecstasy
nitro	speed or nitrous oxide
nix	stranger among the group
Nixon	inferior quality drugs
noble princess of the waters	hallucinogenic mushrooms
nod	to fall asleep for a short period immediately after drug use
nodded out	under the influence of drugs
nods	cough syrup with codeine
noise	heroin
nontoucher	user who does not want to be touched during or after using drugs
noodlelars	methyprylon
nooky, nookie	sexual intercourse
Northern Lights	potent marijuana
nose	any drug that is taken through the nose
nose candy	any drug that is taken through the nose
nose drops	any drug that is taken through the nose
nose powder	any powdered drug that is taken through the nose
nose stuff	any drug that is taken through the nose
noss	nitrous oxide
nox	nitrous oxide
Ns	Darvocet-N
nubs	peyote; mescaline
nugget	crack; high-grade marijuana
number	a marijuana cigarette
number 1	liquid hashish
number 3	cocaine, heroin

number 4	heroin
number 8	heroin
number 9	ecstasy
number 13	morphine
nurse	powdered drugs
O	opium
oboy	marijuana
octane	inhale gasoline
off	withdrawn from drugs
ogoy	heroin
oil	hashish oil
oil burner	an expensive drug habit
oiled	alcohol or drug intoxicated; to be injected with drugs
oink	a police officer
OJ	a marijuana cigarette dipped in opium
old lady White	powdered drugs
old Madge	powdered drugs
old Smoky	the electric chair
old Steve	powdered drugs
olive	cotton used to strain a drug solution as it is pulled into a syringe
on a mission	searching for drugs
on a trip	under the influence of drugs
on ice	in jail
on the bricks	walking the streets; a homeless person
on the lam	to escape from jail or prison
on the nod	under the influence of drugs
on the street	out of jail; public knowledge; a street person; a prostitute
on the stuff	a regular user of drugs; an addict
on the wire	using amphetamines
on top of it	in control
one and one	to use both nostrils when snorting a powdered drug
one hitter	a pipe that is big enough for one use
one way	LSD
one-hit grass	DMT smoked with tobacco, marijuana, or parsley
one-night stand	a casual sexual encounter
one-on-one	Talwin and Pyribenzamine combination
one-toke weed	potent marijuana
OP	opium

ope	opium
operator	a drug supplier or seller
OPP	PCP
optical illusions	LSD
orange bandit	MDMA
orange barrels	LSD
orange bowl	an opium pipe which is fitted with an orange rind
Orange County	Quaaludes
orange crystal	PCP
orange cube	LSD
orange cupcakes	LSD, usually added to other drugs
orange fX rush	1,4-BD
orange haze	LSD
orange micro	LSD3
orange mushrooms	a tablet or blotter impregnated with LSD in the image of a mushroom
orange sunshine	LSD
orange wedges	LSD
oranges	amphetamines
oregano	hashish; marijuana
organic Quaalude	GHB
ounce man	a drug dealer who sells small quantities of drugs
out in left field	under the influence of drugs
out of body	a feeling of separation of the mind from the body one experiences while under the influence of hallucinogens
out of it	alcohol or drug intoxicated; out of touch with reality
out of sight	a pleasurable experience
outer limits	crack and LSD
outfit	equipment used for preparing and using drugs
outside of myself	a feeling of separation of the mind from the body one experiences while under the influence of hallucinogens
overcharged	semiconscious state resulting from too much of a drug
overs and unders	amphetamines and barbiturates
owl	a narcotics agent who works at night
Owsley, Owsley's acid	LSD
oxy	OxyContin
oxy 80's	a semisynthetic opiate

oxycet	a semisynthetic opiate
oxycotton	OxyContin
oyster stew	cocaine
Oz	inhalants
ozone	PCP
Ozzie, Ozzy	LSD
Ozzie's stuff	LSD
P	peyote; PCP; pure heroin
paca lolo, pakalolo	marijuana
pacifier	a homemade hypodermic needle
pack	heroin; marijuana
pack it in	to commit suicide; to give up; to quit
pack of rockets	package of marijuana cigarettes
pack of rocks	crack
pack one's coozie	to place a parcel of drugs into the vagina
pack one's keister	to place a parcel of drugs into the vagina or rectum
pack one's nose	to snort cocaine
packed up	under the influence of drugs
pad	where one resides; where people gather to use drugs
pad money	admission fee to a site where drugs are used
padded	to have drugs concealed on one's body
paid torch	a hired arsonist
painted woman	a prostitute
paisley caps	capsules or pills laced with LSD
Pakistani black	Pakistani marijuana
pan up	to prepare a drug for injection
Panama cut	Panamanian marijuana
Panama gold	gold-color Panamanian marijuana
Panama red	reddish-color Panamanian marijuana
panatela	large marijuana cigarette
pancakes and syrup	combination of glutethimide and codeine cough syrup
pane	LSD
panic	anxiety caused from a shortage of drugs
panic man	an addict who cannot obtain drugs
panic trip	a bad LSD trip
panther piss	raw and inferior quality liquor
paper	paper folded to conceal drugs; a prescription for drugs; paper that is saturated with drugs; money; counterfeit bills
paper acid	LSD consumed from a blotter

paper bag	container for drugs
paper blunts	marijuana within a paper casing rather than a tobacco leaf casing
paper boy	heroin peddler
paper fiend	a drug user who uses amphetamine-soaked paper strips from an amphetamine inhaler
paper hanger	a person who writes worthless checks or passes counterfeit money
parachute down	MDMA after using heroin
parackie	paraldehyde
paradise, paradise white	cocaine
parakeet	paraldehyde
paraphernalia	items involved in drug use
parest	methaqualone
Park Lane No. 2	a type of marijuana sold and used during the Vietnam War
parlay	crack
parsley	marijuana; PCP
pass	a successful drug exchange
passing out game	the choking game
pass-out game	the choking game
paste	to beat
pat	marijuana
pattern	a drug-induced hallucination
pavement princess	a prostitute
pay street	an expensive drug habit
paz	PCP
PCE	synthetic PCP
PCP	phencyclidine
PDA	public display of affection
P-dope	20-30% pure heroin
peace	LSD, PCP
peace pills	PCP, LSD
peace weed	PCP
peaches	orange-colored amphetamines
peanut butter	heroin
peanuts	barbiturates
pearl	cocaine
pearls	amyl nitrite
pearly gates	LSD; morning glory seeds
pears	amyl nitrite
pebbles	crack
peddler	a drug dealer

pee wee	a thin marijuana cigarette
peep	PCP
peepers	users of MDMA
Peg	heroin
pekoe	high-quality opium
pellets	LSD
pen shot	injection of drugs
pen yan	opium
penitentiary highball	a drink made from strained shellac and milk
penitentiary shot	an injection of drugs given from a pin and a medicine dropper
people (the)	influential heroin distributors
pep pills	amphetamines
peppermint swirl	LSD combined with another drug
pepper-uppers	amphetamines
Pepsi habit	occasional use of drugs
per	a prescription for drugs
perfect high	heroin
perform	to have sexual intercourse
period hitter	an occasional drug user
perkers, perkies, perks	oxycodone; Percodan
permafried	an addict
perp	counterfeit crack, made from candle wax and baking soda
Persian brown	brownish-colored heroin from the Middle East
peruvian flake	high-quality cocaine from Peru
peruvian rock	cocaine
Peter	chloral hydrate
Peter Jay	a police officer
Peter Pan	PCP
Peter, Paul, and Mary	ménage à trois
peyote	the cactus from which mescaline is derived
P-funk	synthetic heroin
PG	tincture of opium; paregoric; pregnant
pharming	consuming a mixture of prescription substances
phat rails	lines of powdered drugs
P-head	a phenobarbital user
phennies, phenies, phenos	phenobarbital
Phillies blunt	a cigar hollowed out and filled with marijuana
pianoing	using the fingers to find lost powdered drugs
picking	searching on hands and knees for crack
picking the poppies	an opium addict
pickup	an injection

Slang Terms

piece	a gun; 1 ounce of a drug; the female partner in sexual intercourse
pig	a police officer
pig killer	one who kills a police officer
piggie	opium made into pellets for smoking
piggybacking	the simultaneous injection of 2 drugs
Pikachu	pills containing ecstasy and PCP
pile high and deep	to brag or exaggerate
piles	crack
pill cooker	one who is addicted to opium
pill freak	a user of dangerous drugs; someone who likes to take pills
pill head	a user of dangerous drugs; someone who likes to take pills
pill peddler	a physician
pill pusher	a physician
pillows	knockout drops; opium; methaqualone; a bag containing pills
pimp dust	powdered drugs
pimp your pipe	to lend or rent one's crack pipe
pimp's drug	cocaine
pimpmobile	a customized luxury car that is used by a pimp
pin	a hypodermic needle or pin and medicine dropper used to inject drugs; a very thin marijuana cigarette
pin gon	opium
pin gun	equipment for injecting drugs, made from a pin and a medicine dropper
pin joint	a very thin marijuana cigarette
pin yen	opium
pinch	to arrest; a small amount of marijuana
pinch hitter	one who is hired to inject drugs
pine	marijuana
pine needle oil	1,4-BD
pineapple	a grenade or small bomb
ping a pill	to remove a bit of a pill for a small dose
ping in the wing	an injection of a drug into the arm
pinhead	one who injects drugs with the aid of a pin; an unpleasant, unattractive, or insignificant person
pink blotters	LSD
pink elephants	delirium tremens
pink hearts	amphetamines

pink ladies	barbiturates
Pink Panther	LSD; MDMA
pink robots	LSD
pink spiders	delirium tremens
pink swirl	LSD
pink wedges	LSD
pink witches	LSD
pink, pinks	Seconal; morphine
pinkie	intraarterial injection
pinks and greens	amphetamines
pinned eyes	pinpoint pupils
pinner	small joint of marijuana
pins and needles	morphine
pipe	a large vein; a device used for smoking marijuana or opium
pipe dream	a dream while under the influence of opium
piped	alcohol or drug intoxication
piper	one who snorts powdered drugs
pit	the crease on the inside of the elbow
pixies	amphetamines
pizza toppings	psilocybin, psilocin mushrooms
plant	to hide drugs upon an unsuspecting person; where opium is prepared
play around	to use drugs now and then
playboy bunnies	MDMA
playboys	MDMA
playing the harmonica	inhaling smoke from heated heroin through the rectangular cover of a matchbox
pleasure user	one who uses drugs for pleasure and who is not addicted
plow	marijuana
PMA	synthetic amphetamine, methamphetamine
PO	paregoric
pocket rocket	a marijuana cigarette
pocket shot	internal jugular injection
pod	marijuana
pogo	cocaine
point	a needle
point shot	a shot made with the broken point of a needle or sewing machine needle
poison	heroin; fentanyl
poison people	heroin addicts
poke	marijuana

pokey	jail or prison
pollutant	drug smoke; cigarette smoke
pony	crack
poof	smoking ice
poor man's heroin	Talwin and Ritalin injected to produce effect of heroin mixed with cocaine
poor man's speedball	heroin and methamphetamine
poor man's pot	inhalants
pop	to inject drugs simultaneous
popcorn machine	the lights bar on a police car
poppers	isobutyl nitrite; amyl nitrite
poppy	opium
poppy alley	where opium dens are located
poppy grove	an opium den
poppy puffer	an opium addict
popstick	an opium pipe
pork	police officers
positive	positive attitude before and after drug use
pot	marijuana
potato	LSD
potato chips	crack cut with benzocaine
pothead	a marijuana user
potten bush	marijuana
powder	drugs in powdered form
powder monkey	a supplier or seller of drugs
powder room	a room where drugs are bought or sold
powdered diamonds	cocaine
powdered joy	powdered narcotics
power hitter	a device used to concentrate marijuana
power puller	rubber piece attached to crack stem
pox	opium
PR	Panama Red marijuana
preacher	an informer
predator	heroin
pregnant	a lump in the middle of a marijuana cigarette
press	cocaine; crack
prick	a contemptible person; penis
prime time	crack
primo	crack; marijuana mixed with crack
primos	cigarettes laced with cocaine and heroin
prod	a hypodermic needle
product	oral steroids; LSD that is combined with another drug

Prudential	crack user
prunes	testicles
P-stuff	PCP
psyched up	excited
psychedelic drug	a hallucinogen that produces abnormal psychic effects
puff	to smoke marijuana
puff the dragon	to smoke marijuana
puffer	crack smoker
puffy	PCP
pull a fast one	to rob; to deceive
pump full of lead	to shoot
pumpers	steroids
pumping	selling crack
pumpkin seed	mescaline
puna butter	a variety of Hawaiian marijuana
punchboard	a promiscuous female
puppy	a gun
pure	pure heroin
pure love	pure heroin
purple	LSD; ketamine
purple barrels	LSD
purple flats	LSD
purple haze	LSD
purple hearts	LSD; amphetamines; phenobarbital
purple microdot	LSD
purple ozoline	LSD
purple passion	combination stimulant and depressant
purple rain	PCP
push	to sell drugs
push shorts	to cheat or sell short amounts
pusher	one who sells drugs; metal hanger or umbrella rod used to scrape residue from crack stems
pussy	female partner in sexual intercourse; female genitalia; a weak or timid person
put away	to kill
put it on paper	to saturate a paper with drugs
put on	to intentionally deceive or confuse
put on a circus	to fake withdrawal in an attempt to get drugs
QP	1/4 pound of marijuana
Qs	Quaaludes
quack	methaqualone
quads	barbiturates

quarter	1/4 ounce; $25 drug supply
quarter bag	$25 drug supply
quarter moon	hashish
quarter piece	a fraction of a kilogram
quartermaster	one who sells quarter bag of drugs
quartz	smokable speed
quas	barbiturates
quay	methaqualone
Queen Anne's lace	marijuana
quicksilver	isobutyl nitrite
quill	a matchbook cover used for sniffing cocaine or heroin; heroin, methamphetamine; cocaine
R-2	Rohypnol
racehorse Charlie	cocaine
radical chic	socially prominent people who associate with radicals or minority groups
rag and bones man	a street person
rag picker	a street person
Raggedy Ann	blotter paper stamped with LSD in the character of Raggedy Ann
ragman	a street person
ragweed	inferior quality marijuana
rail	a line of powdered drug
railroad tracks	needle marks along the veins of drug users
railroad weed	inferior quality marijuana
railroader	one who injects drugs intravenously
rainbow roll	various colored barbiturates
rainbows	various colored barbiturates
raincoat	a condom
rainy day woman	marijuana
ram	a male
Rambo	heroin
ran good	marijuana that grows wild
rane	cocaine; heroin
rap	a conversation; to converse; rhythmic vocal expression; arrest or arraignment for a crime
raspberry	female who trades sex for drug money; an injection site that has abscessed
rasta weed	marijuana
rat	an informer
rat pack	a small gang that terrorizes others and vandalizes property
ration	a drug dose or stash

rave	a party designed to enhance a hallucinogenic experience through music and behavior
rave energy	MDMA
raw	crack
raw fusion	heroin
rawhide	heroin
razed	under the influence of drugs
RB	resin bud (marijuana)
RDs	Seconal
reader	a prescription
reader with tail	a forged prescription
ready rock	crack
Reagans	amobarbital
recycle	LSD
red	under the influence of drugs
red and blues	Tuinal
red angelfish	blotter paper saturated with LSD in the character of a red angelfish
red birds	secobarbital
red bullets	barbiturates
red caps	crack
red chicken	heroin
red cross	cross-scored amphetamine tablets
red devils	Seconal
red dimple	LSD combined with another drug
red dirt	marijuana
red dolls	barbiturates
red dot	LSD tablet with a red dot
red dragon	blotter paper saturated with LSD in the character of a red dragon
red eagle	heroin
red flag	something that incites anger
red hots	barbiturates
red jackets	barbiturates
red lilies	barbiturates
red lips	LSD
red phosphorus	smokable speed
red pipe	an artery
red rock	heroin
red-light district	a district in which houses of prostitution are numerous
redneck	a bigoted and ultraconservative person
reds	barbiturates

reefer	a marijuana cigarette
reekstick	tobacco laced with cocaine
register	pulling blood into a syringe or medicine dropper to confirm entry into a vein
regs	marijuana
regular P	crack
reindeer dust	powdered drugs; heroin
RenewTrient	GBL
res	potent residue which is scraped from the pipe and smoked
rest in peace	crack
revitalize plus	1,4-BD
Revivarant	GBL
rhapsody	variation of amphetamine, methamphetamine
rhine	heroin
rhythms	amphetamines
rib	Rohypnol; MDMA
Rice Krispies	amyl nitrite
rich man's aspirin	cocaine
riding a white horse	using powdered heroin
riding a witch's broom	using powdered drugs
riding the poppy train	to smoke opium
riding the thorn	injecting drugs
riding the train	using cocaine
riding the wave	under the influence of drugs
rifle range	where drugs are purchased and injected
rig	equipment used in preparing and using drugs
right croaker	a physician who provides drugs or sells prescriptions to addicts
righteous	superior quality drugs
righteous bush	marijuana
ringer	potent crack
rip off	to steal
ripped	alcohol or drug intoxicated
rippers	amphetamines
rising sun game	the choking game
rits	Ritalin
ritual spirit	MDMA
Ritz and T	Ritalin and Talwin mixture injected
roach	butt of a marijuana cigarette; a police officer; Rohypnol
roach bender	one who smokes marijuana

roach clip a metal clip used to hold the butt of a marijuana cigarette

roach pin a metal pin used to hold the butt of a marijuana cigarette

road dope amphetamines

road rage a driver's anger that results in aggressive behavior on the road

Road Runner a type of ecstasy with the Road Runner's face emblem on it

roasting smoking marijuana

rob the cradle to date or marry someone much younger than yourself

Robbie, Robby cough medicine with codeine

robin eggs blue capsules of LSD

robotripping drinking Robitussin

roche Rohypnol

rock attack crack

rock fiend crack addict

rock house a place where crack is sold and used

rock star female who trades sex for crack or money to buy crack; someone addicted to crack cocaine

rock(s) crystallized form of cocaine or heroin

rocket caps dome-shaped caps on crack vials

rocket fuel PCP

rocket marijuana cigarette

rockette female who uses crack

rocks of hell crack

Rocky III crack

rod a gun

rogues gallery a collection of photos of criminals

roids anabolic steroids

roll ecstasy

roll of reds barbiturates

roll the boy to smoke opium

roller to inject a drug

rollers law enforcement agents; veins that move during the process of injection

rolling MDMA

rolling buzz a drug high of a moderate length of time

rolling stone a person who wanders from place to place

Rolls Royce MDMA

roofies Rohypnol

rook person who can't handle their drugs

rooms	psilocin, psilocybin mushrooms
rooster	crack
root	marijuana
rope	marijuana; Rohypnol
rophies, ropies	Rohypnol
Rose Marie	marijuana
roses	amphetamines
roto rooter	penis
rough stuff	marijuana
row-shay	Rohypnol
rox	crack
royal blues	LSD
Royal Temple Ball	resin mixed with LSD then rolled into a ball
Roz	crack
RPMs	amphetamines; dextroamphetamines
rub out	to kill
Ruffles, ruffies	Rohypnol
rumble	police in the neighborhood; a shakedown or search; a fight
run	the time during which a drug is continuously injected
runners	people who sell or get drugs for dealers
running	MDMA
rupture	PCP
rush	the initial feeling of exhilaration from a drug dose
rush snappers	isobutyl nitrite
Russian sickles	LSD
S&M	sadomasochism
sack	a person who distributes narcotics to small-time dealers
sacrament	LSD that is placed on the tongue in communion wafer form
sacred mushroom	psilocybin, psilocin mushrooms
safety pin mechanic	one who uses a safety pin and medicine dropper to inject drugs
sagebrush whacker	one who smokes marijuana
saidie-maisie	sadomasochism
sak	bag of marijuana
Salmon River quiver	marijuana
salt	heroin
salt and pepper	inferior quality marijuana; black and white police car

salty water marijuana; GHB
Sam federal narcotics agent
Sam and Dave police officers
San Francisco bomb mixture of cocaine, heroin, and LSD
San Pedro mescaline; peyote
San Quentin quail a female below the legal age of sexual consent
sandbag to beat; to assault some; to check a bet, then raise it
sandoz, sandos LSD
sandwich 2 lines of cocaine with a layer of heroin in the middle
sandwich bag $40 bag of marijuana
Santa Marta gold Colombian marijuana
Sassafras marijuana
Satan's secret inhalants
satch paper or clothing that is saturated with a drug and smuggled into a hospital or prison
satch cotton fabric used to filter a solution of narcotics before an injection
satellite an empty paper towel roll used as a pipe to smoke numerous joints
sativa marijuana
Saturday night special a small-caliber revolver; a cheap handgun
sauced alcohol intoxicated
saxophone an opium pipe
scab heroin
scaffle PCP
scag, skag heroin
scagged, skagged addicted to heroin
scarf a joint to swallow a marijuana cigarette in order to avoid getting caught
scat heroin
scate heroin
scattered alcohol or drug intoxicated
schlock drugs; junk
schmack drugs
schmeek heroin
schnozzler a cocaine user
school codeine
school boy paregoric; codeine; a cocaine user
school craft crack
schwillins alcohol
scissors marijuana

Scooby snacks	ecstasy
scoop	a folded matchbook cover used to snort powdered drugs; GHB
scootie	methamphetamines
score	to obtain something, usually drugs or sex; when blood appears in an eyedropper
scorpion	cocaine
Scott	heroin
Scottie, Scotty	cocaine; crack; the high from crack
Scrabble	crack
scramble	worthless or near-worthless heroin
scrape and snort	to share crack by scraping off small pieces to snort
scratch	money
screaming meemies	delirium tremens
screw	sexual intercourse; to cheat someone; a prison guard
scribe	one who can write acceptable forged prescriptions
script	a prescription
script doc	a physician who writes ethically questionable prescriptions
script writer	a sympathetic physician; someone who forges prescriptions
scroll	paper used to roll marijuana cigarettes
scrubwoman's kick	naphtha that is inhaled
scruples	crack
scuffle	PCP
sealed stuff	a can or bottle of opium
sec, seccy, seggy	Seconal
seco-8	secobarbital
second to none	heroin
seconds	second inhalation of a drug from a pipe
second-story man	a thief or burglar
seeds	morning glory seeds
sen	marijuana
send it home	to inject a drug
seni	peyote; mescaline
serenity	chemically related to mescaline and amphetamines; 1,4-BD
serial speedballing	sequencing cough syrup with codeine and heroin over a 1- to 2-day period
sernyl	PCP

serpent	a hypodermic needle
Serpico 21	cocaine
server	crack dealer
ses, sess, sezz	sinsemilla (grade of marijuana)
set	amphetamine and barbiturate mixture; a place where drugs are sold
set up	to arrange for someone to be arrested or caught
Seven Up	cocaine; crack
sewer	the median cephalic vein
sextasy	ecstasy with Viagra
Shabu	freebase cocaine, methamphetamine, PCP
shakes	drug or alcohol withdrawal
shaman	peyote; mescaline
shank	a small quantity of marijuana; a prison-made knife
sharps	needles
sharpshooter	one who most always hits the vein
she	cocaine
shebanging	mixing cocaine with water and squirting it up the nose
sheet rocking	crack and LSD
sheets	PCP
Sherlock Holmes	a police officer
sherm	a cigarette that has been dipped in embalming fluid
shermans	PCP; PCP-laced cigarette
shight, shighty	amphetamines
shill	heroin
shit	heroin
shit-faced	alcohol or drug intoxicated
shmagma	marijuana
shmeck, schmeek	heroin
shoot below the belt	to inject into a vein in the lower part of the body
shoot gravy	to inject a mixture of cooked blood and a dissolved drug
shoot shit	to inject heroin
shoot skin	to miss a vein and inject into the skin
shoot the breeze	nitrous oxide
shoot Yancy	to inject opium
shoot, shoot up	to inject a drug
shooting gallery	where addicts gather to inject drugs
shooting up	to inject drugs

shot	to inject a drug
shot down	under the influence of drugs
shot to the curb	a person who has lost everything due to drug use
shotgun	someone puts the joint or blunt in their mouth backwards and blows the smoke into someones mouth
shovel	equipment used to prepare and use powdered drugs
shrimp	marijuana
shrink	a psychiatrist
shrooms	psilocybin, psilocin mushrooms
shwag	low-grade marijuana
sick dizzies	a reaction to hallucinogenic experience
siddi	marijuana
Sidney	LSD
sightball	crack
silk and satin	amphetamines and barbiturates
Silly Putty	psilocybin, psilocin mushrooms
silo	psilocybin, psilocin mushrooms
Simple Simon	psilocybin, psilocin mushrooms
sinse	marijuana
sinsemilla	potent marijuana
sip	a puff from a marijuana cigarette
sitter	one who coaches another during an LSD trip
sitting well	intoxicated on drugs
sixty-two	2-1/2 ounces of crack
Skag Jones	a heroin addict
skag, scag	heroin
skagged out	alcohol or drug intoxicated
Skagtown	a neighborhood inhabited by addicts
skee	opium
skeegers/skeezers	crack-smoking prostitute
sketch	a bad reaction to LSD or marijuana
sketching	coming down from a speed-induced high
skid	heroin; someone who looks and dresses dirty because of smoking dope
skied	under the influence of drugs
skies	refers to scales used to weigh drugs
skin	paper used for rolling cigarettes
skin flick	a pornographic movie
skin popping	injecting drugs subcutaneously

skin pumping	a subcutaneous or intramuscular injection of drugs
skin search	to examine the skin of a suspected user for needle track marks
skin shooter	a subcutaneous injection of drugs
skin shot	a subcutaneous injection of drugs
skinhead	a person with a shaved head who participates in militant group activities
skinner	a subcutaneous injection of drugs
Skippy	methylphenidate
skirt	a female who trades sex for money and/or drugs
skuffle	PCP
skull buster	a police officer's night stick
skunk	marijuana said to be grown in California
sky river	LSD that is mixed with another drug
skyrockets	amphetamines
slab	a large piece of crack cocaine
slack	a very small amount of drugs
slam	to inject a drug
slammed	to be arrested
slammer	jail or prison
slanging	selling drugs
slanguage	the language of the street
slave	a drug addict
sleep, sleep 500	GHB
sleepers	barbiturates; heroin
sleepwalker	an addict
sleet	crack
sleigh ride	a cocaine party
sleigh rider	cocaine user
slick superspeed	methcathinone
slime	heroin
slinging	dealing drugs
slip the collar	to escape from jail or prison
slits	ecstasy
slow boat	a marijuana cigarette
slum	to use narcotics
slum dump	an opium den
slumber party	a gathering to use drugs
smack	heroin
smack freak	a heroin addict
smackhead	a heroin addict

smart drug	methylphenidate
smash	acetone extracts of marijuana that are added to hashish, rolled in little balls, and smoked
smashed	alcohol or drug intoxicated
smears	LSD
smell it up	to snort powdered drugs
smell the reindeer dust	to snort powdered drugs
smell the stuff	to snort powdered drugs
smizz	heroin
smoke	to smoke drugs that can be smoked
smoke a bowl	to smoke hashish or marijuana
smoke a joint	to smoke a marijuana cigarette
smoke house	a place where one can buy or smoke drugs
smoke joint	a place where one can buy or smoke drugs
smoke you out	smoke marijuana with you
smoked	alcohol or drug intoxicated; killed
smoke-out	a party where attendees smoke drugs
smoking gun	a marijuana or tobacco cigarette that has been laced with heroin and cocaine
smoothie	an undercover agent who is able to pull off a sale from an unsuspecting drug dealer
smudge	a small amount of heroin
Smurf	a cigar dipped in embalming fluid
snakes	delirium tremens
snapped up	intoxicated by drugs
snappers	isobutyl nitrite
snaps	amphetamines
snatcher	a police officer
sniff	to sniff powdered drugs through the nose
sniffer	one who habitually snorts powdered drugs
sniffer bag	$5 bag of powdered drugs
sniffing	spreading compound on piece of wood or cardboard and breathing rapidly through the nose and mouth
sniffing squad	undercover narcotics agents
snipe	a marijuana cigarette butt
snitch	an informer
snite	a lighter used to smoke drugs
snop	marijuana
snort	to sniff powdered drugs
snort a line	to snort cocaine
snorting	intranasal drug use
snot	residue produced from smoking amphetamines

snot balls	rubber cement rolled into balls that are burned and the fumes inhaled
snow	powdered drugs
snow bird	powdered drugs
snow cones	powdered drugs
snow drifter	one who sells powdered drugs
snow eagle	a primary figure in a drug ring
snow flower	a female user of powdered drugs
snow pallets	amphetamines
snow seals	cocaine and amphetamines
snowball	powdered drugs
snowmobiling	using powdered drugs
snowstorm	a large amount of powdered drugs
snozzle	to snort powdered drugs
soap	GHB
soap dope	light pink methamphetamine
soapers	methaqualone
social junker	one who uses drugs only in a social setting
social sniffer	one who uses powdered drugs only in a social setting
society high	one who uses cocaine in a social setting
softballs	barbiturates
soles	hashish
soma	PCP
somatomax	GHB
SomatoPro	1,4-BD
something dreaming game	the choking game
songbird	an informer
soot the chimney	to snort powdered drugs
sophisticated lady	cocaine
soul searching	looking for a vein in which to inject drugs
soup	water bong
source	a drug supplier or wholesaler
space base	cocaine and PCP
space blasting	smoking cocaine and PCP together
space cadet	one who is intoxicated by drugs
space cowboy	the choking game
space dust	crack dipped in PCP
space monkey	the choking game
space ship	glass pipe used to smoke crack
spaced out	altered state of consciousness secondary to prolonged drug use
spangles	Librium

Slang Terms

spare time	possessing marijuana
spark it up	to smoke marijuana
sparking an owl	lighting a joint
Sparkle Plenty	amphetamines
sparklers	amphetamines; ketamine
Sparky	the electric chair
spear	a hypodermic needle
special	superior quality drugs
special K	ketamine
special LA coke	ketamine
speckled eggs	amphetamines
specks	LSD
spectrum	nexus
speed	methamphetamines; amphetamines
speed boat	marijuana, PCP, crack
speed demon	amphetamines; methamphetamines
speed for lovers	ecstasy
speed freak	habitual user of methamphetamines
speed runs	bingeing over several days
speedball	2 drugs injected together
speedster	an amphetamine user
spider blue	heroin
spike	a hypodermic needle
spit ball	a mouthful of freebase vapors puffed into someone else's mouth
splaff	marijuana cigarette laced with acid
splash	amphetamines
splash house	a place where amphetamines or methamphetamines are sold or used
splay	marijuana
spliff	a marijuana cigarette wrapped in newspaper
spliffy	a marijuana cigarette
splim	marijuana
split	to leave
splits	tranquilizers
splivins	amphetamines
spoc	police officers (cops spelled backwards)
spook	a long-time narcotics user
spoon	a utensil used in preparing narcotics for injection; 2 grams of heroin; cocaine measure
spores	psilocin, psilocybin mushrooms
sport of the gods	cocaine use
sporting	to use drugs

spray	inhalants
spread the good news	to share a drug supply
spring	to post bail for someone who is in jail
sprouting	injecting drugs from one syringe to another syringe
sprung	a person who has just started to use drugs
spur	1 gram of a powdered drug
square	a person who uses neither alcohol nor drugs
square dancing tickets	papers laced with LSD
square John	a person who uses neither alcohol nor drugs
square mackerel	marijuana
squat	an abandoned house that has been taken over by homeless people
squirrel	LSD combined with another drug
stack	a pack of marijuana cigarettes
stacking	taking steroids with a prescription
stackola	stacking money
stainless steel ride	lethal injection
stale weed	prison tobacco
stall	a finger cot or condom used as a package for powdered drugs
Stanley's stuff	LSD
star	methcathinone
star stuff	cocaine
stardust	heroin with cocaine
stars	MDMA
star-spangled powder	cocaine
start cooking	to begin injecting drugs into the veins
stash	a supply of concealed drugs
stash bag	a container in which drugs are stored
stash man	a drug dealer or drug runner
stat	methcathinone
steamboat	a device for smoking marijuana
steamroller	pipe used to smoke marijuana
steel and concrete cure	total abstinence from drugs while in prison
steerer	a person who recommends a heroin dealer in return for money or drugs
Stella	paper used to roll marijuana cigarettes
stem	a cylinder used to smoke crack; an opium pipe
stems	marijuana
step on	to dilute drugs
stepping high	alcohol or drug intoxicated
Steve's mission	a place to buy or use drugs

Stevie	a drug-induced hallucination
stick	a marijuana cigarette
stimey	a dime bag of drugs
stinger	a hypodermic needle
stink weed	marijuana
stinky	marijuana
stoms	barbiturates
stone wall horrors	delirium tremens
stoned	under the influence of drugs
stoner	someone who stays under the influence of marijuana
stones	crack
stony bush	marijuana
stoolie	an informer
stoppers	barbiturates
STP	serenity; tranquility; peace; a hallucinogen
straddle the pike	to inject drugs
straight	in possession of narcotics; a person who is not a drug user
straw	a marijuana cigarette
strawberries	barbiturates
strawberry	female who trades sex for drugs or money to buy drugs
strawberry fields	LSD
strawberry hill	LSD
strawberry shortcake	methamphetamine
street ounce	an ounce of diluted heroin for sale on the street
street pusher	one who deals drugs on the street
streetwalker	a prostitute
stretch	to dilute a drug
strike	a dose of drugs
strung out	needing a drug dose because of addiction
stub	a marijuana cigarette butt
stud	a young man, especially one who is promiscuous
stud muffin	a physically fit or handsome male
student	one who is newly addicted to drugs
studio fuel	cocaine
stuff	heroin
stum	marijuana
stumblers	barbiturates
stumbles	inability to walk appropriately as a result of prolonged alcohol or drug use

stung by a viper	addicted to marijuana
stung by the hop	addicted to opium
stung by the white nurse	addicted to powdered drugs
stung by white mosquitoes	addicted to cocaine
submarine	a large marijuana cigarette
suck up	to be excessively attentive in order to gain favor
sucks (it)	something that is extremely objectionable or inadequate
suds	beer
suffocation game	the choking game
suffocation roulette	the choking game
sugar	powdered drugs; LSD
sugar block	crack; LSD
sugar cubes	LSD
sugar daddies	amphetamines
sugar daddy	a man who supports a woman in return for sex; a physician who sells drugs to addicts
sugar down	to dilute powdered drugs with sugar
sugar lumps	LSD
sugar weed	marijuana that has been compressed into a brick with sugar
summer sky	morning glory seeds
sunrise	yellow or orange LSD tablet
sunshine	yellow or orange LSD tablet
super	one person puts the joint in his/her mouth and blows the smoke out for someone else to inhale; PCP
super acid	LSD
super C	cocaine; crack
super flu	withdrawal symptoms
super grass	high-grade or superior quality marijuana
super ice	smokable methamphetamine
super joint	high-grade or superior quality marijuana
super K	ketamine
super kools	PCP
super weed	marijuana or parsley treated with LSD; superior quality marijuana
super X	MDMA
supercharged	intoxicated by drugs
super-jaded	under the influence of drugs

superman	MDMA
supplier	drug source
surfer	PCP
Sustanon 250	injectable steroid
swag	inferior quality marijuana
swans	MDMA
sweatin' me	pressuring me
sweet dreams	morphine
sweet Jesus	morphine
sweet Lucy	marijuana
sweet lunch	marijuana
sweet Mary	marijuana
sweet Morpheus	morphine
sweet stuff	heroin
sweet tooth	a desire for drugs
sweeties, sweets	amphetamines; ecstasy
swell up	crack cocaine
swilly	under the influence of alcohol
swing both ways	to have sex with either men or women
swinger	one who uses a variety of drugs in all forms; one who is sexually promiscuous
swisher	a cigar that has been emptied and filled with marijuana
Swiss purple	LSD
switched on	to be introduced to hallucinogenic drugs
syndicate acid	LSD; PCP
syrup	dark brown Mexican heroin
syrup head	a drug user who uses cough syrup with codeine and a barbiturate
T	PCP
T buzz	PCP
T man	a federal narcotics or treasury agent; a marijuana smoker
tab	a tablet or pill form of a drug
tac	PCP
tag	a euphoric sensation experienced after drug use
tail lights	LSD
taima	marijuana
take	equipment for injecting drugs, usually an eyedropper; money obtained in a robbery; money obtained by selling drugs
take a Brody	to commit suicide
take a dive	to commit suicide

take a Duffy	to fake drug withdrawal
take a fall	to be arrested on drug-related charges
take a powder	to leave; to commit suicide
take a sweep	to snort cocaine
take a trip	to use a hallucinogen
take for a ride	to kill; to cheat
take it in line	to inject drugs into the median cephalic vein
take off	to begin a drug high
take-off artists	addicts who rob other addicts
take-a-too	equipment for injecting drugs, usually an eyedropper
taking a cruise	PCP
taking care of business	addicts' lives and actions on the street
takkouri	marijuana
talcum powder	a bogus powdered drug
tall	under the influence of drugs
tals	Talwin
tamale	a marijuana cigarette that resembles a tamale
tampon	a fat marijuana cigarette
tang	drug addiction
Tango & Cash	heroin laced with methyl fentanyl
tanks	PCP
tapping the bags	removing small amounts of drugs from bags before selling, thus shorting the buyer
tar	opium; heroin
tar dust	cocaine
tarred and feathered	addicted to opium
taste	a small sample of drugs
tattoos	needle track marks
taxing	price paid to enter a crack house; charging more per vial if not a regular customer
tea	marijuana; PCP
tea party	a gathering to smoke marijuana
team meeting	a gathering to smoke marijuana
teardrops	dosage units of crack packaged in the cut-off corners of plastic bags
Teddies and Betties	a mixture of Talwin and pyribenzamine
teddy bears	LSD
teen choking game	the choking game
teenager	1/16 gram methamphetamine
teener	1/16 ounce of crack rock
teeth	bullets
ten sack	marijuana worth $10

tens, 10s	10-mg amphetamine tablets
tension	crack
tester	one who is able to judge the strength of diluted heroin
Texas leaguer	a marijuana smoker
Texas pot	marijuana
Texas shoe shine	inhalant
Texas tea	marijuana
Tex-Mex	marijuana
Thai sticks	bundles of marijuana soaked in hashish oil; marijuana buds bound on short sections of bamboo
Therobolin	injectable steroid
thing	a marijuana cigarette; heroin; main drug interest at the moment
thirst monsters	heavy crack smokers
thirteen, 13	marijuana
thirty-eight, 38	crack sprinkled on marijuana, masturbation
thorn	a hypodermic needle
thoroughbred	drug dealer who sells pure narcotics; a prostitute; a prisoner
threes, 3s	a painkiller that contains 30 mg of codeine
thrill pills	barbiturates
thriller	a marijuana cigarette
thrust	isobutyl nitrite
thrusters	amphetamines
thumb	marijuana
thunder cookie	marijuana
thunder nectar	1,4-BD
thunder weed	marijuana
tia	marijuana leaf
tic	PCP in powder form
tic tac	PCP in powder form
ticket	a hallucinogen
ticket agent	a drug supplier or seller
tie	to inject a drug
tie off	to apply pressure on a vein with a tourniquet
tight	being clean in appearance
tighten up	to give drugs to an individual
tin	container for marijuana; a marijuana pipe made out of aluminum foil
tingling game	the choking game
tish	PCP

tissue crack
titch PCP
tits black tar heroin
toke a pull from a marijuana cigarette
toke pipes pipes used to smoke marijuana
toke up to light a marijuana cigarette
Tom and Jerries MDMA
tom cat a sewing machine needle that is used to open a vein for drug use
Tom Mix an injection of drugs
tomcat a sexually promiscuous male
toncho octane booster which is inhaled
tongue to inject drugs into a vein beneath the tongue
tooies Tuinal capsules
tooles depressant
tools equipment used for injecting drugs; guns
toonies Nexus
toot to snort or sniff cocaine
tooter, tutor a tube used for snorting cocaine
tootsie Tuinal
tootsie roll a marijuana cigarette rolled in brown paper; potent heroin
top gun crack
topi mescaline; peyote
tops peyote; marijuana
tops and bottoms mixture of Talwin and pyribenzamine
torch a marijuana cigarette; to deliberately set a fire
torch cooking smoking cocaine base by using a propane or butane torch as a source of flame
torch up to smoke marijuana
torn up alcohol or drug intoxicated
tornado crack cocaine
torpedo a hired killer; a drink containing chloral hydrate
torture chamber a place of incarceration where drugs are not available
toss up female who trades sex for drugs or money to buy drugs
tossed to be bodily searched for drugs by law enforcement agents
totalled to be intoxicated by drugs
totally spent to have a hangover
toucher drug user who wants affection before, during, or after using drugs

tough	to inject a drug in a vein beneath the tongue
tour guide	one who guides an LSD user through a trip
tout	person who introduces buyers to sellers
toy	a small tin box of prepared opium; equipment used for injecting drugs
TR-6s	amphetamines
tracers	visual effects of hallucinogenics
Track One	area in which houses of prostitution are numerous
Track Two	area in which homosexual houses of prostitution are numerous
tracked up	covered with needle and abscess scars
tracking	repeating a drug-induced hallucination; to repeat words or phrases while under the influence of drugs
tracks	needle marks and abscess scars
trade	a sex partner
tragic magic	crack dipped in PCP
trail	needle marks
trails	LSD-induced perception that moving objects leave multiple images, or trails, behind them
train	gang rape
trained nurse	one who smuggles narcotics into a hospital or prison
trank, tranx, tranq	tranquilizers; depressants
tranquility	a hallucinogenic drug; mescaline; depressants
trap	hiding place for drugs
trash	methamphetamine
trash picker	a street person
trashed	alcohol or drug intoxicated
travel agent	one who guides an LSD user through a trip
tray	a $3 bag of marijuana
trays	vials
tree jumper	a rapist
tree of knowledge	marijuana
trees	drugs in pill and capsule form
triangles	delirium tremens
trick	an act of prostitution or theft
trick track	a prostitute who is addicted to injectable drugs
tricycles and bicycles	mixture of Talwin and pyribenzamine
trip	what a person experiences after using a hallucinogenic drug
trip grass	marijuana mixed with an amphetamine

trip out	to become intoxicated by drugs
triple crowns	MDMA
triple line	superior quality marijuana that is laced with heroin
triple Rolexes	MDMA
triple stacks	MDMA
tripper	a drug user; a person who takes hallucinogens
trips	amitriptyline; LSD
Trojan horse	one who smuggles drugs into a hospital or prison
troll	mixture of LSD and MDMA
troop	crack
truck drivers	amphetamines
Ts and blues	pentazocine
Ts and Rits or Ritz	Talwin and Ritalin injected to produce effect of heroin mixed with cocaine
Ts and Rs	Talwin and Ritalin injected to produce effect of heroin mixed with cocaine
TT1, TT2, TT3	PCP
tubes	water pipes or bongs
tuies	Tuinal
tune in	to experience the effects of a hallucinogenic drug
turbo	a potent form of ecstasy
turd	drugs concealed in a condom in the rectum
turf	the territory gangs consider to be in their control
turkey trots	needle marks from drug injections
turn a cartwheel	to fake a drug withdrawal in an attempt to get drugs
turn a trick	to earn money by theft or prostitution
turn on	to use drugs; to excite sexually
turn out	to introduce someone to drugs or prostitution
turnabout	amphetamine
turned off	withdrawn from drugs
turned on	under the influence of drugs; sexually aroused
turnip greens	marijuana
turps	elixir of terpin hydrate with codeine
tutor, tooter	a straw or something similar to aid in snorting coke
tutti-frutti	flavored cocaine
tutus	MDMA
tweak mission	on a mission to find crack

tweaker	crack user looking for rocks on the floor after a police raid
tweeds	marijuana
Tweety birds	MDMA
twenty, 20	a $20 rock of crack
twenty-five, 25	LSD
twig	a marijuana cigarette
twins	2 smaller particles of rock cocaine that equals a two-O
twirl	to sell drugs
twist	a marijuana cigarette
twisted	intoxication bordering on unconsciousness
twistum	a marijuana cigarette
twisty	a marijuana cigarette
two for nine, 2 for 9	two $5 vials or bags of crack for $9
two-O	$20 piece of rock cocaine, about 1.8 grams gross weight
U boat	a portion of a sealed rubber tube that is filled with drugs and concealed in the rectum
uglies	delirium tremens
ultimate	crack
ultimate Xphoria	MDMA
umbilical cord	methadone
uncle	federal agents
Uncle Fester	a glass pipe
Uncle Milty	barbiturates
Uncle Sid	LSD
under the white cross	under the influence of cocaine
unkie	morphine
up against the stem	addicted to smoking marijuana
up and down	to inject drugs and take pills
up the creek	in trouble
uppers, uppies	amphetamines
ups and downs	amphetamines and barbiturates
uptown	cocaine
utopiates	hallucinogens
uzi	crack; crack pipe
V	Valium
valley	the inside crease of the elbow where drugs are injected
valley dolls	LSD
vals	Valium
Vatican roulette	the rhythm method of birth control

vegetarian	one who smokes marijuana
venom	PCP
Venus	Nexus
vipe	marijuana
viper	one who smokes marijuana
viper's weed	marijuana
vitamin E	ecstasy
vitamin G	GHB
vitamin K	ketamine
vitamin R	Ritalin
vitamins	amphetamines
vivor	a street person who survives
vodka acid	LSD
void	to be under the influence of drugs
volcano 5	red LSD paper
vons	Darvon
vroomed	to be under the influence of drugs
wac, wack	PCP; marijuana or tobacco cigarette dipped in embalming fluid
wacky backy	marijuana
wacky weed	marijuana
wafers	ecstasy; cookies laced with LSD
waffle dust	MDMA
waffles	hits of LSD
wake 'n' bake	to use drugs first thing in the morning
wake-up	amphetamine; the first drug of the day
wakowi	mescaline
Waldorf Astoria	solitary confinement in jail or prison
wall bangers	Quaaludes
warped	intoxicated on drugs
washed up	withdrawn from drugs; one who is no longer successful or needed
waste	to kill
wasted	alcohol or drug intoxicated; exhausted; killed
water	injectable amphetamines
watering hole	a bar where liquor is sold
water-water	marijuana cigarettes dipped in embalming fluid, sometimes laced with PCP
wave	crack
weasel	an informer
wedding bells	LSD; morning glory seeds
wedge series, wedges	LSD-STP combination
weed	marijuana

Slang Terms

weed head	a marijuana user
weed out	weed for sale
weed tea	marijuana
weekend warrior	one who uses drugs on weekends only
weight	the amount of narcotics an addict needs for 1 week
weight belt cleaner	1,4-BD
weight trainers	steroids
weightless	under the influence of drugs
weirded out	one who is disturbed by events which occur while under the influence of drugs
West Coast	Ritalin
West Coast turnarounds	amphetamines
wet	PCP
wet daddy	a marijuana or tobacco cigarette dipped in embalming fluid and laced with PCP
wet dog shakes	delirium tremens
wet-wet	a marijuana or tobacco cigarette dipped in embalming fluid and laced with PCP
whack	to dilute a narcotic; to kill
whacked	intoxicated from drugs; killed
wheat	marijuana
wheels	ecstasy
when-shee	opium
whiff	cocaine
whiffle dust	powdered drugs
whippets	sealed vials containing gases for huffing
whistle blower	an informer
white	cocaine
white angel	a healthcare worker who smuggles drugs to patients or prisoners
white ball	crack
white boy	heroin
white cloud	vapors from drugs that are smoked
white cross	cross-scored amphetamine tablets
white diamonds	MDMA
white domes	LSD
white dove	ecstasy
white dragon	opium
white dust	powdered drugs
white fluff	LSD
white ghost	crack
white girl	cocaine; heroin

white goddess	morphine
white horizon	PCP
white horse	heroin
white junk	heroin
white lady	heroin
white lightning	LSD mixed with another drug; raw liquor
white merchandise	powdered drugs
white mosquito	cocaine
white nurse	powdered drugs
white Owsley	LSD
white powder	cocaine; PCP
white silk	morphine crystals
white stuff	heroin
white sugar	crack
white tornado	freebase cocaine
white-haired lady	heroin
whiteout	isobutyl nitrite
whites, whities	amphetamines
whiz bang	an injected mixture of drugs
whiz	amphetamines
whoops and jangles	symptoms of withdrawal
wicked	potent heroin
wide	under the influence of drugs
widows	amphetamines
wig out	to become psychotic during drug use
wig picker	a psychiatrist
wiggin'	an addict in need of drugs
wild cat	methcathinone and cocaine mixture
wild Geronimo	barbiturates mixed with alcohol
window glass	LSD
window panes	LSD on clear plastic, cellophane, or sheets of gelatin
wings	powdered drugs
wiped out	alcohol or drug intoxicated; exhausted
wired	under the influence of drugs; having a recording device on one's person
wisdom weed	marijuana
witch	powdered drugs; heroin
witch Hazel	heroin
witch's brew	LSD mixed with datura
wizard	1 ounce of marijuana
wizard of Oz	1 ounce of marijuana
wobble weed	marijuana

wokowi	peyote; mescaline
wolf	PCP
wollie	rocks of crack rolled into a marijuana cigarette
wonder star	methcathinone
woodpecker of Mars	Amanita muscaria mushroom
woolas, woolahs	cigarettes laced with cocaine; crack sprinkled on a marijuana cigarette; a hollowed-out cigar refilled with marijuana and crack
woolies	marijuana and crack or PCP mixture
wooly	a cocaine and marijuana cigarette
wooly blunts	marijuana cigarettes laced with crack or PCP
working	selling crack
working half	crack rock weighing 1/2 gram or more
working man's cocaine	methamphetamine
works	equipment for injecting drugs
world traveler	a homeless person who wanders from place to place
wow	PCP
wrangled	to stop using drugs
wrecked	extremely intoxicated from using drugs
wrecking crew	crack
X	MDMA/MDA
X-ing	using ecstasy
Xmas	to be euphoric from drug use
XTC	ecstasy
ya ba	pure form of methamphetamine from Thailand
yahoo, yeaho	crack
yale	crack
yam yam	opium
yanked	arrested
yeh	marijuana
yellow	LSD; barbiturates
yellow bam	methamphetamine
yellow birds	pentobarbital
yellow bullets	pentobarbital
yellow dimples	LSD
yellow dolls	pentobarbital
yellow fever	PCP
yellow jack speed	amphetamines
yellow jackets	depressants
yellow submarines	pentobarbital
yellow sunshine	LSD
yen	desire for drugs

yen shee	opium ash
yen shee suey	opium wine
yen sleep	restless, drowsy state after LSD use
Yerba	marijuana
yesca, yesco	marijuana
yimyom	crack
ying yang	LSD
yuppie flu	the ongoing effects of a cocaine-snorting habit
Z	1 ounce of heroin
Zacatecas purple	potent marijuana grown in the Mexican state of Zacatecas
zambi	marijuana
zap	to kill; to berate an individual
Zen	LSD
zero	opium
zigzag man	LSD; marijuana; marijuana rolling papers
zings	amphetamines
zip	cocaine; 1 ounce of any kind of drug
zip gun	a homemade gun
zol	a marijuana cigarette
zombie	PCP; an addict
zombie buzz	alcohol or drug intoxicated
zombie weed	PCP
zooie	a device that is used to hold the butt of a marijuana cigarette
zoom	ecstasy
zoomers	amphetamines; individuals who sell counterfeit drug, then flees

Appendix 5
Phobias Listed by Clinical Name

Fear is a feeling that is experienced by all humans at one time or another. Phobias take fear a step further than the normal feeling of anxiety one gets when faced with a new adventure, or when one comes face-to-face with something unpleasant. The definition of specific phobia summarizes phobias in general: "specific phobia: (1) a persistent pattern of significant fear of specific objects or situations, manifesting in anxiety or panic on exposure to the object or situation or in anticipation of them, which the person realizes is unreasonable or excessive and which interferes significantly with the person's functioning; (2) a DSM diagnosis that is established when the specified criteria are met." (Source: *Stedman's Medical Dictionary, 28th Edition*)

There is a clinical name for almost every fear. The following pages list phobias in alphabetical order by clinical name and by the fear itself.

CLINICAL NAME(S)	ABNORMAL FEAR OF
A	
ablutophobia	washing or bathing
acarophobia	insects that make one itch
acerophobia	sourness
achluophobia	darkness
acousticophobia	sounds; noise
acrophobia	heights
aeroacrophobia	high open places
aerodromophobia	aircraft; aerodynamics
aeronausiphobia	fear of becoming airsick
aerophobia	air; drafts
agateophobia	insanity
agliophobia	fear of pain
agoraphobia	crowds; open spaces; leaving one's home
agraphobia	sexual abuse
agrizoophobia	wild animals
agyiophobia	streets
aichmophobia	knives; object points
ailurophobia, aelurophobia	cats
albuminurophobia	albumin in urine as sign of kidney disease
alcoholophobia	alcoholism
alektorophobia	chickens
algophobia	pain
alliumphobia	garlic

allodoxaphobia	opinions
altophobia	heights
amathophobia	dust
amaxophobia	riding in vehicles
ambulophobia	walking
amnesiphobia	amnesia
amychophobia	being scratched; scratches
anablephobia	looking upward
ancraophobia	wind
androphobia	men
anemophobia	wind; drafts
anginophobia	sore throat; choking; angina
anglophobia	England or dislike of anything English
angrophobia	becoming angry
ankylophobia	joint immobility
anthrophobia	flowers
anthropophobia	people in society
antlophobia	floods
anuptophobia	remaining single
apeirophobia	infinity
aphephobia	being touched
apiphobia	bees
apotemnophobia	persons with amputations
aquaphobia	water
arachibutyrophobia	peanut butter stuck on roof of mouth
arachnephobia, arachnophobia	spiders
arrhenophobia	men
arsonphobia	fire
ashenophobia	fainting
asthenophobia	weakness
astraphobia, astrapophobia	lightning and thunder
astrophobia	the stars
asymmetriphobia	asymmetry
ataxiophobia	incoordination; ataxia
ataxophobia	disorder
atelophobia	imperfection
atephobia	ruin
athazagoraphobia	being forgotten
atomosophobia	atomic explosion
atychiphobia	failure
aulophobia	flutes or similar wind instruments

aurophobia	gold
auroraphobia	Northern Lights
autodysosmophobia	offensive personal body odor
automatonophobia	ventriloquists' dummies
automysophobia	being dirty
autophobia	self; aloneness; solitude
aviophobia	flying

B

bacillophobia	bacilli
bacteriophobia	bacteria
ballistophobia	missiles; bullets
barophobia	gravity
basiphobia, basophobia	walking
bathophobia	depths
batonophobia	plants
batophobia	high objects
batrachophobia	amphibians
belonephobia	needles; sharp objects
bibliophobia	books
blennophobia	slime; mucus
bogyphobia	demons and goblins
botanophobia	plants and flowers
bromidrosiphobia	having an unpleasant personal body odor
brontophobia	thunder; thunderstorms
bufonophobia	toads

C

cacophobia	ugliness
cainophobia, kainophobia	novelty
caligynephobia	beautiful women
cancerophobia, cancerphobia carcinophobia	cancer; malignancy
cardiophobia	heart disease
carnophobia	meat
catagelophobia, katagelophobia	ridicule; being made fun of
catapedaphobia	jumping from low or high places
cathisophobia, kathisophobia	sitting down
catoptrophobia	mirrors
celtophobia	Celts or dislike of anything Celtic
cenotophobia	anything new
ceraunophobia, keraunophobia	thunder
chaetophobia	hair

cheimaphobia, cheimatophobia	cold
chemophobia	chemicals
cherophobia	gaiety
chionophobia	snow
chiratophobia	being touched
cholerophobia	cholera
chorophobia	dancing
chrematophobia	money; wealth
chromatophobia, chromophobia	colors
chronomentrophobia	clocks
chronophobia	time
cibophobia	food
claustrophobia	confinement; closed spaces
cleisiophobia, cleithrophobia	being locked in an enclosure
cleptophobia	stealing
climacophobia	stairs; climbing
clinophobia	going to bed
clithrophobia	being locked in
cnidophobia	stings; being stung
coitophobia	sexual intercourse
cometophobia	comets
contreltophobia	sexual abuse
coprastasophobia	constipation
coprophobia	excrement
coulrophobia	clowns
counterphobia	seeking out that which is feared
cremnophobia	precipices; cliffs
cryophobia	ice
crystallophobia	glass; crystal
cyberphobia	computers
cyclophobia	bicycles
cymophobia	ocean waves
cynophobia	dogs; rabies
cypridophobia, cypriphobia	venereal disease; sexual intercourse

D

decidophobia	making decisions
defecalgesiophobia	defecating due to pain
deipnophobia	dining; dinner conversation
demonophobia, daemonophobia	demons; the devil
demophobia	crowds

dendrophobia	trees
dentophobia	dentists
dermatophobia, dermatopathophobia, dermatosiophobia	skin disease
dextrophobia	objects to the right
diabetophobia	diabetes
didaskaleinophobia	school
diderodromophobia	railroads; trains
dikephobia	justice
dinophobia	whirlpools
diplopiaphobia	double vision
dipsophobia	drinking
dishabiliophobia	undressing in front of another
domatophobia	houses
doraphobia	fur; skin of animals
dromophobia	crossing streets
dysmorphophobia	deformity
dystychiphobia	accidents

E

ecclesiophobia, ecclesiaphobia	churches
ecophobia	home environment
eisoptrophobia	mirrors
electrophobia	electricity
eleutherophobia	freedom
emetophobia	vomiting
enissophobia	criticism
enochlophobia	crowds
enosiophobia	committing the unpardonable sin
entomophobia	insects
eosophobia	dawn
epistaxiophobia	nosebleeds
epistemphobia	knowledge
equinophobia	horses
eremiophobia, eremophobia	stillness; being alone
ereuthophobia	red; blushing
ergasiophobia	functioning
ergophobia	work
eroticophobia	erotica
erotophobia	sexual love or physical expression
erythrophobia, ereuthophobia	blushing; red
euphobia	hearing good news
eurotophobia	female genitals

F	
febriphobia	fever
felinophobia	cats
fibriophobia	fever
francophobia	France or dislike of anything French
G	
galeophobia	sharks
gallophobia	France; French culture
gamophobia	marriage
gatophobia	cats
geliophobia	laughter
geniophobia	chins
genophobia	sex
genuphobia	knees
gephyrophobia	crossing bridges
gerascophobia	growing old
germanophobia	Germany or German culture
gerontophobia	old age
geumaphobia	tastes
glossophobia	speaking in public
graphophobia	writing
gringophobia	white strangers in Latin countries
gymnophobia	nakedness
gynephobia, gynophobia	women
H	
hadephobia	hell
hagiophobia	saints; holy people
halitophobia	bad breath; halitosis
hamartophobia	sin; error
hamaxophobia	vehicles
haptephobia, haphephobia	being touched
harpaxophobia	robbers
hedonophobia	pleasure
heliophobia	sunlight
hellenologophobia	cumbersome scientific words
hellenophobia	Greece or dislike of anything Greek
helminthophobia	worm infestation
hemophobia, hematophobia	blood
hereiophobia, heresyphobia	radical deviation
herpetophobia	reptiles
heterophobia	the opposite sex

hierophobia	sacred things
hippophobia	horses
hobophobia	beggars; hobos
hodophobia	travel
homichlophobia	fog
homilophobia	sermons
hominophobia	men
homophobia	homosexuals
hoplophobia	firearms
hormephobia	shock
hyalophobia, hyelophobia	glass
hydrargyophobia	mercurial medicines
hydrophobia	water
hydrophobophobia	hydrophobia; rabies or water
hygrophobia	dampness; moisture; liquids
hylephobia	materialism
hylophobia	forests; wood
hypengyophobia	responsibility
hypnophobia	sleep; being hypnotized
hypsiphobia, hypsophobia	high places

I

iatrophobia	doctors
ichthyophobia	fish
iconophobia	worship
ideophobia	ideas
iophobia	poisons
isolophobia	being alone
isopterophobia	termites

J

japanophobia	Japan or dislike of anything Japanese
judeophobia	Jews or dislike of anything Jewish

K

kainotophobia, kainophobia, cainotophobia, cainophobia	anything new; change; novelty
kakorrhaphiophobia	failure; defeat
katagelophobia	ridicule
kenophobia, cenophobia	barren space; emptiness
keraunophobia, ceraunophobia	thunder and lightning
kilobytophobia	computers
kinesophobia	motion

kleptophobia, cleptophobia	stealing; thieves
koniophobia	dust
kopophobia	having a physical or mental exam
L	
lachanophobia	vegetables
lalophobia, laliophobia	speaking; stuttering
leprophobia; lepraphobia	leprosy
leukophobia	the color white
levophobia	objects to the left
ligyrophobia	loud noises
lilapsophobia	tornadoes and hurricanes
limnophobia	lakes
linonophobia	stings; being stung
liticaphobia	lawsuits
lockiophobia	childbirth
logizomechanophobia	computers
logophobia	words
luiphobia	lues; syphilis
lyssophobia	insanity
M	
macrophobia	long waits
mageirocophobia	cooking
maieusiophobia	pregnancy; childbirth
malaxophobia	love play
maniaphobia	insanity
mastigophobia	punishment; being beaten
mechanophobia	machinery
medomalacuphobia	losing an erection
medorthophobia	an erect penis
megalophobia	large objects
melanophobia	the color black
melissophobia	bees
melophobia	music; hatred of music
meningitophobia	meningitis; brain disease
merinthophobia	being bound or tied
mertophobia	poetry
metallophobia	metals
metathesiophobia	change
meteorophobia	meteors
methyphobia	alcohol
microbiophobia	microorganisms; germs

microphobia, mycrophobia	small or minute objects
misophobia, mysophobia	germs; being contaminated
mnemophobia	memories
molysmophobia, molysomophobia	contamination; infection
monopathophobia	definite disease
monophobia	aloneness; being alone
motorphobia	motor vehicles
mottophobia	moths
musicophobia	music
misophobia, mysophobia	contamination; filth
musophobia	mice
mycophobia	mushrooms
mythophobia	myths; stories
myctophobia	darkness
myrmecophobia	ants
myxophobia	slime; mucus

N

namatophobia, nomatophobia	names
nebulaphobia	clouds; fog
necrophobia	corpses; death
nelophobia	glass
neopharmaphobia	new drugs
neophobia	anything new; change; novelty
nephophobia	clouds
noctiphobia	night
nosemaphobia	illness
nosophobia	disease; hospitals
nostophobia	returning home
novercaphobia	stepmother
nucleomitaphobia	nuclear war and weapons
nudophobia, nudiphobia	nudity
numerophobia	numbers
nyctohlophobia	dark wooded areas
nyctophobia	darkness; night

O

obesophobia	weight gain; obesity
ochlophobia	crowds
ochophobia	vehicles
octophobia	number 8
odontophobia	teeth; dental surgery
odynophobia, odynephobia	pain

oecophobia, oikophobia	home environment
oenophobia	wine
oikophobia, oikiophobia, oechophobia	home or home surroundings
olfactophobia	odors
ombrophobia	rain; being rained on
ommatophobia	eyes
oneirophobia	dreams
onomatophobia	hearing certain words or names
ophidiophobia	snakes
ophthalmophobia	being stared at
optophobia	opening one's eyes
ornithophobia	birds
orthophobia	property
osmophobia	odors
osphresiophobia	odors
ostraconophobia	shellfish
ouranophobia	heaven

P

pagophobia	ice; frost
panphobia, panophobia, pantophobia	everything
panthophobia	disease; suffering
papaphobia	the Pope
papyrophobia	paper
paralipophobia	neglect; omission of duty
paraphobia	sexual perversion
parasitophobia	parasites
paraskavedekatriaphobia	Friday the 13th
parthenophobia	young girls; virgins
parturiphobia	pregnancy; childbirth
pathophobia	disease
patriophobia	heredity; hereditary disease
peccatiphobia, peccatophobia	sinning
pediculophobia	lice
pediophobia, pedophobia, paedophobia	dolls; children
peladophobia	bald people
pellagraphobia	pellagra
peniaphobia	poverty
pentheraphobia	mother-in-law
phagophobia	eating; being eaten
phalacrophobia	being bald

phallophobia	the penis
pharmacophobia	medicine
phasmophobia	ghosts
phengophobia	daylight; sunshine
philemaphobia	kissing
philophobia	falling in love
philosophobia	philosophy; philosophers
phobophobia	fearing; phobias
phonophobia	sounds; voices; telephones
photangiophobia	eye pain caused by light
photaugiophobia	bright light
photophobia	light
phronemophobia	thinking
phthiriophobia	lice
phthisiophobia	tuberculosis
placophobia	tombstones
plutophobia	wealth
pluviophobia	rain or being rained on
pneumatiphobia	spirits
pneumatophobia	air
pnigerophobia	smothering
pnigophobia	choking; sore throats
pocresophobia	weight gain
pogonophobia	beards
poinephobia	punishment
poliosophobia	poliomyelitis
politicophobia	politicians
polyphobia	many things
ponophobia	work; fatigue
porphyrophobia	the color purple
potamophobia	rivers; running water
potophobia	drinking
proctophobia	the rectum; rectal disease
prosophobia	progress
proteinphobia	protein foods
psellismophobia	stuttering
pseudohydrophobia	dogs; rabies
psychophobia	the mind
psychrophobia	cold climates or temperatures
pteromerhanophobia	flying
pteronophobia	feathers
pupaphobia	puppets
pyrexiophobia	fever
pyrophobia	fire

R

radiophobia	radiation; x-rays
ranidaphobia	frogs
rectophobia	the rectum; rectal disease
rhabdophobia	being beaten or flogged; magic
rhypophobia, rupophobia	filth
rhytiphobia	getting wrinkles
rupophobia	dirt
russophobia	Russia; anything Russian

S

samhainophobia	Halloween
sarmassophobia	love play
satanophobia	the devil; Satan
scabiophobia	scabies
scatophobia	excrement; obscene language
scelerophobia	bad men; burglars; thieves; robbers
scholionophobia	school
sciophobia, sciaphobia	shadows
scoionophobia	school
scoleciphobia	worms
scopophobia, scoptophobia	being stared at
scotomaphobia	blindness in a visual field
scotophobia	darkness
scriptophobia	writing
selaphobia	flash of light
selenophobia	the moon
seplophobia	decaying matter
sesquipedalophobia	long words
sexophobia	the opposite sex
siderodromophobia	railroad; train travel
siderophobia	stars
sinistrophobia	things to the left
sinophobia	China; anything Chinese
sitophobia, sitiophobia	food
soceraphobia	parents-in-law
sociophobia	society; people
somniphobia	sleep
sophophobia	learning
soteriophobia	dependence on others
spectrophobia	phantoms
spermatophobia, spermophobia	semen (or loss of)
spheksophobia	wasps

stasibasiphobia	standing up and walking
stasiphobia	standing up
staurophobia	crosses; the crucifix
stenophobia	narrow spaces
stygiophobia	hell
suriphobia	mice
symbolophobia	symbolism
symmetrophobia	symmetry
syngenesophobia	relatives
syphilophobia, syphiliphobia	syphilis

T

tabophobia	wasting sickness
tachophobia	speed
taeniophobia, teniophobia	tapeworms
taphephobia, taphophobia	being buried alive
tapinophobia	being contagious
taurophobia	bulls
technophobia	technology
teleophobia	religious ceremonies
telephonophobia	telephones
telophobia	teleology
teratophobia	bearing a deformed child; monsters
testophobia	taking a test
tetanophobia	fear of tetanus
teutophobia, teutonophobia	Germany or German culture
textophobia	fear of certain fabrics
thaasophobia	sitting
thalassophobia	the sea; ocean
thanatophobia	death
theatrophobia	theaters
theologicophobia	theology
theophobia	God
thermophobia	heat
tocophobia	childbirth
tomophobia	surgical operations
tonitrophobia, tonitruphobia	thunder; thunderstorms
topophobia	certain places; performing
toxiphobia, toxicophobia, toxophobia	poison
traumatophobia	physical injury; war
tremophobia	trembling
trichinophobia	trichinosis
trichopathophobia, trichophobia	hair

tridecaphobia, triskaidekaphobia	number 13
tropophobia	moving; making change
trypanophobia	injections
tuberculophobia	tuberculosis
tyrannophobia	tyrants

U

uranophobia	heaven
urophobia	urine; urinating

V

vaccinophobia	vaccination
venereophobia	venereal disease
venustraphobia	beautiful women
verbophobia	words
vermiphobia	worm infestation; germs
vestiphobia	clothing
vitricophobia	stepfather

W

wiccaphobia	witches; witchcraft

X

xanthophobia	the color yellow
xenophobia	strangers; foreigners
xerophobia	arid climates; deserts; dryness
xylophobia	wooden objects; forests

Z

zelophobia	jealousy
zeusophobia	God or gods
zoophobia	animals

Appendix 6
Phobias Listed by Abnormal Fear

ABNORMAL FEAR OF	CLINICAL NAME(S)
accidents	dystychiphobia
air, drafts	aerophobia, pneumatophobia
aircraft; aerodynamics	aerodromophobia
albumin in urine as sign of kidney disease	albuminurophobia
alcohol, alcoholism	methyphobia, alcoholophobia
aloneness; being alone	monophobia, isolophobia
amnesia	amnesiphobia
amphibians	batrachophobia
an erect penis	medorthophobia
animals	zoophobia
ants	myrmecophobia
anything new; change; novelty	cenotophobia, kainotophobia, kainophobia, cainotophobia, cainophobia, neophobia
arid climates; deserts; dryness	xerophobia
asymmetry	asymmetriphobia
atomic explosion	atomosophobia
bacilli	bacillophobia
bacteria	bacteriophobia
bad breath, halitosis	halitophobia
bad men; burglars; thieves; robbers	scelerophobia
bald people	peladophobia
barren space; emptiness	kenophobia, cenophobia
beards	pogonophobia
bearing a deformed child; monsters	teratophobia
beautiful women	caligynephobia, venustraphobia
becoming angry	angrophobia
bees	apiphobia, melissophobia
beggars; hobos	hobophobia
being bald	phalacrophobia
being beaten or flogged; magic	rhabdophobia
being bound or tied	merinthophobia
being buried alive	taphephobia, taphophobia
being contagious	tapinophobia
being dirty	automysophobia
being forgotten	athazagoraphobia
being locked in an enclosure	cleisiophobia, cleithrophobia, clithrophobia
being scratched; scratches	amychophobia

being stared at	scopophobia, scoptophobia, ophthalmophobia
being touched	chiratophobia, haptephobia, haphephobia
bicycles	cyclophobia
birds	ornithophobia
blindness in a visual field	scotomaphobia
blood	hemophobia, hematophobia
blushing; red	erythrophobia, ereuthophobia
books	bibliophobia
bright light	photaugiophobia
bulls	taurophobia
cancer; malignancy	cancerophobia, cancerphobia, carcinophobia
cats	ailurophobia, aelurophobia, elurophobia, felinophobia, gatophobia
Celts; anything Celtic	celtophobia
certain places; performing	topophobia
change	metathesiophobia
chemicals	chemophobia
chickens	alektorophobia
childbirth	lockiophobia, tocophobia
China; anything Chinese	sinophobia
chins	geniophobia
choking; sore throats	pnigophobia
cholera	cholerophobia
churches	ecclesiophobia, ecclesiaphobia
clocks	chronomentrophobia
clothing	vestiphobia
clouds; fog	nebulaphobia, nephophobia
clowns	coulrophobia
cold	cheimaphobia, cheimatophobia
cold climates or temperatures	psychrophobia
colors	chromatophobia, chromophobia
comets	cometophobia
committing the unpardonable sin	enosiophobia
computers	cyberphobia; kilobytophobia; logizomechanophobia
confinement; closed spaces	claustrophobia
constipation	coprastasophobia
contamination; filth; germs	misophobia, mysophobia
contamination; infection	molysmophobia; molysomophobia
cooking	mageirocophobia

corpses; death	necrophobia
criticism	enissophobia
crosses; the crucifix	staurophobia
crossing bridges	gephyrophobia
crossing streets	dromophobia
crowds; open spaces; leaving one's home	agoraphobia; demophobia; enochlophobia; ochlophobia
cumbersome scientific words	hellenologophobia
dampness; moisture; liquids	hygrophobia
dancing	chorophobia
dark wooded areas	nyctohlophobia
darkness; night	nyctophobia; myctophobia; scotophobia achluophobia
dawn	eosophobia
daylight; sunshine	phengophobia
death	thanatophobia
decaying matter	seplophobia
defecating due to pain	defecalgesiophobia
definite disease	monopathophobia
deformity	dysmorphophobia
goblins	bogyphobia
demons; the devil	demonophobia, daemonophobia
dentists	dentophobia
dependence on others	soteriophobia
depths	bathophobia
diabetes	diabetophobia
dining; dinner conversation	deipnophobia
dirt	rupophobia
disease	pathophobia
hospitals	nosophobia
suffering	panthophobia
disorder	ataxophobia
doctors	iatrophobia
dogs; rabies	cynophobia, pseudohydrophobia, hydrophobia
dolls; children	pediophobia, pedophobia, paedophobia
double vision	diplopiaphobia
dreams	oneirophobia
drinking	dipsophobia; potophobia
dust	amathophobia; koniophobia
eating; being eaten	phagophobia
electricity	electrophobia
England or dislike of anything English	anglophobia

erotica	eroticophobia
everything	panphobia, panophobia, pantophobia
excrement; obscene language	scatophobia; coprophobia
eye pain caused by light	photangiophobia
eyes	ommatophobia
failure; defeat	kakorrhaphiophobia; atychiphobia
fainting	ashenophobia
falling in love	philophobia
fear of becoming airsick	aeronausiphobia
fear of certain fabrics	textophobia
fear of pain	agliophobia
fear of tetanus	tetanophobia
fearing; phobias	phobophobia
feathers	pteronophobia
female genitals	eurotophobia
fever	febriphobia, febriophobia; pyrexiophobia
filth	rhypophobia, rupophobia
fire	arsonphobia; pyrophobia
firearms	hoplophobia
fish	ichthyophobia
flash of light	selaphobia
floods	antlophobia
flowers	anthrophobia
flutes or similar wind instruments	aulophobia
flying	pteromerhanophobia; aviophobia
fog	homichlophobia
food	sitophobia, sitiophobia; cibophobia
forests; wood	hylophobia
France or anything French	francophobia; gallophobia
freedom	eleutherophobia
Friday the 13th	paraskavedekatriaphobia
frogs	ranidaphobia
functioning	ergasiophobia
fur; skin of animals	doraphobia
gaiety	cherophobia
garlic	alliumphobia
Germany or anything German	germanophobia; teutophobia; teutonophobia
getting wrinkles	rhytiphobia
ghosts	phasmophobia
glass	hyalophobia, hyelophobia; nelophobia
crystal	crystallophobia
God or gods	zeusophobia; theophobia

going to bed	clinophobia
gold	aurophobia
gravity	barophobia
Greece or anything Greek	hellenophobia
growing old	gerascophobia
hair	trichopathophobia, trichophobia; chaetophobia
Halloween	samhainophobia
music; hatred of music	melophobia
having a physical or mental exam	kopophobia
having an unpleasant personal body odor	bromidrosiphobia
hearing certain words or names	onomatophobia
hearing good news	euphobia
heart disease	cardiophobia
heat	thermophobia
heaven	ouranophobia; uranophobia
heights	acrophobia; altophobia
hell	hadephobia; stygiophobia
heredity; hereditary disease	patriophobia
high objects	batophobia
high open places	aeroacrophobia
high places	hypsiphobia, hypsophobia
home or home surroundings	oikophobia, oikiophobia, oechophobia, ecophobia
homosexuals	homophobia
horses	equinophobia, hippophobia
houses	domatophobia
ice; frost	pagophobia, cryophobia
ideas	ideophobia
illness	nosemaphobia
imperfection	atelophobia
incoordination; ataxia	ataxiophobia
infinity	apeirophobia
injections	trypanophobia
insanity	agateophoia, lyssophobia, maniaphobia
insects	entomophobia
insects that make one itch	acarophobia
Japan or anything Japanese	japanophobia
jealousy	zelophobia
Jews or anything Jewish	judeophobia
joint immobility	ankylophobia
jumping from low or high places	catapedaphobia

justice	dikephobia
kissing	philemaphobia
knees	genuphobia
knives; object points	aichmophobia
knowledge	epistemphobia
lakes	limnophobia
large objects	megalophobia
laughter	geliophobia
lawsuits	liticaphobia
learning	sophophobia
leprosy	leprophobia; lepraphobia
lice	pediculophobia, phthiriophobia
light	photophobia
lightning and thunder	astraphobia, astrapophobia
long waits	macrophobia
long words	sesquipedalophobia
looking upward	anablephobia
losing an erection	medomalacuphobia
loud noises	ligyrophobia
love play	malaxophobia, sarmassophobia
lues, syphilis	luiphobia
machinery	mechanophobia
making decisions	decidophobia
many things	polyphobia
marriage	gamophobia
materialism	hylephobia
meat	carnophobia
medicine	pharmacophobia
memories	mnemophobia
men	androphobia, arrhenophobia, hominophobia
meningitis; brain disease	meningitophobia
mercurial medicines	hydrargyophobia
metals	metallophobia
meteors	meteorophobia
mice	musophobia, suriphobia
microorganisms	microbiophobia
mirrors	catoptrophobia, eisoptrophobia
missiles, bullets	ballistophobia
money; wealth	chrematophobia
mother-in-law	pentheraphobia
moths	mottophobia
motion	kinesophobia

motor vehicles	motorphobia
moving; making change	tropophobia
mushrooms	mycophobia
music	musicophobia
myths; stories	mythophobia
nakedness	gymnophobia
names	namatophobia, nomatophobia
narrow spaces	stenophobia
needles; sharp objects	belonephobia
neglect; omission of duty	paralipophobia
new drugs	neopharmaphobia
night	noctiphobia
Northern Lights	auroraphobia
nosebleeds	epistaxiophobia
novelty	cainophobia, kainophobia
nuclear war and weapons	nucleomitaphobia
nudity	nudophobia, nudiphobia
number 13	tridecaphobia; triskaidekaphobia
number 8	octophobia
numbers	numerophobia
objects to the left	levophobia
objects to the right	dextrophobia
ocean waves	cymophobia
odors	olfactophobia, osmophobia, osphresiophobia
offensive personal body odor	autodysosmophobia
old age	gerontophobia
opening one's eyes	optophobia
opinions	allodoxaphobia
pain	odynophobia, odynephobia, algophobia
paper	papyrophobia
parasites	parasitophobia
parents-in-law	soceraphobia
peanut butter stuck on roof of mouth	arachibutyrophobia
pellagra	pellagraphobia
people in society	anthropophobia
persons with amputations	apotemnophobia
phantoms	spectrophobia
philosophy; philosophers	philosophobia
physical injury; war	traumatophobia
plants and flowers	botanophobia, batonophobia
pleasure	hedonophobia
poetry	mertophobia

poison	toxiphobia, toxicophobia, toxophobia, iophobia
poliomyelitis	poliosophobia
politicians	politicophobia
poverty	peniaphobia
precipices; cliffs	cremnophobia
pregnancy; childbirth	maieusiophobia, parturiphobia
progress	prosophobia
property	orthophobia
protein-rich foods	proteinphobia
punishment; being beaten	mastigophobia, poinephobia
puppets	pupaphobia
radiation; x-rays	radiophobia
radical deviation	hereiophobia, heresyphobia
railroad; train travel, trains	siderodromophobia, diderodromophobia
rain; being rained on	ombrophobia, pluviophobia
red; blushing	ereuthophobia
relatives	syngenesophobia
religious ceremonies	teleophobia
remaining single	anuptophobia
reptiles	herpetophobia
responsibility	hypengyophobia
returning home	nostophobia
ridicule; being made fun of	catagelophobia, katagelophobia
riding in vehicles	amaxophobia
rivers; running water	potamophobia
robbers	harpaxophobia
ruin	atephobia
Russia; anything Russian	russophobia
sacred things	hierophobia
saints; holy people	hagiophobia
scabies	scabiophobia
school	didaskaleinophobia, scholionophobia, scoionophobia
seeking out that which is feared	counterphobia
self; aloneness; solitude	autophobia
semen; loss of semen	spermatophobia, spermophobia
sermons	homilophobia
sex	genophobia
sexual abuse	agraphobia, contreltophobia
sexual intercourse	coitophobia
sexual love or physical expression	erotophobia
sexual perversion	paraphobia

shadows	sciophobia, sciaphobia
sharks	galeophobia
shellfish	ostraconophobia
shock	hormephobia
sin; error	peccatiphobia, peccatophobia, hamartophobia
sitting	thaasophobia
sitting down	cathisophobia, kathisophobia
skin disease	dermatophobia, dermatopathophobia, dermatosiophobia
sleep; being hypnotized	hypnophobia, somniphobia
slime; mucus	blennophobia, myxophobia
small or minute objects	microphobia, mycrophobia
smothering	pnigerophobia
snakes	ophidiophobia
snow	chionophobia
society; people	sociophobia
sore throat; choking; angina	anginophobia
sounds; voices; telephones; noise	phonophobia, acousticophobia
sourness	acerophobia
speaking in public	glossophobia
speaking; stuttering	lalophobia, laliophobia
speed	tachophobia
spiders	arachnephobia, arachnophobia
spirits	pneumatiphobia
stairs; climbing	climacophobia
standing up and walking	stasibasiphobia, stasiphobia
stars	siderophobia
stealing; thieves	kleptophobia, cleptophobia
stepfather	vitricophobia
stepmother	novercaphobia
stillness; being alone	eremiophobia, eremophobia
stings	cnidophobia, linonophobia
strangers; foreigners	xenophobia
streets	agyiophobia
stuttering	psellismophobia
sunlight	heliophobia
surgical operations	tomophobia
symbolism	symbolophobia
symmetry	symmetrophobia
syphilis	syphilophobia, syphiliphobia
taking a test	testophobia
tapeworms	taeniophobia, teniophobia

tastes	geumaphobia
technology	technophobia
teeth; dental surgery	odontophobia
teleology	telophobia
telephones	telephonophobia
termites	isopterophobia
the color black	melanophobia
the color purple	porphyrophobia
the color white	leukophobia
the color yellow	xanthophobia
the devil; Satan	satanophobia
the mind	psychophobia
the moon	selenophobia
the opposite sex	heterophobia, sexophobia
the penis	phallophobia
the Pope	papaphobia
the rectum; rectal disease	proctophobia, rectophobia
the sea; ocean	thalassophobia
the stars	astrophobia
theaters	theatrophobia
theology	theologicophobia
things to the left	sinistrophobia
thinking	phronemophobia
thunder and lightning	keraunophobia, ceraunophobia
thunder; thunderstorms	tonitrophobia, tonitruphobia, brontophobia, ceraunophobia
time	chronophobia
toads	bufonophobia
tombstones	placophobia
tornadoes and hurricanes	lilapsophobia
travel	hodophobia
trees	dendrophobia
trembling	tremophobia
trichinosis	trichinophobia
tuberculosis	phthisiophobia, tuberculophobia
tyrants	tyrannophobia
ugliness	cacophobia
undressing in front of another	dishabiliophobia
urine; urinating	urophobia
vaccination	vaccinophobia
vegetables	lachanophobia
vehicles	hamaxophobia, ochophobia
venereal disease; sexual intercourse	cypridophobia, cypriphobia, venereophobia

ventriloquists' dummies	automatonophobia
vomiting	emetophobia
walking	basiphobia, basophobia, ambulophobia
washing or bathing	ablutophobia
wasps	spheksophobia
wasting sickness	tabophobia
water	hydrophobia, aquaphobia
weakness	asthenophobia
wealth	plutophobia
weight gain; obesity	obesophobia, pocresophobia
whirlpools	dinophobia
white strangers in Latin countries	gringophobia
wild animals	agrizoophobia
wind; drafts	anemophobia, ancraophobia
wine	oenophobia
witches; witchcraft	wiccaphobia
women	gynephobia, gynophobia
wooden objects; forests	xylophobia
words	logophobia, verbophobia
work; fatigue	ponophobia, ergophobia
worm infestation	helminthophobia, vermiphobia
worms	scoleciphobia
worship	iconophobia
writing	graphophobia, scriptophobia
young girls; virgins	parthenophobia

Appendix 7
Psychiatric and Psychological Tests

A Comprehensive Custody Evaluation Standard System (ACCESS)
A Measure of How You Think and Make Decisions
A Structured Addictions Assessment Interview for Selecting Treatment (ASIST)
AAMR Adaptive Behavior Scale Residential and Community, Second Edition
Abbreviated Conners Rating Scale
Abbreviated Conners Teacher Questionnaire
Abbreviated Conners Teacher Rating Scale (ACTRS)
Abbreviated Life Event Questionnaire
ABC Inventory to Determine Kindergarten and School Readiness
Aberrant Behavior Checklist (ABC)
Ability-to-Benefit Admissions Test
Abnormal Involuntary Movements Scale (AIMS)
Abuse Dimensions Inventory
Abuse Risk Inventory for Women, Experimental Edition
Academic Advising Inventory
Academic Alertness Test
Academic Aptitude Test (AAT)
Academic Aptitude Test-Revised (AAT-R)
Academic Instruction Measurement System
Academic Inventory
Academic Orientation Scale
Academic Readiness Scale (ARS)
Acceptance of Disability Scale
Accounting Program Admission Test (APAT)
ACCUPLACER: Computerized Placement Tests
ACER Advanced Test B40
ACER Advanced Test B90
ACER Applied Reading Test
ACER Test of Basic Skills - Blue Series
ACER Test of Basic Skills - Green Series
ACER Test of Reasoning Ability
ACER Word Knowledge Test
Achenbach Child Behavior Checklist
Achenbach Child Behavior Test
Achenbach-Conners-Quay Behavior Checklist (ACQ)
Achievement Checklist
Achievement Test (AT)
Achievement Motivation Profile
Achieving Behavioral Competencies
Achromatic-Chromatic Scale
Ackerman-Schoendorf Scales for Parent Evaluation of Custody (ASPECT)
ACQ Behavior Checklist
ACT Study Power Assessment and Inventory
Act & React Test System (ACTRS)
Activity Pattern Indicator (API)
Acuity of Psychiatric Illness Scale (APIS)
Acute Panic Inventory Adaptability Test
Adaptation of the Wechsler Preschool and Primary Scale of Intelligence for Deaf Children
Adapted Sequenced Inventory of Communication Development (A-SICD)
Adaptive Behavior Evaluation Scale (ABES)
Adaptive Behavior Evaluation Scale-Revised (ABES-R)
Adaptive Behavior Inventory
Adaptive Behavior Inventory for Children (ABIC)

Adaptive Behavior Scale (ABS)
Adaptive Behavior: Street Survival Skills Questionnaire
Adaptive Functioning Index
Adaptive Style Inventory
ADD-H Comprehensive Teacher's Rating Scale
ADD-H Comprehensive Teacher's Rating Scale, Second Edition (ACTeRS)
Addiction Research Center Inventory
Addiction Severity Index (ASI)
Additional Personality Factor Inventory
ADHD Behavior Checklist for Adults
Adjective Checklist, The (ACL)
Adjustment Inventory
Adjustment Scales for Children and Adolescents
Adolescent Alienation Index (AAI)
Adolescent and Adult Psychoeducational Profile
Adolescent Apperception Cards
Adolescent Coping Scale
Adolescent Diagnostic Interview (ADI)
Adolescent Dissociative Experiences Scale (A-DES)
Adolescent Drinking Index (ADI)
Adolescent Drug and Alcohol Diagnostic Assessment (ADAD)
Adolescent Family and Social Life Questionnaire (AFSLQ)
Adolescent Language Screening Test (ALST)
Adolescent Life Change Event Questionnaire (ALCEQ)
Adolescent Multiphasic Personality Inventory (AMPI)
Adolescent Problem Severity Index (APSI)
Adolescent Psychopathology Scale (APS)
Adolescent Risk Behavior Questionnaire
Adolescent Self-Report Trauma Questionnaire
Adolescent Separation Anxiety Test
Adolescent Symptom Inventory-4 (ASI)
Adolescent Coping Orientation for Problem Experiences
Adolescent Family Inventory of Life Events and Changes
Adult Attachment Interview
Adult Attention Deficit Disorder Behavior Rating Scale
Adult Attention Deficit Disorder Evaluation Scale
Adult Basic Learning Examination (ABLE)
Adult Basic Learning Examination-Level I (ABLE-I)
Adult Basic Learning Examination-Level II (ABLE-II)
Adult Career Concerns Inventory (ACCI)
Adult Growth Examination
Adult Language Assessment Scale
Adult Neuropsychological Questionnaire (ANQ)
Adult Personal Data Inventory (APDI)
Adult Personality Inventory (API)
Adult Personality Inventory-Revised
Adult Self-Expression Scale (ASES)
Adult Suicidal Ideation Questionnaire (ASIQ)
Advanced Placement Examination (APE)
Advanced Progressive Matrices
Affective Auditory Verbal Learning Test
Affect Balance Scale (ABS)
Affect Grid Study
Affective Perception Inventory
Affective Perception Inventory-College Level
Affective Style Index
Aged Schizophrenia Assessment Schedule-Cognitive Battery, The

Age Projection Test (APT)
Ages and Stages Questionnaire
Aggregate NeuroBehavioral Student Health and Educational Review (ANSER)
Agoraphobic Cognitions Questionnaire
AGS Early Screening Profile
AH4 Group Intelligence Test
AH5 Group Test of High Grade Intelligence
AH6 Group Tests of High Level Intelligence
Ainsworth Strange Situation Test
Akerfeldt Test
Albany Panic and Phobia Questionnaire
Alberta Essay Scales: Models
Albert's Famous Faces
Alcadd Test
Alcadd Test-Revised Edition
Alcohol Assessment and Treatment Profile
Alcohol Clinical Index
Alcohol Dependence Scale
Alcohol Usage Questionnaire (AUQ)
Alcohol Use Disorders Identification Test (AUDIT)
Alcohol Use Inventory (AUI)
Alphabet Mastery
Alternative Lifestyle Checklist (ALC)
Alzheimer Disease Assessment Scale (ADAS)
Alzheimer Disease Assessment Scale, Cognitive (ADAS-cog)
Ambiguous Intentions Hostility Questionnaire (AIHQ)
Amphetamine Interview Rating Scale (AIRS)
Analysis of Readiness Skills
Analytic Learning Disability Assessment
Analytical Reading Inventory
Andreasen Six-Basic-Factors-Model Questionnaire (A-SBFM)
Animal and Opposite Drawing Technique (AODT)
Animal Naming Test
Ann Arbor Learning Inventory
Annett Hand Preference Scale
Anomalous Sentences Repetition Test, The
Anorectic Attitude Questionnaire
Anorexic Behavior Observation Scale (ABOS)
Anorexic Behavior Scale
Antidepressant Treatment History Form
Anton Brenner Developmental Gestalt Test of School Readiness
Anxiety Disorders Interview Schedule
Anxiety Scale for the Blind (ASB)
Anxiety Scale Questionnaire (ASQ)
Anxiety Scales for Children and Adults (ASCA)
Anxiety Sensitivity Index (ASI)
Anxiety Status Inventory (ASI)
Apathy Evaluation Scale
Aphasia Clinical Battery
Aphasia Diagnostic Profile
Aphasia Language Performance Scale (ALPS)
Applied Knowledge Test
Appraisal of Language Disturbances (ALD)
Apraxia Battery for Adults (ABA)
Apraxia Profile: A Descriptive Assessment Tool for Children
APT Inventory
Aptitude Inventory
Aptitude Interest Inventory
Aptitude Interest Measurement
Aptitude Survey and Interest Schedule-Interest Survey
Aptitude Test for School Beginners (ASB)
Aptitude-Intelligence Test Series
Arithmetic Grade Rating
Arithmetic Skills Assessment Test

Arithmetic Subtest
Arizona Social Support Interview Schedule
Arizona Articulation Proficiency Scale (AAPS)
Arizona Articulation Proficiency Scale, Second Edition
Arizona Battery for Communication Disorders of Dementia (ABCD)
Arizona Sexual Experience Scale
Arlin Test of Formal Reasoning
Armed Services Civilian Vocational Interest Survey
Armed Services Vocational Aptitude Battery
Army Alpha Examination Revised
Army Beta Tests
Army General Classification Test
Arousal Seeking Tendency Scale
Arthur Adaptation of the Leiter International Performance Scale
Arthur Point Scale of Performance Test
Ashland Interest Assessment
ASSESS Personality Battery [Expert System Version 5.X]
Assessing and Teaching Phonological Knowledge
Assessing Linguistic Behaviors: Assessing Prelinguistic and Early Linguistic Behaviors in Developmentally Young Children
Assessing Motivation to Communicate
Assessing Reading Difficulties: A Diagnostic and Remedial Approach
Assessing Specific Competencies
Assessing Specific Employment Skill Competencies
Assessment for Persons Profoundly or Severely Impaired
Assessment in Infancy: Ordinal Scales of Psychological Development
Assessment Inventory
Assessment of Adaptive Areas
Assessment of Basic Competencies (ABC)
Assessment of Bizarre-Idiosyncratic Thinking
Assessment of Career Decision Making (ACDM)
Assessment of Chemical Health Inventory
Assessment of Children's Language Comprehension (ACLC)
Assessment of Core Goals (ACG)
Assessment of Fluency in School-Age Children
Assessment of Qualitative and Structural Dimensions of Object Representations-Revised Edition
Assessment Program of Early Learning Levels (APELL)
Assessment Questionnaire
Association Index
Assigning Structure Stages Test
Association Adjustment Inventory
Athletic Motivation Inventory (AMI)
Attention Deficit Disorder Behavior Rating Scale (ADDBRS)
Attention Deficit Disorder Comprehensive Teacher Rating Scale
Attention Deficit Disorder Evaluation Scale Secondary-Age Student
Attention Deficit Disorder Evaluation Scale, Second Edition
Attention Deficit Disorders Evaluation Scale (ADDES)
Attention Deficit Scales for Adults
Attention-Deficit/Hyperactivity Disorder Test
Attentional and Interpersonal Style Inventory, The
Attitude Inventory
Attitude Survey Program for Business and Industry
Attitude Toward School Questionnaire (ASQ)

Attitudes Toward Disabled Persons (ATDP)
Attitudes Toward Mainstreaming Scale
Attitude Toward Psychiatry Scale
Attitude Toward Serious Mental Illness Scale -Adolescent Version (ATSMI-AV)
Attitudes Toward Working Mothers Scale
Attributional Style Questionnaire
Atypical Depression Index (ADI)
Auditory Apperception Test (AAT)
Auditory Continuous Performance Test
Auditory Discrimination and Attention Test
Auditory Discrimination Test (ADT)
Auditory Selective Attention Test
Autism Behavior Checklist
Autism Diagnostic Interview (ADI)
Autism Diagnostic Interview-Revised
Autism Diagnostic Observation Schedule (ADOS)
Autism Screening Instrument for Educational Planning
Autism Screening Instrument for Educational Planning, Second Edition
Autistic Behavior Composite Checklist and Profile
Autobiographical Memory Test
Azima Battery
Automated Child/Adolescent Social History
Automated MultiTest Laboratory (AML)
Automated Neuropsychological Assessment Metric Battery (ANAM)
Automated Office Battery (AOB)
Bader Reading and Language Inventory
Balanced Emotional Empathy Scale
Ball Aptitude Battery (BAB)
Balthazar Scales for Adaptive Behavior I: Scales of Functional Independence
Balthazar Scales for Adaptive Behavior II: Scales of Social Adaptation
Balthazar Scales of Adaptive Behavior (BSAB)
Bangs Receptive Vocabulary Checklist
Bankson Language Screening Test (BLST)
Bankson Language Test-2 (BLT-2)
Bankson-Bernthal Test of Phonology (BBTOP)
Barber Scales of Self-Regard for Preschool Children
Barbizet and Cany 7/24 Spatial Recall Test
Barclay Classroom Assessment System
Barclay Classroom Climate Inventory (BCCI)
Barclay Early Childhood Skill Assessment Guide
Barclay Learning Needs Assessment Inventory (BLNAI)
Barnes Akathisia Rating Scale (BARS)
BarOn Emotional Quotient Inventory
Barranquilla Rapid Survey Intelligence Test (BRSIT)
Barratt Scale
Barron-Welsh Art Scale (BWAS)
Basic Achievement Skills Individual Screener
Basic Concept Inventory
Basic Educational Skills Test
Basic English Skills Test (BEST)
Basic Inventory of Natural Language
Basic Language Concepts Test
Basic Living Skills Scale
Basic Number Diagnostic Test
Basic Occupational Literacy Test (BOLT)
Basic Personality Inventory (BPI)

Basic Reading Inventory (BRI)
Basic Reading Inventory, Seventh Edition
Basic School Skills Inventory - Diagnostic
Basic School Skills Inventory (BSSI)
Basic School Skills Inventory Battery Test
Basic School Skills Inventory Screen
Basic Skills Assessment Program
Basic Skills Inventory
Basic Visual-Motor Association Test
BASIS-A Inventory
Battelle Developmental Inventory (BDI)
Battelle Developmental Inventory Screening Test
Battery for Health Improvement (BHI)
Bauer Self-Rated Internal State Scale
Bay Area Functional Performance Evaluation
Bay Area Functional Performance Evaluation, Second Edition
Baycrest NeuroCognitive Assessment (BNA)
Bayley II Developmental Assessment
Bayley Scale of Infant Development (BSID)
Bear-Fedio Inventory (BFI)
Bech-Rafaelsen Mania Rating Scale
Beck Anxiety Inventory
Beck Anxiety Inventory, 1993 Edition
Beck Depression Inventory (BDI)
Beck Depression Inventory, 1993 Revised
Beck Depression Inventory-II
Beck Depression Scale
Beck Hopelessness Scale (BHS)
Beck Hopelessness Scale-Revised
Beck Scale for Suicide Ideation
Beck Suicide Intent Scale
Beck Suicide Lethality Scale
Becker Work Adjustment Profile
Bedford Life Events and Difficulties Scale
Bedside Evaluation and Screening Test of Aphasia
Beery Picture Vocabulary Screening (PVS)
Beery Test of Visual Motor Integration
Beery Visual Motor Test
Beery-Buktinica Developmental Test
Beery-Buktinica Developmental Test of Visual Motor Integration
BEHAVE-AD Rating Scale
Behavior Activity Profile (BAP)
Behavior Assessment Battery
Behavior Assessment System for Children
Behavior Assessment System for Children-Revised
Behavior Change Inventory
Behavior Checklist
Behavior Dimensions Scale
Behavior Disorders Identification Scale (BDIS)
Behavior Evaluation Scale
Behavior Evaluation Scale-2 (BES-2)
Behavior Inventory
Behavior Pathology in Alzheimer Disease Rating Scale (BEHAVE-AD)
Behavior Problem Checklist (BPC)
Behavior Rating Profile, Second Edition (BRP-2)
Behavior Rating Scale
Behavior Status Inventory (BSI)
Behavior Style Questionnaire (BSQ)
Behavioral Academic Self-Esteem Scale
Behavioral and Emotional Rating Scale: A Strength-Based Approach to Assessment
Behavioral Assessment of Pain Questionnaire
Behavioral Assessment Test

Behavioral Inattention Test (BIT)
Behavioral Observation Scale for Autism
Behavioral Pathology in Alzheimer Disease Rating Scale
Behavioral Problems Scale
Behavioral Scale for Developmentally Deviant Preschoolers
Behavioural Assessment of the Dysexecutive Syndrome
Behn-Rorschach Test
Bekesy Functionality Detection Test (BFDT)
Belbin Team Roles Self-Perception Inventory
Bell Object Relations and Reality Testing Inventory
Bellevue Index of Depression
Bem Sex Role Inventory (BSRI)
Bender Visual Retention Test
Bender Visual-Motor Gestalt Test (BVMGT)
Bender-Gestalt Test (BGT)
Bender-Gestalt Visual-Motor Test
Bennett Mechanical Comprehension Test
Benton Controlled Oral Word Association
Benton Facial Recognition Test
Benton Judgment Of Line Orientation
Benton Line Orientation Test
Benton Revised Visual Retention Test (BVRT)
Benton Test Of 3-Dimensional Constructional Praxis
Benton Visual Retention Test (BVRT)
Bernreuter Personality Inventory
Berry Visual-Motor Integration Test
Bessell Measurement of Emotional Maturity Scales
Bilingual Home Inventory
Bilingual Syntax Measure II Test (BSM)
Bilingual Verbal Ability Tests
Bingham Button Test (BBT)
Biographical and Personality Inventory, Series II
Biographical Inventory Form U
Bipolar Psychological Inventory (BPI)
Birth-to-Three Developmental Scale
Birth-to-Three Assessment and Intervention System
Black Intelligence Test of Culture Homogeneity (BITCH)
Blessed Behavior Scale
Blessed Dementia Rating Scale (BDRS)
Blessed Information and Concentration Test
Blessed Information-Memory-Concentration Test (BIMC)
Blessed Orientation-Memory-Concentration Test
Blind Learning Aptitude Test
Block Design Subtest
Bloom Analogies Test
Bloom Sentence Completion Test
Bloomer Learning Test
Boder Test of Reading-Spelling Patterns
Body Dysmorphic Disorder Examination-Self Report (BDDE-SR)
Body Dysmorphic Disorder Questionnaire-Dermatology Version (BDDQ-DV)
Body Image and Eating Questionnaire
Body Sensations Questionnaire (BSQ)
Body Shape Questionnaire
Boehm Test of Basic Concepts
Boehm Test of Basic Concepts-Revised
Bolam Test
Bolgar-Fischer Word Test
Bonn Scale for Assessment of Basic Symptoms (BSABS)
Booker Profiles in Mathematics: Numeration and Computation
Booklet Category Test, Second Edition

Boston Assessment of Severe Aphasia (BASA)
Boston Diagnostic Aphasia Examination (BDAE)
Boston Diagnostic Aphasia Examination-Revised (BDAE-R)
Boston Revision of the Wechsler Memory Scale—Mental Control Subtest
Boston Naming Test (BNT)
Botel Reading Inventory
Bracken Basic Concept Scale
Bracken Basic Concept Scale-Revised
Braille Assessment Inventory
Brazelton Neonatal Behavioral Assessment Scale
Bricklin Perceptual Scales
Brief Alcoholism Screening Test
Brief Aphasia Screening Examination (BASE)
Brief Cognitive Rating Scale (BCRS)
Brief Cognitive Test Battery
Brief Disability Questionnaire
Brief Drinker Profile
Brief Impairment Scale (BIS)
Brief Life History Inventory (BLHI)
Brief Neuropsychological Cognitive Examination
Brief Neuropsychological Mental Status Examination (BNMSE)
Brief Outpatient Psychopathology Scale
Brief Pain Inventory
Brief Psychiatric Rating Scale (BPRS)
Brief Psychiatric Rating Scale-Expanded (BPRS-E)
Brief Psychiatric Reacting Scale (BPRS)
Brief Psychiatric Rating Scale for Children (BPRS-C)
Brief Screening Tool and Problem List
Brief Symptom Inventory (BSI)
Brief Test of Attention (BTA)
Brief Test of Head Injury
Brief Visuospatial Memory Test (BVMT)
Brigance Diagnostic Comprehensive Inventory of Basic Skills
Brigance Diagnostic Comprehensive Inventory of Basic Skills-Revised
Brigance Diagnostic Employability Skills Inventory
Brigance Diagnostic Inventory of Basic Skills
Brigance Diagnostic Inventory of Early Development
Brigance Diagnostic Inventory of Essential Skills
Brigance Diagnostic Life Skills Inventory
Brigance Early Preschool Screen for Two-Year-Old and Two-and-a-Half-Year-Old Children
Brigance K & 1 Screen for Kindergarten and First-Grade Children
Brigance Screen
Bristol Achievement Tests
Bristol Language Development Scale (BLADES)
Bristol Social Adjustment Guides
British Ability Scale (BAS)
British Ability Scales: Spelling Scale
Brook Reaction Test (BRT)
Brown and Harris Life Event and Difficulty Schedule
Brown Assessment of Beliefs Scale (BABS)
Brown Attention Deficit Disorder Scale
Brown-Goodwin Scale
Brown-Peterson Distraction Test
Bruininks-Oseretsky Standardized Test
Bruininks-Oseretsky Test
Bruininks-Oseretsky Test of Motor Proficiency
Brunet-Lezine Test
Bryant-Schwan Design Test (BSDT)

Bulimia Test-Revised (BULIT-R)
Bulimic Investigatory Test, Edinburgh (BITE)
Bunney-Hamburg Rating Scale
Burden Interview
Burks Behavior Rating Scale (BBRS)
Burns Brief Inventory of Communication and Cognition
Burns-Roe Informal Reading Inventory
Buschke Selective Reminding Test
Buschke Short-Term Recall Test
Buss-Durkee Hostility Inventory
Buss-Perry Aggression Questionnaire (BPAQ)
Buswell-John Diagnostic Test for Fundamental Processes in Arithmetic
Butcher Treatment Planning Inventory
Bzoch-League Receptive-Expressive Emergent Language Scale
CAGE Alcohol Use Questionnaire
Cain-Levine Social Competency Scale
Calendar of Premenstrual Experiences (COPE)
Calev Recognition/Recall Test
Calgary Depression Scale for Schizophrenia
California Child Q-Set (Q-Set)
California Computerized Assessment Package
California Critical Thinking Dispositions Inventory (CCTDI)
California Critical Thinking Skills Test (CCTST)
California Diagnostic Mathematics Test
California Diagnostic Reading Test
California F Scale
California Infant Scale for Motor Development (CISMD)
California Life Goals Evaluation Schedule
California Motor Accuracy Test, Southern Revised
California Personality Inventory (CPI)
California Preschool Social Competency Scale (CPSCS)
California Psychological Inventory Test (CPIT)
California Psychological Inventory-Revised (CPIT-R)
California Psychotherapy Alliance Scale-Patient Version
California Q-Sort (Q-Sort)
California Short-Form Test of Mental Maturity (CTMM-SF)
California Test of Basic Skills (CTBS)
California Test of Mental Maturity (CTMM)
California Test of Mental Maturity, Short Form
California Test of Personality (CTP)
California Verbal Learning Test
California Verbal Learning Test II (CVLT-II)
California Verbal Learning Test, Research Edition, Adult Version
California Verbal Learning Test for Children
California Word Context Test
Callier-Azusa Scale
Camberwell Family Interview (CFI)
Cambridge Mental Disorders in Elderly Examination
Cambridge Neuropsychological Test Automated Battery (CANTAB)
Cambridge Test Battery
Camelot Behavioral Checklist (CBC)
Campbell Leadership Index (CLI)
Canadian Achievement Survey Tests for Adults
Canadian Achievement Tests, Second Edition
Canadian Cognitive Abilities Test (CCAT)
Canadian Cognitive Abilities Test, Form 7
Canadian Occupational Interest Inventory

Canadian Test of Basic Skills, Forms 7 and 8
Canadian Test of Cognitive Skills
Canadian Tests of Basic Skills (CTBS)
Candidate Profile Record
Canfield Instructional Styles Inventory
Canfield Learning Styles Inventory
Canter Background Interference Procedure for the Bender Gestalt Test
Career Anchors: Discovering Your Real Values-Revised Edition
Career Assessment Inventories for the Learning Disabled
Career Assessment Inventory (CAI)
Career Assessment Inventory, The Enhanced Version
Career Attitudes and Strategies Inventory: An Inventory for Understanding Adult Careers
Career Beliefs Inventory (CBI)
Career Decision Scale
Career Decision-Making Self-Efficacy Scale
Career Development Inventory
Career Directions Inventory
Career Exploration Inventory
Career Factors Inventory
Career Guidance Inventory
Career Interest Inventory
Career Interest Test
Career IQ Test
Career Problem Check List
Career Profile System, Second Edition
Career Thoughts Inventory
Caregiver Strain Index
Caregiver-Teacher Report Form
Carey Temperament Scales
Caring Relationship Inventory (CRI)
Carnegie Interest Inventory (CII)
Carrell Discrimination Test
Carroll Depression Scale (CDS)
Carroll Rating Scale for Depression
Carrow Auditory-Visual Abilities Test
Carrow Elicited Language Inventory (CELI)
Carrow Receptive Language Test
CAT/5 Listening and Speaking Checklist
Category Test (CT)
Category Verbal Fluency Test
Cattell Infant Scale
Cattell Infant Intelligence Scale
Cattell Infant Scale for Intelligence (CISI)
Cattell Infant Scale Inventory (CISI)
Cattell Personality Factor Questionnaire
Cayuga-Onondaga Assessment for Children with Handicaps, Version 7.0 (COACH)
Center for Epidemiologic Studies-Depression Scale (CES-D Scale)
CERAD Assessment Battery
CES-D Scale
CGI Scale
Change Agent Questionnaire (CAQ)
Chart of Initiative and Independence
Charteris Reading Test
Checklist for Autism in Toddlers
Checklist for Child Abuse Evaluation (CCAE)
Checklist of Adaptive Living Skills (CALS)
Chen Internet Addiction Scale (CIAS)
Chestnut Lodge Prognostic Scale for Chronic Schizophrenia
Chicago Word Fluency Test
Child Abuse Inventory
Child Abuse Potential Inventory
Child and Adolescent Adjustment Profile
Child and Adolescent Psychiatric Assessment (CAPA)
Child Anxiety Scale
Child Assessment Schedule (CAS)
Child at Risk for Drug Abuse Rating Scale

Child Behavior Checklist (CBCL)
Child Care Inventory
Child Depression Inventory
Child Development Inventory
Child Dissociative Checklist (CDC)
Child Health Self-Concept Scale
Child Neuropsychological Questionnaire (CNQ)
Child Personality Scale (CPS)
Child Posttraumatic Stress Checklist
Child Posttraumatic Stress Reaction Index
Child Suicide Potential Scale
Child Sexual Behavior Inventory
Child Symptom Inventory-4 (CSI-4)
Childhood Antecedents Questionnaire
Childhood Autism Rating Scale (CARS)
Childhood Maltreatment History Self-Report
Childhood Trauma Questionnaire
Children of Alcoholics Screening Test (CAST)
Children's Academic Intrinsic Motivation Inventory
Children's Adaptive Behavior Scale-Revised
Children's Affective Rating Scale (CARS)
Children's Apperception Test (CAT)
Children's Apperception Test-Human (CAT-H)
Children's Apperceptive Story-Telling Test (CAST)
Children's Articulation Test (CAT)
Children's Auditory Verbal Learning Test-2 (CAVLT-2)
Children's Depression Inventory (CDI)
Children's Depression Rating Scale-Revised (CDRS-R)
Children's Depression Scale (CDS)
Children's Diagnostic Inventory (CDI)
Children's Embedded Figures Test (CEFT)
Children's Exposure to Violence Checklist
Children's Global Assessment Scale (CGAS)
Children's Hypnotic Susceptibility Scale
Children's Inventory of Self-Esteem (CISE)
Children's Language Battery
Children's Manifest Anxiety Scale (CMAS)
Children's Memory Scale (CMS)
Children's Orientation and Amnesia Test (COAT)
Children's Perception of Support Inventory (CPSI)
Children's Perception of Interparental Conflict Scale
Children's Personality Questionnaire (CPQ)
Children's Problems Checklist
Children's Psychiatric Rating Scale (CPRS)
Children's Role Inventory
Children's Self-Concept Scale (CSCS)
Children's Version of the Family Environment Scale
Children's Yale-Brown Obsessive Compulsive Scale (CY-BOCS)
Chinese Polarity Inventory
Christensen Dietary Distress Inventory
CID Phonetic Inventory
CID Preschool Performance Scale
Claridge Schizotypal Personality Scale
Clarke Reading Self-Assessment Survey
Clark-Madison Test of Oral Language
Classroom Atmosphere Questionnaire (CAQ)

Classroom Communication Skills Inventory: Listening and Speaking Checklist
Classroom Environment Index
Classroom Environment Scale, Second Edition
Classroom Environmental Scale (CES)
Classroom Reading Inventory, Seventh Edition
Claybury Selection Battery
Clerical Speed and Accuracy Test
Clifton Assessment Procedures for the Elderly
Clinical Adaptive Test
Clinical Analysis Questionnaire (CAQ)
Clinical Dementia Rating Scale
Clinical Evaluation of Language Fundamentals, 3 Screening Test
Clinical Evaluation of Language Fundamentals, Preschool
Clinical Evaluation of Language Fundamentals, Third Edition
Clinical Evaluation of Language Fundamentals-Revised
Clinical Global Impression-Bipolar (CGI-BP)
Clinical Global Impression of Change (CGIC)
Clinical Global Impression-Improvement
Clinical Global Impressions (CGI)
Clinical Global Impressions Scale
Clinical Global Impressions-Improved (CGI-I)
Clinical Global Improvement (CGI)
Clinical Linguistic Auditory Milestone Scale
Clinical Rating of Drinking Scale (CRDS)
Clinical Rating Scale (CRS)
Clinical Support System Battery
Clinician Global Rating Scale
Clinician Rated Anxiety Scale (CRAS)
Clinician Rated Overall Life Impairment Scale
Clinician-Administered PTSD Scale (CAPS)
Clinician's Global Rating Scale (CGRS)
Clinician's Interview-Based Impression of Change (CIBIC)
Clock Drawing Test, The (CDT)
Cloninger Harm Avoidance Scale
Close Persons Questionnaire (CPQ)
Closed Head Injury Screener
Closed High School Placement Test
Cloze Reading Tests
Clyde Mood Scale (CMS)
Clymer-Barrett Readiness Test
Clymer-Barrett Readiness Test-Revised
Coaching Process Questionnaire
Cocaine Selective Severity Assessment (CSSA)
Code Substitution-Accuracy (CDSACC)
Code Substitution-Efficiency (CDSEFF)
Code Substitution-Immediate Recall-Accuracy (CDSIACC)
Cognistat (The NeuroBehavioral Cognitive Status Examination)
Cognitive Abilities Scale
Cognitive Abilities Test (CAT)
Cognitive Abilities Test, Form 5
Cognitive Assessment Screening Test (CAST)
Cognitive Behavior Rating Scales
Cognitive Capacity Screening Examination (CCSE)
Cognitive Control Battery
Cognitive Diagnostic Battery
Cognitive Laterality Quotient (CLQ)
Cognitive Observation Guide (COG)
Cognitive Performance Test
Cognitive Process Profile
Cognitive Skills Assessment (CSA)
Cognitive Skills Assessment Battery

Cognitive Skills Assessment Battery, Second Edition
Cognitive Symptom Checklists
CogScreen Aeromedical Edition
Cohen-Mansfield Agitation Inventory (CMAI)
Collaborative Study Psychotherapy Rating Scale
College Ability Test (CAT)
College Adjustment Scales
College and University Environment Scales (CUES)
College Characteristics Index (CCI)
College Student Experiences Questionnaire
College Student Questionnaire (CSQ)
College Student Satisfaction Questionnaire (CSSQ)
Collis-Romberg Mathematical Problem Solving Profile
Colorado Educational Interest Battery
Colored Progressive Matrices
Columbia Atypical Depression Diagnostic Scale (CADD)
Columbia Impairment Scale
Columbia Mental Maturity Scale (CMMS)
Columbia Suicide History Form
Combat Exposure Scale (CES)
Common-Metric Questionnaire, The
Communication Abilities Diagnostic Test (CADT)
Communication Activities of Daily Living (CADL)
Communication and Symbolic Behavior Scales
Communication Knowledge Inventory
Communication Profile: A Functional Skills Survey
Communication Response Style: Assessment
Communication Sensitivity Inventory
Communication Skills Profile
Communications Profile Questionnaire
Community College Goals Inventory
Community College Student Experiences Questionnaire
Community College Student Experiences Questionnaire, Second Edition
Community Functioning Scale
Completion, Arithmetic, Vocabulary, and Directions Test
Complex Figure Test (CFT)
Composite International Diagnostic Interview (CIDI)
Composite International Diagnostic Interview-Substance Abuse Module (CIDI-SAM)
Composite Psycholinguistic Age
Composite Risk Index (CRI)
Comprehension of Oral Language
Comprehensive Ability Battery (CAB)
Comprehensive Adult Student Assessment System
Comprehensive Assessment of School Environment
Comprehensive Assessment of Symptoms and History (CASH)
Comprehensive Assessment Program: Achievement Series
Comprehensive Behavior Rating Scale for Children
Comprehensive Career Assessment Scale (CCAS)
Comprehensive Developmental Evaluation Chart
Comprehensive Drinker Profile
Comprehensive Personality Profile
Comprehensive Psychiatric Rating Scale (CPRS)Comprehensive Psychopathological Rating Scale
Comprehensive Qualifying Examination
Comprehensive Receptive and Expressive Vocabulary Test

Comprehensive Scales of Student Abilities: Quantifying Academic Skills and School-Related Behavior Through the Use of Teacher Judgments
Comprehensive Screening Tool for Determining Optimal Communication Mode
Comprehensive Test of Adaptive Behavior
Comprehensive Test of Basic Skills, Forms U and V
Comprehensive Test of Nonverbal Intelligence (CTONI)
Comprehensive Test Of Phonological Processing (CTOPP)
Comprehensive Test of Visual Functioning (CTVF)
Comprehensive Testing Program III
Comprehensive Tests of Basic Skills, Fourth Edition
Compulsive Sexual Disorders Interview
Computer Anxiety Index
Computer Literacy and Computer Science Tests
Computer Programmer Aptitude Battery (CPAB)
Comrey Personality Scale (CPS)
Concentration Performance Test (CPT)
Concept Mastery Test (CMT)
Concept-Specific Anxiety Scale (CAS)
Conceptual Systems Test (CST)
Conflict in Marriage Scale (CIMS)
Conflict Resolution Inventory
Conflict Style Inventory
Conflict Tactics Scale (CTS)
Conners Abbreviated Symptom Questionnaire
Conners Continuous Performance Test
Conners Hyperkinesis Index, Parent Form
Conners Hyperkinesis Index, Teacher Form
Conners Parent and Teacher Symptom Questionnaire
Conners Parent Questionnaire (CPQ)
Conners Parent Rating Scale
Conners Parent-Teacher Rating Scale
Conners Preliminary Parent Report
Conners Rating Scale
Conners Rating Scale-Revised
Conners Teacher Preliminary School Report
Conners Teacher Questionnaire (CTQ)
Conners Teacher Rating Scale (CTRS-28)
Consumer Experience of Stigma Questionnaire (CESQ)
Contextual Memory Test
Continuous Performance Test (CPT)
Continuous Performance Test-Identical Pairs Version
Continuous Visual Memory Test (CVMT)
Continuous Visual Memory Test-Revised
Controlled Oral Word Association Test (COWA)
Controlled Word Association Test
Conversational Skills Rating Scale, The
Cook-Medley Hostility Scale (CMHS)
Coolidge Axis II Inventory
Coolidge Personality and Neuropsychology Inventory for Children
Cooper Assessment for Stuttering Syndromes
Cooperative Primary Test (CPT)
Cooper-Farran Behavioral Rating Scale (CFBRS)
Cooper-MacGuire Diagnostic Word Analysis Test

Coopersmith Self-Esteem Inventories
Coping Inventory for Stressful Situations
Coping Orientations to Problems Experienced (COPE)
Coping Resources Inventory (CRI)
Coping Resources Inventory for Stress
Coping with Stress Test
COPSystem Interest Inventory
Corder-Haizlip Child Suicide Checklist
Cornell Critical Thinking Tests
Cornell Critical Thinking Tests, Level X and Level Z
Cornell Depression Scale
Cornell Dysthymia Rating Scale
Cornell Learning and Study Skills Inventory (CLASSI)
Cornell Medical Index (CMI)
Cornell Scale for Depression in Dementia
Cornell Word Form (CWF)
Correctional Institutions Environment Scale (CIES)
Correctional Institutions Environment Scale, Second Edition
Correctional Officers' Interest Blank
Couples Pre-Counseling Inventory
Couples Pre-Counseling Inventory-Revised Edition
Courtship Analysis
Covi Anxiety Scale
Cowboy Story Test
Craving Analog Scale
Creative Behavior Inventory
Creative Reasoning Test, The
Creative Styles Inventory
Creativity Assessment Packet
Creativity Checklist
Creativity Tests for Children (CTC)
Criterion Test of Basic Skills
Critical Reasoning Tests (CRT)
Croft Readiness Assessment in Comprehension Kit
Cross-Cultural Adaptability Inventory
Crowley Occupational Interests Blank (COIB)
Crown-Crisp Experiential Index
Cues Checklist (CCL)
Cultural Attitude Inventory (CAI)
Cultural Attitude Scale (CAS)
Cultural Inventory
Cultural Literacy Test
Culture Fair Intelligence Test
Culture Shock Inventory
Culture-Free Intelligence Test (CFIT)
Culture-Free Self-Esteem Inventories for Children and Adults
Culture-Free Test
Cumulative Illness Rating Scale
Cumulative Illness Rating Scale-Geriatric (CIRS-G)
Current and Past Psychopathology Scale (CAPPS)
Curtis Completion Form
Curtis Interest Scale
Cybersex Addition List
D/ART Campaign
DABERON-2: Screening for School Readiness (DABERON-2)
Daily Rating Form (DRF)
Daily Rating Scale
Daily Stress Inventory
Dallas Pre-School Screening Test
Dartmouth Assessment of Lifestyle Instrument (DALI)
Das-Naglieri Cognitive Assessment System
Dating Problems Checklist
Davidson Trauma Scale (DTS)
Death Anxiety Scale (DAS)
Death Personification Exercise (DPE)
Decision Making Inventory
Decoding Skills Test
Deductive Reasoning Test
Defense Mechanism Inventory (DMI)
Defense Mechanism Inventory-Revised

Defense Style Questionnaire
Defense Style Questionnaire-40 (DSQ-40)
Defensive Functioning Scale (DFS)
Defining Issues Test
DeGangi-Berk Test of Sensory Integration
Delirium Observation Screening Scale (DOSS)
Delirium Rating Scale (DRS)
Delis-Kaplan Executive Function Scale (DKEFS)
Del Rio Language Screening Test (DRLST)
DeLong Interest Inventory
Dementia Behavior Disturbance Scale
Dementia Mood Assessment Scale (DMAS)
Dementia Rating Scale (DRS)
Dementia Psychosis Scale
Demographic Psychosocial Inventory (DPSI)
Dennis Test of Child Development (DCD)
Denver Articulation Screening Evaluation (DASE)
Denver Articulation Screening Test II
Denver Community Mental Health Questionnaire-Revised
Denver Developmental Screening Test (DDST)
Denver II Test
Depression Adjective Checklist (DACL)
Depression and Anxiety in Youth Scale
Depression Anxiety Stress Scale (DASS)
Depression Inventory
Depression Questionnaire
Depression Questionnaire for Children (DQC)
Depression Rating Scale
Depression Status Inventory (DSI)
Depressive Experiences Questionnaire (DEQ)
Derogatis Affects Balance Scale-Revised
Derogatis Psychiatric Rating Scale
Derogatis Sexual Functioning Inventory
Derogatis Stress Profile
Description of Body Scale
Description Questionnaire
Descriptive Tests of Language Skills
Descriptive Tests of Mathematics Skills
Desert Storm Trauma Questionnaire
Design Fluency Test
Design Judgment Test
Desire for Death Rating Scale
Detroit Test of Learning Aptitude-Primary, Second Edition (DTLA-P:2)
Detroit Test of Learning Aptitude (DTLA)
Detroit Test of Learning Aptitude, Fourth Edition (DTLA-4)
Detroit Test of Learning Aptitude, Third Edition (DTLA-3)
Detroit Test of Learning Aptitude-Adult (DTLA-A)
Developing Cognitive Abilities Test, Second Edition
Developing Skills Checklist (DSC)
Development Inventory
Development Questionnaire
Developmental Activities Screening Inventory (DASI)
Developmental Articulation Test (DAT)
Developmental Assessment of Life Experiences (DALE)
Developmental Assessment of Life Experiences, 2000 Edition
Developmental Assessment of the Severely Handicapped
Developmental Assessment of Young Children
Developmental Behavior Checklist (DBC)

Developmental Hand-Function Test (DHFT)
Developmental Indicators for Assessment of Learning (DIAL)
Developmental Indicators for Assessment of Learning-Revised/AGS Edition (DIAL-R)
Developmental Indicators for Assessment of Learning, Third Edition
Developmental Observation Checklist System
Developmental Profile II
Developmental Sentence Analysis
Developmental Sentence Scoring Test
Developmental Test of Visual Motor Integration (DVMI)
Developmental Test of Visual Perception (DTVP)
Developmental Test of Visual Perception, Second Edition (DTVP-2)
Developmental Test of Visual-Motor Integration, Fourth Edition-Revised
Developmental Test of Visual-Motor Integration, Third Edition
Devereux Adolescent Behavior Rating Scale
Devereux Behavior Rating Scale-School Form
Devereux Elementary School Behavior Rating Scale II (DESBRS-II)
Devereux Scales of Mental Disorders
Devine Inventory, The
Diagnostic Achievement Battery, Second Edition (DAB-2)
Diagnostic Achievement Test for Adolescents
Diagnostic Achievement Test for Adolescents, Second Edition
Diagnostic Achievement Test in Spelling
Diagnostic and Statistical Manual of Mental Disorders (DSM)
Diagnostic and Statistical Manual of Mental Disorders-4th Edition (DSM-IV)
Diagnostic and Therapeutic Technology Assessment (DATTA)
Diagnostic Assessment of Reading (DAR)
Diagnostic Checklist for Behavior-Disturbed Children Form E-2
Diagnostic Employability Profile
Diagnostic Interview for Borderline Patients
Diagnostic Interview for Borderlines (DIB)
Diagnostic Interview for Children and Adolescents
Diagnostic Interview for Children and Adolescents-Computer Version (DICA-IV)
Diagnostic Interview for Children and Adolescents-Child Version (DICA-C)
Diagnostic Interview for Children and Adolescents-Parent Version (DICA-P)
Diagnostic Interview for Children and Adolescents-Revised (DICA-R)
Diagnostic Interview for Genetic Studies (DIGS)
Diagnostic Interview Schedule (DIS)
Diagnostic Interview Schedule for Children (DISC)
Diagnostic Interview For Children And Adolescents (DICA)
Diagnostic Interview Schedule III
Diagnostic Inventory for Screening Children

Diagnostic Mathematics Inventory (DMI)
Diagnostic Mathematics Profiles
Diagnostic Questions for Early or Advanced Alcoholism
Diagnostic Screening Batteries, The
Diagnostic Skills Battery
Diagnostic Spelling Potential Test
Diagnostic Symptom Questionnaire
Diagnostic Test of Arithmetic Strategies
Diagnostic Tests and Self-Helps in Arithmetic
Differential Ability Scales (DAS)
Differential Aptitude Tests (DAT)
Differential Aptitude Tests for Personnel and Career Assessment
Differential Aptitude Tests-Computerized Adaptive Edition
Differential Aptitude Tests, Fourth Edition
Differential Aptitude Tests, Fifth Edition
Differential Test of Conduct and Emotional Problems (DT/CEP)
Digit Span Backward
Digit Span Distractibility Test
Digit Span Subtest
Digit Symbol Substitution Test (DSST)
Digit Vigilance Test
Digital Finger Tapping Test (DFTT)
Dimensional Assessment of Personality Pathology-Basic Questionnaire (DAPP-BQ)
Dimensions of Delusional Experience Scale
Dimensions of Excellence Scales, 1991 Edition
Direct Assessment of Functional Status Scale
Disability Assessment in Dementia Scale
Discourse Comprehension Test
Disinhibition Scale
Disruptive Behavior Disorder Rating Scale
Dissociation Content Scale
Dissociative Disorders Interview Scale
Dissociative Disorders Interview Schedule (DDIS)
Dissociative Experience Scale (DES)
Diversity Awareness Profile (DAP)
Dodd Test of Time Estimation
Dole Vocational Sentence Completion Blank
Domestic Violence Inventory
Dos Amigos Verbal Language Scales
Draw A Person: Screening Procedure for Emotional Disturbance (DAP:SPED)
Draw-A-Bicycle Test
Draw-A-Clock-Face Test
Draw-A-Family Test
Draw-A-Flower Test
Draw-A-House Test
Draw-A-Man Test
Draw-A-Person Test
Draw-A-Picture-From-Memory Test
Driver Risk Inventory (DRI)
Drug Abuse Screening Test (DAST)
Drug Attitude Inventory
Drug Use Screening Inventory (DUSI)
Drug Use Questionnaire
Drug-Taking Confidence Questionnaire
Drumcondra Verbal Reasoning Test 1
Duke Religion Index
Duke Severity of Illness Scale
Durrell Analysis of Reading Difficulty, Third Edition
Dutch Personality Questionnaire (DPQ)
Durham Test
Dyadic Adjustment Scale
Dynamic Personality Inventory (DPI)
Dysfunctional Attitudes Scale (DAS)
Dysfunctional Attitudes and Beliefs About Sleep Questionnaire
Dyslexia Determination Test

Dyslexia Screening Instrument
Dysphagia Evaluation Protocol
Early Child Development Inventory
Early Childhood Attention Deficit Disorders Evaluation Scale
Early Childhood Behavior Scale, The
Early Childhood Environment Rating Scale
Early Childhood Environment Rating Scale-Revised Edition
Early Childhood Physical Environment Observation Schedules and Rating Scales
Early Coping Inventory
Early Development Scale for Preschool Children
Early Intervention Developmental Profile
Early Language Milestone Scale
Early Language Milestone Scale, Second Edition
Early Language: Assessment and Development
Early Mathematics Diagnostic Kit
Early School Assessment (ESA)
Early School Inventory
Early School Personality Questionnaire (ESPQ)
Early Screening Inventory
Early Screening Inventory-Revised
Early Social Communication Scale (ESCS)
Early Speech Perception Test (ESP)
Eating Attitudes Test (EAT)
Eating Disorder Evaluation Scale (EDES)
Eating Disorder Inventory (EDI)
Eating Disorder Inventory for Children
Eating Disorder Inventory, Second Edition (EDI-2)
Eating Disorders Examination (EDE)
Eating Inventory (EI)
Ebbinghaus Curve of Retention Test
Ebbinghaus Test
Eby Elementary Identification Instrument
Eby Gifted Behavior Index
Edinburgh Articulation Test (EAT)
Edinburgh Handedness Inventory
Edinburgh Inventory
Edinburgh Picture Test
Edinburgh Postnatal Depression Scale (EPDS)
Edinburgh Reading Tests
Edinburgh Rehabilitation Status Scale
Education Apperception Test (EAT)
Educational Administrator Effectiveness Profile
Educational Development Series, 1992 Edition
Educational Interest Inventory
Educational Leadership Practices Inventory
Educational Process Questionnaire
Educational Testing Service (ETS)
Edwards Personal Preference Schedule (EPPS)
Effective Reading Test
Effective School Battery, The (ESB)
Egan Bus Puzzle Test, The
Ego Development Scale (EDS)
Ego Function Assessment
Ego State Inventory (ESI)
Ego Strength Test
Egocentricity Index
Ego-Ideal and Conscience Development Test (EICDT)
Eidetic Parents Test (EPT)
Eight State Questionnaire
Einstein Assessment of School-Related Skills
Ekwall/Shanker Reading Inventory, Third Edition
El Senoussi Multiphasic Marital Inventory
Elicited Articulatory System Evaluation

Elihorn Maze Test
Elizur Test of Psycho-Organicity: Children and Adults
Embedded Figures Test (EFT)
Emotional and Behavioral Problem Scale
Emotional and Behavioral Checklist
Emotional or Behavior Disorder Scale
Emotional Problems Scales
Emotions Profile Index
Employability Inventory, The
Employability Maturity Interview
Employee Assistance Program Inventory
Employee Attitude Inventory
Employee Effectiveness Profile
Employee Reliability Inventory (ERI)
Employment Screening Test and Standardization Manual
Employment Values Inventory
Empowerment Inventory
Endicott Work Productivity Scale
Endler Multidimensional Anxiety Scale (EMAS)
Engineering and Physical Science Aptitude Test
English as a Second Language Oral Assessment-Revised
English Language Skills Assessment in a Reading Context
English Skills Assessment
Enhanced ACT Assessment
Ennis-Weir Critical Thinking Essay Test
Entrepreneurial Style and Success Indicator
Environment Scale
Environmental Inventory
Environmental Language Inventory (ELI)
Environmental Pre-Language Battery
Environmental Response Inventory (ERI)
Epworth Sleepiness Scale
ERB Writing Assessment
Erhardt Developmental Prehension Assessment (EDPA)
Erhardt Developmental Vision Assessment (EDVA)
ETS Tests of Applied Literacy Skills
EuroQol Visual Analog Scale
Evaluating Movement and Posture Disorganization in Dyspraxic Children
Evaluation Disposition Environment
Evaluation of Basic Skills
Everyday Worries Scale
Examining for Aphasia Test
Executive Profile Survey
Expressive One-Word Picture Vocabulary Tests (EOWPVT)
Expressive One-Word Picture Vocabulary Tests-Revised (EOWPVT-R)
Expressive One-Word Picture Vocabulary Tests, Upper Extension
Expressive & Receptive One-Word Picture Vocabulary Tests, 2000 Edition
Expressive Vocabulary Test
Extended Merrill-Palmer Scale, The
Extended Personal Attributes Questionnaire (EPAQ)
Extrapyramidal Symptom Rating Scale
Eyberg Child Behavior Inventory (ECBI)
Eysenck Personality Inventory (EPI)
Eysenck Personality Questionnaire (EPQ)
Facial Interpersonal Perception Inventory, The
Facial Recognition Test
Fagerstrom Nicotine Addiction Scale
Fagerstrom Tolerance Questionnaire
Fairview Language Evaluation Test (FLET)

Family Adaptability and Cohesion Evaluation Scale III (FACES III)
Family Apperception Test (FAT)
Family Assessment Device (FAD)
Family Assessment Form: A Practice-Based Approach to Assessing Family Functioning
Family Assessment Measure Version III
Family Attitudes Questionnaire (FAQ)
Family Attitudes Test (FAT)
Family Drawing Depression Scale (FDDS)
Family Environment Scale (FES)
Family Environment Scale, Second Edition
Family Environment Scale, Third Edition Manual
Family Evaluation Form (FEF)
Family History Assessment Module
Family History Research Diagnostic Criteria (FH-RDC)
Family Inventory of Life Events and Changes (FILE)
Family Psychosocial Screening
Family Relations Test (FRT)
Family Relations Test: Children's Version
Family Relationship Inventory
Family Risk Scale
Family Satisfaction Scale
Famous Sayings Test
Famous Writers Aptitude Test
Fast Health Knowledge Test, 1986 Revision
Fatigue Questionnaire
Fazekas Scale
Fear Questionnaire (FQ)
Fear Questionnaire of Marks and Matthews
Fear Survey Schedule (FSS)
Feelings, Attitudes, and Behaviors Scale for Children
Fels Parent Behavior Rating Scale
Figurative Language Interpretation Test (FLIT)
Filipino Work Values Scale
Filtered Audiometer Speech Test (FAST)
Finckh Test
Finger Localization Test
Finger Oscillation Test
Firestone Assessment of Self-Destructive Thoughts
FIRO (Fundamental Interpersonal Relations Orientation) Awareness Scale
First Words and First Sentences Tests
FirstSTEP: Screening Test for Evaluating Preschoolers
Fischer Least Significant Difference Test
Fisher-Logemann Test of Articulation Competence (FLTAC)
Five Ps: Parent Professional Preschool Performance Profile, The
Five Ps: Parent Professional Preschool Performance Profile-Revised, The
Five-Minute Verbal Sampling Test
Fixity of Beliefs Scale
Flanagan Aptitude Classification Tests (FACT)
Flanagan Industrial Tests (FIT)
Flint Infant Security Scale (FISS)
Florida Kindergarten Screening Battery
Flowers Auditory Test of Selective Attention (FATSA)
Fluharty Preschool Speech and Language Screening Test
Follow-Up Drinker Profile
Folstein Mini-Mental Scale
Folstein Mini-Mental Status Examination (MMSE)
Food Choice Inventory
Forer Structured Sentence Completion Test
Forms for Behavior Analysis with Children

Four-Factor Index
Four Picture Test
Four Factor Theory of Etiology
Fournier Test
Franck Drawing Completion Test (FDCT)
Frankfurt Complaint Questionnaire (FCQ)
Freeman Anxiety Neurosis and Psychosomatic Test (FANPT)
Freiburg Personality Inventory (FPI)
Frenchay Activities Index
Frenchay Aphasia Screening Test (FAST)
Frenchay Dysarthria Assessment
Friedman Well-Being Scale
Frost Self-Description Questionnaire (FSDQ)
Frostig Developmental Test of Visual Perception (FDTVP)
Frostig Movement Skills Test Battery (FMSTB)
Fuld Object-Memory Test
Fuld Object-Memory Evaluation
Full Range Picture Vocabulary Test
Full Scale Broad Cognitive Ability
Fullerton Language Test for Adolescents, The
Fullerton Language Test for Adolescents, Second Edition
Full Scale Score Total (FSST)
Functional Activities Questionnaire
Functional Assessment Inventory
Functional Communication Profile (FCP)
Functional Fitness Assessment for Adults over 60 Years
Functional Life Scale (FLS)
Functional Limitation Profile
Functional Linguistic Communication Inventory
Functional Needs Assessment (FNA)
Functional Performance Record (FPR)
Functional Status Index (FSI)
Functional Status Questionnaire (FSQ)
Functional Systems Scale (FSS)
Functional Time Estimation Questionnaire (FTEQ)
Fundamental Achievement Series
Fundamental Interpersonal Relations Orientation-Behavior (FIRO-B)
Fundamental Interpersonal Relations Orientation-Feelings (FIRO-F)
Funkenstein Test
Galveston Orientation and Awareness Test (GOAT)
Gamblers Anonymous 20 Questions
Gambling Symptom Assessment Scale (G-SAS)
GAP Reading Comprehension Test, Third Edition
Gastrointestinal Symptom Rating Scale
Gates-MacGinitie Reading Tests
Gates-MacGinitie Reading Tests, Third Edition
Gates-McKillop-Horowitz Reading Diagnostic Test
Gates-McKillop-Horowitz Reading Diagnostic Test, Second Edition
General Ability Measure for Adults
General Aptitude Test Battery (GATB)
General Aptitude Test Battery, Canadian Edition
General Clerical Test (GCT)
General Cognitive Index (GCI)
General Health Questionnaire (GHQ)
General High Altitude Questionnaire (GHAQ)
General Processing Inventory
General Well-Being Index
Generalized Contentment Scale (GCS)
George Washington University Series
Geriatric Depression Scale (GDS)
Gerontological Apperception Test (GAT)

Gesell Child Development Age Scale, The (GCDAS)
Gesell Developmental Observation, The
Gesell Infant Scale
Gesell Preschool Test
Gesell School Readiness Test
Gibson Spiral Maze, Second Edition
Gifted and Talented Scale
Gifted and Talented Screening Form
Gifted Evaluation Scale (GES)
Gifted Evaluation Scale, Second Edition
Gifted Program Evaluation Survey, The
Gilliam Autism Rating Scale
Glasgow Coma Scale (GCS)
Glasgow Homeopathic Hospital Outcome Scale (GHHOS)
Global Aggression Score
Global Assessment of Functioning Scale (GAF)
Global Assessment of Relational Functioning Scale (GARF)
Global Assessment Scale (GAS)
Global Clinical Judgments Scale
Global Deterioration Scale
Global Obsessive-Compulsive Scale
Global Severity Index (GSI)
Global Sexual Satisfaction Index (GSSI)
Goal Attainment Scale (GAS)
Goldberg Index
Goldman-Fristoe Test of Articulation (G-FTA)
Goldman-Fristoe-Woodcock Auditory Skills Test Battery
Goldman-Fristoe-Woodcock Test
Goldscheider Test
Goldstein-Scheerer Cube Test, The
Goldstein-Scheerer Tests of Abstract and Concrete Thinking
Golombok Rust Inventory of Sexual Satisfaction
Golombok-Rust Inventory of Marital State (GRIMS)
Goodenough Animal Test
Goodenough Draw-A-Man Test
Goodenough Draw-A-Person Test
Goodenough-Harris Drawing Test
Goodenough Intelligence Test
Goodman Lock Box Test, The
Gordon Diagnostic System Test, The
Gordon Occupational Checklist-II (GOCL-II)
Gordon Personal Profile-Inventory (GPI)
Gottfries-Brane-Steen Rating Scale for Dementia
Gottschalk-Gelser Content Analysis Scales
Graded Naming Test
Graded Word Spelling Test
Graduate and Managerial Assessment
Graduate Record Examination Aptitude Test (GREAT)
Grandparent Strengths and Needs Inventory
Grassi Basic Cognitive Evaluation (GBCE)
Grassi Block Substitution Test
Gray Oral Reading Tests
Gray Oral Reading Tests, Third Edition (GORT-3)
Gray Oral Reading Tests-Diagnostic
Gregorc Style Delineator
Grid Test of Schizophrenic Thought Disorder (GTSTD)
Grief Experience Inventory, The (GEI)
Grief Measurement Scale
Griffith Mental Development Scale
Grooved Pegboard Test
Group Diagnostic Reading Aptitude and Achievement Tests, Intermediate Form
Group Embedded Figures Test (GEFT)
Group Encounter Scale (GES)
Group Environment Scale (GES)
Group Environment Scale, Second Edition
Group Inventory for Finding Creative Talent

Group Literacy Assessment
Group Mathematics Test, Third Edition
Group Reading Test (GRT)
Group Reading Test, Fourth Edition
Group Styles Inventory (GSI)
Group Tests of Musical Abilities
Guidance Centre Classroom Achievement Tests
Guide to the Assessment of Test Session Behavior for the WISC-III and the WIAT
Guidelines for Adolescent Preventive Services (GAPS)
Guilford-Zimmerman Aptitude Survey, The
Guilford-Zimmerman Interest Inventory, The (GZII)
Guilford-Zimmerman Personality Test, The (GZPT)
Hachinski Ischemia Scale
Hahnemann Elementary School Behavior Rating Scale
Hahnemann High School Behavior Rating Scale
Hall Occupational Orientation Inventory (HOOI)
Hall-Tonna Inventory of Values
Hallucination Change Scale
Halstead and Reitan Batteries
Halstead Aphasia Test (HAT)
Halstead Category Test
Halstead Impairment Index
Halstead-Russell Neuropsychological Evaluation System (HRNES)
Halstead-Reitan Battery (HRB)
Halstead-Reitan category Subtest
Halstead-Reitan Neurological Battery and Allied Procedures
Halstead-Reitan Neuropsychological Test Battery (HRNTB)
Halstead-Wepman Aphasia Screening Test
Hamburg Obsession/Compulsion Inventory
Hamburg Obsession/Compulsion Inventory-Short Form
Hamburg-Wechsler Intelligence Test for Children (HAWIC)
Hamilton Anxiety Rating Scale (HARS)
Hamilton Depression Inventory
Hamilton Depression Rating Scale (HDRS)
Hamilton Depression Scale (HAM-D)
Hamilton Rating Scale for Anxiety (HAM-A)
Hammill Multiability Achievement Test
Hammill Multiability Intelligence Test (HAMIT)
Hand Test-Revised, The
Handedness Questionnaire
Hanfmann-Kasanin Concept Formation Test
Haptic Intelligence Scale (HIS)
Harding Stress-Fair Compatibility Test
Hare Psychopathy Checklist-Revised (HPCL-R)
Hare Psychopathy Checklist: Screening Version
Harris Test of Lateral Dominance
Harris-Lingoes Subscales
Harter Self-Perception Profile for Children
Harvard Group Scale of Hypnotic Susceptibility (HGSHS)
Harvard Trauma Questionnaire
Hassles and Uplifts Scales, Research Edition
Hausa Speaking Test
Hawaii Early Learning Profile Checklist
Haws Screening Test for Functional Articulation Disorders
Hay Aptitude Test Battery
Hay Aptitude Test Battery-Revised
Health Assessment Questionnaire (HAQ)
Health Attribution Test
Health Behavior Scale (HBS)
Healthcare Questionnaire

Health Problems Checklist
Healy Pictorial Completion Test
Hebrew Speaking Test
Hebrew University Depression Database Questionnaire (HUDD-Q)
HELP Checklist
Henderson-Moriarty ESL/Literacy Placement Test
Henmon-Nelson Ability Test, Canadian Edition
Henmon-Nelson Tests of Mental Ability, The
Herrmann Brain Dominance Instrument
Hess School Readiness Scale (HSRS)
Heston Personality Index (HPI)
High School Personality Questionnaire (HSPQ)
High School Subject Tests
Hill Interaction Matrix (HIM)
Hill Performance Test of Selected Positional Concepts
Hillside Akathisia Scale
Hilson Adolescent Profile
Hilson Personnel Profile/Success Quotient (HPP/SQ)
Hiskey-Nebraska Test of Learning Aptitude (HNTLA)
HIV Risk Assessment Battery
Hodder Group Reading Tests
Hodkinson Mental Test (HMT)
Hogan Personality Inventory
Hogan Personality Inventory-Revised
Hoge 10-Item Intrinsic Religiosity Scale
Holden Psychological Screening Inventory
Hollingshead-Redlich Scale
Holmes and Rahe Social Readjustment Rating Scale
Home Environment Questionnaire
Home Observation for Measurement of the Environment
Home School Situations Questionnaire-Revised
Hooper Visual Organization Test, The
Hopelessness Scale
Hopelessness Scale for Children
Hopkins Symptom Checklist (HSCL)
Hopkins Symptom Checklist-25 (HSCL-25)
Hopkins Symptom Checklist-90 (HSCL-90)
Hopkins Verbal Learning Test (HVLT)
Horn Art Aptitude Inventory
Horn-Hellersberg Drawing Completion Test
Hospital Anxiety and Depression Scale (HADS)
Hostility and Direction of Hostility Questionnaire (HDHQ)
House-Tree Test (HT)
House-Tree-Person Test
Houston Test for Language Development
Houston Test for Language Development-Revised
Howell Prekindergarten Screening Test
How-I-See-Myself Scale (HISMS)
Human Figure Drawing Test (HFD)
Hundred Pictures Naming Test, The (HPNT)
Hunt-Minnesota Test for Organic Brain Damage
Hutchins Behavior Inventory (HBI)
Hymovich Chronicity Impact and Coping Instrument (CICI)
Hypnotic Induction Profile (HIP)
IPI Aptitude-Intelligence Test Series
IDEA Oral Language Proficiency Test II
I-E Scale of Rotter
Illinois Children's Language Assessment Test
Illinois Test of Psycholinguistic Ability (ITPA)

Illness and Symptom History Schedule
Illness Behavior Checklist (IBC)
Illness Behaviour Questionnaire (IBQ)
Illness Perception Questionnaire (IPQ)
Illness Perception Questionnaire-Revised (IPQ-R)
Imagined Process Inventory (IPI)
Impact Message Inventory (IMI)
Impact of Events Scale (IES)
Impact of Events Scale-Revised (IES-R)
Impact of Race-Related Events (IRE)
Importance, Confidence, and Readiness to Quit Ruler
Improving Writing, Thinking and Reading Skills Test
Impulse Control Scale
Impulsive Nonconformity Scale
Inattention/Overactivity with Aggression Conners Scale
Independent Living Behavior Checklist
Index of Adjustment and Values
Index of Potential Suicide
Index of Primitive Thought
Index of Sexual Functioning
Index of Sexuality (IS)
Index of Spouse Abuse
Index of Well-Being (IWB)
Index of Work Satisfaction (IWS)
Individual Learning Disabilities Classroom Screening Instrument (ILDCSI)
Individualized Criterion Reference Testing Mathematics (ICRTM)
Individualized Criterion Reference Testing Reading (ICRTR)
Individualized Criterion Referenced Testing (ICRT)
Infant Behavior Questionnaire
Infant Reading Test, The
Infant/Toddler Environment Rating Scale (ITERS)
Informal Reading Comprehension Placement Test
Inpatient Multidimensional Psychiatric Scale (IMPS)
Insight and Treatment Attitudes Questionnaire (ITAQ)
Insight to Treatment Questionnaire
Insomnia Diagnostic interview
Institutional Functioning Inventory (IFI)
Institutional Goals Inventory (IGI)
Instructional Environment Scale, The (TIES)
Instructional Leadership Inventory
Instrument Timbre Preference Test
Interest Inventory
Interpersonal Sensitivity Measure (IPSM)
Integrated Assessment System (IAS)
Integration Test
Interest Determination, Exploration and Assessment System, Enhanced Version
Intermediate Booklet Category Test
Intermediate Personality Questionnaire (IPQ)
Internal, Personal, and Situational Attributions Questionnaire (IPSAQ)
Internal State Scale (ISS)
International Personality Disorder Examination (IPDE)
International Primary Factors (IPF)
International Primary Factors Test Battery
International Test for Aphasia
International Version of the Mental Status Questionnaire
Inter-Person Perception Test (IPPT)
Interpersonal Communication Inventory (ICI)
Interpersonal Language Skills and Assessment (ILSA)
Interpersonal Perception Scale (IPS)

Interpersonal Reaction Test (IPRT)
Interpersonal Style Inventory
Intra- and Interpersonal Relations Scale
Inventory for Counseling and Development (ICD)
Inventory of Anger Communication (IAC)
Inventory of Complicated Grief
Inventory of Drug-Taking Situations (IDTS)
Inventory of Individually Perceived Group Cohesiveness
Inventory of Peer Influence on Eating Concern
Inventory of Perceptual Skills (IPS)
Inventory of Psychosocial Development (IPD)
Inventory of Suicidal Orientation-30 (ISO-30)
Inwald Personality Inventory (IPI)
Iowa Algebra Aptitude Test (IAAT)
Iowa Conners Rating Scale
Iowa Gambling Task
Iowa Pressure Articulation Test (IPAT)
Iowa Structured Psychiatric Interview (IPSI)
Iowa Stuttering Scale
Iowa Tests of Basic Skills
Iowa Tests of Educational Development, Forms X-8 and Y-8
IPAT Anxiety Scale
IPAT Depression Scale
IPF Test Battery
Irresistible Impulse Test
Irritability Scale
Irritability/Depression and Anxiety Scale
It Scale for Children (ITSC)
Item Counseling Evaluation Test
48-Item Counseling Evaluation Test (ICET)
Jackson Evaluation System
Jackson Personality Inventory (JPI)
Jail Suicide Assessment Tool (JSAT)
James Language Dominance Test
Jansky Screening Index (JSI)
Jarman Underprivileged Area
Jenkins Non-Verbal Test
Jesness Behavior Checklist (JBC)
Jesness Inventory (JI)
Jette Functional Status Index
Jevs Work Sample Battery
Job Attitude Scale (JAS)
Job Content Questionnaire
Job Descriptive Index (JDI)
Job Seeking Skills Assessment
Johns Hopkins Functioning Inventory
Johnson-Kenney Screening Test (JKST)
Johnston Informal Reading Inventory (JIRI)
Jordan Left-Right Reversal Test (JLRRT)
Joseph Pre-School and Primary Self-Concept Screening Test
Jourad Self-Disclosure Questionnaire (JSDQ)
Judgment of Occupational Behavior-Orientation
Jung Association Test
Junior Eysenck Personality Inventory (JEPI)
Kahn Intelligence Test (KIT)
Kahn Test of Symbol Arrangement, The (KTSA)
Karolinska Scales of Personality
Kasanin-Hanfmann Concept Formation Test
Katz Adjustment Scales (KAS)
Katz ADL Index
Kaufman Adolescent and Adult Intelligence Test (KAIT)
Kaufman Assessment Battery for Children (K-ABC)
Kaufman Brief Intelligence Test (K-BIT)
Kaufman Development Scale

Kaufman Infant and Preschool Scale
Kaufman Test of Educational Achievement
Kendrick Cognitive Tests for the Elderly
Kenny Self-Care Evaluation
Kent E-G-Y Test
Kent Infant Development Scale
Kent-Rosanoff Test
KeyMath Revised: A Diagnostic Inventory of Essential Mathematics
Khatena-Torrance Creative Perception Inventory
Kindergarten Auditory Screening Test (KAST)
Kindergarten Language Screening Test (KLST)
Kindergarten Readiness Test (KRT)
Kinetic Family Drawing (KFD)
Knowledge of Occupations Test (KOT)
Knox Cube Test
Kohnstamm Test
Kohs Block-Design Test, The
Kolbe Conative Index (KCI)
Kuder Preference Record
Kuder Preference Record-Vocational (KPR-V)
Kuhlman-Anderson Intelligence Tests
Lambeth Disability Screening Questionnaire
Language Modalities Test for Aphasia (LMTA)
Language Processing Test
Language Screening Test
Laterality Preference Schedule
Launay-Slade Hallucination Scale
Leader Behavior Analysis II (LBAII)
Leader Behavior Description Questionnaire (LBDQ)
Leadership Inventory
Leadership Opinion Questionnaire (LOQ)
Leadership Practices Inventory (LPI)
Leadership Skills Inventory
Learning Accomplishment Profile
Learning and Study Strategies Inventory (LASSI)
Learning Disability Evaluation Scale (LDES)
Learning Efficiency Test-II (LET-II)
Learning Inventory of Kindergarten Experiences (LIKE)
Learning Style Profile (LSP)
Learning Styles Inventory
Leatherman Leadership Questionnaire (LLQ)
Leeds Anxiety Scale
Leeds Scales for the Self-Assessment of Anxiety and Depression
Lehman Quality of Life Interview
Leisure Diagnostic Battery
Leisure Interest Inventory (LII)
Leiter Adult Intelligence Scale (LAIS)
Leiter International Performance Scale (LIPS)
Leiter International Performance Scale-Revised (LIPS-R)
Leiter Recidivism Scale
Let's Talk Inventory for Adolescents
Letter and Category Fluency Test
Letter Cancellation Test
Letter Generation Test
Level of Emotional Awareness Scale (LEAS)
Level of Functioning Scale
Levine-Pilowsky Depression Questionnaire
Leyton Obsessive Inventory (LOI)
Liebowitz Social Anxiety Scale (LSAS)
Life Event Scale - Adolescents
Life Event Scale - Children
Life Experiences Checklist (LEC)
Life History of Aggression Assessment
Life Satisfaction Index (LSI)
Life Skills Profile
Life Skills Profile index

Likert Scale
Limon Self-Image Assessment
Lincoln-Oseretsky Motor Performance Test (LOMPT)
Lindamood Auditory Conceptualization Test (LACT)
Line Bisection Test
Line Cancellation Test
Line Direction Test
Listening Comprehension Test (LCT)
Lock Wallace Short Marital Adjustment Scale
Locus of Control of Behavior Scale
Loevinger's Washington University Sentence Completion Test
Lollipop Test: A Diagnostic Screening Test of School Readiness
Lombard Voice-Reflex Test
London Psychogeriatric Scale (LPS)
Longitudinal Interval Follow-up Evaluation
Lorge-Thorndike Cognitive Abilities Test
Lorge-Thorndike Intelligence Test
Lorr Scale
LOTE Reading and Listening Tests
Louisville Behavior Checklist
Luborsky Health-Sickness Rating Scale
Luria Test
Luria-Nebraska Neuropsychological Battery (LNNB)
Luria Neuropsychological Investigation
Maastricht History and Advice Checklist-Revised (MAAS-R)
Maastricht Interview on Vital Exhaustion (MIVE)
Maastricht Questionnaire (MQ)
MacAndrew Addiction Scale (MAS)
MacArthur Competence Assessment Tool (Mac-CAT)
MacArthur Competence Assessment Tool-Proxy (Mac-CAT-P)
MacArthur Perceived Coercion Scale
Mach Scale
Machover Draw-A-Person Test (MDAP)
Macmillan Graded Word Reading Test
MacQuarrie Test for Mechanical Ability
Major Role Adjustment Scale II
Major Symptoms of Schizophrenia Scale
Management Development Profile
Management Inventory on Leadership, Motivation and Decision-Making (MILMD)
Management Philosophies Scale I-V (MPS)
Management Position Analysis Test
Management Readiness Profile (MRP)
Management Styles Inventory
Management Transactions Audit (MTA)
Manager Profile Record
Managerial Style Questionnaire (MSQ)
Mandel Social Adjustment Scale (MSAS)
Mandsley Personality Inventory (MPI)
Mania 9 Scale
Mania Rating Scale (MRS)
Manic-State Rating Scale
Manifest Anxiety Scale (MAS)
Manipulative Aptitude Test (MAT)
Mann-Whitney U Test
Mantel-Haenszel Test for Linear Trend
Marital Attitudes Evaluation (MATE)
Marital Communication Inventory
Marital Satisfaction Inventory
Marital Satisfaction Inventory
Marks-Sheehan Phobia Scale
Marlowe-Crowne Scale (MCS)
Marlowe-Crowne Scale of Social Desirability Scale (MCSD)
Marriage Adjustment Inventory (MAI)
Marriage Skills Analysis (MSA)
Martin Suicide-Depression Inventory (MSDI)
Martinez Assessment of the Basic Skills

Maslach Burnout Inventory (MBI)
Matching Familiar Figures Test (MFFT)
Maternal Attitude Scale (MAS)
Mathematics Anxiety Rating Scale (MARS)
Mathematics Anxiety Rating Scale-Adolescents (MARS-A)
Matrix Analogies Test
Mattis Dementia Rating Scale
Mattis Organic Mental Status Syndrome Examination (MOMSSE)
Mattis-Kovner Scale
Maudsley Obsessional Compulsive Inventory (MOCI)
Maudsley Personality Inventory (MPI)
Maxfield-Buchholz Social Maturity Scale for Blind Preschool Children
McAndrew Addiction Scale
McAndrew Alcoholism Scale (MAC)
McAndrew Alcoholism Scale-Revised
McCarthy Scales of Children's Ability (MCSA)
McCarthy Screening Test
McGill Pain Assessment Questionnaire (MPAQ)
McGill Pain Questionnaire, The
McGurk Visual Spatial Working Memory Test
McMaster Family Assessment Device
McMaster Health Index Questionnaire
McMaster Structured Interview of Family Functioning
Measurement of Language Development
Measures of Musical Abilities
Measures of Psychosocial Development (MPD)
Medical Fear Survey (MFS)
Medical Investigation of NeuroDevelopmental Disorders (MIND)
Medical Lethality Scale
Medical Outcomes Study Short-Form General Health Survey Physical Functioning Scale
Meeting Street School Screening Test (MSSST)
Meffill-Palmer Scale
Meier Art Judgment Test, The
Memorial Symptom Assessment Scale
Memory Assessment Scales (MAS)
Memory-for-Designs (MFD)
Memory Questionnaire
Menstrual Distress Questionnaire (MDQ)
Mental Alteration Test (MAT)
Mental Deterioration Battery (MDB)
Mental Illness Needs Index (MINI)
Mental Measurements Yearbook (MMY)
Mental Status Questionnaire (MSQ)
Merrill-Palmer Scale
Merrill-Palmer Scale of Mental Tests (MPSMT)
Merrill-Palmer Test of Mental Ability
Mertens Visual Perception Test (MVPT)
Methamphetamine Experience Questionnaire
Metropolitan Achievement Test (MAT)
Metropolitan Achievement Test, Seventh Edition (MAT7)
Metropolitan Language Instructional Test
Metropolitan Readiness Test (MRT)
Meyer-Kendall Assessment Survey (MKAS)
Michigan Alcoholism Screening Test (MAST)
Michigan English Language Assessment Battery
Michigan Picture Inventory
Michigan Picture Test (MPT)
Michigan Picture Test-Revised (MPT-R)
Michigan Screening Profile of Parenting
Michigan Vocabulary Profile Test

Military Environment Inventory
Mill Hill Vocabulary Scale
Miller Analogies Test (MAT)
Miller Assessment for Preschoolers
Miller-Yoder Language Comprehension Test
Millon Adolescent Clinical Inventory (MACI)
Millon Adolescent Personality Inventory (MAPI)
Millon Behavioral Health Inventory (MBHI)
Millon Clinical Multiaxial Inventory (MCMI)
Millon Clinical Multiaxial Inventory II (MCMI-II)
Milwaukee Academic Interest Inventory (MAII)
Mini-Cog
Mini International Neuropsychiatric Interview (MINI)
Mini Inventory of Right Brain Injury (MIRBI)
Mini-Mental State Examination (MMSE)
Minimum Essentials Test (MET)
Minnesota Child Development Inventory (MCDI)
Minnesota Clerical Aptitude Test
Minnesota Clerical Assessment Battery (MCAB)
Minnesota Clerical Test (MCT)
Minnesota Cocaine Craving Scale (MCCS)
Minnesota Differential Diagnosis of Aphasia (MDDA)
Minnesota Importance Questionnaire (MIQ)
Minnesota Impulsive Disorder Interview Model for Compulsive Buying
Minnesota Impulsive Disorders Interview
Minnesota Infant Development Inventory
Minnesota Job Description Questionnaire (MJDQ)
Minnesota Mechanical Assembly Test (MMAT)
Minnesota Multiphasic Personality Inventory (MMPI)
Minnesota Multiphasic Personality Inventory, Adolescent (MMPI-A)
Minnesota Multiphasic Personality Inventory, Second Edition (MMPI-2)
Minnesota Paper Form Board Test (MPFBT)
Minnesota Percepto-Diagnostic Test (MPDT)
Minnesota Preschool Scale
Minnesota Rate of Manipulation Test
Minnesota Satisfaction Questionnaire (MSQ)
Minnesota Satisfaction Scale (MSS)
Minnesota Scholastic Aptitude Test (MSAT)
Minnesota Spatial Relations Test (MSRT)
Minnesota Speed of Reading Test for College Students
Minnesota Teacher Attitude Inventory (MTAI)
Minnesota Test for the Differential Diagnosis of Aphasia (MTDDA)
Minnesota Vocational Interest Inventory (MVII)
Minnesota-Hartford Personality Assay (MHPA)
Miskimins Self-Goal-Other Discrepancy Scale
Mississippi Scale for Combat-Related Posttraumatic Stress Disorder
Missouri Auditory Learning Test
Missouri Kindergarten Inventory of Developmental Skills
Modern Language Aptitude Test

Modern Occupational Skills Test (MOST)
Modified Autonomic Perception Questionnaire
Modified Checklist for Autism in Toddlers
Modified Health Assessment Questionnaire (MHAQ)
Modified Overt Aggression Scale (MOAS)
Modified Rankin Disability Scale
Modified Simpson Dyskinesia Scale
Modified Vigotsky Concept Formation Test
Modified Visual Reproduction Test
Modified Word Learning Test (MWLT)
Money Standardized Road Map Test Of Direction Sense
Monotic Word Memory Test (MWMT)
Montgomery-Asberg Depression Rating Scale (MADRS)
Mood and Physical Symptoms Scale (MPSS)
Mood Disorder Questionnaire
Mooney Faces Closure Test
Mooney Problem Checklists (MPCL)
Mooney Test
Moos Family Environment Scale
Moos Menstrual Distress Questionnaire (MMDQ)
Moral Objections To Suicide Scale (MOSS)
Morbid Anxiety Inventory (MAI)
Morgan-Russell Scale
Mosaic Test
Mother-Child Relationship Evaluation (MCRE)
Mother's Assessment of the Behavior of Her Infant (MABI)
Motivation Analysis Test (MAT)
Motivational Patterns Inventory
Motor Impersistence Test (MIT)
Motor Steadiness Battery
Motor-Free Visual Perception Test (MVPT)
Movement Disorder Questionnaire
Movement Scale
Mullen Scales of Early Learning (MSEL)
Multiaxial Evaluation Report Form
Multidimensional Aptitude Battery
Multidimensional Assessment of Gains in School (MAGS)
Multidimensional Assessment of Philosophy of Education (MAPE)
Multidimensional Health Locus and Control Scale
Multidimensional Pain Inventory (MPI)
Multidimensional Perfectionism Scale
Multidimensional Scale for Rating Psychiatric Patients (MSRPP)
Multidimensional Self Concept Scale (MSCS)
Multifactor Leadership Questionnaire (MLQ)
Multilevel Informal Language Inventory
Multilingual Aphasia Examination (MAE)
Multiphasic Environmental Assessment Procedure (MEAP)
Multiphasic Personality Inventory (MPI)
Multiple Affect Adjective Checklist (MAACL)
Multiple Sleep Latency Test (MSLT)
Multiscore Depression Inventory (MDI)
Multivariate Personality Inventory (MPI)
Murphy-Meisgeier Type Indicator for Children (MMTIC)
Musical Aptitude Profile (MAP)
Myers-Briggs Type Indicator (MBTI)
Myokinetic Psychodiagnosis Test
Names Learning Test (NLT)
Narcotic Addict Treatment Act

National Adult Reading Test (NART)
National Attention Test (NAT)
National Educational Development Test
National Institute of Mental Health-Global Obsessive Compulsive Scale (NIMH-OC)
National Longitudinal Scale of Adolescent Health
National Occupation Competency Testing (NOCT)
National Police Officer Selection Test (POST)
Natural Process Analysis
Naylor-Harwood Adult Intelligence Scale (NHAIS)
Naylor-Harwood Intelligence Scale (NHIS)
Need for Closure Scale (NFCS)
Need for Cognition Scale (NCS)
NEECHAM Confusion Scale
NEO (neuroticism, extroversion, openness to experience) Personality Inventory-Revised (NEO PI-R)
NEO Five-Factor Inventory
NEO Personality Inventory–Revised
Neonatal Behavioral Assessment Scale (NBAS)
Neonatal Behavioral Assessment Scale with Kansas Supplements (NBAS-K)
NeuroBehavioral Cognitive Status Examination
NeuroBehavioral Rating Scale
Neuropsychiatric Inventory (NPI)
Neuropsychiatric Inventory/Nursing Home Version (NPI/NH)
Neuropsychiatric Rating Schedule
Neuropsychological Screening Examination
Neuropsychological Status Examination
Neurotic Personality Factor Test (NPFT)
Neuroticism Scale Questionnaire (NSQ)
Neuroticism-Extroversion-Openness to Experience Personality Questionnaire
Neuroticism-Extroversion-Openness Personality Inventory
New Haven Schizophrenia Index
New Jersey Test of Reasoning Skills
New Mexico Attitude Toward Work Test (NMATWT)
New Mexico Career Planning Test (NMCPT)
New Mexico Job Application Procedures Test (NMJAPT)
New Mexico Knowledge of Occupations Test (NMKOT)
New Sucher-Allred Reading Placement Inventory
New York University Parkinson Disease Scale
NIH Stroke Scale
NIMH Global Obsessive-Compulsive Scale
9-Digit Task
Non-Language Learning Test
Non-Language Multi-Mental Test
Non-Reading Aptitude Test Battery (NATB)
Non-Reading Intelligence Test, Levels 1-3 (NRIT)
Nonverbal Ability Test (NAT)
Normative Adaptive Behavior Checklist
Norris Educational Achievement Test (NEAT)
North American Adult Reading Test (NAART)
North American Depression Inventories for Children and Adults
Northwestern Syntax Screening Test (NSST)
Northwestern University Children's Perception of Speech Test
Northwick Park Index of Independence in ADL

Nottingham Extended ADL Index
Nottingham Health Profile
Nottingham Ten-Point ADL Scale
Novel Memory Task
Novel Recall Task
Numeracy Impact Tests
Numerical Ability Test
Numerical Attention Test (NAT)
Nurses Global Impressions Scale
Nurses Observations Scale for Inpatient Evaluation (NOSIE)
NYLS Adult Temperament Questionnaire
OARS Multidimensional Functional Assessment Questionnaire (OMFAQ)
Object Classification Test (OCT)
Object Sorting Scale (OSS)
Object Sorting Test (OST)
Object Test (OT)
Objective Analytic Battery
Objective Opiate Withdrawal Scale
O'Brien Vocabulary Placement Test
Obsessive-Compulsive Drinking Scale (OCDS)
Obsessive-Compulsive Drinking Scale-Modified for Pathological Gambling (OCDS-PG)
Obsessive-Compulsive Personality Disorder Subscale from Millon Clinical Multiaxial
Obsessive-Compulsive Subscale of the Comprehensive Psychopathological Rating Scale
Occupational Environment Scales, Form E-2
Occupational Roles Questionnaire (ORQ)
Occupational Stress Indicator (OSI)
Occupational Test Series-Basic Skills Test
O'Connor Wiggly Block Test
Offer Parent-Adolescent Questionnaire
Offer Self-Image Questionnaire (OSIQ)
Offer Self-Image Questionnaire for Adolescents
Ohio Work Values Inventory (OWVI)
OISE Picture Reasoning Test (PRT)
Oliphant Auditory Discrimination Memory Test (OADMT)
Oliphant Auditory Synthesizing Test (OAST)
Omnibus Personality Inventory (OPI)
One Word Receptive Picture Vocabulary Test
Opinion Questionnaire
Opinion Toward Adolescents (OTA)
Oral and Written Language Scales (OWLS)
Oral Language Sentence Imitation Diagnostic Inventory (OLSIDI)
Oral Language Sentence Imitation Screening Test (OLSIST)
Oral Verbal Intelligence Test (OVIT)
Oral-Motor/Feeding Rating Scale
Ordinal Scales of Psychological Development
Organic Integrity Test (OIT)
Organizational Climate Exercise II
Organizational Culture Inventory (OCI)
Organizational Value Dimensions Questionnaire (OVDQ)
Orientation Inventory
Orientation-Memory-Concentration Test (OMC)
Orleans-Hanna Algebra Prognosis Test
O'Rourke Mechanical Aptitude Test
Otis Group Intelligence Scale
Otis Quick Scoring Mental Abilities Test
Otis Quick Scoring Mental Abilities Test
Otis Self-Administered Tests of Mental Ability
Otis-Lennon Mental Ability Test (OLMAT)
Otis-Lennon School Ability Test

Ottawa School Behavior Checklist (OSBCL)
Overall Defensive Functioning Score
Overcontrolled Hostility Scale (OHS)
Overt Aggression Scale
Oxford STA Scale
Oxford-Liverpool Inventory of Feelings and Experiences
Paced Auditory Serial Addition Test (PASAT)
PACG Inventory
Pain Apperception Test (PAT)
Pain Perception Profile (PPP)
Pain Questionnaire
Pair Attraction Inventory (PAI)
Panic Control Treatment-Adolescents (PCT-A)
Panic Disorder Severity Scale (PDSS)
Panic-Agoraphobic Spectrum Questionnaire
Pantomime Recognition Test (PRT)
Paranoia 6 Scale
Paranoid Sensitivity Profile
Parent as a Teacher Inventory (PAAT)
Parent Attachment Structured Interview
Parent Attitude Scale (PAS)
Parent Bonding Instrument (PBI)
Parent Interview for Child Syndrome (PICS)
Parent Inventory
Parent Opinion Inventory
Parent Perception of Child Profile (PPCP)
Parent Rating of Student Behavior
Parent-Adolescent Communication Scale
Parental Acceptance-Rejection Questionnaire
Parental Stressor Scale
Parental Stressor Scale: Neonatal Intensive Care Unit (PSS:NICU)
Parenting Stress Index
Parent-Teacher Questionnaire (PTQ)
Partner Relationship Inventory (PRI)
Past Feelings and Acts Of Violence Scale
Pathologic Laughing and Crying Scale (PLACS)
Pathological Gambling Signs Index
Patient Rated Anxiety Scale (PRAS)
Patient Rated Disability Scale
Patient Rated Impairment Scale
Patient Rated Overall Life Impairment
Patient Satisfaction Questionnaire-III
Pattern Misfit Scale
Patterns of Individual Change Scale (PICS)
Paykel Life Events Scale
PDI Employment Inventory
Peabody Developmental Motor Scales and Activity Cards
Peabody Individual Achievement Test (PIAT)
Peabody Mathematics Readiness Test
Peabody Picture Vocabulary Test (PPVT)
Peabody Picture Vocabulary Test–Revised
Peabody Vocabulary Test (PVT)
Pediatric Behavior Scale (PBS)
Pediatric Early Elementary Examination
Pediatric Examination of Educational Readiness at Middle Childhood
Pediatric Extended Examination at Three (PEET)
Pediatric Speech Intelligibility Test
Peer Nomination Inventory of Depression
Peer Profile
Penn State Worry Questionnaire
Perceived Social Support Scale (PSS)
Perception Inventory
Perception of Ability Scale for Students (PASS)

Perception of Illness Scale
Perception-of-Relationships Test (PORT)
Perceptual Maze Test
Performance Assessment of Syntax Elicited and Spontaneous (PASES)
Performance Efficiency Test
Performance Scale Scores
Periodic Evaluation Record (PER)
Peritraumatic Dissociation Index
Peritraumatic Dissociative Experiences Questionnaire
Perkins-Binet Test of Intelligence for the Blind
Perley-Guze Hysteria Checklist
Perley-Guze Symptom Checklist
Personal Adjustment and Role Skills (PARS)
Personal Assessment for Continuing Education (PACE)
Personal Assessment of Intimacy in Relationships (PAIR)
Personal Attributes Questionnaire (PAQ)
Personal Experience and Attitude Questionnaire (PEAQ)
Personal Experience Screening Questionnaire (PESQ)
Personal History Questionnaire
Personal Inventory
Personal Inventory of Needs
Personal Orientation Inventory (POI)
Personal Preference Scale (PPS)
Personal Problems Checklist (PPC)
Personal Problems Checklist for Adolescents
Personal Relationship Inventory (PRI)
Personal Resource Questionnaire (PRQ)
Personal Strain Questionnaire (PSQ)
Personal Style Inventory (PSI)
Personal Values Abstract (PVA)
Personal Values Inventory (PVI)
Personality Adjective Check List (PACL)
Personality Assessment Inventory (PAI)
Personality Diagnostic Questionnaire (PDQ)
Personality Diagnostic Questionnaire-Revised (PDQ-R)
Personality Disorder Examination (PDE)
Personality Factor Questionnaire (PFQ)
16 Personality Factor Questionnaire (16 PF)
Personality Index (PI)
Personality Inventory (PI)
Personality Inventory for Children (PIC)
Personality Questionnaire
Personality Rating Scale (PRS)
Personality Research Form (PRF)
Personnel Reaction Blank
Personnel Selection Inventory
Personnel Tests for Industry (PTI)
Peters et al. Delusions Inventory
Phelps Kindergarten Readiness Scale (PKRS)
Philadelphia Head Injury Questionnaire (PHIQ)
Philadelphia Multilevel Assessment Instrument
Phillips Scale
Phobic Attitude Evaluation
Photoarticulation Test (PAT)
Physical and Architectural Features Checklist
Physical Self-Maintenance Scale
Physical Tolerance Profile (PTP)
Physiognomic Cue Test (PCT)
Picha-Seron Career Analysis
Pictorial Test of Intelligence (PTI)
Picture Anomalies Test
Picture Arrangement Subtest
Picture Articulation and Language Screening Test (PALST)
Picture Completion Subtest
Picture Identification for Children–Standardized Index

Picture Identification Test (PIT)
Picture Interpretation Test
Picture Inventory
Picture Reasoning Test (PRE)
Picture Story Language Test (PSLT)
Picture-World Test
Piers-Harris Children's Self-Concept Scale
Pimsleur Language Aptitude Battery
Pinter-Paterson Performance Test
Pitowsky Illness Behavior Questionnaire
Pittsburgh Sleep Quality Index
Pleasant Events Schedule (PES)
Politte Sentence Completion Test
Polyfactorial Study of Personality
Porch Index of Communicative Ability (PICA)
Porch Index of Communicative Ability in Children (PICAC)
Porteus Maze Test (PMT)
Position Analysis Questionnaire (PAQ)
Positive and Negative Affect Schedule
Positive and Negative Stroke Scale (PANSS)
Positive and Negative Symptom Scale
Positive and Negative Symptoms of Schizophrenia Scale
Positive and Negative Syndrome Scale (PANSS)
Positive Humanitarian Subscale
Positive Military Subscale
Positive Symptom Distress Index
Poststroke Depression Rating Scale
Posttraumatic Stress Disorder Reaction Index
Posttraumatic Stress Disorder Symptom Scale
Potential for Addiction Index
Pragmatics Profile of Early Communication Skills
Pragmatics Screening Test
Predictive Ability Test (PAT)
Predictive Screening Test of Articulation
Preliminary Diagnostic Questionnaire
Premarital Communication Inventory (PCI)
Premenstrual Assessment Form (PAF)
Premorbid Social Adjustment Scale
Pre-Professional Skills Test
Pre-Reading Expectancy Screening Scale (PRESS)
Preschool and Kindergarten Interest Descriptor
Preschool Behavior Checklist
Preschool Development Inventory
Preschool Feelings Checklist
Preschool Language Scale (PLS)
Preschool Language Screening Test
Preschool Screening Test, The
Preschool Speech and Language Screening Test
Prescriptive Reading Inventory (PRI)
Present State Examination (PSE)
Prevocational Assessment and Curriculum Guide (PACG)
Prevocational Assessment Screen (PAS)
Primary Care Evaluation of Mental Disorders
Primary Mental Abilities Test (PMAT)
Primary Self-Concept Inventory (PSCI)
Primary Test of Cognitive Skills (PTCS)
Primary Visual Motor Test (PVMT)
Printing Performance School Readiness Test (PPRST)
Priority Counseling Survey (PCS)
Private Self-Consciousness Scale
Problem Experiences Checklist
Problem Solving Inventory, The
Process Diagnostic (PD)
Process for the Assessment of Effective Student Functioning

Process Skills Rating Scale (PSRS)
Professional and Administrative Career Evaluation/Examination
Professional Employment Test (PET)
Professional Sexual Role Inventory (PSRI)
Proficiency Assessment Report (PAR)
Profile of Adaptation to Life (PAL)
Profile of Mood States (POMS)
Profile of Mood States, Vigor
Profile of Nonverbal Sensitivity (PONS)
Profile of Out-of-Body Experiences (POBE)
Prognostic Scale
Progress Assessment Chart of Social and Personal Development (PAC)
Progressive Achievement Tests of Listening Comprehension (PATLC)
Progressive Achievement Tests of Reading
Progressive Deterioration Scale (PDS)
Projective Assessment of Aging Method
Projective Human Figure Drawing Test
Projective Test
Proteus Maze
PSI Basic Skills Test for Business, Industry and Government
Psychasthenia 7 Scale
Psychiatric Diagnostic Screening Questionnaire (PDSQ)
Psychiatric Epidemiology Research I Interview-Demoralization Scale (PERI-D)
Psychiatric Epidemiology Research Interview (PERI)
Psychiatric Evaluation Form (PEF)
Psychiatric Evaluation Profile (PEP)
Psychiatric Knowledge and Skills Self-Assessment Program (PKSAP)
Psychiatric Status Rating Scale
Psychiatric Status Schedules (PSS)
Psycho-Educational Evaluation
Psychodynamic Psychotherapy Competency Test
Psychoeducational Profile (PEP)
Psychoeducational Profile-Revised (PEP-R)
Psycho-Epistemological Profile (PEP)
Psychogeriatric Dependency Rating Scale
Psycholinguistic Rating Scale
Psychological Distress Inventory
Psychological Inventory
Psychological Screening Inventory (PSI)
Psychopathic Deviance 4 Scale
Psychopathological Rating Scale
Psychopathy Checklist-Revised
Psychosis Screening Questionnaire
Psychosocial Adjustment to Illness Scale (PAIS)
Psychosocial Assessment of Childhood Experiences (PACE)
Psychosocial History Screening Questionnaire (PHSQ)
Psychosocial History Screening Test (PHST)
Psychotherapy Competence Assessment Schedule (PCAS)
Psychotherapy Supervisory Inventory
Psychotic Inpatient Profile (PIP)
Psychotic Reaction Profile (PRP)
PTSD Symptom Scale
Pupil Rating Scale (PRS)
Pupil Rating Scale: Screening for Learning Disabilities
Purdue Industrial Mathematics Test
Purdue Pegboard Dexterity Test
Purdue Student-Teacher Opinionnare (PSTO)
Purdue Teacher Opinionnaire (PTO)
Purdue Teacher Questionnaire (PTQ)
Purpose in Life Test
Pursuit Rotor Task
Quality of Crisis Support Scale

Quality of Life Enjoyment and Satisfaction Questionnaire
Quality of Life Interview (QOLI)
Quality of Life Inventory (QOLI)
Quality of Life Questionnaire (QLQ)
Quality of Life Scale
Quality of Well-Being Scale
Queckenstedt-Stookey Test
Questionnaire on Resources and Stress for Families with Chronically Ill or Handicapped
Quick Picture Vocabulary Test (QPVT)
Quick Screening of Mental Development
Quick Word Test
Quick-Score Achievement Test
Rancho Los Amigos Scale
Race-Related Stressor Scale (RRSS)
Racial Perceptions Inventory (RPI)
Rand Functional Limitations Battery
Rand Patient Satisfaction Questionnaire
Rand Physical Capacities Battery
Rand Social Health Battery
Rand 36-Item Health Survey
Random Letter Test
Random Letter Test Raskin Severity of Depression Scale
Rape Aftermath Symptom Test
Raskin Severity of Depression Scale
Rated Anxiety Scale
Rated Overall Life Impairment
Rathus Assertiveness Test
Rating Inventory for Screening Kindergartners
Rating Scale for Aggressive Behavior in Elderly (RAGE)
Rating Scale of Communication in Cognitive Decline (RSCCD)
Raven Colored Progressive Matrices Test (RCPMT)
Raven Progressive Matrices (RPM)
Raven Standard Progressive Matrices (RSPM)
Raven Test
RBH Test of Learning Ability
Reaction Time Test
Reaction to Loss Inventory
Readiness Inventory
Readiness Scale - Self Rating and Manager Rating Forms
Readiness Test
Reading Comprehension Battery for Aphasia
Reading Comprehension Inventory
Reading Miscue Inventory (RMI)
Reading-Free Vocational Interest Inventory (RFVII)
Reasons for Living Inventory (RLI)
Recent Life Changes Questionnaire (RLCQ)
Receptive One-Word Picture Vocabulary Test (ROWPVT)
Receptive-Expressive Emergent Language Scale (REEL)
Receptive-Expressive Observation Scale
Recognition Memory Test
Reductions in Eating Attitudes Test
Rehabilitation Client Rating Scale (RCRS)
Rehabilitation Indicator (RI)
Reid Report
Reitan Evaluation of Hemispheric Abilities and Brain Improvement Training
Reitan-Indiana Aphasia Screening Test (RIAST)
Reitan-Indiana Neuropsychological Test Battery for Adults
Reitan-Indiana Neuropsychological Test Battery for Children
Reitan-Klove Lateral Dominance Examination
Reitan-Klove Sensory Perceptual Evaluation
Reitan-Klove Sensory Perceptual Examination

Reitan-Klove Tactile Form Recognition Test
Relationship Inventory
Relative Value Scale
Reminding Test
Remote Associates Test (RAT)
Repeatable Battery for Assessment of Neuropsychological Status (RBANS)
Repeated Test of Sustained Wakefulness (RTSW)
Repertory Test
Repression-Sensitization Scale
Resilience: Personal Competence Subscale
Resolution of Delusions Scale (RODS)
Resource-Based Relative Value Scale (RBRVS)
Responsibility and Independence Scale for Adolescents (RISA)
Retirement Descriptive Index (RDI)
Revised Behavior Problem Checklist
Revised Child Anxiety and Depression Scale
Revised Childhood Experiences Questionnaire (CEQ-R)
Revised Children's Depression Scale (RCDS)
Revised Children's Manifest Anxiety Scale
Revised Combat Scale
Revised Denver Prescreening Development Questionnaire (R-PDQ)
Revised Diagnostic Interview for Borderlines
Revised Edinburgh Functional Communication Profile
Revised Evaluating Acquired Skills in Communication
Revised Fear Survey Schedule for Children
Revised Impact of Events Scale (RIES)
Revised NEO Personality Inventory
Revised Ontario Child Health Study Scale
Revised Physical Anhedonia Scale (PAS)
Revised Token Test
Revised Ways of Coping Checklist
Rey and Taylor Complex Figure Test
Rey Auditory Verbal Learning Tool (RAVLT)
Rey Complex Figure Test
Reynell Developmental Language Scales
Reynell-Zinkin Scales: Developmental Scales for Young Handicapped Children
Reynolds Adolescent Depression Scale (RADS)
Reynolds Adolescent Scale
Reynolds Child Depression Scale (RCDS)
Rey-Osterrieth Complex Figure Test
Rey-Osterrieth Complex Figure Copy and Delayed Recall Test
Rey-Osterrieth Complex Figure Design
Rhode Island Pupil Identification Scale (PIPIS)
Right-Left Orientation Test (RLO)
Right-Wing Authoritarianism Scale
Riley Articulation and Language Test (RALT)
Riley Inventory of Basic Learning Skills (RIBLS)
Riley Motor Problems Inventory
Riley Preschool Developmental Screening Inventory (RPDSI)
Ring and Peg Tests of Behavior Development
Risk Assessment Battery
Risk Behavior Index
Risk Inventory
Risk of AIDS Behavior Scale
Risk-Taking, Attitude, Values Inventory (RTAVI)

Ritvo-Freeman Real Life Rating Scale for Autism
Rivermead ADL Test
Rivermead Behavioral Memory Test (RBMT)
Rivermead Mobility Index (RMI)
Rivermead Motor Assessment
Rivermead Perceptual Assessment Battery
Robert Apperception Test for Children (RATC)
Roeder Manipulative Aptitude Test
Rogers Criminal Responsibility Scale
Role Construct Repertory Test
Rorschach Content Test (RCT)
Rorschach Index of Primitive Thought
Rorschach Inkblot Test
Rorschach Test
Rosen Drawing Test
Rosenberg Self-Esteem Scale (RSES)
Ross Information Processing Assessment
Ross Test of Higher Cognitive Processes
Rotter Sentence Completion Test (RSCT)
Rucker-Gable Educational Programming Scale (RGEPS)
Rule Eleven Psych Evaluation
Russell Version Wechsler Memory Scale
Rust Inventory of Schizotypal Cognitions
Rutler-Graham Psychiatric Interview
Rutter Child Behaviour Questionnaire
Rutter-B Questionnaire
Safran Student's Interest Inventory (SSII)
Salamon-Conte Life Satisfaction in the Elderly Scale (LSES)
Sales Personality Questionnaire (SPQ)
Salience Inventory, The (SI)
Sandler-Hazari Scale
Santa Ana Form Board Test
Sarason General Anxiety and Test Anxiety Scale
Satisfaction Inventory
SCAL Scale
Scale for Assessment of Thought, Language, and Communication
Scale for Emotional Blunting (SEB)
Scale for the Assessment of Negative Symptoms (SANS)
Scale for the Assessment of Positive Symptoms (SAPS)
Scale for Assessment of Thought, Language, and Communication
Scale for the Assessment of Unawareness of Mental Disorder (SUMD)
Scale of Independent Behavior
Scale of Social Development
Scale to Assess Narrative Development
Scale to Assess Unawareness of Mental Disorder (SUMD)
Scaled Curriculum Achievement Levels Test (SCALE)
Scales of Creativity and Learning Environment (SCALE)
Schaie-Thurstone Adult Mental Abilities Test
Schedule for Affective Disorders and Schizophrenia for School-Age Children (KIDDIE-SADS)
Schedule for Affective Disorders and Schizophrenia for School-Age Children-Epidemiologic Version (K-SADS-E)
Schedule for Affective Disorders and Schizophrenia for School-Age Children-Present Episode (K-SADS-P)
Schedule for Assessment of Insight (SAI)
Schedule for Attitudes Toward Hastened Death
Schedule for the Assessment Negative Symptoms
Schedule of Affective Disorders

Schedule of Recent Experience (SRE)
Schedules for Clinical Assessment in Neuropsychiatry (SCAN)
Schizophrenia 8 Scale
Schizophrenia-Mania Rating Scale
Scholastic Abilities Test for Adults (SATA)
School Ability Test (SAT)
School Assessment Survey (SAS)
School Atmosphere Questionnaire (SAQ)
School Attitude Test (SAT)
School Climate Inventory
School Handicap Condition Scale (SEH)
School Interest Inventory
School Library/Media Skills Test
School Motivation Analysis Test (SMAT)
School Problem Screening Inventory (SPSI)
School Readiness Screening Test
School Social Skills Rating Scale
Schubert General Ability Battery
Schwab and England Activities of Daily Living Scale
Scott Mental Alertness Test
Screen for Caregiver Burden
Screening Assessment for Gifted Elementary Students, Primary (SAGES-P)
Screening for learning disabilities
Screening for Learning Disabilities, Pupil Rating Scale
Screening Inventory
Screening Kit of Language Development (SKOLD)
Screening Questionnaire
Screening Test for Auditory Comprehension of Language (STACL)
Screening Test for Educational Prerequisite Skills (STEPS)
Screening Test for the Assignment of Remedial Treatment (START)
Screening Test of Academic Readiness
Screening Test of Adolescent Language
Screening Tests for Young Children and Retardates (STYCAR)
S-D Proneness Checklist
SEARCH: A Scanning Instrument for the Identification of Potential Learning Disability
Seashore Rhythm Test (SRT)
Self-Administered Questionnaire
Seasonal Pattern Assessment Questionnaire (SPAQ)
Seeking of Noetic Goals Test, The
Selective Reminding Test
Self-Administered Dependency Questionnaire (SADQ)
Self-Assessment Depression Scale
Self-Assessment in Writing Skills
Self-Concept and Motivation Inventory (SCAMI)
Self-Concept as a Learner Scale
Self-Concept Scale
Self-Consciousness Scale
Self-Control Inventory
Self-Control Scale (SCS)
Self-Description Inventory
Self-Description Questionnaire II (SDQII)
Self-Esteem Index (SEI)
Self-Esteem Inventory, The (SEI)
Self-Esteem Questionnaire
Self-Perception Inventory (SPI)
Self-Perception Profile for Children
Self-Rating Depression Scale (SDS)
Self-Report Personality Inventory
Self-Report Psychological Inventory
Self-Report Questionnaire
Semi-Structured Assessment for the Genetics of Alcoholism
Senior Apperception Technique, The (SAT)

Senoussi Multiphasic Marital Inventory (SMMI)
Sensation-Seeking Scale (SSS)
Sense of Coherence Questionnaire
Sensory Integration and Praxis Tests (SIPT)
Sentence Closure Test
Sentence Completion Test (SCT)
Separation Anxiety Symptom Inventory (SASI)
Sequenced Inventory of Communication Development (SICD)
Sequenced Inventory of Language Development (SILD)
Sequential Assessment of Mathematics Inventories: Standardized Inventory
Sequential Tests of Educational Progress, Series III (STEP-III)
Series of Emergency Scales
7-Minute Screen for Dementia
Severity of Event Scale
Severity of Psychiatric Illness Scale
Severity of Psychosocial Stressors Scale
Sex Inventory (SI)
Sex Knowledge and Attitude Test (SKAT)
Sexual Abuse Interview
Sexual and Physical Abuse Questionnaire
Sexual Compatibility Test (SCT)
Sexual Desire Index (SDI)
Sexual Experience Survey (SES)
Sexual Experiences Questionnaire
Sexual Functioning Index (SFI)
Sexual Risk Index
Sexuality Preference Profile (SPP)
Shapes Analysis Test (SAT)
Shedler-Western Assessment Procedure-200 (SWAP-200)
Sheehan Disability Scale
Sheltered Care Environment Scale
Shipley Abstraction Test
Shipley Institute of Living Scale (SILS)
Shipley Institute of Living Scale for Measuring Intellectual Impairment
Shipley Personal Inventory (SPI)
Shipley-Hartford Scale
Shipman Anxiety Depression Scale (SADS)
Short-Form Health Survey
Short Form Test of Academic Aptitude (SFTAA)
Short Form 36-Item Questionnaire (SF36)
Short Form McGill Pain Questionnaire
Short Imaginal Processes Inventory (SIPI)
Short Increment Sensitivity Index (SISI)
Short Michigan Alcoholism Screen Test
Short Michigan Alcoholism Screening Test (SMAST)
Short Orientation-Memory-Concentration Test (SOMC)
Short Portable Mental Status Questionnaire (SPMSQ)
Short Test for Use with Cerebral Palsy Children
Short Test of Mental Status
Shortened Edinburgh Reading Tests
Sickness Impact Profile (SIP)
Side Effect and Life Satisfaction Inventory
Similarities Subtest
Similarities Test of Verbal Abstract Reasoning
Simple Choice Reaction Time Task
Simpson Scale
Simpson-Angus Scale (SAS)
Singer-Loomis Inventory of Personality (SLIP)
Single and Double Simultaneous Stimulation Test

Situational Attitude Scale (SAS)
Situational Confidence Questionnaire (SCQ)
Six-Hour Retarded Child Test
Sixteen Personality Factor Questionnaire
Skill Inventory
Skill Scan for Management Development
Slavson Activity Interview Therapy
Sleep and Breathing Problems Scale
Sleep Screening Questionnaire for Parents
Sleepiness Scale
Slingerland Screening Tests (SST)
Slosson Children's Version Family Environment Scale
Slosson Drawing Coordination Test
Slosson Intelligence Test-Primary (SIT-P)
Slosson Intelligence Test-Revised (SIT-R)
Slosson Test of Reading Readiness (STRR)
Smell Identification Test
Smith-Johnson Nonverbal Performance Scale
Smoking Behavior Questionnaire (SBQ)
Snaith-Hamilton Pleasure Scale
Social Adequacy Index (SAI)
Social Adjustment Scale
Social Adjustment Scale II
Social Adjustment Self-Report Questionnaire
Social Adjustment Self-Report Scale (SASRS)
Social and Health Assessment
Social and Occupational Functioning Assessment Scale (SOFAS)
Social and Prevocational Information Battery (SPIB)
Social Avoidance and Distress Scale
Social Behavior Assessment Inventory (SBAI)
Social Behavior Assessment Schedule
Social Climate Scale (SCS)
Social Constraints Scale (SCS)
Social Disability Scale
Social Dysfunction and Aggression Scale
Social Function Index (SFI)
Social Intelligence Test
Social Interaction Scale
Social Maladjustment Schedule
Social Problem-Solving Inventory-Revised, Short Form
Social Readjustment Rating Scale (SRRS)
Social Reintegration Scale
Social Relations Test (SRT)
Social Relationships Index (SRI)
Social Reticence Scale
Social Stress And Functionality Inventory (SSFI)
Social Support Questionnaire
Social Support Scale
Social Thoughts and Beliefs Scale (STABS)
Social Ties Checklist
Social-Emotional Dimension Scale
Sociodemographic Information Checklist and Referral/Intake Form-McGill Couple and Family Clinic
SOI-Learning Abilities Test: Screening Form for Gifted
Somatic 3 Scale
Somatic Inkblot Series
Sorting of Figures Test (SOFT)
South Oaks Gambling Screen (SOGS)
South Oaks Gambling Screen-Revised for Adolescents (SOGS-RA)
Southern California Postrotary Nystagmus Test
Southern California Sensory Integration Tests

Spadafore Diagnostic Reading Test
SPAR Spelling and Reading Test
Spatial Orientation Memory Test (SOMT)
Special Aptitude Test Battery (SATB)
Specific Aptitude Test Battery
SPECTRUM-I: A Test of Adult Work Motivation
Speech and Language Screening Questionnaire (SLSQ)
Speech Questionnaire
Speech with Alternating Masking Index (SWAMI)
Speech-Language Pathology Evaluation Assessment
Speech-Sounds Perception Test
Spelling Grade Equivalent
Spelling Scale
Spielberger Anger-Out Scale
Spielberger Anxiety Inventory
Spielberger State-Trait Anger Expression Inventory
Spielberger State-Trait Anxiety Inventory
Spiritual Well-Being Scale (SWBS)
Spondee Picture Test (SPT)
S-R Inventory of Anxiousness
SRA Arithmetic Test
SRA Pictorial Reasoning Test
SRA Reading Test
SRA Verbal
St. George Anxiety Questionnaire
St. Paul-Ramsey Scale
Staff Burnout Scale for Health Professionals
Standard Progressive Matrices
Standardized Assessment of Depressive Disorders (SADD)
Standardized Clinical Outcome Rating Scale for Depression
Standardized Test of Computer Literacy (STCL)
Stanford Achievement Test (SAT)
Stanford Acute Stress Reaction Questionnaire
Stanford Diagnostic Arithmetic Test
Stanford Diagnostic Reading Test (SDRT)
Stanford Early School Achievement Test
Stanford Hypnotic Clinical Scale and Children
Stanford Hypnotic Susceptibility Scale (SHSS)
Stanford Sleepiness Scale
Stanford-Binet Intelligence Scale (SBIS)
Stanford-Binet Profile
Stanford-Binet Scale
Stanford-Binet Scale-Revised
Stanford-Binet Test
State Shame And Guilt Scale (SSGS)
State-Trait Anger Expression Inventory (STAXI)
State-Trait Anger Scale (STAS)
State-Trait Anxiety Index
State-Trait Anxiety Inventory (STAI)
State-Trait Anxiety Inventory for Children (STAIC)
State-Trait Anxiety Inventory for Stein Sentence Completion Test
State-Trait Personality Inventory (STPI)
Status Questionnaire
Stein Sentence Completion (SSC)
Stem Completion Test
Stephens Oral Language Screening Test (SOLST)
Stimulus Recognition Test
Stoelting Brief Intelligence Test (S-BIT)
Stone and Neale Daily Coping Assessment
Strauss and Carpenter Revised Outcome Criteria Scale
Strauss-Carpenter Scale
Street Survival Skills Questionnaire
Stress and Functionality Inventory

Stress Evaluation Inventory
Stress Impact Scale (SIS)
Stress Response Scale
Strong-Campbell Interest Inventory (SCII)
Stroop Color-Word Test
Stroop Color Interference Test
Stroop Color-Word Interference Test
Structure of Intellect Learning Abilities Test, From P
Structured and Scaled Interview to Assess Maladjustment (SSIAM)
Structured Clinical Interview for DSM-III-R (SCID)
Structured Clinical Interview for DSM-III-R Dissociative Disorders (SCID-D)
Structured Clinical Interview for DSM-III-R Non-Patient Edition (SCID-NP)
Structured Clinical Interview for DSM-III-R Personality Disorders (SCID-II)
Structured Clinical Interview for DSM-III-R Psychotic Disorders (SCID-PD)
Structured Clinical Interview for DSM-III-R Dissociative Disorders
Structured Clinical Interview for DSM-III-R Psychotic Disorders
Structured Clinical Interview for DSM-III-R-Patient Version (SCID-P)
Structured Clinical Interview for DSM-IV (SCID)
Structured Clinical Interview for DSM-IV Axis I Disorders: Clinician Version (SCID-CV)
Structured Clinical Interview for DSM-IV Axis II Personality Disorders (SCID-II)
Structured Clinical Interview for DSM-IV Dissociative Disorders (SCID-D)
Structured Clinical Interview for DSM-IV Patient Edition
Structured Clinical Interview for the Panic-Agoraphobic Spectrum
Structured Composite International Diagnostic Interview for Psychological Disorders
Structured Interview for Assessing Perceptual Anomalies
Structured Interview of Reported Symptoms (SIRS)
Structured Photographic Expressive Language Test-II (SPELT-P)
Structured Trauma Interview
Student Adaptation to College Questionnaire (SACQ)
Student Adjustment Inventory (SAI)
Student Opinion Inventory (SOI)
Student Reactions to College (SRC)
Student Talent and Risk Profile
STYCAR Hearing Test (SHT)
STYCAR Language Test (SLT)
STYCAR Vision Test (SVT)
Styles of Management Inventory
Style of Mind Inventory (SMI)
Subject Treatment Emergent Symptom Scale
Subjective High Assessment Scale
Subjective Opiate Withdrawal Scale (SOWS)
Subjective Response Questionnaire
Subjective Symptoms Scale
Subjective Treatment Emergent Side Effects Scale
Subjective Units of Distress Scale (SUDS)
Substance Abuse and Mental Health Administration (SAMHA)
Substance Abuse Problem Checklist
Substance Abuse Questionnaire (SAQ)
Substance Abuse Subtle Screening Inventory (SASSI)
Suicide Intent Scale
Suicide Intervention Response Inventory
Suicide Opinion Questionnaire (SOQ)
Suicide Probability Scale

Suicide Risk Scale
Suicide-Depression Proneness Checklist (SDPC)
Suinn Test Anxiety Behavior Scale (STABS)
Supervisory Practices Inventory
Supervisory Practices Test (SPT)
Supervisory Profile Record
Suprathreshold Adaptation Test (STAT)
Survey of School Attitudes
Survey of Study Habits and Attitudes (SSHA)
Surveys of Achievement
Survival and Coping Beliefs Scale (SCBS)
Swanson, Nolan, and Pelham Rating Scale
Swinging Story Test
Symbol Digit Modalities Test (SDMT)
Symbolic Play Test (SPT)
Symptom Checklist 90-Revised Global Severity Index
Symptom Checklist-90 (SCL)
Symptom Checklist-90-Revised (SCL-90-R)
Symptom Rating Scale (SRS)
Synthetic Sentence Identification Test
System for Testing and Evaluation of Potential
System of Multicultural Pluralistic Assessment (SOMPA)
Systematic Assessment for Treatment of Emergent Events (SAFTEE)
Tactile Finger Recognition Test (TFRT)
Tactile Form Recognition Test (TFRT)
Tactile Perception Test
Tactile Performance Test (TPT)
Taiwan Earthquake Experience Questionnaire
Talbieh Brief Distress Inventory (TBDI)
TARC Assessment System
Task Assessment Scale
Taylor Manifest Anxiety Scale (TMAS)
Taylor-Johnson Temperament Analysis
Teacher and Parent Separation Anxiety Rating Scales for Preschool Children
Teacher Assessment of Social Behavior (TASB)
Teacher Attitude Inventory
Teacher Evaluation Scale (TES)
Teacher Feedback Questionnaire
Teacher Inventory
Teacher Opinion Inventory
Teacher's School Readiness Inventory (TSRI)
Teacher Stress Inventory
Teaching Styles Inventory
Teen Addiction Severity Index (T-ASI)
Temperament and Character Inventory (TCI)
Temperament and Values Inventory
Temperament Assessment Battery for Children
Tennessee Self-Concept Scale (TSCS)
Test Anxiety Inventory (TAI)
Test Anxiety Profile
Test Anxiety Scale
Test for Auditory Comprehension of Language (TACL)
Tests for Auditory Comprehension of Language-Revised (TACL-R)
Test for Examining Expressive Morphology (TEEM)
Test of Adolescent Language (TOAL)
Test of Adolescent/Adult Word Finding (TAWF)
Test of Articulation Performance - Diagnostic (TAP-D)
Test of Articulation Performance, Screen (TAP-S)
Test of Attentional Style
Test of Attitude Toward School (TAS)
Test of Auditory Discrimination (TAD)
Test of Cognitive Style in Mathematics (TCSM)
Test of Concept Utilization (TCU)

Test of Creative Potential
Test of Early Language Development (TELD)
Test of Early Language Development, Second Edition (TELD-2)
Test of Early Mathematics Ability, Second Edition (TEMA-2)
Test of Early Reading Ability, Second Edition (TERA-2)
Test of Early Written Language, Second Edition (TEWL-2)
Test of Economic Literacy (TEL)
Test of Functional Health Literacy in Adults (TOFHLA)
Test of Kindergarten/First Grade Readiness Skills (TKFGRS)
Test of Language Competence (TLC)
Test of Language Competence for Children (TLC-C)
Test of Language Development-Intermediate, Second Edition (TOLD-I:2)
Test of Language Development-Primary, Second Edition (TOLD-P:2)
Test of Language Development (TOLD)
Test of Listening Accuracy in Children (TLAC)
Test of Memory and Learning (TOMAL)
Test of Memory Malingering (TOMM)
Test of Nonverbal Auditory Discrimination (TENVAD)
Test of Nonverbal Intelligence (TONI)
Test of Nonverbal Intelligence-3 (TONI-3)
Test of Pragmatic Language (TOPL)
Test of Problem Solving
Test of Social Inferences (TSI)
Test of Variables of Attention
Test of Visual Motor Integration
Test of Visual Perception
Test of Word Finding (TWF)
Test of Word Finding in Discourse (TWFD)
Test of Work Competency and Stability (TWCS)
Test of Written Language (TOWL)
Test of Written Language-3 (TOWL-3)
Test of Written Spelling
Tests of Fundamental Abilities in Visual Art
Tests of Mechanical Comprehension
Tests of Perception of Scientists and Self (TOPOSS)
Texas Revised Inventory of Grief
Thackray Reading Readiness Profile (TRRP)
Thematic Apperception Test (TAT)
Thematic Aptitude Test (TAT)
This I Believe Test (TIB)
Thorndike Handwriting Scale
Thought Disorder Index
Three-Minute Reasoning Test
Three-Dimensional Block Construction Test
Three-Factor Eating Questionnaire
Three-Item Delirium Scale
Thurstone Scale
Thurstone Attitude Scale
Thurstone Interest Schedule
Thurstone Temperament Schedule
Time and Change Test
Time Perception Inventory
Time Problems Inventory
Time Sense Test
Time-Sample Behavioral Checklist, The (TSBC)
Time Use Analyzer
Timed Stereotypes Rating Scale
Tinker Toy Test
TLC-Learning Preference Inventory
TOEFL Test of Written English
Token Test for Aphasia, The
Token Test for Children, The

Token Test for Receptive Disturbances in Aphasia
Tomkins-Horn Picture Arrangement Test
Toronto Alexithymia Scale (TAS)
Toronto Functional Capacity Questionnaire (TFCQ)
Torrance Tests of Creative Thinking (TTCT)
Tourette Syndrome Global Scale
Tourette Syndrome Questionnaire
Tourette Syndrome Severity Scale
Tower of Hanoi Test
Tower of Hanoi Puzzle
Tower of Toronto Test
Trail Making Test
Trainer's Assessment of Proficiency (TAP)
Trait Evaluation Index
Transition Behavior Scale (TBS)
Transitional Object Questionnaire
trauma Assessment for Adults-Self Report
Trauma Symptom Checklist for Children Ages 8–15
Traumatic Antecedents Questionnaire
Treatment Appraisal Questionnaire
Tridimensional Personality Questionnaire (TPQ)
Trier Social Stress Test (TSST)
Trites Neuropsychological Test Battery
Twenty Statements Test (TST)

Unified Huntington Disease Rating Scale
Unified Psychogeriatric Biopsychosocial Evaluation and Treatment (UPBEAT)
Unpleasant Events Schedule (UES)
Utah Test of Language Development (UTLD)
Uzgiris-Hunt Scale

Validity Indicator Profile
Valpar Work Sample Battery
Values Inventory
Values Inventory for Children (VIC)
Vane Evaluation of Language Scale (VELS)
Verbal and Oral Language Ability
Verbal Fluency Test
Verbal Language Development Scale
Verbal Meaning Test
Verbal Scale Scores
Verbal Subtest
Verbal-Auditory Screen for Children (VASC)
Verbalizer-Visualization Questionnaire (VVQ)
Verdun Depression Rating Scale (VDRS)
Verdun Target Symptom Rating Scale (VTSRS)
Vigotsky Concept Formation Test, Modified
Vigotsky Test
Vineland Adaptive Behavior Scale
Vineland Social Maturity Scale (VSMS)
Visual Analogue Scales
Visual Form Discrimination Test (VFDT)
Visual Motor Test
Visual Neglect Test
Visual Pattern Completion Test
Visual Perception Test
Visual Retention Test
Visual Search and Attention Test (VSAT)
Visual Subtest
Visual-Auditory Screen for Children (VASC)
Visual-Motor Gestalt Test (VMGT)
Visual-Motor Integration Test (VMIT)
Visual-Motor Sequencing Test (VMST)
Vocabulary Comprehension Scale

Vocational Apperception Test (VAT)
Vocational Evaluation and Work Adjustment (VEWA)
Vocational Interest and Sophistication Assessment (VISA)
Vocational Interest Inventory
Vocational Interest Inventory and Exploration Survey
Vocational Interest Questionnaire (VIQ)
Vocational Interest, Experience, and Skill Assessment (VIESA)
Vocational Opinion Index (VOI)
Vocational Planning Inventory (VPI)
Vocational Preference Inventory (VPI)
Voc-Tech Quick Screener (VTQS)
von Zerssen Self-Rating Scale
Vulpe Assessment Battery-Revised
Wahler Physical Symptoms Inventory
Wahler Self-Description Inventory (WSDI)
WAIS-R Block Design Test
Wakefield Self-Assessment Depression Inventory
Waldrop Scale
Walker-McConnell Scale of Social Competence and School Adjustment
War Zone Exposure Subscale
Ward Atmosphere Scale (WAS)
Ward Behavior Rating Scale (WBRS)
Waring Intimacy Questionnaire (WIQ)
Washington Psychosocial Seizure Inventory
Washington Speech Sound Discrimination Test (WSSDT)
Washington University Sentence Completion Test (WUSCT)
Watson-Glaser Critical Thinking Appraisal (WGCTA)
Watts-Vernon Reading Test
Way of Coping Checklist (WOC)
Ways of Coping Scale
Weak Opiate Withdrawal Scale (WOWS)
Wechsler Adult Intelligence Scale (WAIS)
Wechsler Adult Intelligence Scale-Revised
Wechsler Adult Intelligence Test-Revised-Hong Kong Version
Wechsler Individual Achievement Test (WIAT)
Wechsler Individual Achievement Test, Second Edition (WIAT-II)
Wechsler Intelligence Scale
Wechsler Intelligence Scale for Children (WISC)
Wechsler Intelligence Scale for Children–Revised (WISC-R)
Wechsler Intelligence Scale for Children-Revised Version and Version III
Wechsler IQ Scale
Wechsler Memory Scale (WMS)
Wechsler Memory Scale, Russell Version
Wechsler Memory Scale, Standard and Russell Versions
Wechsler Memory Scale/Memory Quotient (WMS-MQ)
Wechsler Preschool Primary Scale of Intelligence (WPPSI)
Wechsler-Bellevue Scale (WBS)
Weiss Comprehensive Articulation Test
Weiss Intelligibility Test
Weller-Strawser Scales of Adaptive Behavior for the Learning Disabled
Welsh Figure Preference Test
Wender Utah Rating Scale
Wepman Auditory Discrimination Test
Wesman Personnel Classification Test
Western Aphasia Battery (WAB)
Western Personality Inventory

What I Like to Do: An Inventory of Students' Interest (WILD)
Wheatley Stress Profile
Whitaker Index of Schizophrenic Thinking (WIST)
White Bear Suppression Inventory
Who Are You? Test
WHO Handicap Scale
Wide Range Achievement Test, The (WRAT)
Wide Range Achievement Test-Revised, The (WRAT-R)
Wide Range Achievement Test, Third Edition, The (WRAT-3)
Wide Range Assessment of Memory and Learning, The (WRAML)
Wide Range Employment Sample Test, The (WREST)
Wide Range Intelligence and Personality Test, The (WRIPT)
Wide Range Interest-Opinion Test, The (WRIOT)
Wide Range Vocabulary Test
Wiggins Content Scale (WCS)
Wiggly Block Test, The
Wilson-Patterson Attitude Inventory (WPAI)
Wing Negative Symptom Scale
WISC-III Companion
Wisconsin Card-Sorting Test (WCST)
Wisconsin Motor Battery
Wisconsin Psychosocial Pain Inventory
Wisconsin Scoring Test
Within Session Rating Scale for Cocaine
Wittenborn Psychiatric Rating Scale (WITT)
Wittenborn Psychiatric Rating Scale Test
Wonderlic Personnel Test (WPT)
Wood Assessment Scale
Woodcock Language Proficiency Battery
Woodcock Reading Mastery Test
Woodcock-Johnson Achievement Test (WJAT)
Woodcock-Johnson Psycho-Educational Battery-Revised (WJPB-R)
Word Association Test
Word Finding Test
Word Fluency Test
Word Intelligibility by Picture Identification (WIPI)
Word Processing Test
Word Processor Assessment Battery
Word Recognition Test
Word-in-Context Test
Wordlist Learning Test
Work and Social Adjustment Scale
Work Attitudes Questionnaire (WAQ)
Work Behavior Inventory
Work Environment Preference Schedule (WEPS)
Work Environment Scale (WES)
Work Information Inventory (WII)
Work, Home, and Leisure Activities Scale
Work Interest Index
Work Motivation Inventory (WMI)
Work Personality Profile
Work Sample Battery
Work Values Inventory (WVI)
World of Work Inventory (WWI)
World Health Organization Composite International Diagnostic Interview
World Health Organization Quality of Life – BREF (WHOQOL-BREF)
Worry Scale for Children
Worse Premorbid Adjustment Scale
Wortman Social Support Scale
Writing Skills Test
Written Language Assessment

Yale-Brown Obsessive-Compulsive Scale (Y-BOCS)
Yale-Brown Obsessive Compulsive Scale, Modified for Pathological Gambling (PG-YBOCS)
Yale Global Tic Severity Scale
Yale Revised Developmental Schedule
Yale Schedule for Tourette Syndrome and Other Behavioral Disorders
Yale Schedule for Tourette Syndrome and Other Behavioral Disorders, Hebrew Version
Yale Tic Severity Scale
Yale-Brown Obsessive Compulsive Scale (YBOCS)
Young Adult Behavior Checklist
Young Mania Rating Scale (YMRS)
Ziegler Mania Rating Scale
Zung Anxiety Scale
Zung Depression Scale (ZDS)
Zung Self-Rating Anxiety Scale
Zung Self-Rating Depression Scale

Drugs by Indication

ACETAMINOPHEN POISONING

Mucolytic Agent
- Acetadote® (US)
- acetylcysteine
- Mucomyst® (US/Can)
- Parvolex® (Can)

ALCOHOLISM TREATMENT

Aldehyde Dehydrogenase Inhibitor Agent
- Antabuse® (US)
- disulfiram

Antidote
- naltrexone
- ReVia® (US/Can)

ALCOHOL WITHDRAWAL (TREATMENT)

Alpha-Adrenergic Agonist
- Apo-Clonidine® (Can)
- Catapres® (US)
- clonidine
- Dixarit® (Can)
- Duraclon™ (US)
- Novo-Clonidine (Can)
- Nu-Clonidine® (Can)

Antihistamine
- Apo-Hydroxyzine® (Can)
- Atarax® (US/Can)
- hydroxyzine
- Novo-Hydroxyzin (Can)
- PMS-Hydroxyzine (Can)
- Vistaril® (US/Can)

Benzodiazepine
- alprazolam
- Alprazolam Intensol® (US)
- Alti-Alprazolam (Can)
- Apo-Alpraz® (Can)
- Apo-Chlordiazepoxide® (Can)
- Apo-Clorazepate® (Can)
- Apo-Diazepam® (Can)
- Apo-Oxazepam® (Can)
- chlordiazepoxide
- clorazepate
- Diastat® (US/Can)
- Diazemuls® (Can)
- diazepam
- Diazepam Intensol® (US)
- Gen-Alprazolam (Can)
- Librium® (US)
- Novo-Alprazol (Can)
- Novo-Clopate (Can)
- Novoxapram® (Can)
- Nu-Alprax (Can)
- oxazepam
- Oxpram® (Can)
- PMS-Oxazepam (Can)
- Serax® (US)
- Tranxene® SD™-Half Strength (US)
- Tranxene® SD™ (US)
- Tranxene® (US)
- T-Tab® (US)
- Valium® (US/Can)
- Xanax TS™ (Can)
- Xanax® (US/Can)
- Xanax XR® (US)

Beta-Adrenergic Blocker
- Apo-Atenol® (Can)
- Apo-Propranolol® (Can)
- atenolol
- Gen-Atenolol (Can)
- Inderal® LA (US/Can)
- Inderal® (US/Can)
- InnoPran XL™ (US)
- Novo-Atenol (Can)
- Nu-Atenol (Can)

Nu-Propranolol (Can)
PMS-Atenolol (Can)
propranolol
Propranolol Intensol™ (US)
Rhoxal-atenolol (Can)
Tenolin (Can)
Tenormin® (US/Can)

ALZHEIMER DISEASE

Acetylcholinesterase Inhibitor
- Aricept® (US/Can)
- Cognex® (US)
- donepezil
- Exelon® (US/Can)
- rivastigmine
- tacrine

Acetylcholinesterase Inhibitor (Central)
- galantamine
- Reminyl® (US/Can)

Cholinergic Agent
- Exelon® (US/Can)
- rivastigmine

Ergot Alkaloid and Derivative
- ergoloid mesylates
- Hydergine® (Can)

N-Methyl-D-Aspartate Receptor Antagonist
- memantine
- Namenda™ (US)

AMMONIA INTOXICATION

Ammonium Detoxicant
- Acilac (Can)
- Apo-Lactulose® (Can)
- Cholac® (US)
- Constilac® (US)
- Constulose® (US)
- Enulose® (US)
- Generlac® (US)
- Kristalose™ (US)
- lactulose
- Laxilose (Can)
- PMS-Lactulose (Can)

ANTIFREEZE POISONING

Antidote
- Antizol® (US)
- fomepizole

ANXIETY

Antianxiety Agent
- Apo-Buspirone® (Can)
- BuSpar® (US/Can)
- Buspirex (Can)
- buspirone
- Gen-Buspirone (Can)
- Lin-Buspirone (Can)
- Novo-Buspirone (Can)
- Nu-Buspirone (Can)
- PMS-Buspirone (Can)

Antianxiety Agent, Miscellaneous
- meprobamate
- Miltown® (US)
- Novo-Mepro (Can)

Antidepressant/Phenothiazine
- amitriptyline and perphenazine
- Etrafon® (Can)
- Triavil® (US/Can)

Antidepressant, Tetracyclic
- maprotiline
- Novo-Maprotiline (Can)

Antidepressant, Tricyclic (Secondary Amine)
- amoxapine

Antidepressant, Tricyclic (Tertiary Amine)
- amitriptyline and chlordiazepoxide
- Apo-Doxepin® (Can)
- doxepin
- Limbitrol® DS (US)
- Limbitrol® (US/Can)
- Novo-Doxepin (Can)
- Prudoxin™ (US)
- Sinequan® (US/Can)
- Zonalon® (US/Can)

Antihistamine
- Aler-Dryl (US-OTC)

Allerdryl® (Can)
AllerMax® (US-OTC)
Allernix (Can)
Apo-Hydroxyzine® (Can)
Atarax® (US/Can)
Banophen® (US-OTC)
Benadryl® Allergy (US-OTC/Can)
Benadryl® Dye-Free Allergy (US-OTC)
Benadryl® Gel Extra Strength (US-OTC)
Benadryl® Gel (US-OTC)
Benadryl® Injection (US)
Compoz® Nighttime Sleep Aid (US-OTC)
Diphen® AF (US-OTC)
Diphen® Cough (US-OTC)
Diphenhist (US-OTC)
diphenhydramine
Diphen® (US-OTC)
Genahist® (US-OTC)
Hydramine® Cough (US-OTC)
Hydramine® (US-OTC)
hydroxyzine
Hyrexin-50® (US)
Novo-Hydroxyzin (Can)
Nytol® Extra Strength (Can)
Nytol® Maximum Strength (US-OTC)
Nytol® (US-OTC/Can)
PMS-Diphenhydramine (Can)
PMS-Hydroxyzine (Can)
Siladryl® Allergy (US-OTC)
Silphen® (US-OTC)
Simply Sleep® (Can)
Sleepinal® (US-OTC)
Sominex® Maximum Strength (US-OTC)
Sominex® (US-OTC)
Tusstat® (US)
Twilite® (US-OTC)
Unisom® Maximum Strength SleepGels® (US-OTC)
Vistaril® (US/Can)

Barbiturate
butabarbital sodium
butalbital, aspirin, caffeine, and codeine
Butisol Sodium® (US)
Fiorinal®-C 1/2 (Can)
Fiorinal®-C 1/4 (Can)
Fiorinal® With Codeine (US)
Phrenilin® With Caffeine and Codeine (US)
Tecnal C 1/2 (Can)
Tecnal C 1/4 (Can)

Benzodiazepine
alprazolam
Alprazolam Intensol® (US)
Alti-Alprazolam (Can)
Apo-Alpraz® (Can)
Apo-Bromazepam® (Can)
Apo-Chlordiazepoxide® (Can)
Apo-Clorazepate® (Can)
Apo-Diazepam® (Can)
Apo-Lorazepam® (Can)
Apo-Oxazepam® (Can)
Apo-Temazepam® (Can)
Ativan® (US/Can)
bromazepam (Canada only)
chlordiazepoxide
clorazepate
CO Temazepam (Can)
Diastat® (US/Can)
Diazemuls® (Can)
diazepam
Diazepam Intensol® (US)
Gen-Alprazolam (Can)
Gen-Bromazepam (Can)
Gen-Temazepam (Can)
Lectopam® (Can)
Librium® (US)
lorazepam
Lorazepam Intensol® (US)
Novo-Alprazol (Can)
Novo-Bromazepam (Can)

Novo-Clopate (Can)
Novo-Lorazem® (Can)
Novo-Temazepam (Can)
Novoxapram® (Can)
Nu-Alprax (Can)
Nu-Bromazepam (Can)
Nu-Loraz (Can)
Nu-Temazepam (Can)
oxazepam
Oxpram® (Can)
PMS-Lorazepam (Can)
PMS-Oxazepam (Can)
PMS-Temazepam (Can)
ratio-Temazepam (Can)
Restoril® (US/Can)
Riva-Lorazepam (Can)
Serax® (US)
temazepam
Tranxene® SD™-Half Strength (US)
Tranxene® SD™ (US)
Tranxene® (US)
T-Tab® (US)
Valium® (US/Can)
Xanax TS™ (Can)
Xanax® (US/Can)
Xanax XR® (US)

General Anesthetic
Actiq® (US/Can)
Duragesic® (US/Can)
fentanyl
Sublimaze® (US)

Neuroleptic Agent
Apo-Methoprazine® (Can)
methotrimeprazine (Canada only)
Novo-Meprazine (Can)
Nozinan® (Can)

Phenothiazine Derivative
Apo-Trifluoperazine® (Can)
Novo-Trifluzine (Can)
PMS-Trifluoperazine (Can)
Terfluzine (Can)
trifluoperazine

Sedative
Apo-Bromazepam® (Can)
bromazepam (Canada only)
Gen-Bromazepam (Can)
Lectopam® (Can)
Novo-Bromazepam (Can)
Nu-Bromazepam (Can)

ARSENIC POISONING

Chelating Agent
BAL in Oil® (US)
dimercaprol

ATTENTION DEFICIT HYPERACTIVITY DISORDER (ADHD)

Amphetamine
Adderall® (US)
Adderall XR™ (US)
Desoxyn® (US/Can)
Dexedrine® (US/Can)
dextroamphetamine
dextroamphetamine and amphetamine
Dextrostat® (US)
methamphetamine

Central Nervous System Stimulant, Nonamphetamine
Concerta® (US/Can)
Cylert® (US)
dexmethylphenidate
Focalin™ (US)
Metadate® CD (US)
Metadate™ ER (US)
Methylin™ ER (US)
Methylin™ (US)
methylphenidate
PemADD® CT (US)
PemADD® (US)
pemoline
PMS-Methylphenidate (Can)
Ritalin® LA (US)

Ritalin-SR® (US/Can)
Ritalin® (US/Can)
Norepinephrine Reuptake Inhibitor, Selective
atomoxetine
Strattera™ (US)

AUTISM

Antidepressant, Selective Serotonin Reuptake Inhibitor
Alti-Fluoxetine (Can)
Apo-Fluoxetine® (Can)
CO Fluoxetine (Can)
fluoxetine
FXT® (Can)
Gen-Fluoxetine (Can)
Novo-Fluoxetine (Can)
Nu-Fluoxetine (Can)
PMS-Fluoxetine (Can)
Prozac® (US/Can)
Prozac® Weekly™ (US)
Rhoxal-fluoxetine (Can)
Sarafem™ (US)
Antipsychotic Agent, Butyrophenone
Apo-Haloperidol® (Can)
Apo-Haloperidol LA® (Can)
Haldol® Decanoate (US)
Haldol® (US)
haloperidol
Haloperidol-LA Omega (Can)
Haloperidol Long Acting (Can)
Novo-Peridol (Can)
Peridol (Can)
PMS-Haloperidol LA (Can)

BARBITURATE POISONING

Antidote
Actidose-Aqua® (US-OTC)
Actidose® with Sorbitol (US-OTC)
Carcocaps® (US-OTC)
Charcadole® Aqueous (Can)
Charcadole® (Can)
Charcadole® TFS (Can)
CharcoAid® G (US-OTC)
charcoal
Charcoal Plus® DS (US-OTC)
EZ-Char™ (US-OTC)
Kerr Insta-Char® (US-OTC)

BENZODIAZEPINE OVERDOSE

Antidote
Anexate® (Can)
flumazenil
Romazicon® (US/Can)

BIPOLAR DEPRESSION DISORDER

Anticonvulsant
Alti-Divalproex (Can)
Apo-Divalproex® (Can)
Depacon® (US)
Depakene® (US/Can)
Depakote® Delayed Release (US)
Depakote® ER (US)
Depakote® Sprinkle® (US)
Epival® ER (Can)
Epival® I.V. (Can)
Gen-Divalproex (Can)
Novo-Divalproex (Can)
Nu-Divalproex (Can)
PMS-Valproic Acid (Can)
PMS-Valproic Acid E.C. (Can)
Rhoxal-valproic (Can)
valproic acid and derivatives
Antimanic Agent
Apo-Lithium® (Can)
Carbolith™ (Can)
Duralith® (Can)
Eskalith CR® (US)
Eskalith® (US)
Lithane™ (Can)
lithium
Lithobid® (US)
PMS-Lithium Carbonate (Can)
PMS-Lithium Citrate (Can)

Antipsychotic Agent
Clopixol-Acuphase® (Can)
Clopixol® (Can)
Clopixol® Depot (Can)
zuclopenthixol (Canada only)

BROMIDE INTOXICATION

Diuretic, Loop
Edecrin® (US/Can)
ethacrynic acid

CACHEXIA

Progestin
Apo-Megestrol® (Can)
Lin-Megestrol (Can)
Megace® OS (US)
Megace® (US/Can)
megestrol acetate
Nu-Megestrol (Can)

CURARE POISONING

Cholinergic Agent
edrophonium
Enlon® (US/Can)
Reversol® (US)

CYANIDE POISONING

Antidote
Cyanide Antidote Package
methylene blue
sodium nitrite, sodium thiosulfate, and amyl nitrite
sodium thiosulfate
Vasodilator
amyl nitrite

DEMENTIA

Acetylcholinesterase Inhibitor
Aricept® (US/Can)
donepezil
Antidepressant, Tricyclic (Tertiary Amine)
Apo-Doxepin® (Can)
doxepin
Novo-Doxepin (Can)
Prudoxin™ (US)
Sinequan® (US/Can)
Zonalon® (US/Can)
Benzodiazepine
Apo-Diazepam® (Can)
Diastat® (US/Can)
Diazemuls® (Can)
diazepam
Diazepam Intensol® (US)
Valium® (US/Can)
Ergot Alkaloid and Derivative
ergoloid mesylates
Hydergine® (Can)

DEPRESSION

Antidepressant
Celexa™ (US/Can)
citalopram
Antidepressant, Alpha-2 Antagonist
mirtazapine
Remeron® SolTab® (US)
Remeron® (US/Can)
Antidepressant, Aminoketone
bupropion
Wellbutrin SR® (US)
Wellbutrin® (US/Can)
Wellbutrin XL™ (US)
Antidepressant, Miscellaneous
Apo-Nefazodone® (Can)
nefazodone
Antidepressant, Monoamine Oxidase Inhibitor
Alti-Moclobemide (Can)
Apo-Moclobemide® (Can)
isocarboxazid
Manerix® (Can)
Marplan® (US)
moclobemide (Canada only)
Nardil® (US/Can)

Novo-Moclobemide (Can)
Nu-Moclobemide (Can)
Parnate® (US/Can)
phenelzine
PMS-Moclobemide (Can)
tranylcypromine

Antidepressant, Phenethylamine
Effexor® (US/Can)
Effexor® XR (US/Can)
venlafaxine

Antidepressant/Phenothiazine
amitriptyline and perphenazine
Etrafon® (Can)
Triavil® (US/Can)

Antidepressant, Selective Serotonin Reuptake Inhibitor
Alti-Fluoxetine (Can)
Alti-Fluvoxamine (Can)
Apo-Fluoxetine® (Can)
Apo-Fluvoxamine® (Can)
Apo-Sertraline® (Can)
CO Fluoxetine (Can)
escitalopram
fluoxetine
fluvoxamine
FXT® (Can)
Gen-Fluoxetine (Can)
Gen-Sertraline (Can)
Lexapro™ (US)
Luvox® (Can)
Novo-Fluoxetine (Can)
Novo-Fluvoxamine (Can)
Novo-Sertraline (Can)
Nu-Fluoxetine (Can)
Nu-Fluvoxamine (Can)
Nu-Sertraline (Can)
olanzapine and fluoxetine
paroxetine
Paxil® CR™ (US/Can)
Paxil® (US/Can)
Pexeva™ (US)
PMS-Fluoxetine (Can)
PMS-Fluvoxamine (Can)
PMS-Sertraline (Can)
Prozac® (US/Can)
Prozac® Weekly™ (US)
ratio-Sertraline (Can)
Rhoxal-fluoxetine (Can)
Rhoxal-fluvoxamine (Can)
Rhoxal-sertraline (Can)
Sarafem™ (US)
sertraline
Symbyax™ (US)
Zoloft® (US/Can)

Antidepressant, Tetracyclic
maprotiline
Novo-Maprotiline (Can)

Antidepressant, Triazolopyridine
Alti-Trazodone (Can)
Apo-Trazodone® (Can)
Apo-Trazodone D®
Desyrel® (US/Can)
Gen-Trazodone (Can)
Novo-Trazodone (Can)
Nu-Trazodone (Can)
PMS-Trazodone (Can)
trazodone

Antidepressant, Tricyclic (Secondary Amine)
Alti-Desipramine (Can)
Alti-Nortriptyline (Can)
amoxapine
Apo-Desipramine® (Can)
Apo-Nortriptyline® (Can)
Aventyl® (Can)
Aventyl® HCl (US)
desipramine
Gen-Nortriptyline (Can)
Norpramin® (US/Can)
nortriptyline
Norventyl (Can)
Novo-Desipramine (Can)
Novo-Nortriptyline (Can)
Nu-Desipramine (Can)
Nu-Nortriptyline (Can)
Pamelor® (US)

PMS-Desipramine
PMS-Nortriptyline (Can)
protriptyline
Vivactil® (US)

Antidepressant, Tricyclic (Tertiary Amine)
amitriptyline
amitriptyline and chlordiazepoxide
Apo-Amitriptyline® (Can)
Apo-Doxepin® (Can)
Apo-Imipramine® (Can)
Apo-Trimip® (Can)
doxepin
imipramine
Levate® (Can)
Limbitrol® DS (US)
Limbitrol® (US/Can)
Novo-Doxepin (Can)
Novo-Tripramine (Can)
Nu-Trimipramine (Can)
PMS-Amitriptyline (Can)
Prudoxin™ (US)
Rhotrimine® (Can)
Sinequan® (US/Can)
Surmontil® (US/Can)
Tofranil-PM® (US)
Tofranil® (US/Can)
trimipramine
Zonalon® (US/Can)

Antipsychotic Agent, Thienobenzodiaepine
olanzapine and fluoxetine
Symbyax™ (US)

Benzodiazepine
alprazolam
Alprazolam Intensol® (US)
Alti-Alprazolam (Can)
Apo-Alpraz® (Can)
Gen-Alprazolam (Can)
Novo-Alprazol (Can)
Nu-Alprax (Can)
Xanax TS™ (Can)
Xanax® (US/Can)
Xanax XR® (US)

DRUG DEPENDENCE (OPIOID)

Analgesic, Narcotic
Dolophine® (US/Can)
Metadol™ (Can)
methadone
Methadone Intensol™ (US)
Methadose® (US/Can)

INSOMNIA

Antihistamine
Aler-Dryl (US-OTC)
Allerdryl® (Can)
AllerMax® (US-OTC)
Allernix (Can)
Apo-Hydroxyzine® (Can)
Atarax® (US/Can)
Banophen® (US-OTC)
Benadryl® Allergy (US-OTC/Can)
Benadryl® Dye-Free Allergy (US-OTC)
Benadryl® Injection (US)
Compoz® Nighttime Sleep Aid (US-OTC)
Diphen® AF (US-OTC)
Diphenhist (US-OTC)
diphenhydramine
Diphen® (US-OTC)
doxylamine
Genahist® (US-OTC)
Hydramine® (US-OTC)
hydroxyzine
Hyrexin-50® (US)
Novo-Hydroxyzin (Can)
Nytol® Extra Strength (Can)
Nytol® Maximum Strength (US-OTC)
Nytol® (US-OTC/Can)
PMS-Diphenhydramine (Can)
PMS-Hydroxyzine (Can)
Siladryl® Allergy (US-OTC)
Silphen® (US-OTC)
Simply Sleep® (Can)

Sleepinal® (US-OTC)
Sominex® Maximum Strength (US-OTC)
Sominex® (US-OTC)
Tusstat® (US)
Twilite® (US-OTC)
Unisom® Maximum Strength SleepGels® (US-OTC)
Vistaril® (US/Can)

Barbiturate
amobarbital
amobarbital and secobarbital
Amytal® (US/Can)
butabarbital sodium
Butisol Sodium® (US)
Luminal® Sodium (US)
Nembutal® Sodium (Can)
Nembutal® (US)
pentobarbital
phenobarbital
PMS-Phenobarbital (Can)
secobarbital
Seconal® (US)

Benzodiazepine
Apo-Diazepam® (Can)
Apo-Flurazepam® (Can)
Apo-Lorazepam® (Can)
Apo-Temazepam® (Can)
Apo-Triazo® (Can)
Ativan® (US/Can)
CO Temazepam (Can)
Dalmane® (US/Can)
Diastat® (US/Can)
Diazemuls® (Can)
diazepam
Diazepam Intensol® (US)
Doral® (US/Can)
estazolam
flurazepam
Gen-Temazepam (Can)
Gen-Triazolam (Can)
Halcion® (US/Can)
lorazepam
Lorazepam Intensol® (US)
nitrazepam (Canada only)
Novo-Lorazem® (Can)
Novo-Temazepam (Can)
Nu-Loraz (Can)
Nu-Temazepam (Can)
PMS-Lorazepam (Can)
PMS-Temazepam (Can)
ProSom™ (US)
quazepam
ratio-Temazepam (Can)
Restoril® (US/Can)
Riva-Lorazepam (Can)
temazepam
triazolam
Valium® (US/Can)

Hypnotic
Alti-Zopiclone (Can)
Apo-Zopiclone® (Can)
Gen-Zopiclone (Can)
Imovane® (Can)
Nu-Zopiclone (Can)
Rhovane® (Can)
zopiclone (Canada only)

Hypnotic, Nonbarbiturate
Ambien® (US/Can)
Aquachloral® Supprettes® (US)
chloral hydrate
PMS-Chloral Hydrate (Can)
Somnote™ (US)
zolpidem

Hypnotic, Nonbenzodiazepine (Pyrazolopyrimidine)
Sonata® (US/Can)
Starnoc® (Can)
zaleplon

IRON POISONING

Antidote
deferoxamine
Desferal® (US/Can)
PMS-Deferoxamine (Can)

MANIA

Anticonvulsant
- Alti-Divalproex (Can)
- Apo-Divalproex® (Can)
- Depacon® (US)
- Depakene® (US/Can)
- Depakote® Delayed Release (US)
- Depakote® ER (US)
- Depakote® Sprinkle® (US)
- Epival® ER (Can)
- Epival® I.V. (Can)
- Gen-Divalproex (Can)
- Novo-Divalproex (Can)
- Nu-Divalproex (Can)
- PMS-Valproic Acid (Can)
- PMS-Valproic Acid E.C. (Can)
- Rhoxal-valproic (Can)
- valproic acid and derivatives

Antimanic Agent
- Apo-Lithium® (Can)
- Carbolith™ (Can)
- Duralith® (Can)
- Eskalith CR® (US)
- Eskalith® (US)
- Lithane™ (Can)
- lithium
- Lithobid® (US)
- PMS-Lithium Carbonate (Can)
- PMS-Lithium Citrate (Can)

Phenothiazine Derivative
- Apo-Chlorpromazine® (Can)
- chlorpromazine
- Largactil® (Can)
- Novo-Chlorpromazine (Can)

METHANOL POISONING

Pharmaceutical Aid
- alcohol (ethyl)

METHOTREXATE POISONING

Folic Acid Derivative
- leucovorin

MUSCARINE POISONING

Anticholinergic Agent
- atropine

NARCOTIC DETOXIFICATION

Analgesic, Narcotic
- Dolophine® (US/Can)
- Metadol™ (Can)
- methadone
- Methadone Intensol™ (US)
- Methadose® (US/Can)

OBSESSIVE-COMPULSIVE DISORDER (OCD)

Antidepressant, Selective Serotonin Reuptake Inhibitor
- Alti-Fluoxetine (Can)
- Alti-Fluvoxamine (Can)
- Apo-Fluoxetine® (Can)
- Apo-Fluvoxamine® (Can)
- Apo-Sertraline® (Can)
- CO Fluoxetine (Can)
- fluoxetine
- fluvoxamine
- FXT® (Can)
- Gen-Fluoxetine (Can)
- Gen-Sertraline (Can)
- Luvox® (Can)
- Novo-Fluoxetine (Can)
- Novo-Fluvoxamine (Can)
- Novo-Sertraline (Can)
- Nu-Fluoxetine (Can)
- Nu-Fluvoxamine (Can)
- Nu-Sertraline (Can)
- paroxetine
- Paxil® CR™ (US/Can)
- Paxil® (US/Can)
- Pexeva™ (US)
- PMS-Fluoxetine (Can)
- PMS-Fluvoxamine (Can)
- PMS-Sertraline (Can)
- Prozac® (US/Can)

Prozac® Weekly™ (US)
ratio-Sertraline (Can)
Rhoxal-fluoxetine (Can)
Rhoxal-fluvoxamine (Can)
Rhoxal-sertraline (Can)
Sarafem™ (US)
sertraline
Zoloft® (US/Can)

Antidepressant, Tricyclic (Tertiary Amine)
Anafranil® (US/Can)
Apo-Clomipramine® (Can)
clomipramine
CO Clomipramine (Can)
Gen-Clomipramine (Can)
Novo-Clopramine (Can)

OPIOID POISONING

Antidote
nalmefene
naloxone
naltrexone
Narcan® (US/Can)
Revex® (US)
ReVia® (US/Can)

PANIC ATTACKS

Benzodiazepine
alprazolam
Alprazolam Intensol® (US)
Alti-Alprazolam (Can)
Apo-Alpraz® (Can)
Apo-Temazepam® (Can)
CO Temazepam (Can)
Gen-Alprazolam (Can)
Gen-Temazepam (Can)
Novo-Alprazol (Can)
Novo-Temazepam (Can)
Nu-Alprax (Can)
Nu-Temazepam (Can)
PMS-Temazepam (Can)
ratio-Temazepam (Can)
Restoril® (US/Can)
temazepam
Xanax TS™ (Can)
Xanax® (US/Can)
Xanax XR® (US)

PANIC DISORDER (PD)

Antidepressant, Selective Serotonin Reuptake Inhibitor
paroxetine
Paxil® CR™ (US/Can)
Paxil® (US/Can)
Pexeva™ (US)

PREMENSTRUAL DYSPHORIC DISORDER (PMDD)

Antidepressant, Selective Serotonin Reuptake Inhibitor
Alti-Fluoxetine (Can)
Apo-Fluoxetine® (Can)
CO Fluoxetine (Can)
fluoxetine
FXT® (Can)
Gen-Fluoxetine (Can)
Novo-Fluoxetine (Can)
Nu-Fluoxetine (Can)
PMS-Fluoxetine (Can)
Prozac® (US/Can)
Prozac® Weekly™ (US)
Rhoxal-fluoxetine (Can)
Sarafem™ (US)

PSYCHOSES

Antipsychotic Agent
Clopixol-Acuphase® (Can)
Clopixol® (Can)
Clopixol® Depot (Can)
olanzapine
quetiapine
Seroquel® (US/Can)
zuclopenthixol (Canada only)
Zyprexa® (US/Can)
Zyprexa® Zydis® (US/Can)

Antipsychotic Agent, Benzisoxazole
- Risperdal Consta™ (US)
- Risperdal® (US/Can)
- risperidone

Antipsychotic Agent, Butyrophenone
- Apo-Haloperidol® (Can)
- Apo-Haloperidol LA® (Can)
- droperidol
- Haldol® Decanoate (US)
- Haldol® (US)
- haloperidol
- Haloperidol-LA Omega (Can)
- Haloperidol Long Acting (Can)
- Inapsine® (US)
- Novo-Peridol (Can)
- Peridol (Can)
- PMS-Haloperidol LA (Can)

Antipsychotic Agent, Dibenzoxazepine
- Apo-Loxapine® (Can)
- loxapine
- Loxitane® C (US)
- Loxitane® (US)
- Nu-Loxapine (Can)
- PMS-Loxapine (Can)

Antipsychotic Agent, Dihydroindoline
- Moban® (US/Can)
- molindone

Phenothiazine Derivative
- Apo-Chlorpromazine® (Can)
- Apo-Fluphenazine® (Can)
- Apo-Fluphenzaine Decanoate® (Can)
- Apo-Perphenazine® (Can)
- Apo-Prochlorperazine® (Can)
- Apo-Trifluoperazine® (Can)
- chlorpromazine
- Compazine® (Can)
- Compro™ (US)
- fluphenazine
- Largactil® (Can)
- mesoridazine
- Modecate® (Can)
- Moditen® Enanthate (Can)
- Moditen® HCl (Can)
- Novo-Chlorpromazine (Can)
- Novo-Trifluzine (Can)
- Nu-Prochlor (Can)
- pericyazine (Canada only)
- perphenazine
- PMS-Fluphenazine Decanoate (Can)
- PMS-Trifluoperazine (Can)
- prochlorperazine
- Prolixin Decanoate® (US)
- Serentil® (Can)
- Stemetil® (Can)
- Terfluzine (Can)
- trifluoperazine
- Trilafon® (Can)

Thioxanthene Derivative
- Navane® (US/Can)
- thiothixene

PYRIMETHAMINE POISONING

Folic Acid Derivative
- leucovorin

SCHIZOPHRENIA

Antipsychotic Agent
- Clopixol-Acuphase® (Can)
- Clopixol® (Can)
- Clopixol® Depot (Can)
- Fluanxol® (Can)
- flupenthixol (Canada only)
- Geodon® (US)
- olanzapine
- quetiapine
- Seroquel® (US/Can)
- ziprasidone
- zuclopenthixol (Canada only)
- Zyprexa® (US/Can)
- Zyprexa® Zydis® (US/Can)

Antipsychotic Agent, Benzisoxazole
- Risperdal Consta™ (US)
- Risperdal® (US/Can)
- risperidone

Antipsychotic Agent, Dibenzodiazepine
- clozapine
- Clozaril® (US/Can)
- Fazaclo™ (US)
- Gen-Clozapine (Can)
- Rhoxal-clozapine (Can)

Antipsychotic Agent, Quinolone
- Abilify™ (US)
- aripiprazole

Neuroleptic Agent
- Apo-Methoprazine® (Can)
- methotrimeprazine (Canada only)
- Novo-Meprazine (Can)
- Nozinan® (Can)
- thioproperazine (Canada only)

Thioxanthene Derivative
- Fluanxol® (Can)
- flupenthixol (Canada only)

SMOKING CESSATION

Antidepressant, Monoamine Oxidase Inhibitor
- Alti-Moclobemide (Can)
- Apo-Moclobemide® (Can)
- Manerix® (Can)
- moclobemide (Canada only)
- Novo-Moclobemide (Can)
- Nu-Moclobemide (Can)
- PMS-Moclobemide (Can)

Smoking Deterrent
- Commit™ (US-OTC)
- Habitrol® (Can)
- NicoDerm® (Can)
- NicoDerm® CQ® (US-OTC)
- Nicorette® Plus (Can)
- Nicorette® (US-OTC/Can)
- nicotine
- Nicotrol® (Can)
- Nicotrol® Inhaler (US)
- Nicotrol® NS (US)
- Nicotrol® Patch (US-OTC/Can)

TOXICITY, NONSPECIFIC (TREATMENT)

Antacid
- Dulcolax® Milk of Magnesia (US-OTC)
- magnesium hydroxide
- magnesium oxide
- Mag-Ox® 400 (US-OTC)
- Phillips'® Milk of Magnesia (US-OTC)
- Uro-Mag® (US-OTC)

Antidote
- Actidose-Aqua® (US-OTC)
- Actidose® with Sorbitol (US-OTC)
- Carcocaps® (US-OTC)
- Charcadole® Aqueous (Can)
- Charcadole® (Can)
- Charcadole® TFS (Can)
- CharcoAid® G (US-OTC)
- charcoal
- Charcoal Plus® DS (US-OTC)
- EZ-Char™ (US-OTC)
- ipecac syrup
- Kerr Insta-Char® (US-OTC)

Diuretic, Osmotic
- mannitol

Electrolyte Supplement, Oral
- sodium phosphates

Laxative
- Citro-Mag® (Can)
- magnesium citrate

VALPROIC ACID POISONING

Dietary Supplement
- Carnitor® (US/Can)
- levocarnitine

Notes

Notes

Notes

Notes

Notes

Notes

Notes

Notes

Notes

Notes

Notes

Notes

Notes

Notes

Notes

Notes

Notes